Lecture Notes in Electrical Engineering

Volume 1008

The book series *Lecture Notes in Electrical Engineering* (LNEE) publishes the latest developments in Electrical Engineering—quickly, informally and in high quality. While original research reported in proceedings and monographs has traditionally formed the core of LNEE, we also encourage authors to submit books devoted to supporting student education and professional training in the various fields and applications areas of electrical engineering. The series cover classical and emerging topics concerning:

- Communication Engineering, Information Theory and Networks
- Electronics Engineering and Microelectronics
- Signal, Image and Speech Processing
- Wireless and Mobile Communication
- Circuits and Systems
- Energy Systems, Power Electronics and Electrical Machines
- Electro-optical Engineering
- Instrumentation Engineering
- Avionics Engineering
- Control Systems
- Internet-of-Things and Cybersecurity
- Biomedical Devices, MEMS and NEMS

For general information about this book series, comments or suggestions, please contact leontina.dicecco@springer.com.

To submit a proposal or request further information, please contact the Publishing Editor in your country:

China

Jasmine Dou, Editor (jasmine.dou@springer.com)

India, Japan, Rest of Asia

Swati Meherishi, Editorial Director (Swati.Meherishi@springer.com)

Southeast Asia, Australia, New Zealand

Ramesh Nath Premnath, Editor (ramesh.premnath@springernature.com)

USA, Canada

Michael Luby, Senior Editor (michael.luby@springer.com)

All other Countries

Leontina Di Cecco, Senior Editor (leontina.dicecco@springer.com)

**** This series is indexed by EI Compendex and Scopus databases. ****

Triwiyanto Triwiyanto · Achmad Rizal ·
Wahyu Caesarendra
Editors

Proceeding of the 3rd International Conference on Electronics, Biomedical Engineering, and Health Informatics

ICEBEHI 2022, 5–6 October, Surabaya, Indonesia

Springer

Editors
Triwiyanto Triwiyanto
Department of Electromedical Engineering
Poltekkes Kemenkes Surabaya
Surabaya, Indonesia

Achmad Rizal
School of Electrical Engineering
Telkom University
Indonesia, Indonesia

Wahyu Caesarendra
Faculty of Integrated Technologies
Universiti Brunei Darussalam
Gadong, Brunei Darussalam

ISSN 1876-1100 ISSN 1876-1119 (electronic)
Lecture Notes in Electrical Engineering
ISBN 978-981-99-0247-7 ISBN 978-981-99-0248-4 (eBook)
https://doi.org/10.1007/978-981-99-0248-4

This Springer imprint is published by the registered company Springer Nature Singapore Pte Ltd.
The registered company address is: 152 Beach Road, #21-01/04 Gateway East, Singapore 189721, Singapore

Organization

Organizing Committee

Dr. Triwiyanto, Poltekkes Kemenkes Surabaya (Chairman)
Dr. Endro Yulianto, Poltekkes Kemenkes Surabaya (Technical Program Committee Chair)
Sari Luthfiyah, Poltekkes Kemenkes Surabaya (Secretary I)
Anita Miftahul Maghfiroh, Poltekkes Kemenkes Surabaya (Secretary II)
Triana Rahmwati, Poltekkes Kemenkes Surabaya
M. Prastawa Assalim T. P., Poltekkes Kemenkes Surabaya
Ridha Mak'ruf, Poltekkes Kemenkes Surabaya
Priyambada Cahya Nugraha, Poltekkes Kemenkes Surabaya
Farid Amrinsani, Poltekkes Kemenkes Surabaya
Syaifudin, Poltekkes Kemenkes Surabaya
Syevana Dita Musvika, Poltekkes Kemenkes Surabaya
Levana Forra Wakidi, Poltekkes Kemenkes Surabaya
Singgih Yudha Setiawan, Poltekkes Kemenkes Surabaya
Lusiana, Poltekkes Kemenkes Surabaya
Deenda Putri Duta Natalia, Poltekkes Kemenkes Surabaya

Proceeding Editorial Board

Dr. Triwiyanto, Poltekkes Kemenkes Surabaya, Indonesia
Dr. Achmad Rizal, Telkom University, Bandung, Indonesia
Wahyu Caesarendra, Ph.D., Universiti Brunei Darussalam, Brunei Darussalam

Scientific Program Committee

Achmad Rizal, Telkom University, Indonesia
Agung Triayudi, Universitas Nasional, Indonesia
Anggara Trisna Nugraha, Politeknik Perkapalan Negeri Surabaya, Indonesia
Alfin Hikmaturokhman, IT Telkom Purwokerto, Indonesia
Alfian Pramudita Putra, Biomedical Engineering, Faculty Science and Technology, Universitas Airlangga, Indonesia
Alfian Ma'arif, Universitas Ahmad Dahlan, Indonesia
Anilkumar Suthar, Rajasthan Technical University, India
Bambang Guruh Irianto, Poltekkes Kemenkes Surabaya, Indonesia
Candra Zonyfar, Universitas Buana Perjuangan Karawang, Indonesia
Devi Handaya, Politeknik Negeri Jakarta, Indonesia
Dwi Ely Kurniawan, Politeknik Negeri Batam, Indonesia
Deyby Huamanchahua Canchanya, Tecnológico de Monterrey, Mexico
Eka Legya Frannita, Universitas Gadjah Mada, Indonesia
Eko Supriyanto, Universiti Teknologi Malaysia, Malaysia
Ejay Nsugbe, Cranfield University, Cranfield, United Kingdom
Faheem Reegu, Jazan University, Saudi Arabia
Haresh Pandya, Saurashtra University, India
Hasanain Al-Behadili, University of Misan, Iraq
Harikrishna Parikh, Saurashtra University, India
Henderi, Universitas Raharja, Indonesia
Jasten Keneth D. Treceñe, Eastern Visayas State University, Tanauan Campus, Philippines
Johan Reimon Batmetan, Universitas Negeri Manado, Indonesia
Joseph Bamidele Awotunde, University of Ilorin, Ilorin, Kwara State, Nigeria
Kharudin Ali, UC TATI, Malaysia
Mas Aly Afandi, Institut Teknologi Telkom Purwokerto, Indonesia
Manas Kumar Yogi, Pragati Engineering College (Autonomous), India
Mera Kartika Delimayanti, Politeknik Negeri Jakarta, Indonesia
Michael G Albino., President Ramon Magsaysay State University, Philippines
Nada Fitrieyatul Hikmah, Institut Teknologi Sepuluh Nopember, Indonesia
Phuoc-Hai Huynh, An Giang University, Vietnam
Pradeep N, Bapuji Institute of Engineering and Technology, Davangere, India
Raja Siti Nur Adiimah Raja Aris, UC TATI, Malaysia
Ramen A Purba, Politeknik Unggul LP3M, Medan, Indonesia
Rendra Gustriansyah, Universitas Indo Global Mandiri, Indonesia
Riky Tri Yunardi, Universitas Airlangga, Indonesia
Rismayani, STMIK Dipanegara Makassar, Indonesia
Sidharth Pancholi, Indian Institute of Technology Delhi, India
Shajedul Islam, Health Sciences University of Hokkaido, Japan
Suzanna Ridzuan Aw, University College TATI, Malaysia
Vishwajeet Shankhwar, National Institute of Technology Jalandhar, India

Vijay Anant Athavale, Walchand Institute of Technology, India
Wahyu Pamungkas, Institut Teknologi Telkom Purwokerto, Indonesia
Wan Faizura Wan Tarmizi, UC TATI, Malaysia
Yohanssen Pratama, Institut Teknologi Del, Indonesia
Yuant Tiandho, Universitas Bangka Belitung, Indonesia

Preface

3rd ICEBEHI 2022, the 3rd International Conference on Electronics, Biomedical Engineering, and Health Informatics, took place during October 4–5, 2022, on virtual platforms (Zoom app). The conference was organized by Department of Medical Electronics Technology, Health Polytechnic Ministry of Health Surabaya (Poltekkes Kemenkes Surabaya), Surabaya, Indonesia, and co-organized by Institut Teknologi Telkom Purwokerto, Indonesia; Institut Teknologi Telkom Surabaya, Indonesia; Walchand Institute of Technology, India; Vocational Faculty, Universitas Muhammadiyah Yogyakarta, Indonesia; STIKES Semarang, Indonesia; and Universitas Trisakti, Indonesia, with aims of bringing together as a family all leading scientists, academicians, educationist, young scientists, research scholars, and students to present, discuss, and exchange their experiences, innovation ideas, and recent developments in the field of electronics, biomedical engineering, and health informatics.

The ICEBEHI-2022 conference was held online through the Zoom application. More than 100 participants (presenters and non-presenters) attended the conference; they were from Taiwan, India, Vietnam, Cameroon, Iran, Brunei Darussalam, Poland, South Korea, Nigeria, Thailand, Saudi Arabia, and Indonesia. The scientific program of this conference included many topics related to electronics and biomedical engineering as well as those in related fields. At this conference, three distinguished keynote speakers and one invited speaker delivered their research works in the area of Biomedical Engineering. Each keynote speech lasted 50 minutes.

ICEBEHI-2022 conference collects the latest research results and applications on electronics, biomedical engineering, and health informatics. It includes a selection of 44 papers from 133 papers submitted to the conference from universities all over the world. All of the accepted papers were subjected to strict peer-reviewing by 2–3 expert referees. All articles have gone through a plagiarism check. The papers have been selected for this volume because of their quality and relevance to the conference.

We are very grateful to the committee which contributed to the success of this conference. Also, we are thankful to the authors who submitted the papers; it was the quality of their presentations and communication with the other participants that really made this web conference fruitful. Last but not the least, we are thankful to the Lecture Note in Electrical Engineering (Springer) Publishing for their support; it was not only the support but also an inspiration for the organizers. We hope this conference can be held every year to make it an ideal platform for people to share views and experiences in electronics, biomedical engineering, health informatics, and related areas. We are expecting you and more experts and scholars around the globe to join this international event next year.

Surabaya, Indonesia Dr. Triwiyanto Triwiyanto

Contents

About the Editors

Dr. Triwiyanto Triwiyanto received the B.S. degree in Physics from Airlangga University, Indonesia, M.S. degree in Electronic Engineering from the Institut Teknologi Sepuluh Nopember Surabaya, Indonesia, in 2004, and the Ph.D. degree in Electrical Engineering from Gadjah Mada University, Yogyakarta, Indonesia, in 2018. From 1998 to 2004, he was Senior Lecturer with the Microcontrollers Laboratory. Since 2005, he has been Assistant Professor with the Medical Electronics Technology Department, Health Polytechnic Ministry of Health Surabaya, Indonesia. In 2018, Triwiyanto received the best Doctoral Student Award from Gadjah Mada University. Additionally, he is Editor-in-Chief in several peer review journals, Chairman, and Technical Programme Committee in several international conferences. His current research interests include microcontroller, electronics, biomedical signal processing, machine learning, rehabilitation engineering, and surface electromyography (sEMG)-based physical human–robot interactions.

Dr. Achmad Rizal received bachelor of engineering in telecommunication engineering from STT Telkom (now, Telkom University), Bandung, Indonesia, in 2000. He received master degree in biomedical engineering from Institut Teknologi Bandung, Bandung, Indonesia, in October 2006. He received Ph.D. degree from Universitas Gadjah Mada, Yogyakarta, Indonesia. His research interests include biomedical signal processing, biomedical image processing, biomedical instrumentation, and telemedicine. Now, he is Associate Professor in School of Electrical Engineering, Telkom University.

Dr. Wahyu Caesarendra is Assistant Professor at the Faculty of Integrated Technologies, Universiti Brunei Darussalam, since October 2018. He received Doctor of Philosophy degree from the University of Wollongong in 2015. He worked as Postdoctoral Research Fellow in Rolls-Royce@NTU Corp Lab, School of Mechanical and Aerospace Engineering, Nanyang Technological University, Singapore, from February 2017 to September 2018. In 2011, Wahyu Caesarendra was awarded of University Postgraduate Award and International Postgraduate Tuition Award from the University of Wollongong. He worked in the automotive and electrical company prior to joining Diponegoro University as Lecturer in 2007. He was Visiting Assistant Professor at the National Taiwan University of Science and Technology from August 5 to 11, 2019. He has authored more than 130 research articles in journals and conference proceedings. He is also Academic and Guest Editor in peer-reviewed journals. His research interest includes vibration condition monitoring, fault diagnosis and prognosis, mechatronics and robotics, machine learning and deep learning, mechanical design and 3D printing, smart manufacturing, and IoT.

A Preliminary Study of Vehicle License Plate Detection and Identification

Ahmad Sanmorino and Samsuryadi

Abstract In this study, the authors would like to propose vehicle license plate detection and identification using machine learning approaches. The goal of this study is to pave the way for more in-depth research on vehicle license plate detection and identification using machine learning approaches. A license plate is the vehicle's unique identity that serves as proof of the legitimacy of the vehicle's operation. It is typically in the form of a plate or other material with specific specifications issued by the police. This plate is installed on each vehicle and contains the area code, registration number, and validity period. This study begins with a review of several related publications, with a focus on license plate detection and identification for each method. The investigation is furthered by identifying and comprehending the benefits of each method. Finally, the authors attempt to propose a vehicle license plate detection and identification model based on the advantages of each method previously discussed. The proposed model is simulated using Python programming. The simple simulation results show a 99% accuracy rate. Based on the simulation results, it is shown that the contribution of this study is that the Faster RCNN-based model is proven to be used for vehicle license plate detection and identification with fair accuracy. This model, however, is still conceptual and needs to be improved. It will be fully tested and discussed in future work.

Keywords Plate detection · Number-plate recognition · Faster R-CNN

1 Introduction

The detection and identification of vehicle license plates are critical in smart transportation systems. They have a wide range of potential applications, from speed

A. Sanmorino (✉)
Universitas Indo Global Mandiri, Palembang, Indonesia
e-mail: sanmorino@uigm.ac.id

Samsuryadi
Universitas Sriwijaya, Palembang, Indonesia

T. Triwiyanto et al. (eds.), *Proceeding of the 3rd International Conference on Electronics, Biomedical Engineering, and Health Informatics*, Lecture Notes in Electrical Engineering 1008, https://doi.org/10.1007/978-981-99-0248-4_1

monitoring, traffic monitoring, and parking management to security systems, so they have attracted a lot of attention in recent years. This is understandable because, as the number of vehicles increases, so does the number of crimes committed against vehicle owners, such as theft, or robbery. There are several studies with various methods related to vehicle license plate detection and identification. Most existing methods are only effective under specific conditions or with sophisticated image capture systems. In an uncontrolled environment, recognizing vehicle license plates accurately remains a difficult task. The tasks of plate detection and identification, on the other hand, are always linked. The methods used in these two phases should complement one another. The detection accuracy can be used to improve identification accuracy, and the outcome can be used to eliminate errors in vehicle number plate identification.

As an input medium, the vehicle license plate detection mechanism can utilize closed-circuit television cameras (CCTV) that are already installed along the highways. There are high-tech CCTV cameras with ultra HD systems with the best capture results. For component protection, this high-tech CCTV is protected by a special metal that is resistant to extreme weather, such as hot temperatures or corrosion due to rain. This can be the best solution to get a clear vehicle license plate on the highway.

Through this short paper, the author would like to discuss several studies related to vehicle license plate detection and identification. The discussion focuses on license plate detection, character segmentation, and character recognition for each method. The study is furthered by identifying and comprehending the benefits of each method. Finally, the authors attempt to propose vehicle license plate detection and identification method based on the advantages of each method that are already discussed.

2 Related Works

In general, the topic of vehicle license plate detection and identification has been discussed for a long time and is still evolving. Kakani et al. [1] propose automatic number-plate recognition (ANPR) method based on optical character recognition (OCR) that improves performance with trained neural network features. Localization of license plates, character segmentation, and character recognition are the three layers of methods that have been implemented. 300 license plates from India and other countries were tested. The accuracy score for plate localization is 96.7%, and character recognition is 92.2%, according to the test results. The overall accuracy of plate detection is 94.45%. Furthermore, Nayak et al. [2] applied the ANPR methodology to make it easier to detect stolen vehicle number plates. The ANPR methodology is applied using edge finding and Window Filtering methods. The progress of this study shows that ANPR with the Edge Finding method and the Window Filtering method obtained quite good results.

Yogheedha et al. [3] also used the ANPR technique with the template matching method in their research. The results of this study show a 92% accuracy rate, with the ability to correctly detect 13 plates out of a total of 14 vehicle license plates tested. This ANPR method was proposed to support Universiti Malaysia Perlis' smart parking system. Sharma [4] investigated the performance of a vehicle number plate recognition system using an ANPR method based on template matching. Several layers of algorithms are used, including morphological operations, edge recognition, smoothing and filtering, plate localization, and character segmentation. According to Selmi et al. [5], a complicated hardware specification is required to obtain a high-quality plate image. Different treatments should be implemented for high-speed vehicles and vice versa. The author employs a variety of image pre-processing and convolution neural network approaches to divide images into two categories: vehicle plate and non-plate. In this study, the author used two datasets, Caltech and AOLP, each with 126 images and 2,049 vehicle license plates. According to the evaluation results, the approach proposed by the author achieves an accuracy score of 94.8% when tested using the Caltech dataset.

The output of a CCTV camera is typically in the form of videos (moving objects) or images. This video or image is fed into detection and identification algorithms. The following discussion will center on research into detection and identification methods. The object on the vehicle plate image is isolated into a square shape using the detection method. Color-based detection, texture-based detection, edge-based detection, and character-based detection are the four types of detection methods [6–8].

Color-based detection methods are based on the observation that the color of the license plate is typically different from the color of the background. Chang et al. [9] proposed a method for detecting Taiwan license plates in RGB images using the difference between the foreground and background. They created a color detector mechanism that detects the edges of red-white, black-white, and green-white objects. Another study looked at the pixels of object color to develop a plate detection method [10]. A strip search was used to isolate vehicle license plates using the color-geometric template. To detect inclined or deformed license plates, color-based detection methods can be used. However, in natural scene conditions, this method is very sensitive to various lighting effects and cannot distinguish other objects in the image that are similar in size and color to the license plates.

Texture-based detection methods attempted to detect license plates based on pixel intensity distributions in plate localizations. Giannoukos et al. [11] proposed a Sliding Concentric Window (SCW) technique for identifying license plates in images based on the texture of local irregularities. To increase detection speed, Operator Context Scanning (OCS) was used. Yu et al. [12] used a wavelet transform to extract the plate image's horizontal and vertical details. The projection data was then processed using Empirical Mode Decomposition (EMD) to locate the desired wave crest, which indicates the position of texture in a license plate image. Texture-based detection methods outperform color-based detection methods but have a higher computational complexity. Vehicle license plates are typically rectangular in shape with a specific aspect ratio, and they have a higher edge density than the rest of the image, so this edge shape is widely used to detect license plates. Yuan et al. [13] proposed a novel line density filter approach for connecting high-edge-density regions and removing low-edge-density regions in each row and column of a license plate image. Another study [14] developed an edge-based method for plate detection. Edge clustering was performed using Expectation–Maximization (EM), which extracts regions with a high density of edges and shapes similar to plates as candidate license plates. Edge-based detection methods are quick to compute, but there is a problem if the input is a complex image with many irregular edges.

A character-based detection method contains more detailed information than color, texture, or edge detection methods. Initially, Li et al. [15] used the Maximally Stable Extreme Region (MSER) to extract candidate characters from license plate images, and continued with the Conditional Random Field (CRF) method to develop the relationship between license plate characters. Finally, license plates were located using the sum-product message sent over CRF. License plate detection was approached as a visual matching problem by Zhou et al. [7]. For each character, the Principal Visual Word (PVW) was used to obtain geometric properties such as orientation, characteristic scale, and relative position. This property is used to extract license plates. To detect localized character regions, Llorca et al. [16] combined the Maximally Stable Extreme Regions (MSER) and the Stroke Width Transform (SWT). Finally, the Hough transform was used to localize the regions with characters on license plates. Character-based detection methods are more relevant and can be improved further, most notably by implementing deep learning techniques.

Other studies on license plate identification usually break down the characters in the plate first and then identify each selected character using Optical Character Recognition (OCR) methods. Maximally Stable Extreme Region (MSER) was used for character segmentation by Hsu et al. [14]. For feature extraction, a Local Binary Pattern (LBP) was used. The authors then used Linear Discriminant Analysis (LDA) to classify the characters. In other research, Hou et al. [17] proposed an SWT-based method for segmenting characters on license plates. Characters on reverse license plates can also be identified using this method. MSER was used by Gou et al. [18] to break characters in license plates and determine character location on license plates. The characters on the plate were identified using Restricted Boltzmann Machines (RBM) in the following stage.

To be honest, character segmentation is a difficult job. This job is influenced by illumination, shadow, or blur in the license plate image. It has an immediate impact on license plate recognition. It immediately affects plate recognition. Even with a great method, the character cannot be correctly identified if the segmentation is incorrect. Deep learning enhancements allow for direct identification of the entire license plate without character segmentation. This reduces overall time complexity. Moon et al. [19] use Hidden Markov Models (HMMs) in conjunction with the Viterbi algorithm for label sequence determination to perform character segmentation. Another study, Goodfellow et al. [20], used a large distributed method with a deep layered neural network to propose a probabilistic model for reading arbitrary multi-digit numbers without character segmentation. According to Li and Shen [21], sequence labeling is a major issue in license plate identification. Convolutional Neural Networks (CNNs) were selected to be used in a sliding window fashion to extract a sequence of feature vectors from the license plate localize box.

3 Proposed Method

The authors proposed a license plate detection and identification model by studying and comprehending the benefits and limitations of several related methods that have been discussed. For detection and identification, this conceptual model employed character-based enhancement. We call it 'enhancement' because deep learning algorithms are used to improve the performance of this character-based detection [22–24]. The detection and identification of license plates are accomplished using a single deep learning method, a deep neural network. This was chosen in order to be more effective in the detection and identification process [25–27]. Figure 1 depicts detailed explanations of the proposed model.

We used Faster Region Convolutional Neural Network (Faster R-CNN) as a backbone in this conceptual model for license plate detection and identification. The main part of the Faster R-CNN model is the convolutional layers. The main purpose of the convolutional layer is to detect local anomalies of a feature from the previous

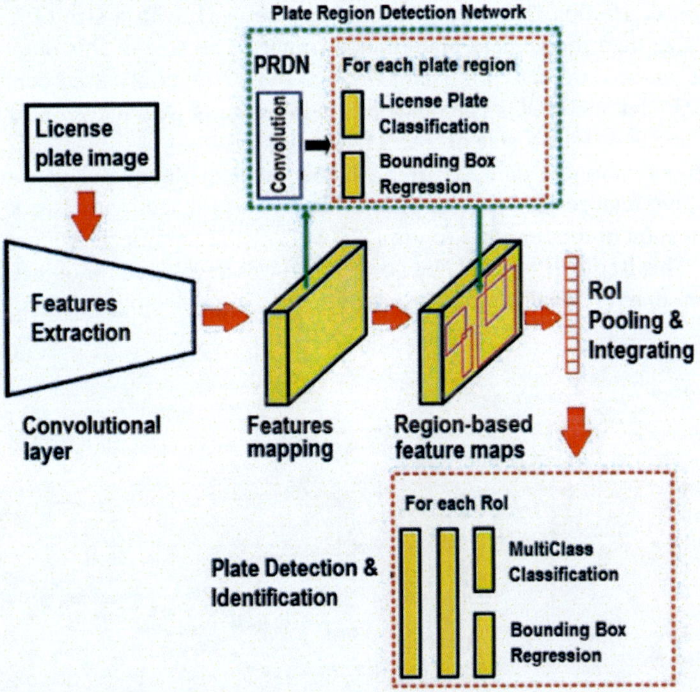

Fig. 1 Conceptual model

layer and map the results. In each convolution layer, there are several m_1 filters. The number of filters used in one convolution screen is equal to the size of the feature map volume from the previous layer. Each filter can detect a specific feature at each location on the vehicle plate based on the feature mapping. The output of $Y_{(l)}{}^{i}$ from the first layer $m_{(l)}{}^{1}$ is a feature map of size $m_{(l)}{}^{3} \times m_{(l)}{}^{3}$. For the ith feature map, more popularly known as $Y_{(l)}{}^{i}$, the score can be calculated using Eq. 1:

$$Y_i^{(l)} = B_i^{(1)} + \sum_{j=1}^{m_1^{(l-1)}} K_{i,j}^{(1)} * Y_j^{(l-1)} \tag{1}$$

where $K_{i,j}^{(l)}$ is a filter of size $2h_1^{(1)} + 1 \times 2h_2^{(1)} + 1$ which brings together the jth feature map in layer $(l - 1)$ with the feature map in layer and $B_i^{(1)}$ shows the bias matrix. The path of the convolution layer that meets the following layer produces the classified vehicle plate image information as shown. All pixels are then assembled into edges, all edges are assembled into motifs, all motifs are assembled into parts, all parts are assembled into objects, and all objects are assembled into scenes [28–30]. Figure 2 depicts a detailed explanation of the Faster R-CNN convolution layers.

The region proposal network (RPN) begins with the input of a vehicle plate image entered into the core of the convolutional neural network. First, the vehicle plate image is resized so that it has a minimum side size of 600px and the longest side a maximum of 1000px. The output of the core network with a size of h × w has a smaller size than the vehicle plate image (input). The size of this output is very dependent on the core network used. The two most commonly used core network types are ZF-Net and VGG. The convolution layer starts with a layer size of 3 × 3 (64 units) and ends with a size of 3 × 3 (512 units).

The proposed model consists of a number of convolutional layers to extract discriminative features for license plates. Plate region detection network (PRDN) is a modification of the Region Proposal Network (RPN) approach proposed by Ren et al. [31]. This Region Proposal Network (RPN) was developed for object detection applications that rely on the region proposal method to predict object locations. They

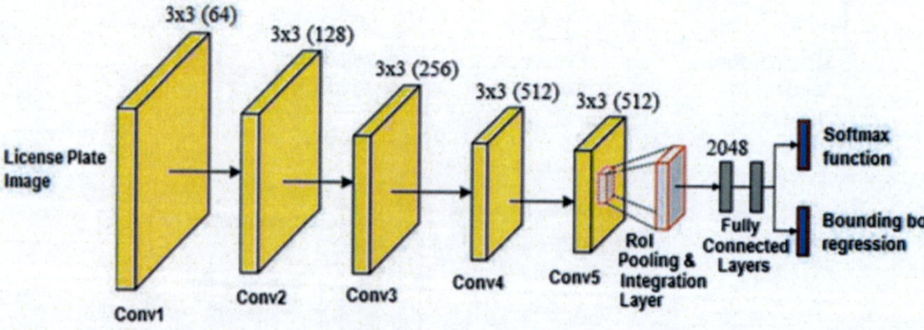

Fig. 2 The faster R-CNN convolution layers

used a single network for RPN, which generates region operation proposals, and Fast R-CNN, which categorizes regions. For license plate detection and identification, a plate region detection network tailored specifically for car license plates, a Region of Interest (RoI) pooling and integrating layer, a deep learning classifier, and bounding box regression are used [32, 33]. Faster R-CNN shares a full-image convolutional layer with fast R-CNN for feature mapping, resulting in low complexity and cost-free region proposals. Faster R-CNN uses the high-quality region proposal performed by PRDN after it has been trained end-to-end for region detection. A PRDN is a fully connected network that detects plate bounds as well as scores at the same time.

This procedure speeds up plate detection and identification. A PRDN takes any size plate image as input and outputs a set of rectangular image plates, each with a plate score. Begin with m x m reference boxes for each sliding window, which is initialized by PRDN to have different aspect ratios and scales at each convolution feature map location. Each sliding window is converted into a lower-dimensional vector, which is then fed into two pairs of fully connected layers, a multiclass classification layer, and a bounding box regression layer [34].

4 Results

The Faster RCNN-based model has been simulated in Python programming using less than 100 license plate images. The simple simulation results show a 99% accuracy rate. Table 1 shows the results of testing the recognition of letters and numbers contained in license plate images.

Classification using Faster R-CNN succeeded in predicting almost 100% (average score of 99%) letters or numbers correctly (precision and recall scores). Faster R-CNN produces an average comparison of precision and recall of letters or numbers that have been identified by 99% (F1-score). When compared to other deep learning algorithms, detection using Faster R-CNN has a better accuracy score and test time. Details of the results of the comparison are shown in Table 2.

Table 2 shows a brief comparison between the proposed identification method and other related deep learning methods. The author deliberately chooses the deep learning method with many similarities as a comparison so that the comparison results are relevant and based on the same theory. Based on the comparison, it can be seen that the use of Faster R-CNN proved to have better accuracy (99%) than R-CNN and SPP-Net (78% and 92%). When viewed from the test time (s), the comparison results put Faster R-CNN in the fastest position, which is only 2.3 s, while R-CNN and SPP-Net are 49.2 s and 4.4 s. The results of this comparison show that the selection of Faster R-CNN as the core for the vehicle plate detection and identification method is the right and relevant choice. However, the author realizes that it is still very early to state that the proposed method is better overall than other detection methods; the real conditions in the field greatly affect the outcome. Testing involving various factors is needed so that when implemented it can accommodate all unexpected conditions in the field.

Table 1 Testing for letters and numbers

Letters/numbers	Precision	Recall	F1-score
B	0.99	1.00	1.00
D	1.00	0.99	1.00
G	1.00	0.99	0.99
0	0.99	0.99	0.99
1	1.00	0.99	0.99
4	0.99	1.00	1.00
5	1.00	1.00	1.00
6	1.00	1.00	1.00
8	1.00	0.99	1.00
9	1.00	1.00	1.00
H	1.00	1.00	1.00
J	1.00	1.00	1.00
L	0.99	0.99	0.99
T	1.00	1.00	1.00
W	0.99	1.00	1.00

Table 2 Accuracy and test-time comparison

Model	Accurary (%)	Miss (%)	Test time (s)
R-CNN	78	22	49,2
Faster R-CNN	99	1	2,30
SPP-Net	92	8	4,40

5 Discussion

If Table 2 shows the results of the comparison of the accuracy of the Faster R-CNN-based method that the author proposes to several other methods, then Table 3 shows a comparison of the results of the identification of our proposed method against the identification method proposed by several other authors.

Table 3 Accuracy comparison to other related studies

Authors	Method	Accuracy (%)
Kakani et al. [1]	Feed-forward ANN-based OCR algorithm	94.45
Yogheedha et al. [3]	ANPR technique	92.00
Selmi et al. [5]	CNN approaches	94.80
Sanmorino et al. (this study)	Faster R-CNN	99.00

Table 3 shows Kakani et al. [1]'s proposed identification method using feed-forward ANN-based OCR algorithm that succeeded in getting an accuracy score of 94.45%. Another author, namely Yogheedha et al. [3], managed to get a score of 92.00%, while Selmi et al. [5] use Convolution Neural Network approaches as the core for the proposed method to identify vehicle plates, obtaining an accuracy score of 94.80%. It can be understood based on this comparison that the accuracy score obtained by the author in this study is at a fairly good level (99.00%). The author does not say that our proposed method is the best because the identification process is also influenced by various factors so it requires more comprehensive testing in the future.

The author realizes that the results of this test are not final, in the sense that the accuracy score obtained can still decrease. The limited number of datasets used in the test is one of the obstacles in this study. However, this does not mean that the results of this test will be in vain, because from the beginning the author considered that what had been done in this study was still preliminary, according to the title that we carried on the first page. For a more comprehensive comparison against other related methods, a factor to consider is the similarity of the variables used in the test. In our view, there will always be differences in the use of variables, but the conditions should not exceed the generally agreed-upon threshold. So for the similarity of the variables used, the closer to 100% the better; if it cannot be met then more than or equal to 90% is still acceptable. This figure is still acceptable because there are various factors in the field, such as difficulties in obtaining data or at least references to a variable.

6 Conclusion

There have been numerous studies and discussions about vehicle license plate detection and identification. The advantages and limitations of each method are known as a result of the discussion and comparison. By understanding the benefits of the methods discussed, the author proposes a vehicle license plate detection and identification model. This proposed model used a Faster R-CNN approach with modifications to the Region Proposal Network (RPN). This proposed model appears to be relevant in terms of reducing test time while also being more accurate. It is evident from the test results that obtained a score of 99% for accuracy, better than other related CNN methods. The test time(s) for the proposed method is also better than that of R-CNN and SPP-Net. The proposed method only takes 2.3 s. In the future, the author will increase the amount of image data as an input convolutional layer and involve several external factors in the field (real conditions) so that the accuracy that has been obtained can be maintained.

References

1. Kakani BV, Gandhi D, Jani S (2017) Improved OCR based automatic vehicle number plate recognition using features trained neural network. In: 8th international conference on computing, communication and networking technologies. ICCCNT 2017
2. Nayak V et al (2020) Automatic number plate recognition. Int J Adv Trends Comput Sci Eng 9(3):3783–3787
3. Yogheedha K et at (2018) Automatic vehicle license plate recognition system based on image processing and template matching approach. In: 2018 international conference on computational approach in smart systems and design and applications. ICASSDA 2018, pp 1–8
4. Sharma G (2018) Performance analysis of vehicle number plate recognition system using template matching techniques. J Inf Technol Softw Eng 08(02)
5. Selmi Z, Halima MB, Alimi AM (2018) Deep learning system for automatic license plate detection and recognition. In: Proceedings of the international conference on document analysis and recognition, vol 1. ICDAR, pp 1132–1138
6. Anagnostopoulos CNE et al (2006) A license plate-recognition algorithm for intelligent transportation system applications. IEEE Trans Intell Transp Syst 7(3):377–392
7. Zhou W et al (2012) Principal visual word discovery for automatic license plate detection. IEEE Trans Image Process 21(9):4269–4279
8. Du S et al (2013) Automatic license plate recognition (ALPR): a state-of-the-art review. IEEE Trans Circ Syst Video Technol 23(2):311–325
9. Chang S-L et al (2004) Automatic license plate recognition. IEEE Trans Intell Transp Syst 5(1):42–53
10. Ashtari AH, Nordin MJ, Fathy M (2014) An Iranian license plate recognition system based on color features. IEEE Trans Intell Transp Syst 15(4):1690–1705
11. Giannoukos I et al (2010) Operator context scanning to support high segmentation rates for real time license plate recognition. Pattern Recognit 43(11):3866–3878
12. Yu S et al (2015) A novel license plate location method based on wavelet transform and EMD analysis. Pattern Recognit 48(1):114–125
13. Yuan Y et al (2017) A robust and efficient approach to license plate detection. IEEE Trans Image Process 26(3):1102–1114
14. Hsu G-S, Chen J-C, Chung Y-Z (2013) Application-oriented license plate recognition. IEEE Trans Veh Technol 62(2):552–561
15. Li B et al (2013) Component-based license plate detection using conditional random field model. IEEE Trans Intell Transp Syst 14(4):1690–1699
16. Llorca DF et al (2016) Two-camera based accurate vehicle speed measurement using average speed at a fixed point. In: Proceedings of 19th international conference on intelligent transportation systems, pp 2533–2538
17. Hou Y et al (2015) License plate character segmentation based on stroke width transform. In: Proceedings of the 8th international congress on image signal processing, pp 954–958
18. Gou C et al (2016) Vehicle license plate recognition based on extremal regions and restricted boltzmann machines. IEEE Trans Intell Transp Syst 17(4):1096–1107
19. Bulan O et al (2017) Segmentation and annotation-free license plate recognition with deep localization and failure identification. IEEE Trans Intell Transp Syst 18(9):2351–2363
20. Goodfellow IJ et al (2014) Multidigit number recognition from street view imagery using deep convolutional neural networks. In: Proceedings of the international conference on learning and representations, pp 1–13
21. Li H, Shen C (2016) Reading car license plates using deep convolutional neural networks and LSTMs
22. Sihang W et al (2020) Precise detection of Chinese characters in historical documents with deep reinforcement learning. Pattern Recogn 107
23. Alshehri M et al (2022) Character-level word encoding deep learning model for combating cyber threats in phishing URL detection. Comput Electr Eng 100

24. Boukthir K et al (2022) Reduced annotation based on deep active learning for arabic text detection in natural scene images. Pattern Recogn Lett 157
25. Mimura M (2022) Evaluation of printable character-based malicious PE file-detection method. Internet Things 19
26. Hevia-Tuero C et al (2021) Does English orthography influence bilingual Spanish readers? The effect of grapheme crosslinguistic congruency and complexity on letter detection. Cogn Dev 59
27. Zhang Y et al (2015) Text string detection for loosely constructed characters with arbitrary orientations. Neurocomputing 168
28. Ma Y et al (2005) An invitation to 3-D vision: from images to geometric models. Springer, New York
29. LeCun Y et al (2010) Convolutional networks and applications in vision. In: Circuits and systems, international symposium on, pp 253–256
30. LeCun Y et al (2015) Deep learning. Nature 251:436–444
31. Ren S et al (2015) Faster R-CNN: Towards realtime object detection with region proposal networks. Proc Adv Neural Inf Process Syst, pp 91–99
32. Liao C et al (2021) Deep learning for registration of region of interest in consecutive wireless capsule endoscopy frames. Comput Methods Programs Biomed 208
33. Mitra A et al (2018) The region of interest localization for glaucoma analysis from retinal fundus image using deep learning. Comput Methods Programs Biomed 165
34. Marini F (2020) Non-linear modeling: neural networks, 2nd edn, vol 3. Elsevier

Feature Selection Using Extra Trees Classifier for Research Productivity Framework in Indonesia

Ahmad Sanmorino, Luis Marnisah, and Hastha Sunardi

Abstract In this study, the authors succeeded in proving the Extra Trees Classifier reliable as a feature selection mechanism for the research productivity framework. In order to find features that significantly impact research output in higher education institutions, the selection was carried out. The eight selected features are Scientific Article (Gain: 0.36), Number of Citations (Gain: 0.22), Number of Conferences Attended (Gain: 0.17), Intellectual Property Right (Gain: 0.04), Education Qualification (Gain: 0.03), Grant Awardee (Gain: 0.27), Number of Grants (Gain: 0.05), and Lecturer Grade (Gain: 0.05). For the testing phase, the Naive Bayes (NB) classifier and K-Nearest Neighbors classifier are used. The selected features successfully passed it with a high accuracy score, for K-NN by 87%, and NB by 81%. These features are used as variables for the research productivity framework. Up to this point, the variables that construct the framework that the authors propose can go through a testing phase with results as expected, with an accuracy score of more than 70%, which is categorized as relevant or acceptable results. For future work, the univariate selection and correlation matrix will be added as a feature selection with the Extra Trees Classifier, so the selected features are more relevant and are used as a construct for the research productivity framework.

Keywords Feature selection · Extra trees classifier · Research productivity framework

1 Introduction

The purpose of this study is to prove that Extra Trees Classifier can be used as a feature selection mechanism for the research productivity framework. Producing usable results from a research endeavor is referred to as research productivity. Research performance and productivity are correlated, with higher research performance being

A. Sanmorino (✉) · L. Marnisah · H. Sunardi
Universitas Indo Global Mandiri, Palembang, Indonesia
e-mail: sanmorino@uigm.ac.id

T. Triwiyanto et al. (eds.), *Proceeding of the 3rd International Conference on Electronics, Biomedical Engineering, and Health Informatics*, Lecture Notes in Electrical Engineering 1008, https://doi.org/10.1007/978-981-99-0248-4_2

produced with better productivity. A country's level of knowledge and technological advancement can be shown in its research productivity. Lecturers are the major players who play a significant part in the advancement of science and technology in a university setting. Research is one of the three pillars of higher education, and instructors are expected to engage in it. The processes required to obtain the pertinent features make up the feature selection mechanism [1]. Extra Trees Classifier (ETC) is a form of ensemble learning technique that integrates the classification outcomes from various decision trees, which are then gathered in a forest [2, 3]. Feature selection is used to determine the degree of relationship between independent features and dependent features. The selected features are used as variables that construct the framework for research productivity in higher education institutions (HEI). The framework is used as a guide for research managers in improving research productivity at HEI. To prove whether the selected variables are relevant to use, a test is carried out involving the data mining classifier [4], K-Nearest Neighbors [5], and Naïve Bayes [6]. The evaluation of the classification results is explained by the confusion matrix table [7, 8], equipped with accuracy score, precision, recall, and Receiver Operating Characteristic (ROC) curve [9, 10].

2 Related Works

This research is related to the previous project that has been done [11, 12]. A brief survey of research productivity is shown in Table 1.

3 Materials and Methods

The dataset was obtained from Sinta (Science and Technology Index), which is run by the Republic of Indonesia's Ministry of Research and Technology. A portal called Sinta offers data about Indonesian research performance. The datasets collected from the Sinta portal are Scientific Article (A), Number of Citations (C), Number of Conferences Attended (CO), Intellectual Property Right (IPR), Nationality (N), Gender (G), Education Qualification (D), Grant Awardee (RG), Number of Grants (GT), Lecturer Status (WT), and Lecturer Grade (R). Research design in order to select the variables that construct the framework is shown in Fig. 1. During preprocessing, the raw data is transformed into statistical data. This statistical data is numerical data for the needs of variable selection mechanisms and data mining modeling. The Extra Trees algorithm is used in the feature importance selection phase. A sort of ensemble learning technique called Extra Trees Classifier (ETC) mixes the output of various decision trees [17–19]. Important variables were extracted from the generated dataset in this study using the Extra Trees Classifier [20]. Information gain is the criterion used to make the decision [21].

Table 1 Short survey of publications related to research productivity

Author	Feature name	Feature selection mechanism
Ramli et al. [13]	Research article, conference article, lecturer age, gender, status of marital, educational qualification, work experience, position, work division, number of citation, and target variable (research performance status)	Not mentioned
Henry et al. [14]	Work achievement, work policy, monthly payment, leadership in research, supervision in research, lecturer age, educational qualification, cluster, lecturer track	Chi-square, Nagelkerke R square, Lemeshow test
Wichian et al. [15]	Management of research, communication skills, work with team, higher education policy, library cost, lab facility, lecturer age, academic level, creative thinking, contribution in research, vision-ambition, international meeting, good method in research, research endowment	Chi-square, R-square, Cronbach alpha
Nazri et al. [16]	Amount of research grant, department, administrative post, number of doctorate students, faculty member, invitation as guest speaker, research article, lecturer age, designation, win of research grant, lecturer gender, research performance, status of marital, job status	Spearman Rho correlation

To get the value of information gain, we must first find the entropy of the dataset feature. For the Entropy Eq. (1) [21]:

$$\text{Entropy}(S) = \sum\nolimits_{i=1}^{C} p_i \log_2(p_i) \tag{1}$$

where c is the number of unique class labels and p_i is the proportion of rows with output label i. After the entropy is obtained, the information gain Eq. (2):

$$\begin{aligned} \text{Gain}(S, A) = {} & \text{Entropy}(S) \\ & - \sum\nolimits_{v \epsilon \text{Values}(A)} \frac{|S_v|}{|S|} \text{Entropy}(S_v) \end{aligned} \tag{2}$$

where S is the set of instances, A is the attribute, S_v is the subset of S with $A = v$, and Values (A) is the set of all possible values of A.

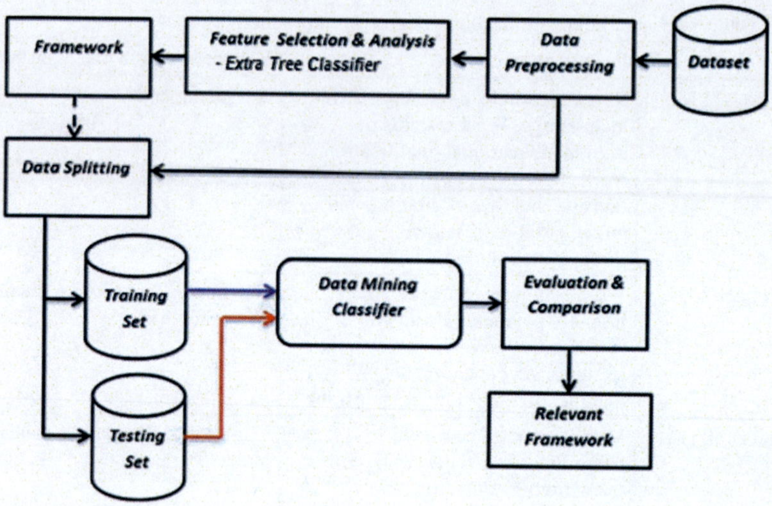

Fig. 1 Research design

The Gain score obtained by each feature will be compared and analyzed, ranked in order. Based on this ranking, the selected features are used as variables that construct the research productivity framework [22–24]. In the next stage, the framework is tested using a data mining classifier. The data mining classifiers involved are K-Nearest Neighbors (K-NN) and Naïve Bayes (NB). The reason for choosing these two classifiers is because the data used is supervised (categorical datasets) [25, 26]. So the use of K-NN and NB classifiers for testing is the right choice.

For the evaluation and analysis of the classification results [27], the confusion matrix approach (True Positive, False Positive, True Negative, False Negative), accuracy, precision, recall, F1-score [28, 29], and Receiver Operating Characteristic curve (ROC) are used [30, 31]. Based on the evaluation results, the feasibility of the variables that construct the framework is assessed, whether they have an acceptable score and are relevant for use.

4 Result and Discussion

The feature importance calculation is shown in Fig. 2.

Figure 2 shows the gain score for each feature; the Article and Citation scores occupy the highest position. A detailed explanation of the gain score for each feature is in Table 2. The calculation of gain scores for the overall dataset (302 records) is done using the Extra Trees Classifier library in Python Programming. A detailed explanation of the gain scores for each feature is shown in Table 2.

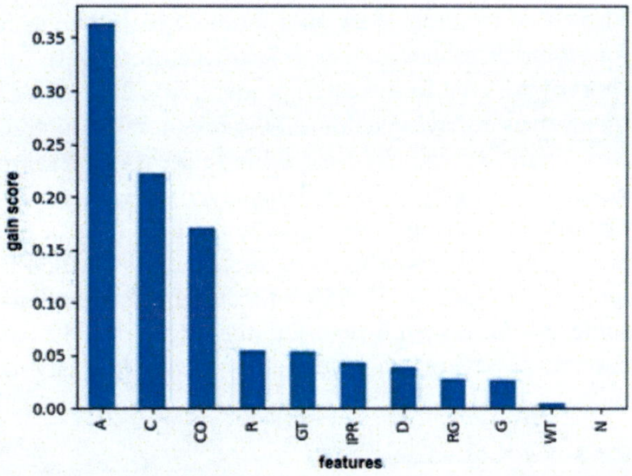

Fig. 2 Feature importance selection using extra trees classifier

Table 2 The gain scores for each feature

No	Features	Gain score
1	Scientific article (A)	0.362
2	Number of citations (C)	0.222
3	Conferences attended (CO)	0.170
4	Lecturer grade (R)	0.054
5	Number of grants (GT)	0.052
6	Intellectual property right (IPR)	0.042
7	Education qualification (D)	0.038
8	Grant awardee (RG)	0.270
9	Gender (G)	0.259
10	Lecturer status (WT)	0.004
11	Nationality (N)	0.000

The more relevant or significant a feature is to the target feature, the greater its gain score. The Article has the highest gain score toward Research Productivity, which is 0.362, followed by Citation at 0.222. Analyze this because the Articles have a very good spread of data. Most lecturers already have Scopus-indexed articles. Even the top quartile score equals the maximum score, although there are still lecturers who have not published their scientific articles (min = 0). The two features that have the lowest scores are Nationality and Lecturer Status. For the Nationality, it is dominated by 'Indonesian', while the Lecturer Status is more dominated by 'Permanent Lecturer'.

Based on this selection, Gender (G), Lecturer Status (WT), and Nationality (N) were not used in building the framework. The chosen feature then turns into variables that build the suggested framework. The testing phase using the data mining classifier comes after receiving the input variables. Figure 3 displays the evaluation outcomes using the K-NN algorithm. Figure 3 shows the K-NN algorithm Confusion Matrix.

61.54% of lecturers were appropriately identified as having fallen short of the goal for research production. 9.89% of lecturers were mistakenly classified as falling short of the goal for research productivity. 25.27% of lecturers accurately identified themselves as having achieved the research productivity target. 3.30% of academics were mistakenly counted as having achieved the research productivity target. The NB classifier Confusion Matrix is displayed in Fig. 4. 63.74% of lecturers were accurately identified as having fallen short of the goal for research production. There was zero percent of lecturers who were mistakenly classified as falling short of the goal for research production. 17.58% of lecturers accurately identified themselves as having achieved the research productivity target. 18.68% of academics were mistakenly counted as having achieved the research output target.

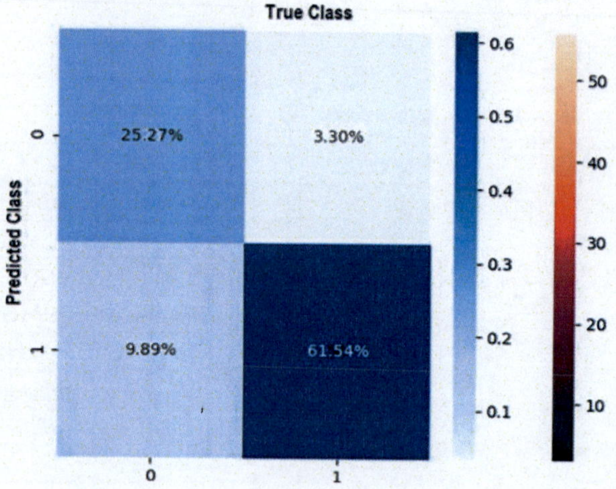

Fig. 3 K-NN confusion matrix

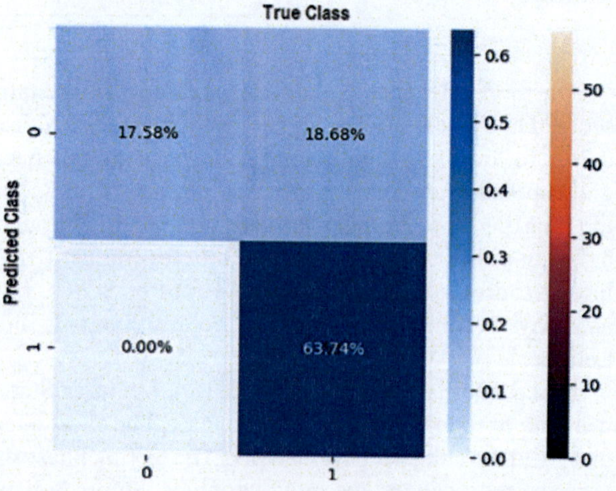

Fig. 4 Naïve Bayes confusion matrix

Table 3 Classifier performance comparison

Classifier	Accuracy (%)	Misclassification (%)
K-nearest neighbors	87	13
Naïve Bayes	81	19

Table 4 Accuracy scores comparison

Author	Algorithm used	Accuracy scores (%)
Ramli et al. [13]	Artificial neural network	82.24
	Support vector machine	80.47
	Logistic regression	80.31
	Decision tree	83.40
Henry et al. [14]	Logistic regression	78.2
Wichian et al. [15]	Neural network (back propagation)	90.72
Nazri et al. [16]	J-48	75.30
	C4.5	70.20
	Decision tree	70.30
	PART	75.00
Sanmorino et al. (this study)	K-nearest neighbors	87.00
	Naïve Bayes	81.00

The comparison of the performance of K-NN and NB classifier is shown in Table 3.

The K-NN algorithm has the highest accuracy score, which is 87%, followed by NB at 81%. This test's essence is not to get the highest score, but whether the components that construct the proposed framework could go through the evaluation phase with relevant results. A good or acceptable outcome is one that has a categorization score of more than 70%. When compared with other related research, the accuracy score is quite good. The accuracy comparison of the study with other methods is presented in Table 4; although using different datasets, the characteristics of the dataset that the author uses are similar to the datasets used by other researchers.

5 Conclusion

Based on the feature selection using Extra Trees Classifier, eight input variables were obtained, namely Scientific Article (Gain: 0.36), Number of Citations (Gain: 0.22), Number of Conferences Attended (Gain: 0.17), Intellectual Property Right (Gain: 0.04), Education Qualification (Gain: 0.03), Grant Awardee (Gain: 0.27), Number of Grants (Gain: 0.05), and Lecturer Grade (Gain: 0.05). The next stage is testing the selected features; two data mining algorithms were involved, KN Neighbors and Naïve Bayes algorithm. The accuracy score for each classifier is K-NN by 87%, and NB by 81%. These features are used as variables for the research productivity framework. Up to this point, the variables that construct the framework that the researcher proposes can go through a testing phase involving two data mining classifiers with results as expected, with an accuracy score of more than 70%, which is categorized as relevant or acceptable results.

References

1. Theodoridis S (2020) Classification: a tour of the classics
2. Kaisar S, Chowdhury A (2022) Integrating oversampling and ensemble-based machine learning techniques for an imbalanced dataset in dyslexia screening tests. ICT Express
3. Anand M et al (2022) Deep learning and natural language processing in computation for offensive language detection in online social networks by feature selection and ensemble classification techniques. Theor Comput Sci
4. Anns H (2018) Basic classification concepts 13
5. Urso A et al (2018) Data mining: prediction methods, pp 1–18
6. Berrar D (2018) Bayes theorem and Naive Bayes classifier, vol 1
7. Kotu V, Deshpande B (2015) Predictive analytics and data mining—chapter3: data exploration. Predictive analytics and data mining
8. Xu J, Zhang Y, Miao D (2019) Three-way confusion matrix for classification: a measure driven view. Inf Sci
9. Combined M (2012) Risks, odds, and ROC curves, no 1
10. Riffenburgh RH (2012) Statistic in medicine. ScienceDirect
11. Sanmorino A, Ermatita S, Rini DP (2020) A robust framework using gamification to increase scientific publication productivity. In: Proceedings—2nd international conference on informatics, multimedia, cyber, and information system, ICIMCIS 2020, pp 29–33
12. Sanmorino A, Ermatita S (2019) The preliminary results of the kms model with additional elements of gamification to optimize research output in a higher education institution. Int J Eng Adv Technol 8(5):554–559
13. Ramli NA, Nor NHM, Khairi SSM (2019) Prediction of research performance by academicians in local universities using data mining approach, vol 040021
14. Henry C, Md Ghani NA, Hamid UMA, Bakar AN (2020) Factors contributing towards research productivity in higher education. Int J Eval Res Educ 9(1):203–211
15. Na Wichian S, Wongwanich S, Bowarnkitiwong S (2009) Factors affecting research productivity of faculty members in government universities: LISREL and neural network analyses. Kasetsart J Soc Sci 30(1):67–78
16. Nazri MZA, Ghani RA, Abdullah S, Ayu M, Samsiah RN (2019) Predicting academic publication performance using decision tree, no 2, pp 180–185
17. Nussbaum M (2022) Machine learning and processing of large data. Reference module in earth systems and environmental sciences
18. Zucco C (2019) Multiple learners combination: introduction. Encycl Bioinform Comput Biol 1:519–524
19. Challapalli A, Li G (2022) Machine learning guided optimization of biomimetic polymeric lattice structures. Encycl Mater Plast Polym 2:280–299
20. Kaur K, Mittal SK (2020) Classification of mammography image with CNN-RNN based semantic features and extra tree classifier approach using LSTM. Mater Today Proc

21. Kareva I, Karev G (2020) Replicator dynamics and the principle of minimal information gain. Model Evol Heterog Popul 129–154
22. Ebrahimi B et al (2022) A cross-inefficiency approach based on the deviation variables framework. Omega 111
23. Wan X, Xu F, Luo X (2022) Economic optimization for process transition based on redundant control variables in the framework of zone model predictive control. Energy 241
24. Wang J, Chen Y, Zhu S, Xu W (2022) Depth feature extraction-based deep ensemble learning framework for high frequency futures price forecasting. Digit Signal Process 127
25. Ababneh AH (2022) Investigating the relevance of Arabic text classification datasets based on supervised learning. J Electron Sci Technol 20(issue 2)
26. Janjua F et al (2021) Textual analysis of traitor-based dataset through semi supervised machine learning. Futur Gener Comput Syst 125:652–660
27. Evaluating F, To P, Model P (2015) Model evaluation
28. Derczynski L (2013) Complementarity, F-score, and NLP evaluation, pp 261–266
29. Berrar D (2018) Performance measures for binary classification. Encycl Bioinform Comput Biol ABC Bioinform 1–3(1):546–560
30. Urso A, Fiannaca A, La Rosa M, Ravì V, Rizzo R (2018) Data mining: classification and prediction. Encycl Bioinform Comput Biol ABC Bioinform 1–3:384–402
31. Brown SD, Myles AJ (2020) Decision tree modeling, 2nd edn. Elsevier Inc.

A Survey on Big Data Analytics for Load Prediction in Smart Grids

Seemant Tiwari

Abstract Big data analytics has lately gained favor in energy management systems (EMS). EMS is in charge of overseeing, optimizing, as well as administering the electricity industry's activities. Energy utilization estimation is essential in EMS since it aids in generation planning, administration, and energy discussion. Advanced Technology, telecommunication, and automation systems are used in intelligent power grids, or "smart grids," which have become a popular trend worldwide. A challenging issue giving smart energy intelligence is predicting future network demand (energy demand). A huge number of data information is being composed through smart meters on a regular basis. Large number of analytics can aid trendy the development of intelligent energy management solutions. With this type of activity, power analysis is crucial. It is the act of gathering data since smart meters in the real period as well as since archival supplies besides smearing about the form of data investigation approach to uncover relevant relationships, tendencies, and themes. Precise predicting will permit a utility provider to strategize the resources and also to take controller actions to balance the supply and the electricity demand. The computation complexity of our investigation makes it possibly helpful for cases utilizing large-scale load prediction. Our work is capable of generating a more precise inquiry than a current prediction model, which is thought to be among the finest, according to numerous experimental results. In addition, the prediction methodologies are examined from both big data as well as traditional data perspectives.

Keywords Big data · Intelligent grid · Predicting the load · Analytical statistics

1 Introduction

The need for electricity has multiplied as a result of the most recent scientific improvements and developments. Additionally, overpopulation has an impact on energy consumption [1]. The conventional infrastructure is responsible for energy

S. Tiwari (✉)
Southern Taiwan University of Science and Technology, Tainan City 71005, Taiwan
e-mail: da82b203@stust.edu.tw

T. Triwiyanto et al. (eds.), *Proceeding of the 3rd International Conference on Electronics, Biomedical Engineering, and Health Informatics*, Lecture Notes in Electrical Engineering 1008, https://doi.org/10.1007/978-981-99-0248-4_3

production to fulfill the request of both producers and consumers [2]. The input that is available on the source besides demand sides can be effectively sensed by a smart grid. Utilizing devices and systems, authentic information is collected from multiple sites. Large data mentions the vast capacity of this information that is collected. Big data, or the enormous volume of information it contains, is utilized for a variety of analytical tasks [3]. The smart grid's multiple connectivities among customers and providers guarantees effective resource use [4]. Modern-day smart grids' biggest difficulties are lowering electrical costs and increasing customer convenience [5].

Present social and financial trends are driving up power requirements, and emerging businesses need effective design and operation. As a result, traditional electricity generation networks are finding it difficult to increase capacity. Electrical infrastructure is nothing like that as the maximum significant systems will be in charge of transporting the energy across the overhead transmission lines between distant power generations to existing clients. Such horizontal and coordinated processes are now out-of-date and inadequate to handle the durability, operational excellence, and sustainable development demands postured by such adjustments as a result of the existence of ecological and financial worries, the beginnings of substitute power sources, hybrid cars, or other technical advances, that in flip compelled necessity designing systems of electricity connectivity [6].

The advent of such a smart grid period and also the greater accessibility of renewables machinery allowed homes and smaller firms, which were previously thought of as recipients of services, to proactively donate the extra power they produced for including others [7]. The foundation of this technique is two-way monitoring and connectivity among suppliers and users, allowing for simple transmission including both electricity and information. Two factors are implied through this new product: firstly, such a smart grid will produce a significant quantity of information as part of its operations, and secondly, the big data idea will be used in smart metering. The concept of energy analysis is established there. It involves gathering sensor information in real time as well as from historical data sources, then using some kind of statistical technique to discover significant connections, tendencies, and anomalies.

To deliver smart grid expertise, grid demand forecasts are a crucial responsibility. An energy supplier will be able to prepare supplies like gasoline ahead and perform measures like turning on and offloading management equipment and changing power rates, among other things, with the use of precise predictions. Projecting a quantity supplied institution's "peak load"—or highest energy use—for a later time step is the issue at hand. The questioned customer identity may be of different granularities. A smart device for a home, a group of smart appliances for a community, an energy station for a village or town, or a power plant are a few examples (for a whole grid casing a huge environmental zone). The duration of the time step in the issue can vary, too. It could be 6 min, 15 min, hours, one day, the first week, and so on.

In the 1990s, scientists have been attempting to find a solution to the issue of anticipating power load [50]. Numerous methodologies, including time series studies like the ARIMA approach, fuzzy logic, the neuro-fuzzy approach, artificial neural networks (ANN), and support vector regression were developed. Among the most recent breakthroughs among these many tactics is the use of hybrid methodologies. It was shown that hybrid models would produce superior outcomes to more traditional techniques such as artificial neural networks.

An in-depth treatment of the use of big data with smart grids is given in this report, which also discusses load estimation in smart grids. The remaining document is prepared in the following manner: the foundation material and introduction of all significant themes and theories are accessible in Sect. 2. The phases of power analytics are defined in Sect. 3. Forecasting methods are deliberated in Sect. 4. The issues besides alternative solutions that its sector faces are discussed in Sect. 5. The discussion is in Sect. 6. Section 7 is an evaluation of load prediction techniques currently in use. Section 8 eventually brings the article to a close.

2 Foundation

Univariate models as well as multivariate models are the first two levels of the categorization architecture for estimation techniques. Split statistical models and AI models for univariate models primarily into two categories; statistical models include ARIMA and LR. NARX and LSTM AI model.

Statistical models and AI models are the two categories of multivariate models. Decision tree, classification and regression tree (CART), and Naïve Bayesian statistical models. The three categories of AI models are ensemble, hybrid, and deep learning. The methodology for ensemble models is described: Tree Bagger as well as Random Forest. RNN and CNN are two deep learning models. Hybrid models include ANN + PSO and SVM + PSO.

2.1 Big Data

Big data is currently a buzzword that everybody used. Furthermore, nobody is aware of the origin of the idea. Alvin Toffler introduced big data in the 1980s with their book The Third Wave. The utilization of a lot of data as well as its advantages for culture was also addressed by several Chinese investigators throughout the following ten years [8], resulting in noteworthy technical advancement, acquiring a really large amount of data became impossible. The usefulness of digitizing and information technology in the industry, though, began to be considerably highlighted in the trade and industrial realms also with advances in computer tools and gadgets like the websites, cellphones, and iPads. Those activities produced a significant amount of value is created, called "big data," as they are also known.

Big data's worth can be challenging to comprehend. The key seems to be that big data refers to more than just the quantities of information. It does have several qualities including worth, quantity, variety, speed, and honesty. The information gathered is helping manufacturing businesses decide things that will increase overall income. Knowledge about company activities has been further analyzed for previous errors, modeled for operational plans, and exposed to probabilistic recurrence assessment [9].

2.2 Smart Grid

Contingency grids served as the primary electricity generation for several years. Nevertheless, the state of affairs is changing significantly. The sensor network is a great illustration. A younger group of networks known as "smart grids" are comprised of equipment, technology, and telecommunication systems. The primary goals of such a smart grid are increased network stability and adaptability. Additionally, the smart grid can lessen energy losses caused by electricity distribution procedures. Additionally, over the past ten years, the appeal of renewables has grown steadily. The innovative aspect of modern networks is whether renewables, such as wind turbines and solar panels, could be quickly added to a distributed process to minimize grid congestion [10]. The present increased consumption of energy sources causes traditional electricity systems to be overloaded. System failures are consequently occurring quite regularly. Such factors have an influence on the structure of the electricity supply and also the economy in some locations. In additional terms, the smart grid presents a chance for the development of renewable energy causes.

In [10], renewable research is encouraged by the smart grid. As a result, a novel idea for power production emerged. Power service's exposure to electricity, solar, biowaste, and groundwater is growing. Nevertheless, for a myriad of purposes, these power sources could be unpredictable. For instance, solar panels cannot make electricity during foggy days. The advantage of the smart grid is that it can address dispersed generating issues besides enhancing the excellence of energy systems. Additionally, monitors and monitoring devices in smart grid organizations keep an eye on renewable activities. The evolution in the energy business concluded the historical few ages is what led to the advancements in smart grid organizations that are now available. In addition to revising and redesigning the production, transmitting, distributing, and consuming procedures to operate more efficiently, sensing and metering plans have also been added to monitor the functioning of the grid.

2.3 Big Data and Smart Grid

Several researchers across a variety of fields utilize the traditional 5 V model to explain the idea of big data.

Volume—Data becomes large mostly because of its enormous volume. Every day, readings from smart meters are collected in terabytes. Devices and monitoring devices, which are concentration measurement devices, can readily produce a large number of information sampling in smart grids. The need to store these huge amounts of information has become a major issue. Various storage options are offered for such a circumstance. Additionally, such places are software-connected to each other, enabling easy access to the information in one store by some other.

Velocity—Information is logged at a real frequency. Measured data by smart meters are taken at incredibly brief periods. A continual broadcasting method is being used. The place where the data is created and conveyed is determined by movement. Each sample seems to have a different weight, resulting in the issue. The coming does seem to hold some serious challenges for data transmission and storage.

Variety—Data from monitors, smart meters, and other relays, for example, might have a range of configurations. Data that is together organized and unorganized is gathered. To render the dataset intelligible as well as practical, it is regulated. Additionally, diversity denotes a vast range of data resources. Different data inputs, including wearable sensors and movies, can now be analyzed to produce more accurate findings than in the past.

Veracity—Data's validity is its ability to be trusted and recognized for what it is. The captured data could contain inaccurate or noisy values. The inaccurate results may be the result of device failure. Additionally, authenticity relates to the caliber of acquired data. Given the enormous amount of data acquired, there is a very high likelihood that this knowledge will have an impact on that analysis's findings.

Value—It is the removing of useful information from a set of information. The following stage is to comprehend the significance of information and how it will become beneficial. The problem is that even if the collection of data grows, less critical data is recorded. Nevertheless, the quantity of useful data increases as more precise smart measuring equipment is used.

2.4 Sources of Data for Smart Grids

The smart grid is just a sophisticated mechanism that eliminates a large amount of information from technology operating procedures. Further specifically, data is being collected again from point of electricity production to the point of client usage. Additionally, these data include measurements via smart meters. In [11], various types of devices which are deployed in the systems and digital metering in users' houses, workplaces, or industries handle a large portion of the gathering of information. A measuring collection of information is what it is. Details relating to industrial policy failures can be found in the company data provider. While it is impossible to assemble knowledge just on climate or vacations, the functioning of the electricity grid is impacted by such exterior sources of information.

3 Power Analytics

3.1 Data Gathering, Sharing, and Filtering

As has been indicated in the preceding section, several methods of data collecting are used according to the foundation of the information. For illustration, information about components beyond the smart grids is typically gathered from a variety of external sources, whereas quantitative research about electricity in smart grids is gathered besides that distributed through the aid of smart meters, which are implemented together with electricity firms and consumers. Such devices measure using varying degrees of precision and collecting precision based on the style. These observations often contain information about the feeder flow, energies more than any amount of time, node voltages, voltage level, harmonic distortion, active/reactive, and load profile. After the information has been composed, it is crucial to create reliable and affordable telecommunication services which would enable the connection of datasets that are dispersed across vast areas. Such networks can be connected to the network, but each offers advantages and disadvantages within itself. The cordless connection enables the inexpensive transmission of data from many edge devices to data centers, even when the data may be contaminated by interference. But at the additional point, traditional wired equipment, including Power Line Communication (PLC), has now been positively executed [11].

In [12], the three different connection configurations make up the smart grid's telecommunications network. Home Area Network, inside a modern house or apartment, is a system of smart meters as well as other gadgets. It is mostly used for native power monitoring and has a data transfer amount of fewer than 1 Kbps. Neighborhood Area Network is a system of many home-based routers whose primary purpose is to gather and store information on energy use in the load system infrastructure. Wide Area Network is a connection of every part of the smart grid. It is capable of transmitting a lot of data across a wide region.

In [13], through this point, it was clear that it was not the best course of action to acquire and analyze all the information which the smart grid produces since it would only result in higher transaction cost, computational burden, and computer storage capacity use. Data preparation is necessary to prevent such undesirable effects and boost the speed and effectiveness of predictive analytics. Data preparation is the method of dividing the size of the dataset to generate better condensed, intelligible representations of the generative model or to further classify the data with fewer actual errors. Three general types of data preparation approaches were identified. Data Integration: This aims to discover characteristics that are identical but have various terms, or separate characteristics having high similarity, and reduce the range of data by eliminating such "additional" characteristics that resulted from the combination of all smart meter data collections. Additionally, characteristics that are strongly linked are covered. Data Purification: It discusses how to handle information that is incomplete or unexpected. Usually, typically, removal or approximation procedures are utilized when there are null data. Contrarily, unusual numbers must either be regarded as information loss or left in the information source because they represent a recently occurring extremely rare occurrence. Transformation of Data: It deals with edge detection, where a group of fresh characteristics is produced by combining and transforming old ones. These methods are provided comprehensively and based on the specifications for particular tasks as well as the characteristics of the data gathering; they may be utilized solely or in groups.

3.2 Data Analytics

The aim of data analysis or machine learning would be to extract meaningful information from such a lot of structured research to determine patterns, and tendencies, including correlations that will reveal the untapped potential for the effective use of possessions already available. A thorough data analysis methodology is just what gives intelligent networks their intelligence; without it, establishing a pure, dependable, as well as effective grid is only a daft idea. The two most popular methods within machine learning were supervised besides unsupervised intelligence. These 2 vary in that category association is the emphasis on supervised learning whereas the emphasis on unsupervised learning is indeed the inherent patterns of the material. To obtain any information from the data, it is vital to consider data specificity because in supervised learning the information is categorized whereas in unsupervised learning it was not [14]. To obtain any information about the data, it is vital to consider data classification performance because even in supervised learning the information is categorized whereas it is not done in unsupervised learning.

4 Forecasting Methods

The estimation techniques are divided into two categories inside this segment: univariate models as well as multivariate models.

4.1 Forecasting Loads Utilizing Time Series Models

Electricity usage time series are records of electrical use made over a steady rhythm that is distributed uniformly. Time series forecasting makes predictions about upcoming outcomes depending on observations from the past. Here are a few well-known time series prediction methods that have been used to anticipate energy usage.

Autoregressive Integrated Moving Average. Probably the greatest widely used technique aimed at predicting time series data is ARIMA. ARIMA, often called the

Jenkins-Box technique, was first developed by Jinkens et al. [15]. This could determine the likelihood that a potential value will fall inside a given range of outcomes. ARIMA stands for Auto-Regression (AR) plus Moving Average (MA). According to the AR method, the present value of both sequences is dependent on their prior readings. The MA method goes under the premise that now the past dispersion from a sequence' mean affects the present variance of a number. The given form of ARIMA is (p, d, q,), whereby p signifies the number of autoregressive components, d is the amount of inter-annual variations, and q is the amount of delay prediction error. Pattern selection, statistical inference, and validation of the model are the three fundamental ARIMA processes.

Modify the time series into a stationary one if it is not already one. The mathematical model helps as the basis for emerging the predicting formula of ARIMA [42] as in Eqs. (1) and (2):

$$y_t = x_t' = x_t - x_{t-1} \tag{1}$$

where x_t' is first-order differencing; suppose x_t= series, and x_{t-1} = simply subtract the prior value, and y_t = create the new series:

$$x_t'' = x_t' - x_{t-1}' \tag{2}$$

where x_t'' is second-order differencing, x_t'= first-order differencing, and x_{t-1}' = first-order differencing on x_{t-1}:

$$\begin{aligned} xt'' &= x_t' - x_{t-1}' \\ &= (x_t - x_{t-1}) - (x_{t-1} - x_{t-2}) \\ &= x_t - 2x_{t-1} + x_{t-2} \end{aligned} \tag{3}$$

where xt'' = second-order differencing which can be identified by Eq. (3).

The extended formula for the ARIMA predictor can be expressed as follows using the equations mentioned above:

$$\text{ARIMA }(1, 1, 1)\, y_t = x_t\text{-}x_{t\text{-}1}$$

$$y_t = \emptyset_1 y_{t-1} + \theta_1 e_{t-1} + e_t \tag{4}$$

where e_t represents noise; $\emptyset_1$ and θ_1 represent parameters

Therefore, Eq. (4) gives us one AR parameter, one MA parameter, as well as the noise term.

Artificial Neural Network. Influenced by biological neurons, ANN is a group of networks of tiny computer units named neurons. Time series and multivariate data could both be predicted using ANN models. NARX and LSTM are two examples of well-liked time series ANN estimation techniques [16].

Human minds store information that they learn to memorize. Both the mind and the computers are capable of storing knowledge, but they do it through fundamentally various techniques. The information is saved in a certain area in computers, but the mind changes the connections between its neurons to store it because a neuron cannot store anything; it can only relay signals from one neuron to another.

Researchers could describe the mind as a vast neuronal network where the connections between the neurons create special information. Since this neural net mimics the functioning of the brain, we are referring to the brain. The neural network is comprised of linkages between nodes, much as the brain is made up of neuronal connections. Since the neural net imitates the connection of neurons, being the most major factor of the mind, what constitutes a neuron inside a neural net is a node. Human brains employ neuron associations, whereas neural networks utilize neuron weights of the connections.

Think about a node [44]. Signals x_1, x_2, x_3 are the nodes, while y represents the outputs. The values for the signals are w_1, w_2, and w_3, while b is biased, which would be connected to storing information. Consequently, we could state that weights and bias are the means through which the neural network stores its data. Upon accessing the node, the input signals are amplified by the weights:

$$u = (w_1 \times x_1) + (w_2 \times x_2) + (w_3 \times x_3) + b \tag{5}$$

$$u = wx + b \tag{6}$$

where x_1, x_2, and x_3 are signals

w_1, w_2, and w_3 are the signal's associated weights.

Bias, represented by the letter b, is related to the storage of information.

The sum is the node's output. Equation (5) clearly illustrates that the more weight, the more impact. The value function equation may be expressed in matrix notation.

$$w = [w_1\ w_2\ w_3] \tag{7}$$

$$x = \begin{bmatrix} x_1 \\ x_2 \\ x_3 \end{bmatrix} \tag{8}$$

where x_1, x_2, x_3 are signals, and w_1, w_2,w_3 are the signal's associated weights. The weighted sum Eq. (7) and Eq. (8) can be expressed in matrix form.

The node's output is analyzed using the "activation function:"

$$y = \emptyset\,(u) \tag{9}$$

Activation function is referred to as ø, which controls how a node behaves.A neural network node's result is given in Eq. (10):

$$y = \emptyset\,(u)$$

Value of u, by Eq. (6), is

$$y = \emptyset\,(wx + b) \tag{10}$$

where y is the output of a neural network node, b is biased, x is signal, w is signal-associated weight, and ø is activation function; a node's behavior is determined by its activation function.

Non-Linear Autoregressive Network with Exogenous Variable. A non-linear autoregressive recurrent neural network is called NARX. This has a response structure, where the platform's hidden layers are interconnected to the output nodes. Because it has a feedback link that includes multiple hidden layers rather than just the input layer, it differs from backpropagation ANN. Through the use of the previous relationship with the future or capture data, NARX additionally makes use of memories. It simulates a non-linear function using repetition again from the time series' historical values.

The changes and improvements in the time series are predicted using this transformation function. The previous delayed elements with the same time series serve as the channel's input. A popular dynamics neural design for input–output analysis of non-linear systems is the NARX circuit.

The NARX connection is made as a feedback control time-delayed neural network for use in time series forecasting. Without the feedback mechanism of delayed results, its prediction accuracy would be significantly worse. In [43], the extended formula in Eq. (11) for NARX looks like this:

$$y_t = f(y_{t-1}, y_{t-2}, y_{t-3}, y_{t-4}, \ldots\ldots u_{t-1}, u_{t-2}, u_{t-3}, u_{t-4}) \tag{11}$$

where f is the function, the relevant variable is y, the measured variable is u, and u assists in predicting y.

Long Short-Term Memory. A machine learning technique called LSTM is an RNN version. In [16], the primary goal of the LSTM proposal was to circumvent the disappearing gradients issue that arises during the learning of deep recurrent neural networks.

Each hidden unit neuron in LSTM is a storage cell with conscience recurring edges. Since these edges have a strength of 1, the gradients can traverse over several levels before bursting or disappearing.

Recurrent neural networks of the Long Short-Term Memory (LSTM) kind can acquire ordering dependent on classification predictive issues.

The inputs weight w, recurring weights r, and biases b of an LSTM layer are its learning weights. Provided by indicates, the cell state at time step t is

$$c_t = f_t * c_{t-1} + i_t * g_t \tag{12}$$

$$h_t = o_t * \sigma_c(c_t) \tag{13}$$

where * represents the vectors' component multiplication.

σ_c represents the state activation function indicated.

From [41], the elements at time step t are defined through the next set of Eqs. (14), (15), (16), and (17):

$$f_t = \sigma_g\left(w_f x_t + r_f h_{t-1} + b_f\right) \tag{14}$$

$$i_t = \sigma_g(w_i x_t + r_i h_{t-1} + b_i) \tag{15}$$

$$o_t = \sigma_g(w_o x_t + r_o h_{t-1} + b_o) \tag{16}$$

$$g_t = \sigma_c\left(w_g x_t + r_g h_{t-1} + b_g\right) \tag{17}$$

Here, σ_g represents the gate activation function, f_t represents forget gate, i_t represents input gate, o_t represents output gate, and g_t represents the cell candidate.

Analyzing Time Series Forecasting Approaches Comparatively. In [17], while ANN methods function superior at long-term prediction, ARIMA is best adapted toward short-term prediction. ANNs can represent non-stationary time series because they can understand the fundamental trends in the information with the aid of hidden layer nodes [18]. The flexibility with which neural networks may generate non-linear mappings among extracted features is one of its key advantages. These do a great job of capturing the non-linear behavior of the time series.

4.2 Predicting Loads Using Multivariate Models

Several inputs are used in multivariate models. Those sources, also known as independent factors, are the elements that have an impact on how much power is consumed. Such factors can include aspects of the climate (such as temperatures, moisture, cloud cover, and wind velocity), aspects of the schedule (such as the hours of the day and the day after), and even the charge of fuel. The three primary kinds of multivariate predicting techniques are ensemble, hybrid, and deep learning models.

Prediction of Load Using Ensemble Models. The forecast models known as ensemble methods integrate several learners to make superior efficiency. Ensemble models are methods for supervised learning. A powerful and efficient architecture is created by combining several ineffective learning strategies. The ensemble method combines several concepts to assist reduce generalization problems that may not be addressed by a singular programming strategy.

Suppose that there are 3 estimate representations A, B, and C each of which has an average accuracy of 89, 82, and 75 percent. Assume that A and C have a high degree of correlation and that model B does not. Mixing modeling A and C in this situation will not lower the estimation error, but adding model B to either model A or model C will result in more accuracy. Each prediction technique is given a specific value. Conventional approaches are used to give those weights.

The following are a few methods for distributing weight. Collinearity calculation: to choose the basic models, determine the covariance for every model with everyone. To make the final design sufficiently generic to provide minimal prediction error, eliminate the strongly associated models. Weight assignment by ANN: it is possible to employ neural networks to choose the proper values for the estimation techniques. Weight assignment by Bayesian: determining the likelihood function of each scenario assigns weights.

One of the 2 methods is possible: (1) an in-sample method is Bayesian model averages. (2) Predicting probability scale is a method that is not predetermined. Equal weight assignment: provide each model with the same amount of weight. Compared to more requirements for optimum, this one is the cheapest and frequently produces good results. It cannot, therefore, evaluate the algorithms according to their effectiveness. Additional methods involve learner-forward choice, bagged, and input sample enhancing.

Random Forest. The best ensemble learning methods are random forest (RF). Models are selected from a large set of data via substitution those are selections of the data's characteristics. Decision trees (DT) are created using a random selection of the data. With all of these examples of randomly picked data, multiple DTs are created, creating a random forest. Whatever tree-generating technique can produce DT. The RF method characteristics include a splitting criterion for decision trees as well as the number of trees in the method. For instance, data is used to construct 90 trees. Each tree develops a reaction to the test sample after receiving a test piece, resulting in 90 forecasts again for sample material. The ultimate anticipated number of the random forests is a biased sum of such replies. Since nearby are numerous trees in the forest created from various data sources, the projection system is particularly generic and cannot possibly be the majority of the cases.

In [19], researchers used the random forest to anticipate the short-term electrical load of an academic campus building. Regarding load forecasting, a two-staged framework is proposed. In the early phase, the moving average approach is used to analyze the trends in electricity usage. The best super variable, such as the trees, the splitting criterion for decision trees, and the minimal divide, is learned on RF in the second phase. Test and error are used to choose the parameter settings. In regards to MAPE besides RMSE, our suggested model performs better than SVR as well as ANN.

In [45], the generic bagging method is applied to tree learners by the random forest optimization technique. Provided a practice set, x = $x_1, x_2, \ldots. x_n$ with responses y = y_1, $y_2, \ldots. y_n$, after replacing the training dataset with such a random selection, bagging repeatedly (B times) fitting trees to such sampling. For b = 1....B, (1) n training instances from x and y are sampled with substitution; refer to these as x_b, y_b. (2) construct a regression and classifier tree f_b on x_b, y_b.

By summing the forecasts from each separate regression tree on x' after training, forecasts for unobserved observations x' can be generated by Eq. (18):

$$f = \frac{1}{B}\sum_{b=1}^{B} f_b(x') \tag{18}$$

where the bootstrapped data is represented by the random forest tree f_b, $x^{'}$ represents the sample, and B is a free variable; an optimal number of trees B can be found using cross-validation. Since the model's variance is reduced while raising the bias, this technique improves predictive accuracy.

Hybrid Systems Are Used for Load Forecasting. Approaches toward hybrid predicting combine approaches like regression as well as information filtering. Hybrid systems mitigate each product's obvious weaknesses while combining inherent advantages from two or more different techniques. Typically, a predicting technique is paired with such a metaheuristic optimization procedure to fine-tune the forecaster's model limitations. The hyper-parameters of the system should be selected following the trained data to develop an appropriate prediction. For all inputs, the standard hyper-parameters do not always ensure successful training. Through the integration of the most effective statistical as well as machine learning techniques, hybrid approaches promise to improve time series prediction.

Hybrid Support Vector Machine. SVM is a very effective estimate procedure. Among the most used approaches for forecasting, because of its reliability and precision of computing SVM was first suggested [20]. SVM develops an ideal hyperplane to categorize training samples into appropriate groups. Expense penalties, hypersensitive error function value, as well as sigma kernel parameters are the three primary hyper-parameters in SVM.

In [21], the researchers use a customized ABC optimization method to tune the model parameters of the least square SVM. Numerous estimation techniques are outperformed by the hybrid approach. The outcomes of the predictions demonstrate how well the hybrid model works. It surpasses several estimation methods, including ANN and ARMA. SVM [48], implementation in overall. Assume we have an n-sample training dataset. (x_i, y_i), (i = 1, 2,….,n), using the binary class labels y_i that belong to the input data vector x_i. In [49], the parameters construct the SVM classifier:

$$w.\emptyset(x_i) + b \geq 1 \quad if\ y_i = +1 \tag{19}$$

$$w.\emptyset(x_i) + b \leq 1 \quad if\ y_i = -1 \tag{20}$$

That is a single condition that can be expressed:

$$y_i(w.\emptyset(x_i) + b) \geq 1 \quad i = 1, \ldots, n \tag{21}$$

where ø(x) is a non-linear element's source space to a high-dimensional space transformation matrix. The separating hyper lane is defined by the weight matrix w. b is a deviation from the architecture of the separating hyper lane (0, 0).

If the provided dataset cannot be separated, a slack constant ξ_i is added such that, Eqs. (22) and (23),

$$y_i(w.\emptyset(x_i) + b) \geq 1 - \xi_i \quad i = 1, \ldots, n \tag{22}$$

$$\xi_i \geq 0 \qquad i = 1, \ldots, n \tag{23}$$

Hybrid ANN. The degree to which the algorithm is suited to the training data determines how much an ANN performs. The number of neurons, hidden layers, learning rate, velocity, and biases are the hyper-parameters of an ANN. In [22], a mixed predictive framework is proposed. The biological algorithm has employed the hyper-parameters of ANN. The outcomes demonstrate the suggested model's effectiveness and a high degree of precision in comparison to existing models.

Load Forecasting Based on DNN Models. In [23], DNNs are ANN variations with deep structures and numerous hidden units that are concatenated into the system. DNN's automatic image learning capabilities enable the learning algorithm to complicated non-linear functions and produce input-to-output mappings without manually creating characteristics [16].

A feed forward neural network, or autoencoder, is an unsupervised method of learning [47]. As implied by the name, autoencoders use an encoding algorithm to encrypt the data y = f(x). A decoding function is used to recreate the encoded information on the output node $x^{'}$= g(x). It is possible to write the rebuilt out as $x^{'}$= g (f(x)). In essence, hidden layers are used to copy the I/P to the O/P nodes. Autoencoders are used to reduce the size of inputs. Several encoding levels are layered with each other as hidden layers in a layered autoencoder. An autoencoder formula is shown in Eq. (24):

$$x' = g(wx + b) \tag{24}$$

Here, $x^{'}$ is the input that was rebuilt. The encoding factor is g. The weights are w, and b is the bias.

Convolution Neural Network. CNN is an intake ANN that applies the convolutional matrix multiplication to enter information. In essence, CNN uses three fundamental levels to construct its networks. Convolution, rectified linear unit (ReLU), and dumping level are these structures. Convolutional filtering is used in the convolution operation to excerpt the structure's information [23]. In [46], the following formula defines the convolution operation in Eq. (25):

$$y(t) = (x * w)(t) = \int x(a)w(t - a)da \tag{25}$$

where the input is x, w stands for kernel filter, and y is the outcome. That is the original input image at time t.

Evaluation of Multivariate Forecasting Techniques in Comparison. The strengths and weaknesses of the estimation techniques covered in the preceding part are briefly summarized in this section. This article also provides a relative examination of different models. The fundamental problem with RF is that a high number of trees is used to estimate the brand the method is extremely computationally and computationally intensive. As a result, this method won't be useful for making projections instantaneously. Although RF is quick to train, the learned model's predicting process takes longer.

In the occurrence of sufficient data, a large model, and powerful computing, DNN produces accurate forecasting predictions. Compared to other classifiers, DNN has the enormous benefit of not requiring feature extraction. It is a framework that is very adaptable to new issues.

5 Issues and Alternative Solutions

Big data is a crucial development in the modern day. It has numerous uses in numerous industrial fields. Big data analytics does have many benefits, but there are also several potential drawbacks when working with large datasets. The fact that information comes from a variety of smart grid devices such as sensors is among the key issues with datasets. Data aggregation is a viable alternative for handling a particular collection of information that comes in several forms.

Sometimes while using the smart grid, the network needs to react right away. An illustration of it may be an electrical network failure. Real-time analysis is necessary to identify unusual network activity. It includes several positive aspects, including quick data handling and a specific system's methodology to handle large datasets to prevent errors in the functioning of smart grids.

Electricity analysis of large data problems can be overcome in a variety of ways. Multiple software solutions may be able to resolve the problems of data amount and variety. The Apache Hadoop technology stage is by far the maximum dependable of them all. The computer's primary functions involve working with large amounts of data and dividing it up across components so that it may be processed quickly.

6 Discussion

The in-depth analysis of current load prediction models resulted in the following conclusions: These findings may aid in better load prediction understanding. If an optimization technique is modified, a decline in the locally optimal and an instability result could result. DNN requires a lot of computing power.

The number of neurons in hidden units, in addition to the total interlayer, should rise in very modest, sequential steps while choosing the best network settings, whereas a rise in the number of layers of neurons results in a surge across both integration time difficulties. A sufficient amount of data should be used as input variables since load data involves periodicity.

To create a reliable and comprehensive prediction system, sufficient data input that covers the entire periodicity trend must be collected. The majority of load forecasting studies does not take big data into account. Big data analysis helps to determine previously undiscovered insights that help manage and organize trading activities.

As demonstrated by the research study, load monitoring may identify periods of high-power usage. It is feasible to control power infrastructure, lessen grid congestion, or save revenue on investments. It is among the potential applications in the area of energy analysis. Investigators are indeed looking at the upcoming issues and difficulties in big data applications that are connected to managing data, data processing, as well as network issues.

We plan to investigate autonomous feature extraction in a research plan that will further enhance the precision of their regression model. Additionally, we intend to thoroughly evaluate our technology using numerous smart grid demand datasets from various nations and businesses and then perfect it to guarantee its applicability in all situations. Last but not the least, we believe that utility companies may find my study to be beneficial for their large-scale load forecasting applications for customer organizations at various resolution ranges.

We may say that several studies find that LSTM-based load power prediction is more accurate and less error-prone than conventional statistics-based prediction methods like AR, ARMA, and ARIMA. Therefore, using LSTM to estimate power requirements with some more hyper-tuned variables and optimizations could be successful and produce superior outcomes.

7 Comparative Load Prediction Techniques Currently in Use

The enormous amount and complexity of big data make it impossible for standard estimation techniques to manage it. By using small volumes of training data to create models, deep neural network (DNN) efficiently maintains storage. It divides the data into portions and does simultaneous training on several CPU cores. Table 1 displays the fundamental characteristics of the various prediction techniques.

Table 1 Characteristics of the various prediction techniques

Parameters	Structure	Prediction range	Area	Prediction technique	Elements
Historical energy needs and usage	Amusement facilities' everyday, hour, and 15-min power use	Medium period	Ontario, Canada	ANN, SVR [24]	Fit for handling massive amounts of information
Past loads and meteorological data	1.2 million customers (home, governmental) use the actual distribution model on an hourly basis	Short-term and one week from now	Not brought up	Regression tree, segmentation, and hierarchical clustering [25]	Computer illiterate
Weather and traffic data from the past	A national road from Goyang to Paju was seen to include hourly traffic and meteorological data	Short-term, tomorrow	South Korea	The decision tree [26]	Simple
Previous load	Three Intelligent homes are loaded per second into the dataset	Short-term, daily, and next week	Umass Trace Online Repository	Adaptive Neuro-Fuzzy Inference System [27]	Good precision, ease of
Previous consumption	Usage of the Budweiser Gardens exhibition space for 15 min	Short-term, daily, and next week	Ontario, Canada	SVR [28]	Easy and fast
Data on past temperatures and power usage	National Penghu University of Science and Technology's Hartcourt North Building	Short term	Taiwan	Multipoint fuzzy prediction [29]	High precision

(continued)

Table 1 (continued)

Parameters	Structure	Prediction range	Area	Prediction technique	Elements
Outside temperature, humidity levels, and the temperature of the supply and returns of cold water	Information from the university buildings of the Hong Kong Polytechnic University covering a year's worth of operations	Short term	Hong Kong	Association rule mining, decision tree model [30]	Simple
Weather information and electricity use	Details on 5000 families' usage at 15-min interludes from a project with the Chattanooga Electric Power Board	Future days, weeks, and short-term	Chattanooga, U.S.A	Sparse coding, ridge regression [31]	High precision
A temperature within and outside, humidity, solar radiation, calendar characteristics, and usage	Climate and usage at a Girona University office	Future day, week, and short-term	Girona University	ANN, SVR [32]	Regression models are less precise than ANN but easier and quicker
Previous load	5 cities' hourly usage	Short term	FARS electric power company	SVR [33]	High precision
Past load information	Belsito Prisciano feeder Azienda Comunale Energia e Ambiente (ACEA) power grid load time is 10 min; the distance to Rome is 10,490 km	Short-term, a day, and ten minutes	Rome	Echo State Network [34]	High precision

(continued)

Table 1 (continued)

Parameters	Structure	Prediction range	Area	Prediction technique	Elements
Historical cost and meteorological characteristics	HVAC system usage statistics for a five-star hotel in Hangzhou City, China	Short-term, tomorrow	State Grid Corporation of China Hangzhou, China	SVR [35]	Simple
Previous load	Data about NSW State's hourly consumption in real-time	Short-term, daily, and next week	Australia	RBFNN [36]	High precision
Temperature, kind of date	3000 Irish homes' Smart meters' worth of data from the Irish Social Science Data Archive (ISSD) took 30 min to load	Short term	Ireland	K-mean [37]	A quick learner
Previous load	15 min are needed to load each household's meter data	Short term	Taipei, Taiwan	The decision tree [38]	Accuracy, robustness to noise information
Lagged burdens, calendar, and weather elements	Irish Social Science Data Archive's "Smart Metering Customer Behavior Trial" used 5000 houses for a 15-min power load (ISSDA)	Quite Short-term, between 15 and 1 h in the future	Ireland	ANN [39]	Engineered automatically, robustness to noisy data
Temperature and humidity	2012 Global Energy Predicting Contest, temperature, and hourly load	Short-term, upcoming day and week	USA regions, 21	Recency effect [40]	Effective use of big data

8 Conclusion

This study is anticipated to act as a starting point for such inexperienced investigators involved in the arena of electricity ingesting estimating. The majority of the investigation focuses on predicting short-term or medium-term loads. A place that requires further investigation is long-term load prediction. The method used to estimate the electricity consumed varies depending on the circumstance and forecasting timeframes. It is stated that while univariate classifiers work well on minor datasets, multivariate estimate models are appropriate for big datasets.

Concerning effectiveness, deep learning projection approaches perform better than any traditional or computational intelligence predictive model. In addition, their great processing capacity gives computers the best option for big data analytics including projection, when other machine learning techniques struggle to deliver satisfactory results. DNN has also been shown to be a successful tool for long-term prediction.

References

1. Aslam S, Herodotou H, Mohsin SM, Javaid N, Ashraf N, Aslam S (2021) A survey on deep learning methods for power load and renewable energy forecasting in smart microgrids. Renew Sustain Energy Rev 144
2. Rabiya K, Nadeem J (2020) A survey on hyperparameters optimization algorithms of forecasting models in smart grid. Sustain Cities Soc 61
3. Syed D, Zainab A, Ghrayeb A, Refaat SS, Abu-Rub H, Bouhali O (2021) Smart grid big data analytics: Survey of technologies, techniques, and applications. IEEE Access 9:59564–59585
4. Lei C, Qu Y, Gao L, Xie G, Yu S (2020) Detecting false data attacks using machine learning techniques in smart grid: a survey. J Netw Comput Appl 170
5. Salkuti SR (2020) A survey of big data and machine learning. Int J Elect Comput Eng 10(1):575–580
6. Ancillotti E, Bruno R, Conti M (2013) The role of communication systems in smart grids: architectures, technical solutions, and research challenges. Comput Commun 36(17–18):1665–1697
7. Da Silva PG, Dejan I, Karnouskos S (2014) The impact of smart grid prosumer grouping on forecasting accuracy and its benefits for local electricity market trading. IEEE Trans Smart Grid 5(1):402–410
8. Zhang H, Li Y, Shen C, Sun H, Yang Y (2015) The application of data mining in finance industry based on big data background. In: IEEE 17th international conference on high performance computing and communications. IEEE 7th international symposium on cyberspace safety and security. IEEE 12th international conference on embedded software and systems. New York, pp 1536–1539
9. Yang L, Zhang J-J (2017) Realistic plight of enterprise decision-making management under big data background and coping strategies. In: IEEE 2nd international conference on big data analysis. Beijing, pp 402–405
10. Guner S, Ozdemir A (2011) Turkish power system: from conventional past to smart future. In: 2011 2nd IEEE PES International conference and exhibition on innovative smart grid technologies. Manchester, pp 1–4
11. Zhang Y, Huang T, Bompard EF (2018) Big data analytics in smart grids: a review. Energy Inf 1

12. Baimel D, Tapuchi S, Baimel N (2016) Smart grid communication technologies-overview, research challenges and opportunities. In: International symposium on power electronics, electrical drives, automation and motion. Capri, pp 116–120
13. Diamantoulakis PD, Kapinas VM, Karagiannidis GK (2015) Big data analytics for dynamic energy management in smart grids. Big Data Res 2(3):94–101
14. Zhao Z, Liu H (2007) Spectral feature selection for supervised and unsupervised learning. In: Proceedings of the 24th international conference on machine learning, pp 1151–1157
15. Box G, Jenkins G, Reinsel G, Ljung G (2008) Time series analysis: forecasting and control. Wiley, Hoboken, NJ, USA
16. Zheng H, Yuan J, Chen L (2017) Short-term load forecasting using EMD-LSTM neural networks with a Xgboost algorithm for feature importance evaluation. Energies 10(8):1168
17. Wei Z, Li X, Li X, Hu Q, Zhang H, Cui P (2017) Medium-and long-term electric power demand forecasting based on the big data of smart city. J Phys Conf Series 887, China.
18. Ertugrul OF (2016) Forecasting electricity load by a novel recurrent extreme learning machines approach. Int J Electr Power Energy Syst 78:429–435
19. Moon J, Kim KH, Kim Y, Hwang E (2018) A Short term electric load forecasting scheme using 2-stage predictive analytics. In: IEEE International Conference on Big Data and Smart Computing. Shanghai, pp 219–226
20. Cortes C, Vapnik V (1995) Support-vector networks. Mach Learn 20:273–297
21. Shayeghi H, Ghasemi A, Moradzadeh M, Nooshyar M (2015) Simultaneous day-ahead forecasting of electricity price and load in smart grids. Energy Convers Manage 95:371–384
22. Xiao L, Wang J, Hou R, Wu J (2015) A combined model based on data pre-analysis and weight coefficients optimization for electrical load forecasting. Energy 82:524–549
23. Dong X, Qian L, Huang L (2017) Short-term load forecasting in smart grid: a combined CNN and K-means clustering approach. In: IEEE International Conference on Big Data and Smart Computing. Jeju, p. 119–125
24. Katarina G, Alexandra L, Miriam A, Luke S (2016) Energy forecasting for event venues: big data and prediction accuracy. Energy Build 112:222–233
25. Zhang P, Wu X, Wang X, Bi S (2015) Short-term load forecasting based on big data technologies. CSEE J Power Energy Syst 1(3):59–67
26. Arias MB Bae S (2016) Electric vehicle charging demand forecasting model based on big data technologies. Appl Energy 183:327–339
27. Sulaiman SM, Jeyanthy PA, Devaraj D (2016) Big data analytics of smart meter data using adaptive neuro fuzzy inference system (ANFIS). In: International conference on emerging technological trends (ICETT), pp 1–5
28. Grolinger K, Capretz MAM, Seewald L (2016) Energy consumption prediction with big data: balancing prediction accuracy and computational resources. In: IEEE international on congress big data, pp 157–164
29. Chang HH, Chiu W-Y, Hsieh T-Y (2016) Multipoint fuzzy prediction for load forecasting in green buildings. In: International conference on control, automation and systems. Gyeongju, pp 562–567
30. Xiao F, Wang S, Fan C (2017) Mining big building operational data for building cooling load prediction and energy efficiency improvement. In: IEEE international conference on smart computing (SMARTCOMP). Hong Kong, pp 1–3
31. Yu C-N, Mirowski P, Ho TK (2017) A sparse coding approach to household electricity demand forecasting in smart grids. IEEE Trans Smart Grid 8(2):738–748
32. Massana J, Pous C, Burgas L, Melendez J, Colomer J (2015) Short-term load forecasting in a non-residential building contrasting models and attributes. Energy Build 92:322–330
33. Kavousi-Fard A, Samet H, Marzbani F (2014) A new hybrid modified firefly algorithm and support vector regression model for accurate short-term load forecasting. Expert Syst Appl 41(13):6047–6056
34. Bianchi FM, De Santis E, Rizzi A, Sadeghian A (2015) Short-term electric load forecasting using echo state networks and PCA decomposition. IEEE Access 3:1931–1943

35. Chen Y, Tan H, Song X (2017) Day-ahead forecasting of non-stationary electric power demand in commercial buildings: hybrid support vector regression based. Energy Procedia 105:2101–2106
36. Lu Y, Zhang T, Zeng Z, Loo J (2017) An improved RBF neural network for short-term load forecast in smart grids. In: IEEE international conference on communication systems (ICCS). Shenzhen, China, pp 1–6
37. Li Y, Guo P, Li X (2016) Short-term load forecasting based on the analysis of user electricity behavior. Algorithms 9(4):80
38. Hsiao Y-H (2015) Household electricity demand forecast based on context information and user daily schedule analysis from meter data. IEEE Trans Ind Inf 11(1):33–43
39. Quilumba FL, Lee WJ, Huang H, Wang DY, Szabados RL (2015) Using smart meter data to improve the accuracy of intraday load forecasting considering customer behavior similarities. IEEE Trans Smart Grid 6(2):911–918
40. Wang P, Liu B, Hong T (2016) Electric load forecasting with recency effect: a big data approach. Int J Forecast 32(3):585–597
41. Hochreiter S, Schmidhuber J (1997) Long short-term memory. Neural Comput 9(8):1735–1780
42. Box GEP, Jenkins GM, Reinsel GC, Ljung GM (2015) Time series analysis: forecasting and control. Wiley
43. Saeed A, Amirreza T, Ali C (2022) Fault detection and isolation of gas turbine using series-parallel NARX model. ISA Trans 120:205–221
44. Xu A, Li R, Huimin C, Xu Y, Li X, Lin G, Yan Z (2022) Artificial neural network (ANN) modeling for the prediction of odor emission rates from landfill working surface. Waste Manag 138:158–171
45. James G, Witten D, Hastie T, Tibshirani R (2013) An introduction to statistical learning. Springer Second Edition
46. Aslam S, Ayub N, Farooq U, Alvi MJ, Albogamy FR, Rukh G, Haider SI, Azar AT, Bukhsh R (2021) Towards electric price and load forecasting using CNN-based ensembler in smart grid. Sustainability 13(22):12653
47. Wang X, Liu H (2018) Soft sensor based on stacked auto-encoder deep neural network for air preheater rotor deformation prediction. Adv Eng Inform 36:112–119
48. Aung Z, Toukhy M, Williams J, Sanchez A, Sergio H (2012) Towards accurate electricity load forecasting in smart grids. In: Fourth international conference on advances in databases, knowledge, and data applications, pp 51–57
49. Vapnik VN (2000) The nature of statistical learning theory. Information Science and Statistics Springer, New York
50. Adams G, Allen PG, Morzuch BJ (1991) Probability distributions of short-term electricity peak load forecasts. Int J Forecast 7(3):283–297

Analysis of Three-Phase Induction Motor Speed Performance with Load Torque Changes Using Inverter Space Vector Pulse Width Modulation (SVPWM) Control

Setiyono and Bambang Dwinanto

Abstract This paper presents an analysis of the Space Vector Pulse Width Modulation method which is applied to an inverter for controlling asynchronous alternating current motors or three-phase induction motors through modeling simulations using Simulink MATLAB tools. Induction motors have complex rotational speed control characteristics. Its performance is influenced by several things, including the number of poles, and the frequency setting of the input voltage. To get a wide frequency setting, generally an inverter switch is use which is regulated by controlling the switch gate trigger pulse. This modeling is also used to determine the control pattern of the inverter switch trigger, the characteristics of the voltage curve, torque current, and speed of a three-phase induction motor. This study is also expected to help researchers in solving problems related to the Space Vector Pulse Width Modulation programming algorithm more concisely and easily because the inverter trigger pattern can be directly implemented into electronic control programming. The simulation results show that the induction motor can work on load changes with small torque ripples, stator, and rotor currents with small ripples and is followed by a linear rotational speed setting.

Keyword Space vector pulse width modulation · Inverter · Three-phase induction motor

1 Introduction

Induction machines as electric power equipment are widely used in various fields, including industry, transportation, offices, and households. Besides having the advantages offered, this machine also has a weakness in setting the rotational speed. The rotational speed of an induction motor can be controlled in two ways, namely direct and indirect starting. Starting directly is done by connecting the motor to the grid voltage. This method has the disadvantage of causing power losses when the motor

Setiyono (✉) · B. Dwinanto
Department of Electrical Engineering, Gunadarma University, Jakarta, Indonesia
e-mail: setiyono@staff.gunadarma.ac.id

T. Triwiyanto et al. (eds.), *Proceeding of the 3rd International Conference on Electronics, Biomedical Engineering, and Health Informatics*, Lecture Notes in Electrical Engineering 1008, https://doi.org/10.1007/978-981-99-0248-4_4

is initially connected to a power source, because at that time the motor draws a very large starting current. The starting method is indirectly by adjusting the supply voltage, input current, stator field flux, and frequency using an electronic device known as a Variable Speed Drive (VSD), especially Inverter [1] [2]. The use of VSD in induction motors has an effect on the improvement of torque, speed, and current drawn by the motor. The study begins with modeling the character control of speed, rotor current, and motor torque [3–7]. Ahmed J. Ali1 modeled the transient regulation approach of a cage-rotor induction motor based on the winding function (WFA) which assumes the MMF coupling between the rotor and stator is sinusoidal and non-sinusoidal. The result is that the second model approach is better [4]. Babak Kiani in his paper writes a Limited Set Model Predictive Direct Torque control method (FS—MPDTC) to reduce torque and flux ripples, by implementing two or more Space Vector Pulse Modulation (SVPWM) voltage vectors [8]. Yassine Zahraoui said space vector modulation is a very appropriate solution to reduce high ripple levels regardless of its complexity [9]. Mihoub Youcef implemented RST and adaptive fuzzy controller (AFC) to increase variable speed Induction motor drive control system [10]. Arkan A. Kadum presents a new adaptive hysteresis band control approach used in direct torque control (DTC) of induction motor drive (IM) with a switching pattern for PWM signal generation; the simulation results under different operating conditions over a wide speed range show the validity, effectiveness, and feasibility of the proposed design [11]. Several other researchers developed induction motor drives with space vector control to obtain lower torque ripple and wider speed regulation [12–19]. Control with VSD is generally done by setting the ignition pattern of the inverter switch using switch control or vector control. Switch ignition settings with vector control have advantages such as more efficient use of energy, and produce a wide rotational speed setting. This study describes a study of induction motor control testing on various changes in load torque using the Space Vector Pulse Width Modulation method to see the character of the stator current, rotor current, and speed of a three-phase induction motor through modeling using the Simulink MATLAB tool. Previous researchers used a lot of Sinusoidal Pulse Width Modulation (SPWM) control method, but in the article the method of generating a gate ignition signal using the Space Vector Modulation (SVPWM) method has a smaller harmonic distortion and a higher output voltage than the SPWM method. The simulation results show that the design of the induction motor speed regulation using SVPWM can work well and is able to operate at changes in load torque. This design can be a technological contribution and a reference for advanced researchers to be implemented into electronic circuits.

2 Space Vector Concept

The representation of the time function of a balanced three-phase system of a voltage and current can be shown in Eq. (1):

$$v_a + v_b + v_c = 0 \tag{1}$$

The magnitude and direction of the vector $[v_a 00]^T$ of a three-phase system is placed along the coordinates of the d-axis; the vector $[0 v_b 0]^T$ is shifted by 120^0 and the vector $[00 v_c 0]^T$ is shifted by 240^0. Figure 1 is an illustration of this vector in imaginary coordinates d-q.

$$\alpha = tg^{-1}\left(\frac{V_d}{V_q}\right) = \omega = 2\pi f \tag{2}$$

where $f =$ fundamental frequency for Eq. (2).

If v_a, v_b, v_c is specified as a reference, the vector v_{ref} can be determined by Eq. (3):

$$v_{ref} = \frac{2}{3}\left[v_a + v_b e^{j(2/3)\pi} + v_c e^{-j(2/3)\pi}\right] \tag{3}$$

The vector v_{ref} (three-dimensional space) is then transformed into a two-dimensional d-q space base system into an algebra for the sum of real elements and imaginary elements in Eq. (4):

$$\begin{bmatrix} v_d \\ v_q \end{bmatrix} = \frac{2}{3}\begin{bmatrix} 1 & \frac{-1}{2} & \frac{-1}{2} \\ 0 & \frac{\sqrt{3}}{2} & \frac{-\sqrt{3}}{2} \end{bmatrix}\begin{bmatrix} v_a \\ v_b \\ v_c \end{bmatrix} \tag{4}$$

The next step is the transformation of the d-q coordinate space to the $\alpha - \beta$ coordinates obtained by Eq. (5):

$$\begin{bmatrix} v_\alpha \\ v_\beta \end{bmatrix} = \begin{bmatrix} \cos(\omega t) & \cos\left(\frac{\pi}{2} + \omega t\right) \\ \sin(\omega t) & \sin\left(\frac{\pi}{2} + \omega t\right) \end{bmatrix}\begin{bmatrix} v_d \\ v_q \end{bmatrix} = \begin{bmatrix} \cos(\omega t) & -\sin(\omega t) \\ \sin(\omega t) & \cos(\omega t) \end{bmatrix}\begin{bmatrix} v_d \\ v_q \end{bmatrix} \tag{5}$$

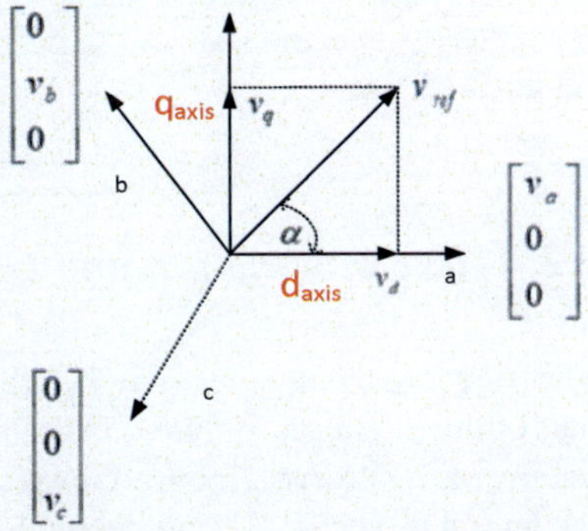

Fig. 1 Placement of the Vector of a three-phase to d-q Coordinate

If v_a, v_b, v_c is a three-phase voltage-balanced system with a maximum value of V_m, then the vector $v(t)$ can be denoted by Eq. (6):

$$v(t) = V_m e^{j\omega t} \quad (6)$$

Thus, $v(t)$ is a vector with a maximum amplitude of V_m rotating at a constant angular velocity of ω rad/sec.

2.1 Eight Vector Switching Inverter Combinations in Space Vector Pulse Modulation (SVPWM)

The performance of the three-phase inverter switch can be grouped into eight states. Switches a, b, and c have complementary switch pairs a', b', and c' where when switch a is connected or ON then the complementary switch pair a' is open or OFF. Likewise, switch b and switch c work in reverse with their complementary switches b' and c'.

Figure 2 describes a three-phase inverter having eight switching conditions that can be formed in eight binary compositions from 000 to 111. Each composition is denoted by V_0, V_1, V_2, V_3, V_4, V_5, V_6, and V_7 hereinafter referred to as vector switching. V_1, V_2, V_3, V_4, V_5, and V_6 are called non-zero vectors because they produce an output voltage that is not equal to zero, while V_0 and V_7 are called zero vectors where this vector produces an output voltage equal to zero.

Figure 3 shows 6 vectors mapped to six sectors (sectors 1 to 6) in a position around the central point forming a hexagonal shape while two vectors are mapped to the center point (origin) [9, 20–22]. Each sector has a vector angular distance of 60^0. In one rotation on the complex coordinate plane d-q, V_{ref} will pass through the six non-zero vectors and zero vectors. The inverter output voltage is also affected by the SVPWM modulation index. Selection of the right modulation index will assist in the production of the rated voltage. If the modulation index is less, the pulse duration on time will be less and therefore, the device conduction time will also be less, so the inverter output voltage is reduced [23, 24].

Table 1 shows the state of the output voltage (V_0–V_7) at various switch conditions for each sector.

2.2 Time Calculation and Gate Trigger Pattern

The trigger of the inverter switch gate with the SVPWM method is the most important part of this research. Figure 4 explains the basis for calculating the trigger timing of the inverter gate switch based on vector analysis in sector 1. V_{ref} is the resultant of the length of vector V_A and vector V_B, and can be represented by Eq. (7):

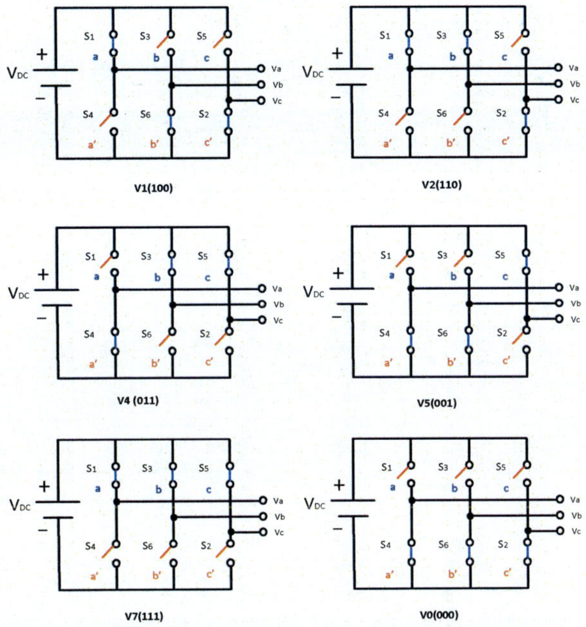

Fig. 2 Eight combinations of inverter switch conditions

Fig. 3 The position of each vector on the coordinate plane of two-dimensional space, d-q

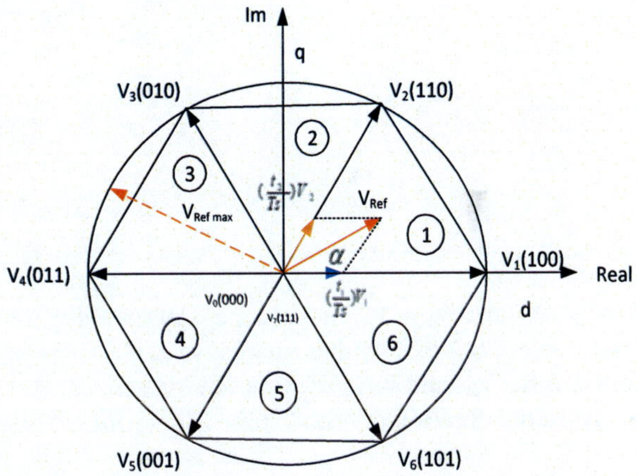

$$V_{\mathrm{ref}} = V_{\mathrm{A}} + V_{\mathrm{B}} \tag{7}$$

In each sector, the value of is always in the interval $0 \leq \alpha \leq \frac{\pi}{3}$. The voltage V_{ref} in sector 1 is of angle 60^0, the value $V_{\mathrm{A}} = V_1$, $V_{\mathrm{B}} = V_2$, then the voltage V_{ref} in sector

Table 1 Inverter output voltage in vector switching state

Voltage vectors	Sector	Switching vector			Line to neutral voltage			Line-to-line voltage		
		a	b	c	V_{an}	V_{bn}	V_{cn}	V_{ab}	V_{bc}	V_{ac}
V_0	0 (origin)	0	0	0	0	0	0	0	0	0
V_1	1	1	0	0	2/3	– 1/3	– 1/3	1	0	– 1
V_2	2	1	1	0	1/3	1/3	– 2/3	0	1	– 1
V_3	3	0	1	0	– 1/3	2/3	– 1/3	– 1	1	0
V_4	4	0	1	1	– 2/3	1/3	1/3	– 1	0	1
V_5	5	0	0	1	– 1/3	– 1/3	2/3	0	– 1	1
V_6	6	1	0	1	1/3	– 2/3	1/3	1	– 1	0
V_7	0 (Origin)	1	1	1	0	0	0	0	0	0

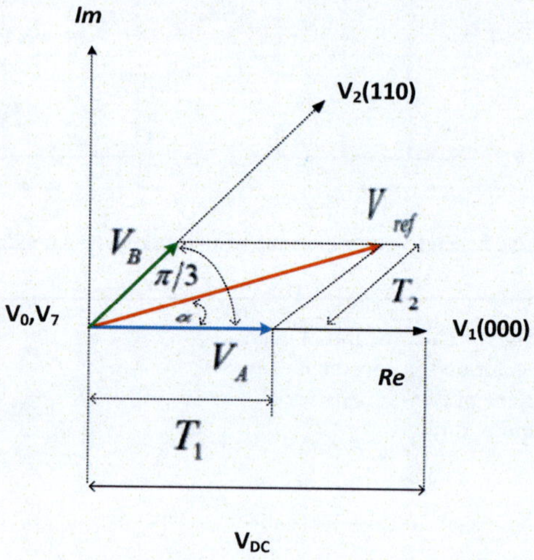

Fig. 4 Calculation of V_{ref}, T_1, and T_2 in sector 1

2, $V_A = V_2$ and $V_B = V_3$. In the same way for every other sector, V_{ref} shifts or moves left counterclockwise with a time lapse of T_z. T_1 is the time lapse for V_A, T_2 is the time lag for V_B, and T_0 is the time interval for V_0 and V_7. In sector 1 mathematical analysis, the duration of each T time is determined by Eq. (8), Eq. (9), and Eq. (10):

$$T_1 = T_z.a.\frac{\sin\left(\frac{\pi}{3} - \alpha\right)}{\sin\left(\frac{\pi}{3}\right)} \tag{8}$$

$$T_2 = T_z.a.\frac{\sin(\alpha)}{\sin\left(\frac{\pi}{3}\right)} \tag{9}$$

$$T_z = T_1 + T_2 + T_0 \tag{10}$$

where $0 \leq \alpha \leq 60^0$; $T_z = \frac{1}{f_z}$; and $a = \frac{|\overline{V}_{ref}|}{\frac{2}{3}V_{dc}}$

Figure 4 explains each sector the value of is always in the interval $0 \leq \alpha \leq \frac{\pi}{3}$, in sector 1 V_{ref} angle of $\alpha = 0^0$ is the same as V_1, for angle of $\alpha = \frac{\pi}{3}$ is parallel to V_2. In sector 2, V_{ref} angle of $\alpha = 0^0$ is the same as V_2, for angle of $\alpha = \frac{\pi}{3}$ is parallel to V_3. And so on for calculations in other sectors [25] using Eq. (11) and Eq. (12).

Time duration in sector *n*

$$T_1 = \frac{\sqrt{3}T_z|\overline{V}_{ref}|}{V_{dc}}\left(sin\left(\frac{\pi}{3} - \alpha + \frac{n-1}{3}\pi\right)\right) \quad (11)$$

$$T_2 = \frac{\sqrt{3}T_2|\overline{V}_{ref}|}{V_{dc}}\left(\sin\left(\alpha - \frac{n-1}{3}\pi\right)\right) \quad (12)$$

where n = 1, 1 through 6 (that is, sectors 1 through 6, $0 \leq \alpha \leq 60^0$).

3 Method

The working method with the tool of Simulink MATLAB software through analyses parameters of each section in this paper such as voltage, gate pulse, stator currents, rotor currents, and much more positively impacted this study. It is the result of the design developed by the researcher (space vector modulation), which also produces various effects that can be used as a reference for other researchers due to the data analyzed.

Some of the parameters analyzed in this paper include the generation of reference voltages, the turn-on time of the inverter switch for each sector, gate pulses, stator currents, rotor currents, and the relationship between torque and DC motor speed. Figure 5 describes the research method used by building a path or wiring step from the designed system design. The working steps are as follows: The three-phase power source is a three-phase sine wave generator at a frequency of 50 Hz, and variable amplitude with a phase difference of 1200 for each wire. These three voltages are then transformed into a 2-coordinate system or abc—αβ which is called the park transformation. The reference voltage and the sector selection angle are used to determine the sector of the plane on the d-q coordinate axis where the stress vector is selected. There are six sectors in the d-q coordinate axis; each sector is 600. The next step is to determine the values of T_z, T_1, T_2, and T_0 using Eqs. 7, 8, 9, and 10 to get the timing pattern of the inverter ignition pulse. The inverter pulse generator is obtained by comparing the space vector modulator signal with a triangular carrier signal with a frequency of 4 kHz. The inverter is composed of 3 leg pairs of IGBT switches as Variable Speed Driver (VSD) activated by a pulse ignition pulse. A three-phase induction motor as a load is simulated with parameters 54 HP (4 kW), 400 V, 50 Hz, and 1430 rpm. The value of the DC link voltage on the inverter is 400 V. When the position vector is at V_0 and V_7 then no current flows in the load or $I_{inv} = 0$ A. All

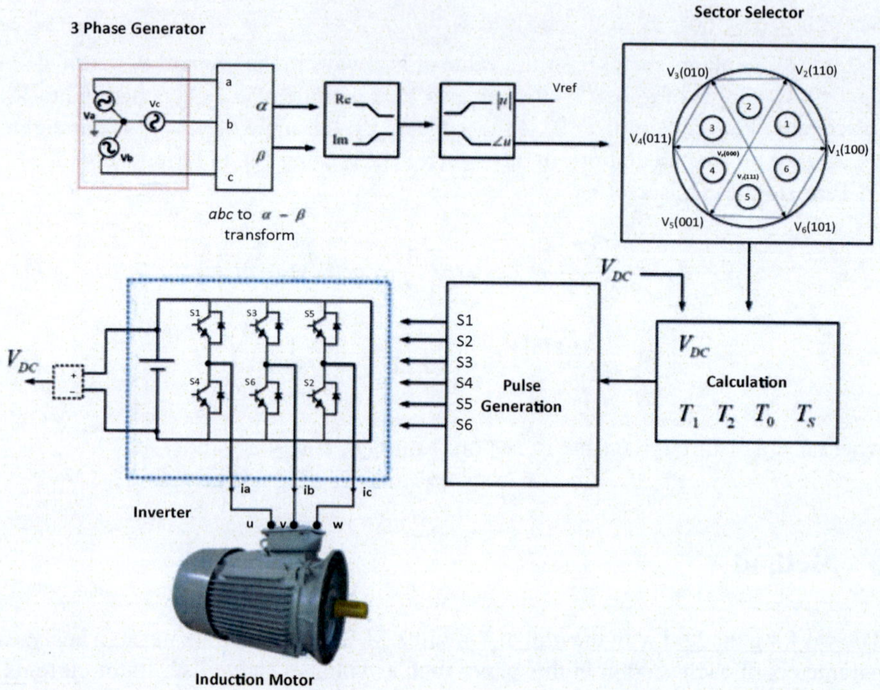

Fig. 5 Design of a space vector modulation system for control of a three-phase induction motor

voltages in each sector are multiplied by V_{dc}. To change the magnitude of $abc—\alpha\beta$ or better known as park transformation, the three-phase source voltage is lowered to a level of 1 V, 50 Hz with different phase angles of 0^0, 120^0, and 120^0. The system design in Fig. 5 is then modeled in Simulink MATLAB. The results of the modeling shown in Fig. 6 is a three-phase two-level inverter with a three-phase induction motor load.

4 Results and Discussion

Observations were made by running the modeling and then analyzing the simulated waves at the observed modeling image points. Using Eq. (1), the angle can be obtained in degrees in the form of a sawtooth wave with an amplitude of 3 $V_{(p-p)}$ (in the top figure). Figure 10 is the center of the angle in radians with an amplitude of 180 $V_{(p-p)}$, while the bottom picture is the value of V_{beta}/V_{alpha} in the form of a sinusoidal wave with an amplitude of 1 $V_{(p-p)}$ with a phase difference of 900. Figure 7 is a graph of changes in load torque, electromagnetic torque, and induction motor speed with time. In the model built, the induction motor bears the load at different times. Load

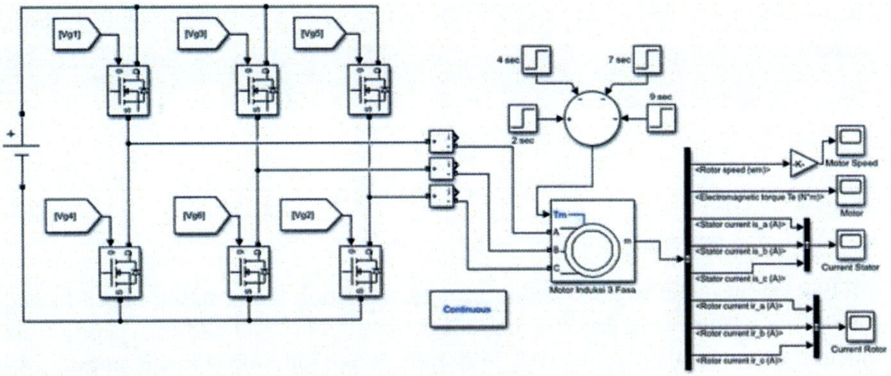

Fig. 6 MOSFET two-level inverter as a three-phase induction motor drive

of three-phase induction motor with parameters 54 HP (4 kW), 400 V, 50 Hz, and 1430 rpm. So the relationship between motor torque and load torque can be analyzed as follows using Eq. (13):

$$T_a = T_L + T_{sh} \tag{13}$$

T_a = torque (armature) or motor torque.

T_{sh} = shaft torque = net power shaft torque.

T_L= torque (loss).

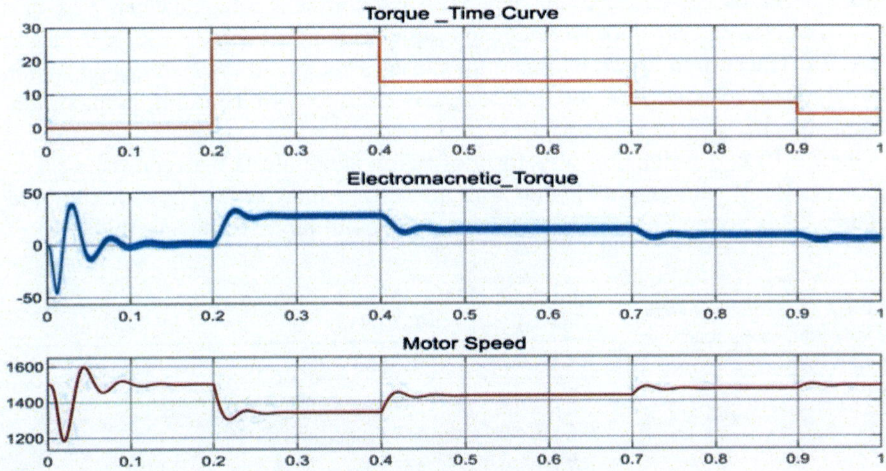

Fig. 7 Load torque curve, electromagnetic torque, and induction motor speed

$T_{sh} = \frac{P_{out}}{\omega}$,
where $\omega = \frac{2\pi N}{60}$

N = full load motor speed.

so $\omega = \frac{2\times3.14\times1430}{60} = 149.62$ rad/s.

$T_{sh(max)} = \frac{4000}{149.62}$

$T_{sh(max)} = 26.73$ Nm.

Table 2 shows that between 0 and 0.2 s the induction motor has not been loaded or when the motor is starting the load torque is at zero level and the speed of the induction motor is at a maximum of 1499 rpm. When the time is in the range 0.2 s–0.4 s, the motor is loaded and the maximum torque is 26.73 Nm; at this time, the speed of the induction motor drops and is at a minimum speed of 1334 rpm. The time is between 0.4 s and 0.7 s and between 0.7 s and 0.9 s the load is reduced so that the speed increases according to the decrease in load torque.

Figure 8 describes the change in stator current at the start, zero loads, maximum load and 1/2 maximum load, 1/4 maximum load torque, and 1/8 maximum load torque. It appears that at the start of the motor running, the motor draws a large current of about 50 $A_{(p-p)}$. After the motor rotates for a while, the current approaches zero when the time is between 0.1 s and 0.2 s at which time the motor has not been loaded and rises to a maximum when it is at 0.2 s < t < 0.4 s maximum load torque. The current decreases over time between 0.4 s and 0.9 s following the decrease in load torque. The stator current pattern is in the form of a sinusoid with the same amplitude for each phase, and this magnitude affects the load torque.

Figure 9 shows the rotor current waveform when starting the motor, zero loads, 1/2 peak load, 1/4 peak load, and 1/8 peak loads. When starting the rotor current, a large current of about 45 $A_{(p-p)}$isdrawn, and then it drops to zero at zero loads. The rotor current reaches the maximum when full load torque is obtained when 0.2 s < t < 0.4 s. Then the current slopes as the load torque decreases when 0.4 s < t < 0.7 s and t > 0.9 s. The current drawn by this rotor causes a change in the load torque. When the minimum rotor current, the load torque is close to zero, resulting in maximum motor speed.

Figure 10 is a simulation waveform of two voltage levels between three-phase lines V_a, V_b, V_c and amplitude 400 $V_{(p-p)}$ at a frequency of 50 Hz with SVPWM control. This voltage has a THD which is still quite large. Reducing this level of

Table 2 Net torque change of induction motor load against time

Time (s)	Tsh (N.m)	Speed (rpm)
0 < t < 0.2	0	1499
0.2 < t < 0.4	$T_{sh\ (max)} = 26.72$	1435
0.4 < t < 0.7	1/2 $T_{sh\ (max)} = 13.36$	1468
0.7 < t < 0.9	1/4 $T_{sh\ (max)} = 6.68$	1484
t > 0.9	1/8 $T_{sh\ (max)} = 3.34$	1492

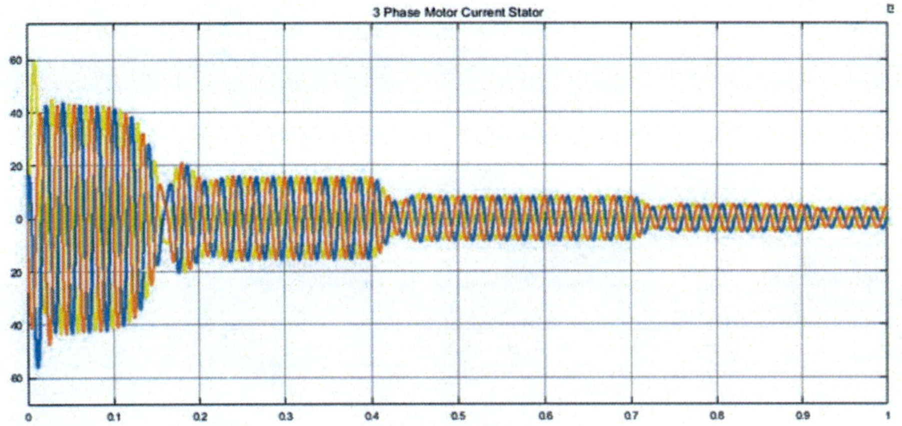

Fig. 8 Stator current against changes in load torque at various times

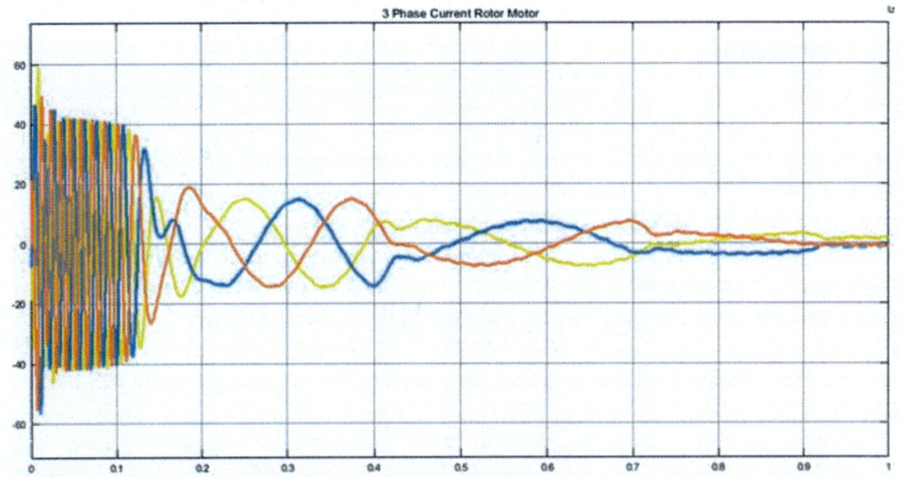

Fig. 9 Rotor current at various load torque changes

harmonics can be overcome by increasing the number of levels at the output voltage by adding an inverter arranged in a cascade.

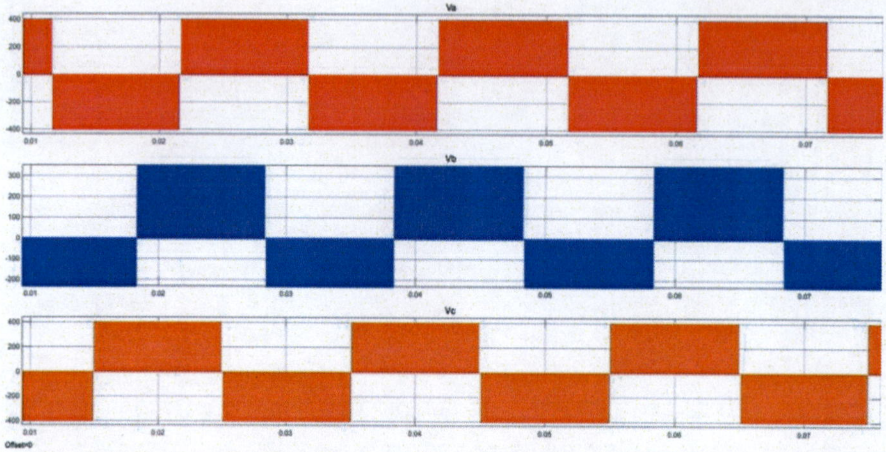

Fig. 10 Inverter output voltage V_a, V_b, V_c with SVPWM control

5 Conclusion

The Space Vector Pulse Width Modulation method is a pulse width modulation technique that is very effective in controlling the performance of asynchronous machines. Inverter trigger pulse generation is based on the performance component of the inverter switch which is divided into 6 sectors to get the reference voltage and sector angle values. The difference in the angle of the sector is 60^0 for each sector. The duration and time pattern of the switching on of the inverter switch is the same, but the phase is different by 60^0. The load torque of the induction motor is influenced by the rotor current which has ripples when the load changes at the start and when the motor experiences a load change. The two inverter output voltage levels still have a high Total Harmonics Distortion (THD) level, so a higher number of levels is needed so that the THD content can be reduced. This model is easy to implement into the actual circuit so that it can help researchers to make Variable Speed Drives (VSD) for induction motors with good control.

References

1. Vashishtha S, Rekha KR (2021) Modified digital space vector pulse width modulation realization on low-cost FPGA platform with optimization for 3-phase voltage source inverter. Int J Electr Comput Eng 11, 3629–3638. https://doi.org/10.11591/ijece.v11i4.pp3629-3638
2. Strankowski P, Guzinski J, Morawiec M, Lewicki A, Wilczynski F (2020) Sensorless five-phase induction motor drive with third harmonic injection and inverter output filter. Bull Polish Acad Sci Tech Sci 68, 437–445. https://doi.org/10.24425/bpasts.2020.133369
3. Algamluoli AF, Abbas NH (2021) Speed controller design for three-phase induction motor based on dynamic adjustment grasshopper optimization algorithm. Int J Electr Comput Eng

11, 1143–1157. https://doi.org/10.11591/ijece.v11i2.pp1143-1157
4. Ali AJ, Khalaf LA, Ahmed AH (2021) Modeling and simulation of a 3-ϕ induction motor based on two types of WFA. Int J Electr Comput Eng 11, 1105–1113. https://doi.org/10.11591/ijece.v11i2.pp1105-1113
5. Al-Yoonus MA, Al-Deen Alyozbaky OS (2021) Detection of internal and external faults of single-phase induction motor using current signature. Int J Electr Comput Eng. 11, 2830–2841. https://doi.org/10.11591/ijece.v11i4.pp2830-2841
6. Benbouhenni H (2019) A comparison study between fuzzy PWM and SVM inverter in NSMC control of stator active and reactive power control of a DFIG based wind turbine systems. Int J Appl Power Eng. 8, 78 https://doi.org/10.11591/ijape.v8.i1.pp78-92
7. Wróbel KT, Szabat K, Serkies P (2019) Long-horizon model predictive control of induction motor drive. Arch Electr Eng 68, 579–593. https://doi.org/10.24425/aee.2019.129343
8. Kiani B, Mozafari B, Soleymani S, Mohammadnezhad Shourkaei H (2021) Predictive torque control of induction motor drive with reduction of torque and flux ripple. Bull Polish Acad Sci Tech Sci 69, 1–13. https://doi.org/10.24425/bpasts.2021.137727
9. Zahraoui Y, Akherraz M, Fahassa C, Elbadaoui S (2020) Induction motor harmonic reduction using space vector modulation algorithm. Bull Electr Eng Informatics 9, 452–465. https://doi.org/10.11591/eei.v9i2.1682
10. Youcef M, Djilali T, Moreau S, Said H, Bachir D (2021) Dsp improvement of a vector speed induction motor control with a rst and adaptive fuzzy controller. Bull Electr Eng Informatics 10, 1232–1244. https://doi.org/10.11591/eei.v10i3.1798
11. Kadum AA (2020) New adaptive hysteresis band width control for direct torque control of induction machine drives. Int J Power Electron Drive Syst 11, 1908–1917. https://doi.org/10.11591/ijpeds.v11.i4.pp1908-1917
12. Fang J, Wang G, Li R, Liu S, Wang S (2021) Improved virtual space vector modulation for neutral point voltage oscillation and common-mode voltage reduction in neutral point clamped three-level inverter. Arch Electr Eng 70, 203–218. https://doi.org/10.24425/aee.2021.136062.
13. Elkholi OA, Enany MA, Abdo AF, Eid M (2020) Novel approach for svpwm of two-level inverter fed induction motor drive Int J Power Electron Drive Syst 11, 1750–1758. https://doi.org/10.11591/ijpeds.v11.i4.pp1750-1758
14. Kadum AA (2020) PWM control techniques for three phase three level inverter drives. Telkomnika (Telecommunication Comput Electron Control 18, 519–529. https://doi.org/10.12928/TELKOMNIKA.V18I1.12440
15. Shashibhushan S, Sonoli S (2019) Starting torque and torque ripple reduction using SVPWM based vector control of induction motor with nine-level cascaded multilevel inverter fed with solar PV power. Int J Power Electron Drive Syst 10, 1123. https://doi.org/10.11591/ijpeds.v10.i2.pp1123-1132
16. Hasoun M, Afia A, El Khafallah M, Benkirane, K (2020) A pwm strategy for dual three-phase pmsm using 12-sector vector space decomposition applied on electric ship propulsion. Int J Power Electron Drive Syst 11, 1701–1710. https://doi.org/10.11591/ijpeds.v11.i4.pp1701-1710
17. Tomasov V, Usoltsev A, Zolov P, Gribanov P (2017) The effect of space vector modulation algorithm on characteristics of three-phase voltage inverter for drives of optical telescopes. Bull Polish Acad Sci Tech Sci 65:629–637. https://doi.org/10.1515/bpasts-2017-0068
18. Bouziane M, Abdelkader M (2019) Direct space vector modulation for matrix converter fed dual star induction machine and neuro-fuzzy speed controller. Bull Electr Eng Informatics. 8, 818–828. https://doi.org/10.11591/eei.v8i3.1560
19. Shults TE, Husev O, Blaabjerg F, Roncero-Clemente C, Romero-Cadaval E, Vinnikov D (2019) Novel space vector pulsewidth modulation strategies for single-phase three-level NPC impedance-source inverters. IEEE Trans Power Electron 34:4820–4830. https://doi.org/10.1109/TPEL.2018.2859194
20. Vashishtha S, Rekha KR (2018) A survey: Space vector PWM (SVPWM) in 3φ voltage source inverter (VSI). Int J Electr Comput Eng. 8, 11–18. https://doi.org/10.11591/ijece.v8i1.pp11-18

21. Mahsahirun SN, Idris NRN, Yusof ZM, Sutikno T (2020) Fundamental elements of constant volt/hertz induction motor drives based on dspace ds1104 controller. Int J Power Electron Drive Syst 11, 1670–1685. https://doi.org/10.11591/ijpeds.v11.i4.pp1670-1685
22. Selvakumar K, Palanisamy R, Stalin AR, Gopi P, Ponselvin P, Saravanan K (2019) Simulation of 3-phase matrix converter using space vector modulation. Int J Electr Comput Eng 9, 909. https://doi.org/10.11591/ijece.v9i2.pp909-916
23. Sharma A, Anandh N, Gao S (2020) Modulation index effect on inverter based induction motor drive. Int J Power Electron Drive Syst 11, 1785–1798. https://doi.org/10.11591/ijpeds.v11.i4.pp1785-1798.
24. Pongiannan CB, Yusuff RK, Tariq A, Maddileti M, Tharwinkumar TT (2019) A simple switching on-time calculation revision in multilevel inverter-space vector modulation to achieving extended voltage boundary operation. Int J Power Electron Drive Syst 10, 653. https://doi.org/10.11591/ijpeds.v10.i2.pp653-661
25. Porwal A, Baria K, Deshpande A (2014) Modeling and simulation of svpwm based application. 3:140–148

Assessing the Effect on Cognitive Workload Index, EEG Band Ratios, and Band Frequencies Using Band Power and Implementing Machine Learning Classification

Gunda Manasa, Krashana D. Nirde, Suhas S. Gajre, and Ramchandra Manthalkar

Abstract Cognitive resource theory combines individual differences in attentional resources and task demands to predict variance in task performance. Mind wandering, on the other hand, refers to the occurrence of thoughts that are both stimulus-independent and task unrelated. In order to analyze the cognitive load, band ratios during a mental arithmetic task can be identified by electroencephalogram. In this paper, the dataset is collected from publicly available online sources and consists of 36 subjects performing eyes closed or relaxed state tasks of 180 s and mental arithmetic tasks (series of subtraction) of 60 s. Based on the count quality of the subtraction task, subjects are divided into two groups: "Bad" and "Good". The main aim of the research is to assess the cognitive workload by analyzing different band ratio indices obtained from the band power which is calculated using the wavelet decomposition function. Individual frequency band variations show the performance of the subjects in doing the task. Finally, Binary classification with various classifiers is used to classify the performance of the classifier. The classification was done with six different classifiers in that only three classifiers obtained the same results like Support Vector Machine, Gaussian Naïve Bayes, and Logistic Regression with 73%.

Keywords Mind wandering · Cognitive workload index (CWI) · Binary classification · Support vector machine (SVM) · Gaussian Naïve Bayes (GNB) · Logistic regression

G. Manasa (✉) · K. D. Nirde · S. S. Gajre · R. Manthalkar
Department of Electronics and Telecommunication Engineering, SGGSIE&T, Nanded 431606, India
e-mail: gundamanasa89@gmail.com

K. D. Nirde
e-mail: nirde.krishna@gmail.com

S. S. Gajre
e-mail: suhasgajre@gmail.com

R. Manthalkar
e-mail: rmanthalkar@gmail.com

T. Triwiyanto et al. (eds.), *Proceeding of the 3rd International Conference on Electronics, Biomedical Engineering, and Health Informatics*, Lecture Notes in Electrical Engineering 1008, https://doi.org/10.1007/978-981-99-0248-4_5

1 Introduction

In general we studied human brain functions performing different cognitive loads. In this contribution we want to explore the effect of load on the brain using band power, band frequencies by performing different band ratios. Normally implementing machine learning algorithms for classification of good and bad subjects [1].

Cognitive workload based on electroencephalography (EEG) is an important marker of brain activity for workload analysis (mental effort). Cognitive workload is a measurement of the load placed on memory and other executive functions that are used to demonstrate cognitive abilities. Memory load was investigated using EEG signals during cognitive tasks inducing seven levels of workload using arithmetic tasks [2, 3]. The variations in brain lobes for different load levels are investigated [4].

The total electrical oscillations in layer potentials created by the interconnection of the principal inhibitory and excitatory neurons are represented by the EEG signal [5, 6]. Mind wandering (MW) episodes, like concern, are characterized by the appearance of task-unrelated feelings and ideas that divert attention away from the current task [7]. Mind Wandering can happen when you're doing something else, and it shows up as you think about something else [8]. Prospection and future planning [9], creativity [10], and mental breaks, which can help you get out of a bad mood [11], have all been linked to Mind Wandering. Others have consistently viewed Mind Wandering as a condition of diminished working memory and attentional control [12, 13] and as a predictor of performance errors, in addition to its relationship with these more positive processes. Mind Wandering has also been linked to a reduction in attention and focus [14, 15]. Increase in EEG theta band power and decrease in EEG beta band power were linked to a state of Mind Wandering in a proof-of-concept study; [16] reported that a condition of Mind Wandering was associated with high EEG theta band power and low EEG beta band power. When you're awake and close your eyes, your alpha waves are higher than when you're awake and open your eyes [17].

Power has been found to predict various aspects of cognitive performance on other tasks. Many such research has found that good memory performance is linked to higher resting power [18], and that a higher ERD is correlated with better effectiveness on a semantic search task [19]. External stimulus, such as task-relevant visual pictures or warning signs, suppresses alpha waves during cognitive activities [20]. During brief waiting times between task attempts [21, 22] and mental imagery, which demands inward-directed thought [23], alpha waves are increased. Decreases in perceptual discrimination have been linked to enhanced alpha activity prior to an incoming stimulus [24]. The task-related power variations show that alpha activity is sensitive to cognitive demands: it is repressed in response to sensory stimulation and boosted during periods of no stimulation [25].

The role of alpha power in the suppression of sensory processes to protect thinking from continuing distraction has been demonstrated in numerous studies [26, 27], and it is a promising metric to describe Mind Wandering [28]. Although some studies have observed the contrary tendency, our findings are consistent with multiple earlier findings that connect greater alpha power with Mind Wandering in the frontal, occipital, and posterior parts of the brain [29–31]. When compared to episodes of focused attention, a high in theta and a low in beta power have been reported during Mind Wandering [32].

In [33], researchers have calculated different EEG band ratios for evaluating the cognitive load indices of the subjects in pre- and post meditation. In this paper, we have evaluated the subject's performance before the task and while doing the task to know the variations among cognitive load and EEG band ratios [33].

The key contribution of the proposed work is to analyze the band ratios, cognitive load index, individual band frequencies, prefrontal electrode of the subjects, and finally applied the binary classification with different classifiers like Support Vector Machine (SVM), K-nearest neighbor (KNN), Decision Tree, Random Forest, Gaussian Naïve Bayes (GNB), and Logistic Regression. The paper is arranged into four sections. Section 2 includes materials and methods, Sect. 3 includes results and analysis, Sect. 4 includes discussion, and Sect. 5 includes a conclusion.

2 Materials and Methods

2.1 Recording and Selection of the EEG Signals

The EEG signals were recorded from Neurocom Monopolar EEG 23-channel system (Ukraine, XAI-MEDICA). All 23 electrodes are mounted on the scalp of the subject according to the International 10–20 scheme. The electrodes mounted on the scalp recorded the signals from different parts of the brain, which is divided into different lobes like frontal, temporal, parietal, and occipital. The placement of electrodes which are used to measure the frontal, temporal, parietal, occipital and central lobes of the brain are shown in Fig.1. The interconnected ear reference electrodes are used to reference all electrodes. The inter-electrode impedance was kept below 5 k, and the sampling rate was 500 Hz. A 0.5 Hz cutoff frequency HPF, a 45 Hz cutoff frequency LPF, and a 50 Hz power line notch filter are used.

Recording of each EEG signal includes artifact-free EEG segments of 180 s (resting state) and 60 s (mental counting). Out of 66 participants, 30 were removed from the database due to imprudent artifacts present with eyes and muscles. So overall we found 36 subjects best. The task includes both Females and Males marked as "F" and "M": 27 female and 9 male subjects with ages ranging 17–26 with no physical and mental disorders.

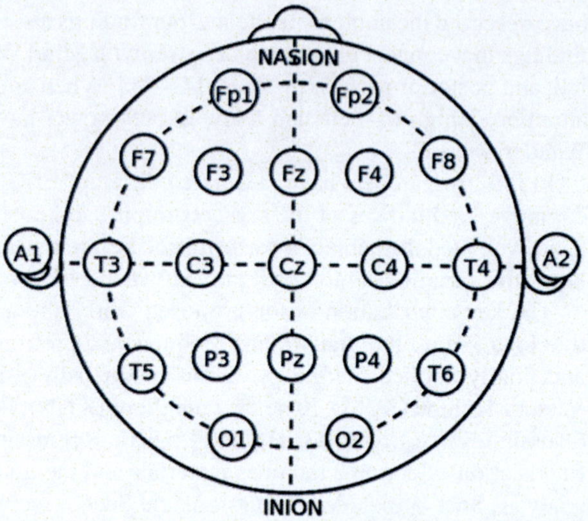

Fig. 1 10–20 international system of EEG 21 channel electrode placement

2.2 *Attribute of Subject Participation in the Protocol*

During the recording of the EEG signal, subjects were asked to sit in a dark soundproof chamber with reclined armchair; they were asked to relax during the resting state or before the task and informed about the arithmetic task; this relaxation state was recorded for 3 min duration. After the relaxation, subjects performed the arithmetic task for 4-min duration but for analyzing the changes that occur in the load, the dataset was considered 1 min arithmetic task, and the remaining 3 min are excluded. Based on the count of subtractions done by the subjects, they were divided into 2 groups: "Bad" and "Good". A total of 26 subjects' performance was under "Good" and 10 subjects' performance was under "Bad".

Participation in the protocol includes a series of subtraction or number of subtractions. It includes the process of first taking the difference between the four-digit number and the result of subtracting, divided by the subtrahend. More information can be found in the paper [34].

2.3 *Wavelet Decomposition*

The nature of the EEG signal has a time-varying property; in order to convert the time domain signal to the frequency domain, we used wavelet transform. Wavelet transform can provide the time and frequency signals simultaneously. A wavelet family with mother wavelet ψ (t) consisting of functions $\psi_{a,b}(t)$ of the form are taken from [35]

$$\psi_{a,b}(t) = \frac{1}{\sqrt{a}}\psi\left(\frac{t-b}{a}\right) \quad (1)$$

where a is positive and defines the scale and b is any real number that defines the shift. When $|a| > 1$ then $\psi_{a,b}(t)$ has a larger time width than ψ(t) and corresponds to a lower frequency, whereas $|a| < 1$ then the wavelet obtained from Eq. (1) is the compressed version of mother wavelet and corresponds to higher frequency [36].

The continuous wavelet transforms (CWT) of a function $x(t)$, introduced by Morlet, is defined by

$$\text{CWT}(a, b) = \int_{-\infty}^{\infty} x(t)\ \psi_{a,b}(t)dt \quad (2)$$

CWT(a, b) is a function of 2 variables: Eq. (1) variable a determines the amount of time scaling or dilation, and from Eq. (2) variable b represents the shift $\psi_{a,0}(t)$ by an amount b along the time axis and indicates the location of the wavelet window along it [37].

By breaking down the signal into a rough approximation and finer details, the DWT analyzes the signal at various frequency bands with various resolutions. Scaling functions and wavelet functions, which are related to lowpass and highpass filters, respectively, are two sets of functions used by DWT. The time domain signal is simply subjected to consecutive highpass and lowpass filtering to obtain the signal's decomposition into various frequency bands. First, a half-band highpass filter (g[n]) and a lowpass filter (h[n]) are applied to the original signal $x[n]$. Therefore, the signal can be subsampled by two by simply removing every other sample. This is a single level of decomposition and may be stated mathematically as follows using Eqs. (3) and (4):

$$\text{Y}_{\text{high}}[\text{k}] = \sum\nolimits_{n} x[n] \cdot \text{g}[2\text{k} - n] \quad (3)$$

$$\text{Y}_{\text{low}}[\text{k}] = \sum\nolimits_{n} x[n] \cdot \text{h}[2\text{k} - n] \quad (4)$$

where $\text{Y}_{\text{high}}[\text{k}]$ and $\text{Y}_{\text{low}}[\text{k}]$ are the outputs of highpass and lowpass filters.

Figure 2 illustrates this procedure, where $x[n]$ denotes the original signal to be decomposed, and h[n] and g[n] are low pass and high pass filters, respectively. The obtained frequency bands are analyzed to acquire the band power.

Band power considers the energy distribution in the signal and is computed as a sum of the squares of the signal data points [38] using Eq. (4):

$$\text{BP} = \sum\nolimits_{n=1}^{N} |x_n|^2 \quad (5)$$

where x_n are signal data points from 1 to N.

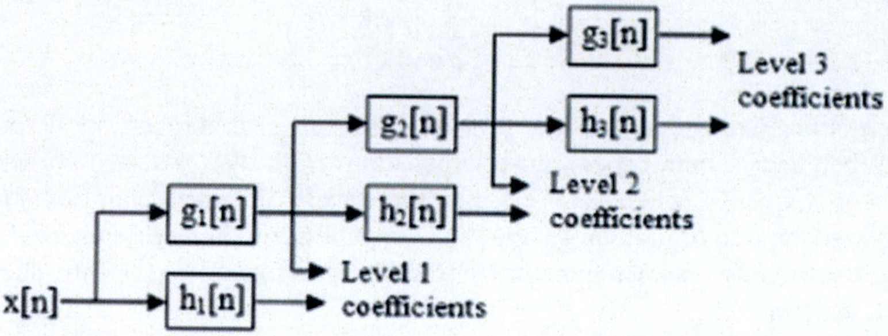

Fig. 2 1-D wavelet decomposition

3 Results and Analysis

The band frequencies obtained from Fig. 2 were used to analyze cognitive load among the "Good" and "Bad" when subjects performed eyes closed and mental arithmetic tasks.

3.1 Individual Band Frequencies

The subjects are divided into 2 groups: "Good" and "Bad"; the task involves performing resting state and mental arithmetic task. Individual band frequencies are used to assess the performance of the subject by considering the resting state and mental arithmetic task.

From Figs. 3, 4, 5 and 6 subjects above the line represents the while doing task (mental arithmetic task-1 min), line below represents before the task (resting state-3 min).

We compared both groups (i.e., "Good" and "Bad") and cannot conclude for the Delta band in Figs. 3a and 4a. Individual groups performance-wise, we found that "Good" participants were more (line above) and felt sleepy in the moments before the task (resting state), but "Bad" subjects were less (line below) and did not feel drowsy in the moments before the task (resting state). While doing a task (line above) of both groups, we found a smaller number of "Good" subjects (did not feel sleepy) and a greater number of "Bad" subjects (due to sleepiness).

Figures 3b and 4b show the response of the "Good" and "Bad" subjects for the Theta band. Individual group performance-wise, we found an equal number (line above and below) of "Good" subjects, which is due to relaxation in both the tasks, whereas less number (line above) of "Bad" subjects due to difficulty found while doing the task and more number (line above) due to relaxation before the task (resting state).

Figures 3c and 4c show the response of the "Good" and "Bad" subjects for the Alpha band; we compared both groups (line above), more "Good" subjects and less

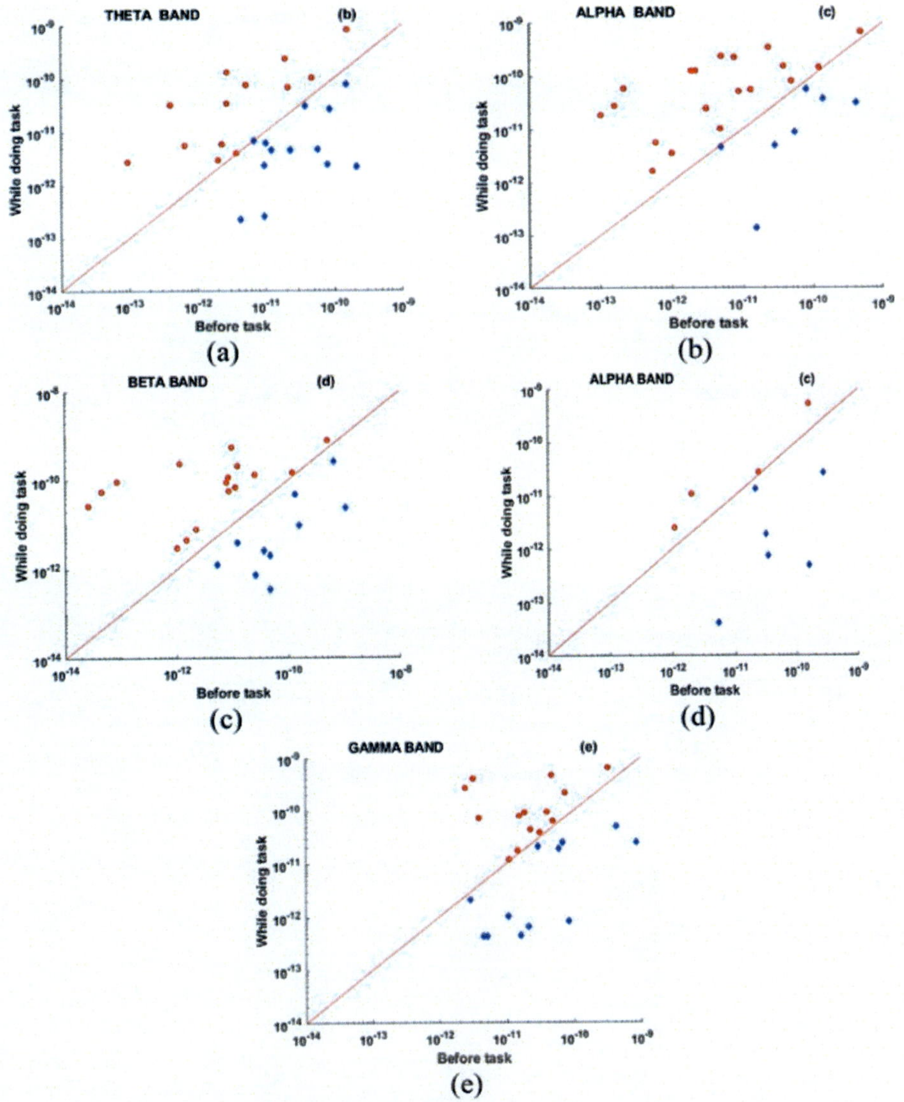

Fig. 3 Analysis of "Good" subjects performing before and while doing tasks: **a** Delta band, **b** Theta band, **c** Alpha band, **d** Beta band, and **e** Gamma band

"Bad" subjects and vice versa for the line below. Individual group performance-wise, we found more (line above) "Good" subjects due to being awake and relaxed while doing the task, and less (line above) "Bad" subjects due to difficulty while doing the task. In the line below, we see less "Good" subjects awakened and relaxed, and more "Bad" subjects relaxed.

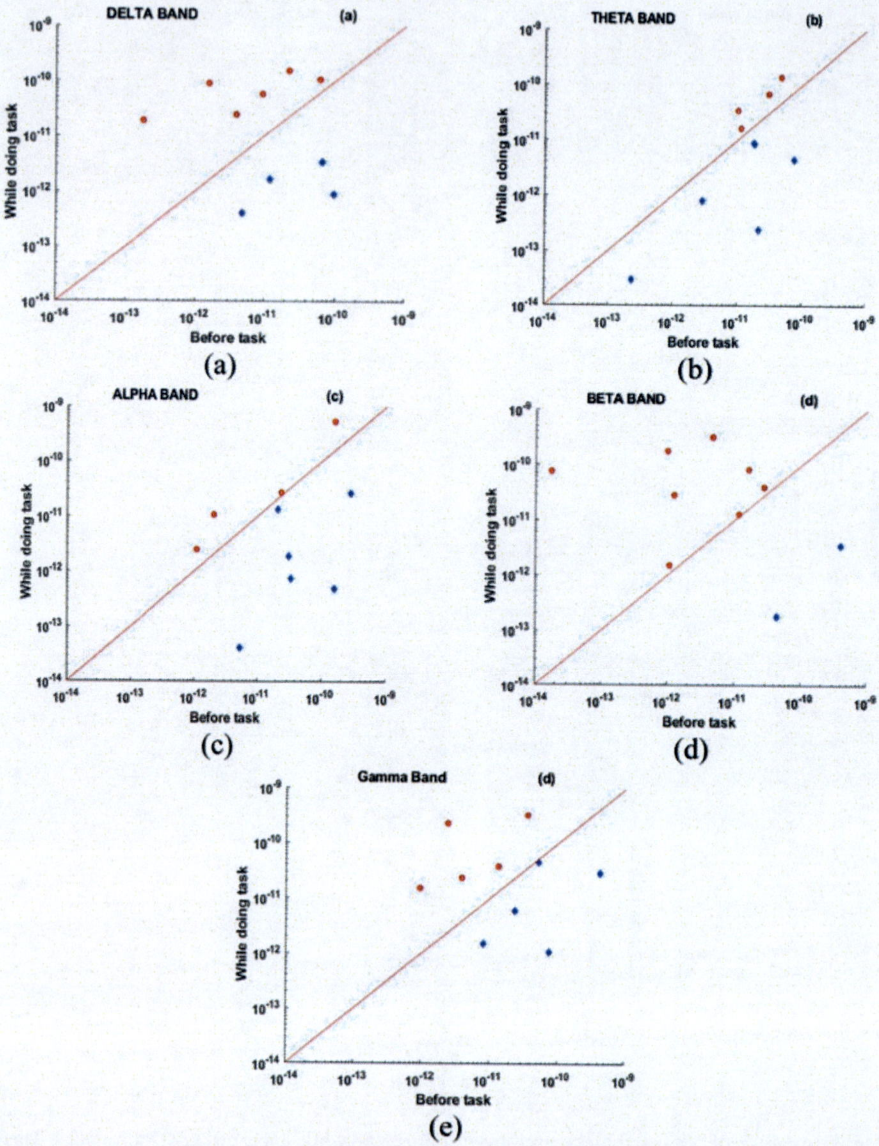

Fig. 4 Analysis of "Bad" subjects performing before and while doing tasks: **a** Delta band, **b** Theta band, **c** Alpha band, **d** Beta band, and **e** Gamma band. **Note* All the graphs in this paper are log scaled ($x = y$) for easy prediction of the subjects among the 2 tasks, i.e., before the task and while doing the task, and red line is used to show the separation among the performance of the task

We compared both groups in the line above and cannot conclude the beta band in Figs. 3d and 4d. Individual group performance-wise, we found more number (line above) of "Good" and "Bad" subjects due to consciousness while doing a task. Subjects of both groups in the line below are less conscious before the task.

In Figs. 3e and 4e, we compare the responses of the "Good" and "Bad" subjects for the Gamma band, and we cannot conclude for the gamma band (due to equal distribution of subjects among line below and above). Individual group performance-wise, we have more "Good" subjects in the line above, indicating concentration. We are unable to reach a conclusion for "Bad" subjects (due to an equal distribution before and while doing the task).

3.2 *Cognitive Load Indices (EEG Band Ratios)*

EEG cognitive load indices which represent the different EEG band ratios are analyzed using mean and standard deviation and are shown in Table 1 using Eq. (6):

$$\text{Mean} = \frac{1}{n} \sum\nolimits_{i=1}^{n} a_i \tag{6}$$

where n = number of values; a_i= dataset values. Standard Deviation using Eq. (7):

$$\sigma = \sqrt{\frac{\sum (x_i - \mu)^2}{N}} \tag{7}$$

where σ = standard deviation, N = size of elements, x_i = each value from the element, and μ = the element means.

Table 1 Comparison of different EEG band ratios between bad and good subjects performing before (3 min) and while doing (1 min) task using mean and standard deviation (mV)

EEG band ratio (Hz)	Activity index	Bad (3 min)	Bad (1 min)	Good (3 min)	Good (1 min)
		Before (mV)	While doing (mV)	Before (mV)	While doing (mV)
α/θ	Performance enhancement	2.99 ± 4.09	2.17 ± 3.69	1.55 ± 2.14	1.49 ± 0.90
β/α	Arousal index	0.72 ± 1.34	1.22 ± 0.62	1.94 ± 2.07	1.16 ± 1.23
β/θ	Neural activity	2.17 ± 5.51	2.65 ± 2.31	3.02 ± 4.45	1.74 ± 1.12
$\beta/\alpha + \theta$	Engagement	0.54 ± 1.08	0.83 ± 0.49	1.18 ± 1.41	0.69 ± 0.59
θ/α	Load index	0.33 ± 0.24	0.46 ± 0.27	0.64 ± 0.46	0.66 ± 1.10
$\alpha + \theta/\beta$	Alertness	1.83 ± 0.92	1.19 ± 2.03	0.84 ± 0.70	1.43 ± 1.69
$\frac{(\beta+\gamma)}{(\alpha+\theta)}$	CWI	1.21 ± 2.19	1.64 ± 1.03	2.08 ± 2.44	1.32 ± 1.12

The load on memory increases when task difficulty increases. The performance enhancement in "Bad" subjects refers to an increase in alpha frequency which indicates mind wandering; while doing a task, the same alpha frequency has decreased which shows less mind wandering, as alpha frequency increases when eyes are closed whereas it decreases when eyes are open (relaxation). The same performance of alpha frequency is observed for "Good" subjects that increased before the task (more relaxation) and decreased while doing the task (less relaxation) due to eyes closing and opening.

The arousal index represents the excitement in the subjects; we can see an increase in arousal index for "Bad" subjects from before the task to while doing the task, while a decrease in the arousal index from before to while doing the task for "Good" subjects; this represents that "Good" subjects showed less excitement when compared to "Bad" subjects.

The neural activity represents an improvement in cognitive skills, increase in neural activity for "Bad" subjects from before to while doing, while decrease before to while doing the task for "Good" subjects, shows "Good" subjects stressed to task and showed decrement.

The engagement activity, if it increases in "β", shows alertness and focus, while a decrease in "θ" shows cognitive load; from the above table, we see an increase in engagement before the task for "Bad" subjects and decrease while doing the task for "Good" subjects, decrease in "θ" represents the cognitive load had effect on "Good" subjects (increased β, less θ). Load index represents the stress, increment is observed in both "Bad" and "Good" subjects, and stress is observed while doing the task. There is a decrease in alertness activity from before the task to while doing the task in "Bad" subjects, whereas decrease to an increase in "Good" subjects, which showed alertness while doing the task.

The CWI (Cognitive Workload Index) ratio based on EEG band power [35] was obtained using mean and standard deviation of the band power. It shows decrease to increase in "Bad" subjects, whereas increase to decrease in "Good" subjects. Load showed the effect on "Bad" subjects while doing the task which decreased the performance, whereas "Good" subjects did not feel difficulty while doing the task.

CWI performance for "Good" and "Bad" subjects with band power is shown in Fig. 5a, b. CWI represents the load on subjects in which there are more (line below) "Bad" subjects than "Good" subjects (line above). Due to the load, the "Bad" subjects had difficulty in performing the task (while doing the task), whereas the "Good" subjects were more conscious, concentrated, and relaxed (while doing the task).

3.3 *Prefrontal Electrode Analysis*

The prefrontal electrodes were used to assess the effect of load on the skull; we examined the individual data of Fp1 and Fp2 electrodes for the subjects before and while doing the task as shown in Fig. 6. Various cognitive skills can be analyzed,

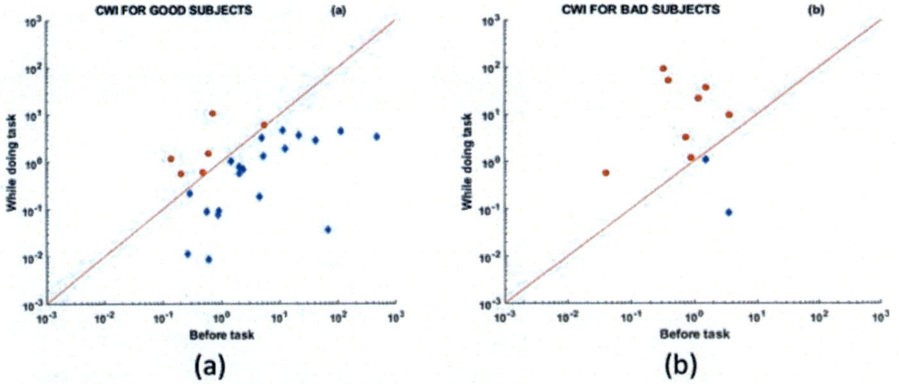

Fig. 5 CWI for subjects performing before, while doing task, **a** "Good" **b** "Bad"

but we evaluated only cognitive load on subjects performing the task. Band powers of Fp1 and Fp2 for "Good" and "Bad" subjects are more while doing the task (line above), whereas less before the task (line below).

3.4 Binary Classification

Different methods were used to obtain the binary classification results like Support Vector Machine (SVM), K-Nearest Neighbor (KNN), Decision Tree, Random Forest, Gaussian Naïve Bayes (GNB), and Logistic Regression. The binary classification is done by taking the mean of individual (Fp1, Fp2, F3, F4, Fz, F7, F8, C3, C4, Cz, P3, P4, Pz, O1, O2, T3, T4, T5, T6) electrodes and calculating overall mean of 19 electrodes for one subject; this process is repeated for all subjects and finally the obtained mean results are divided into 2 parts: 1."Bad" before mental arithmetic (3 min) and while doing the mental arithmetic task (1 min); 2."Good" subjects before mental arithmetic (3 min) and while doing the mental arithmetic task (1 min).

The obtained mean using Eq. (5) of all the subjects considered is divided between "Bad" and "Good". The subjects' mean is merged (before, while doing the mental arithmetic task of "Bad") and labeled as "0" (zero). The same is repeated for "Good" subjects and labeled as "1" (one). Finally, testing and training are done and classification techniques applied. Different classifier results can be seen in Fig. 7. Support Vector Machine (SVM), Gaussian Naïve Bayes (GNB), and Logistic Regression obtained 73%.

Frequency bands were extracted using wavelet decomposition and band power of each frequency band was calculated individually. Individual frequency bands like delta, theta, alpha, beta, and gamma showed the separation among the subjects (below and above the line) in performing the resting state and arithmetic state which can be seen in Figs. 1 and 2. EEG band ratios were analyzed between "Bad" and "Good"

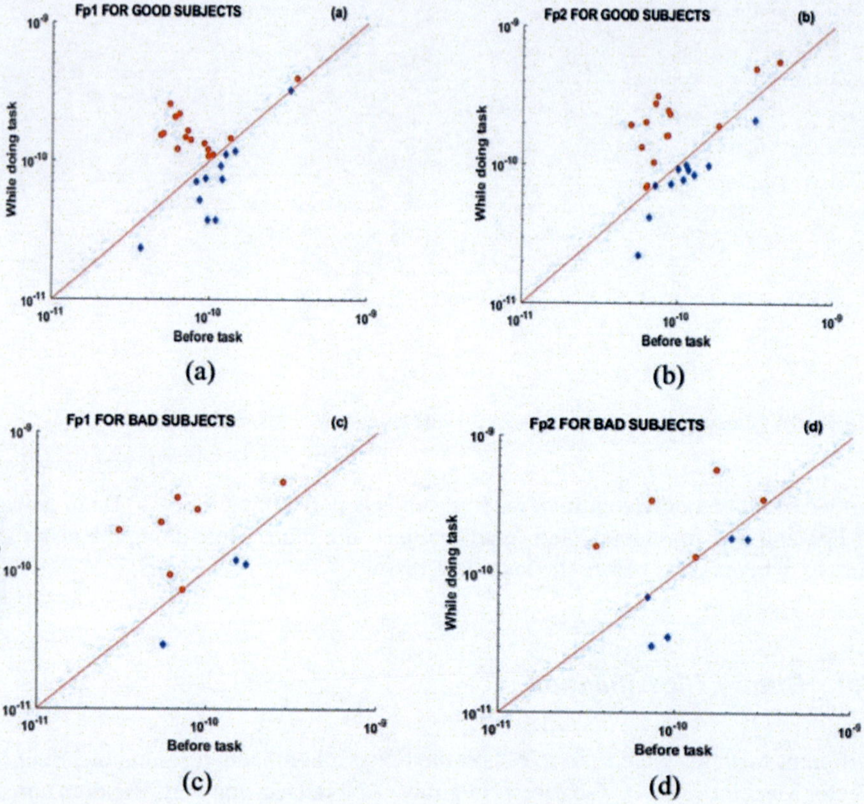

Fig. 6 Fp1 and Fp2 for subjects performing before and while doing the task: **a**, **b** "Good"; **c**, **d** "Bad"

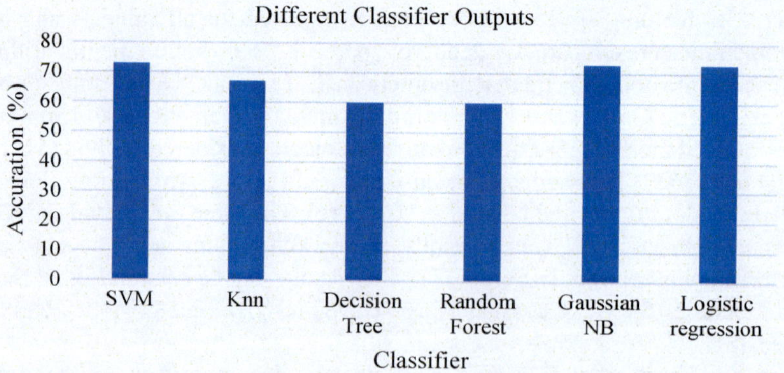

Fig. 7 Different classifier outputs: SVM (Support Vector Machine), KNN (K-Nearest Neighbor), DT (Decision Tree), RT (Random Forest Tree), Gaussian NB (Naive Bayes), and Logistic Regression

when both the groups performed resting state and arithmetic task; from these, variations in the different activity index can be seen in Table 1; cognitive load was observed among 2 groups and found more in "Bad" subjects when compared with "Good" subjects because the "Good" subjects didn't find difficulty in the task whereas "Bad" subjects found difficulty in the task. Cognitive skills are analyzed at the prefrontal electrodes of the brain, hence we found that "Good" subjects are above the line, while "Bad" subjects are below the line which can be seen in Fig. 6. Finally, binary classification was applied classification among the "Bad" and "Good" subjects and obtained 73% for Support Vector Machine, Gaussian Naïve Bayes, and Logistic Regression.

4 Discussion

The techniques here used to interpret the cognitive workload index, different bands ratios, and prefrontal electrodes using the wavedec function, from Fig. 3 (analysis of "Good" subjects) and Fig. 4 (analysis of "Bad" subjects) comparisons among 2 groups when subjects performing while doing the task and before the task with 5 frequency bands are seen. When analyzed the individual frequency bands, "Good" subjects' performance was better observed while doing the task of alpha and beta bands whereas as theta, delta, and gamma are not that much better. "Bad" subjects while doing task did not performed better which can be seen from the delta, theta, alpha, and gamma bands; only the beta band has better performance which states that "Bad" subjects felt difficulty while doing the task (mental arithmetic task). EEG band ratio variations show the subjects' performance. Results can be compared with the previous research [33], but our paper considered 2 groups performing 2 individual tasks: one resting state and another arithmetic task. Variations among the pre- and post meditation were seen previously; here, we saw variations among subjects' performance among "Good" and "Bad" with different frequency band ratios. Figure 5 shows the variations in cognitive workload that occurred in the two groups while doing and before the task. Different activity indices are analyzed with band ratios when subjects performed two tasks, i.e., while doing and before. "Bad" group subjects performed before and while doing the task and variations in the activity indices can be seen; performance enhancement has increased when subjects were resting and decreased while doing the task; arousal index showed a decrease in resting state whereas increased while doing the task, neural activity shows the decrease while resting and increase while doing the task, engagement of the subjects has decreased in resting state whereas it increased while doing task, load index decreased when resting task and increased while doing the task, alertness has seen an increase in resting task whereas a decrease while doing the task, and cognitive workload index decreased in resting task and increased while doing the task. "Bad" subjects have low engagement, load index, and cognitive workload index when resting task was performed and increased while doing the task. In "Good" group subjects, performance enhancement, arousal, and neural activity band ratios show increase in resting task when compared to while doing the task, in engagement and cognitive workload index (CWI) band ratios shows increase in resting task and decrease in while doing task can be seen, whereas in load index and alertness has shown decreased in resting state and increased in while doing the task. In Fig. 6, prefrontal electrodes of the brain are considered, i.e., Fp1 and Fp2; these two electrodes are used to assess cognitive skills. Here, machine learning classifiers are used for binary classification.

The limitation includes variation in delta and theta frequency bands did not show better performance, when individual band performance was considered in "Good" subjects, whereas in "Bad" subjects alpha and theta frequency bands did not show better performance.

5 Conclusion

This paper used the decomposition technique to observe the variations in frequency band when subjects performed resting tasks and while doing tasks. From the results, we observed that cognitive load on subjects increased while doing the task, and increase in beta band and decrease in alpha band can be observed. EEG band power ratios used to know the variations in frequency bands and their effects on the subjects' performance, prefrontal electrodes, and binary classification showed differences among the "Good" and "Bad" subjects performing the task. The future scope includes the advanced techniques for assessing the cognitive load when subjects perform yoga and meditation.

Acknowledgements Here, we have used an online public dataset from Ukraine, XAI-MEDICA; we would like to thank Bioethics Commission of Educational and Scientific Centre, "Institute of Biology and Medicine", Taras Shevchenko National University of Kyiv. We want to thank all research scholars and professors of the E&TC Engineering department from SGGSIE&T, Nanded, Maharashtra, India.

References

1. Gupta SS, Manthalkar RR, Gajre SS (2021) Mindfulness intervention for improving cognitive abilities using EEG signal. Biomed Signal Process Control 70:103072
2. Wang S, Gwizdka J, Chaovalitwongse WA (2015) Using wireless EEG signals to assess memory workload in the $ n $-back task. IEEE Trans Hum Mach Syst 46(3):424–435
3. Zarjam P, Epps J, Lovell NH (2015) Beyond subjective self-rating: EEG signal classification of cognitive workload. IEEE Trans Auton Ment Dev 7(4):301–310
4. Zander TO, Kothe C (2011) Towards passive brain–computer interfaces: applying brain–computer interface technology to human–machine systems in general. J Neural Eng 8(2):025005
5. Gordon N (2000) Review cognitive functions and epileptic activity. Seizure 9(3):184–188
6. Nunez PL (1995) Experimental connections between EEG data and the global wave theory. Neocort Dyn Hum EEG Rhythms 534–590
7. Smallwood J, Schooler JW (2006) The restless mind. Psychol Bull 132(6):946

8. Mason MF, Norton MI, Van Horn JD, Wegner DM, Grafton ST, Macrae CN: Wandering minds: the default network and stimulus-independent thought. Science 315(5810):393–395
9. Baumeister RF, Masicampo EJ, Vohs KD (2011) Do conscious thoughts cause behavior? Annu Rev Psychol 62:331–361
10. Baird B, Smallwood J, Mrazek MD, Kam JW, Franklin MS, Schooler JW (2012) Inspired by distraction: mind wandering facilitates creative incubation. Psychol Sci 23(10):1117–1122
11. Ruby FJ, Smallwood J, Engen H, Singer T (2013) How self-generated thought shapes mood—the relation between mind-wandering and mood depends on the socio-temporal content of thoughts. PloS One 8(10):e77554
12. McVay JC, Kane MJ (2009) Conducting the train of thought: working memory capacity, goal neglect, and mind wandering in an executive-control task. J Exp Psychol Learn Memory Cogn 35(1):196
13. Unsworth N, McMillan BD (2014) Similarities and differences between mind-wandering and external distraction: a latent variable analysis of lapses of attention and their relation to cognitive abilities. Acta Psychol 150:14–25
14. Smallwood J, Nind L, O'Connor RC (2009) When is your head at? An exploration of the factors associated with the temporal focus of the wandering mind. Conscious Cogn 18(1):118–125
15. Stawarczyk D, Majerus S, Catale C, D'Argembeau A (2014) Relationships between mind-wandering and attentional control abilities in young adults and adolescents. Acta Psychol 148:25–36
16. Braboszcz C, Delorme A (2011) Lost in thoughts: neural markers of low alertness during mind wandering. Neuroimage 54(4):3040–3047
17. Adrian ED, Matthews BH (1934) The Berger rhythm: potential changes from the occipital lobes in man. Brain 57(4):355–385
18. Klimesch W, Vogt F, Doppelmayr M (1999) Interindividual differences in alpha and theta power reflect memory performance. Intelligence 27(4):347–362
19. Doppelmayr M, Klimesch W, Hödlmoser K, Sauseng P, Gruber W (2005) Intelligence related upper alpha desynchronization in a semantic memory task. Brain Res Bull 66(2):171–177
20. Thut G, Nietzel A, Brandt SA, Pascual-Leone A (2006) α-Band electroencephalographic activity over occipital cortex indexes visuospatial attention bias and predicts visual target detection. J Neurosci 26(37):9494–9502
21. Carp J, Compton RJ (2009) Alpha power is influenced by performance errors. Psychophysiology 46(2):336–343
22. Compton RJ, Arnstein D, Freedman G, Dainer-Best J, Liss A (2011) Cognitive control in the intertrial interval: evidence from EEG alpha power. Psychophysiology 48(5):583–590
23. Cooper NR, Croft RJ, Dominey SJ, Burgess AP, Gruzelier JH (2003) Paradox lost? Exploring the role of alpha oscillations during externally vs. internally directed attention and the implications for idling and inhibition hypotheses. Int J Psychophysiol 47(1):65–74
24. Van Dijk H, Schoffelen JM, Oostenveld R, Jensen O (2008) Prestimulus oscillatory activity in the alpha band predicts visual discrimination ability. J Neurosci 28(8):1816–1823
25. Compton RJ, Gearinger D, Wild H (2019) The wandering mind oscillates: EEG alpha power is enhanced during moments of mind-wandering. Cognit Affect Behav Neurosci 19(5):1184–1191
26. Benedek M (2018) Internally directed attention in creative cognition
27. Klimesch W (2012) Alpha-band oscillations, attention, and controlled access to stored information. Trends Cogn Sci 16(12):606–617
28. Arnau S, Löffler C, Rummel J, Hagemann D, Wascher E, Schubert AL (2020) Inter-trial alpha power indicates mind wandering. Psychophysiology 57(6):e13581
29. Baldwin CL, Roberts DM, Barragan D, Lee JD, Lerner N, Higgins JS (2017) Detecting and quantifying mind wandering during simulated driving. Front Hum Neurosci 11:406
30. Macdonald JS, Mathan S, Yeung N (2011) Trial-by-trial variations in subjective attentional state are reflected in ongoing prestimulus EEG alpha oscillations. Front Psychol 2:82
31. Baird B, Smallwood J, Lutz A, Schooler JW (2014) The decoupled mind: mind-wandering disrupts cortical phase-locking to perceptual events. J Cogn Neurosci 26(11):2596–607

32. van Son D, de Rover M, De Blasio FM, van der Does W, Barry RJ, Putman P (2019) Electroencephalography theta/beta ratio covaries with mind wandering and functional connectivity in the executive control network. Ann N Y Acad Sci 1452(1):52–64
33. Jadhav N, Manthalkar R, Joshi Y (2017) Assessing effect of meditation on cognitive workload using EEG signals. In: Second international workshop on pattern recognition 2017 Jun 19, vol 10443. SPIE, pp 269–273
34. Zyma I, Tukaev S, Seleznov I, Kiyono K, Popov A, Chernykh M, Shpenkov O (2019) Electroencephalograms during mental arithmetic task performance. Data 4(1):14
35. Al-Fahoum AS, Al-Fraihat AA (2014) Methods of EEG signal features extraction using linear analysis in frequency and time-frequency domains. International Scholarly Research Notices
36. Sifuzzaman M, Islam MR, Ali MZ (2009) Application of wavelet transform and its advantages compared to Fourier transform
37. Ezra YB, Lembrikov BI, Schwartz M, Zarkovsky S (2018) Applications of wavelet transforms to the analysis of superoscillations. Wavelet theory and its applications, vol 195
38. Gupta SS, Taori TJ, Ladekar MY, Manthalkar RR, Gajre SS, Joshi YV (2021) Classification of cross task cognitive workload using deep recurrent network with modelling of temporal dynamics. Biomed Signal Process Control 70:103070
39. Choi MK, Lee SM, Ha JS, Seong PH (2018) Development of an EEG-based workload measurement method in nuclear power plants. Ann Nuclear Energy 111:595–607

Fetal ECG Signal Processing Using One-Dimensional Convolutional Neural Network (1D CNN) for Fetal Arrhythmias Detection

Nurul Aulia Fitri, Yunendah Nur Fu'adah, and Rita Magdalena

Abstract Arrhythmia is a condition in which the heart beats faster or beats slower. In the fetus, arrhythmia is a fairly rare condition. However severe arrhythmias can lead to death and birth defects if not detected and treated properly. The early stages of detecting arrhythmias in the fetus can be done using an electrocardiogram (ECG). A normal ECG signal consisting of PQRST waves and an estimated heart rate can be used to diagnose arrhythmias. Manual examination of fetal arrhythmias is often impractical. Therefore, this study proposes a more effective and simple automatic detection system to detect fetal arrhythmias using segmentation of the ECG signal waveform in the form of PQRST waves with the One-Dimensional Convolutional Neural Network (1D CNN) method. This study uses 3 hidden layers with output channels of 16, ReLU activation, fully connected layer, flatten layer, dropout 0.5, and sigmoid activation. The dataset used is non-invasive fetal ECG arrhythmia from Physionet with two categories: Normal and arrhythmias. The best results obtained from this study are with the following parameters: AdaMax optimizer with fixed parameters learning rate of 0.001, epoch of 100, and batch size of 64 provide better performance with an accuracy of 96%. Based on the result, the proposed system has the potential to be used as a non-invasive tool for the early detection of arrhythmia in the fetus so that it can assist medical personnel in providing appropriate treatment.

Keywords Convolutional Neural Network (CNN) · Electrocardiogram (ECG) · Fetal arrhythmias

1 Introduction

Arrhythmia is a condition in which there is abnormal electrical activity in the heart [1]. Arrhythmias do not only occur in adults but can also occur in fetuses. Fetal arrhythmia is a disorder of the fetal heart such as tachyarrhythmias and bradyarrhythmias. The normal fetal heart rate ranges from 110–180 beats per minute, in the case

N. A. Fitri (✉) · Y. N. Fu'adah · R. Magdalena
School of Electrical Engineering, Telkom University, Bandung 40257, Indonesia
e-mail: nurulauliaf@student.telkomuniversity.ac.id

T. Triwiyanto et al. (eds.), *Proceeding of the 3rd International Conference on Electronics, Biomedical Engineering, and Health Informatics*, Lecture Notes in Electrical Engineering 1008, https://doi.org/10.1007/978-981-99-0248-4_6

of tachyarrhythmias, the fetal heart rate is more than 180 beats per minute, while in bradyarrhythmias, the fetal heart rate is less than 110 beats per minute [2]. Fetal arrhythmias can be found in approximately 1% of fetuses and up to 49% of all fetal referrals for echocardiography [3][4]. Approximately, 10% of pregnancies complicated by fetal arrhythmias can lead to death [5]. At 21 weeks of age with a high risk of pregnancy, fetal arrhythmias occurred in 16.6% [6][7]. Benign fetal arrhythmias are common but severe arrhythmias such as Ventricular Tachycardia, Supra-ventricular Tachycardia (SVT), Bradiarrhythmia, Junctional and Atrial Flutter (AF) are relatively rare but can lead to death [7]. Fetal ECG can be used for the early detection of fetal arrhythmias.

Electrocardiogram (ECG) is a tool to record the cardiac cycle through electrical signals from the heart. ECG is an important tool and is often used to diagnose cardiovascular disease [8]. The ECG will produce a signal consisting of PQRST waves [9]. To diagnose a disease in the heart, an ECG signal is needed to represent each condition of the ECG signal, extracting the ECG features is the most challenging aspect [10]. Figure 1, shows the normal PQRST waveform.

ECG of fetuses with arrhythmia conditions can be seen through changes in the QRS complex wave or QT interval. The QRS complex is an important part of the ECG signal because it describes the electrical activity of the heart during ventricular contraction. The waveform and timing of the QRS complex can provide information about the condition of the heart [11].

Several studies related to the detection of fetal arrhythmias with non-invasive fetal ECG arrhythmia datasets for normal and arrhythmia categories have been developed

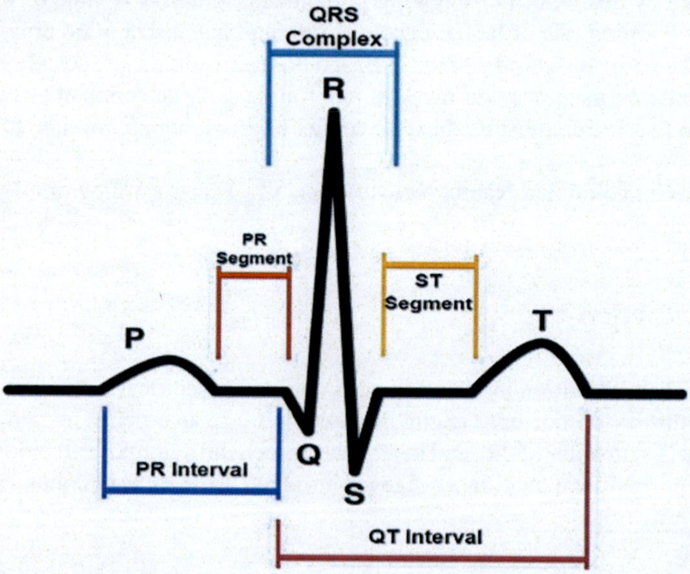

Fig. 1 PQRST waveform

using various methods. In 2017, Apsana. S et al. propose a study about "A Novel Algorithm For Early Detection of Fetal Arrhythmia Using ICA". This study used the Blind Signal Separation (BSS) and Independent Component Analysis (ICA) methods to extract fetal ECG signals. Then, using a novel algorithm to detect arrhythmias, Peak Detection Algorithm (PDA) to extract features and Bayesian classifier to classify normal and arrhythmia categories. This study obtained an accuracy of 93.71% [12]. In 2019, Md. S. R. Pavel et al. proposed a study about "Fetal Arrhythmia Detection Using Fetal ECG Signal". This study uses the Support Vector Machine (SVM) classifier, Gaussian Kernel to detect affected fetuses' arrhythmias, and the Leave One Out (LOO) method for model testing. This study obtained an accuracy of 83.33% [13]. In 2020, Biswarup Gangguly et al. proposed a study about "A Non-invasive Approach for Fetal Arrhythmia Detection and Classification". This study used 1D convolution with Kernel Wavelet as a classifier to extract time domain features from subjects with arrhythmias and normal categories. The acquired time domain features are sent to the Artificial Neural Network (ANN) to be identified and classified. This study obtained an accuracy of 96% [14].

In this study, a non-invasive fetal ECG arrhythmia dataset will be used for the arrhythmia and normal categories. Optimization methods such as Adam, AdaMax, Nadam, and RMSprop will be used to find out which optimizer provides the best results. Based on the previous study, the weakness is that the method is done manually and separately. For example, feature extraction and classification in ANN are done separately. Therefore, this study uses the One-dimensional CNN (1D CNN) method because the feature extraction and classification process is simpler and not done separately. Manual examination takes more time to be interpreted by doctors and there are still errors and differences of opinion between doctors in interpreting ECG signals [15]. Therefore, an automatic detection system is needed to assist medical personnel in providing appropriate treatment for the early detection of arrhythmia in the fetus.

2 Material and Method

2.1 Dataset

The dataset used in this study is a non-invasive fetal ECG arrhythmia obtained from Physionet [1]. There are 500 ECG and NIFECG recordings from mothers and pregnant women collected during routine check-up. There were 12 fetal arrhythmia ECG data recordings, 14 normal rhythm ECG data recordings, and 6 channel recordings, namely 1 maternal chest channel and 5 abdominal channels from 26 female subjects. Each recording has a duration that varies from 7–32 min with a sampling frequency of 500 Hz or 1 kHz. Data with normal conditions were obtained when the fetal age ranged from 20–36 weeks with an average age of 21 weeks, while data with arrhythmia conditions was obtained when the fetal age ranged from 22–41 weeks

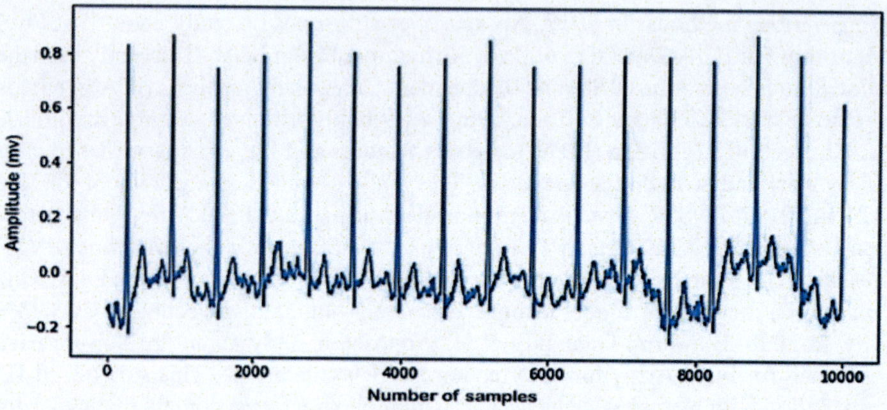

Fig. 2 Form of fetal arrhythmias ECG signal

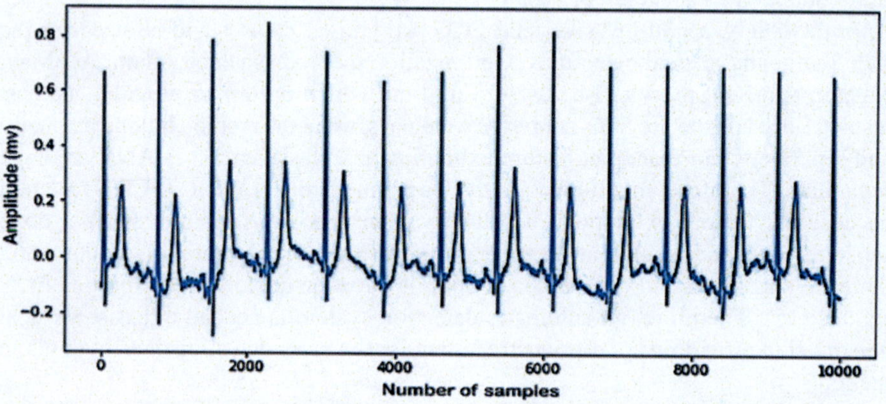

Fig. 3 Normal rhythm of fetal ECG signal

with an average age of 36 weeks [2]. This study uses 11 arrhythmia ECG data and 14 normal ECG data, the dataset is segmented so that 17,384 data are obtained which will be used for the training process and data validation. As much as 80% of the data for the training process and 20% of the data for the validation process. Figure 2 is a form of fetal arrhythmia ECG signal, while Fig. 3 is a form of normal rhythm ECG signal.

2.2 *Convolutional Neural Network (CNN)*

Convolutional Neural Network is another form of Artificial Neural Network (ANN) model that has better generalization capabilities compared to other networks that use a fully connected layer with a feed-forward architecture [3]. CNN can extract unique features in digital data such as images or signals from low-level patterns to high-level patterns [4].

Based on Fig. 4, it can be seen that 1D CNN consists of input and output signals and two main stages, namely: Feature extraction and classification. Feature extraction consists of convolution layer, pooling layer, and ReLU activation [5]. Classification consist of a fully connected layer. This research will use the convolutional layer, maxpooling layer, ReLU activation, flatten layer, fully connected layer, and sigmoid activation.

Feature Extraction. Feature extraction is the process of taking unique characteristics and providing a pattern from an object to be processed [6]. Feature extraction consists of two stages: The convolutional layer, and the pooling layer.

Convolutional Layer. The convolutional layer is the first layer where every convolution in the input data subregion with the kernel is calculated, coupled with the bias, then inputted through the activation function to generate a feature map in the next layer [7]. CNN method can be divided into 1D CNN and 2D CNN. 1D CNN can be used to process time series data, while 2D CNN can be used to process image data [8]. The convolutional Layer is defined in the following Eq. (1) [9, 10]:

$$h^{l,k} = f\left(b_i^{l,k} + \sum_{n=1}^{N} w_{n,i}^{l,k} \times x_{i+n-1}^{i+1,k}\right). \tag{1}$$

Based on Eq. 1, $h^{l,k}$ is the output of $i^{t,h}$ neurons in layer l, f () is the activation function, $b_i^{l,k}$ bias term for feature map $i^{t,h}$ in layer l, $x_{i+n-1}^{i+1,k}$ is the neuron output in layer l - 1, and $w_{n,i}^{l,k}$ is kernel convolution $k^{t,h}$ in the $l^{t,h}$ layer.

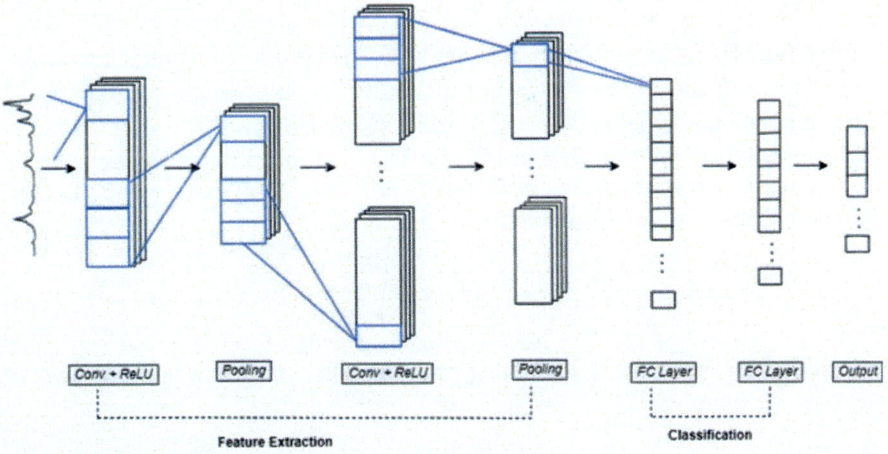

Fig. 4 The architecture of CNN

ReLU Activation. Relu is an activation layer that can convert all input values to positive numbers by minimizing errors. The activation RELU is defined in the following Eq. (2) [3]:

$$f(x)_{\text{ReLU}} = max(0, x) \tag{2}$$

In Eq. 2, ReLU can convert $x = 0$ and $x < 0$ to $x = 0$ while still maintaining the original value for $x > 0$.

Pooling Layer. In this layer, the feature map dimensions are reduced from large dimensions to smaller dimensions by maintaining the most dominant information to obtain a feature map subsample [3]. The pooling Layer is defined in the following Eq. (3) [9]:

$$\sigma_i^{l,k} = f\left(\sigma_i^{l,k} pool\left(x_i^{l-1,k}\right) + b_i^{l,k}\right). \tag{3}$$

From Eq. (3), $\sigma_i^{l,k}$ is the output of $i^{t,h}$ in layer l, $f()$ is the activation function, $b_i^{l,k}$ the term bias for feature map $i^{t,h}$ in layer l, $\sigma_i^{l,k}$ is the equation of sampling weight, $\left(x_i^{l-1,k}\right)$ is the neuron output in layer l - 1, and the pool is a function of pooling.

Classification. Classification is used to identify data that has been processed from feature extraction. This stage consists of a fully connected layer.

Fully Connected Layer. In this layer, the feature map from the convolutional layer or pooling layer is used as input by going through the flattening process to become a 1D vector so that it can be input into the fully connected layer [3][11]. The fully connected layer is defined in the following Eq. (4) [9]:

$$\sigma_i^{l,k} = f\left(\left(w_i^{l,k} x_i^{l-1,k}\right) + b_i^{l,k}\right). \tag{4}$$

From Eq. (4), $\sigma_i^{l,k}$ is the output of $i^{t,h}$ at layer l, $f()$ is the activation function, $b_i^{l,k}$ is bias term for feature map $i^{t,h}$ at layer l, $\sigma_i^{l,k}$ is the sampling weight equation, $x_i^{l-1,k}$ is the neuron output at layer l—1, $w_i^{l,k}$ is the network weight.

Sigmoid Activation. An activation function that describes a characteristic s-shaped curve by taking a real number as input and binding the output in the range [0,1] [3]. Sigmoid activation is defined in the following Eq. (5) [12]:

$$f(x)_{sigm} = \frac{1}{1 + e^{-x}}. \tag{5}$$

Equation (5) shows the function that transforms the value of x into the range of 0–1.

2.3 Proposed CNN

In this study, the proposed 1D CNN model consisted of fetal ECG signal as input and consists of two main stages, namely: Feature extraction and classification. At the feature extraction stage, there are 3 convolution layers with 16 output followed by kernel size and ReLU in each layer, then 3 layers of maxpool with a length of 2 in each layer. The classification layer consists of flattened layer, dropout 0.5 [13], 3 dense layers [14], and sigmoid activation. Each dense layer consists of a different number of neurons, the first layer has 256 neurons, the second layer has 100, and the third layer has 3 neurons.

Figure 5 contains the details of the proposed 1D CNN model. In addition, this study uses normalization to minimize signal differences due to the recording process [15] and the fivefold cross validation method to assess the generalizability of a system [16] by re-sampling the data 5 times with the same size.

2.4 System Performance

This study uses precision, recall, and f1-score to assess the performance of the system as measured in Eq. (6), (7), (8), and (9) [12].

$$\text{Accuracy} = \frac{\text{TP} + \text{TN}}{\text{TP} + \text{TN} + \text{FP} + \text{FN}}. \tag{6}$$

$$\text{Precision} = \frac{\text{TP}}{\text{TP} + \text{FP}} \tag{7}$$

$$\text{Recall} = \frac{\text{TP}}{\text{TP} + \text{FN}} \tag{8}$$

$$\text{F1} - \text{score} = 2 \times \frac{\text{recall} \times \text{precision}}{\text{recall} + \text{precision}} \tag{9}$$

True Positive (TP) is the data that deserves to be arrhythmia and it is predicted to be arrhythmia, True Negative (TN) is the data that deserves to be normal and it is predicted to be normal, False positive (FP) is the data that deserves to be normal and it is predicted to be arrhythmia, False Negative (FN) is the data that has an arrhythmia value but it is predicted to be normal.

Fig. 5 Proposed 1D CNN for fetal arrhythmia detection

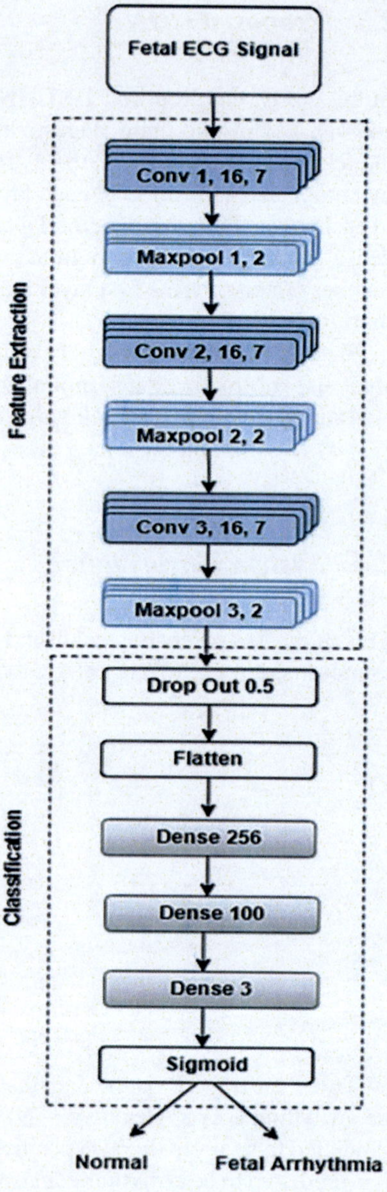

Table 1 Comparison of performance system in various optimizer

Optimizer	Accuracy (%)	Precision (%)	Recall (%)	F1-Score (%)
Adam	0.9431	0.94	0.94	0.94
AdaMax	0.9600	0.96	0.96	0.96
Nadam	0.7100	0.70	0.71	0.70
RMSprop	0.9816	0.98	0.98	0.98

3 Result and Discussion

3.1 Result

In this study, the segmentation process is carried out to obtain 17.384 segmented data, wherein 80% of the data was used for training data and 20% was used for validation. This study uses 1D CNN with fixed parameters namely: Learning rate of 0.001, epoch of 100, and batch size of 64. Then, the variable parameters include Adam, Nadam, AdaMax, and Rmsprop optimizer. And the other following parameters are precision, recall, and f1-score.

Table 1 shows the results of the various optimizer. The highest result is on the RMSprop optimizer with an accuracy of 98%. But based on the shape of the graph obtained in Fig. 6, the RMSprop optimizer has more spikes compared to other optimizers tested.

Table 2 shows the result of the system performance of each class from the best optimizer. Precision, Recall, and F1-score for each class is more than 90%. This shows that the model proposed in this study can classify normal conditions and fetal arrhythmias conditions quite well.

Based on Fig. 6, it can be found that the best result of the graph is obtained with AdaMax optimizer because there is only a slight spike in the AdaMax curve compared to the graph curves of other optimizers. The best Result can be seen in Fig. 6c, d. Then in Fig. 7, it can be seen that the results obtained by each class are quite good.

3.2 Discussion

In this study, we developed a fetal arrhythmia detection system with a different method than the conventional method used in previous studies. The method we use is simpler because it can minimize the processing steps, such as the feature extraction and classification process. The two processes are still in the same method. While in previous studies, different methods were needed for the feature extraction and classification process. The best results obtained in this study are based on the accuracy value and the shape of the graph obtained from the optimizer variation

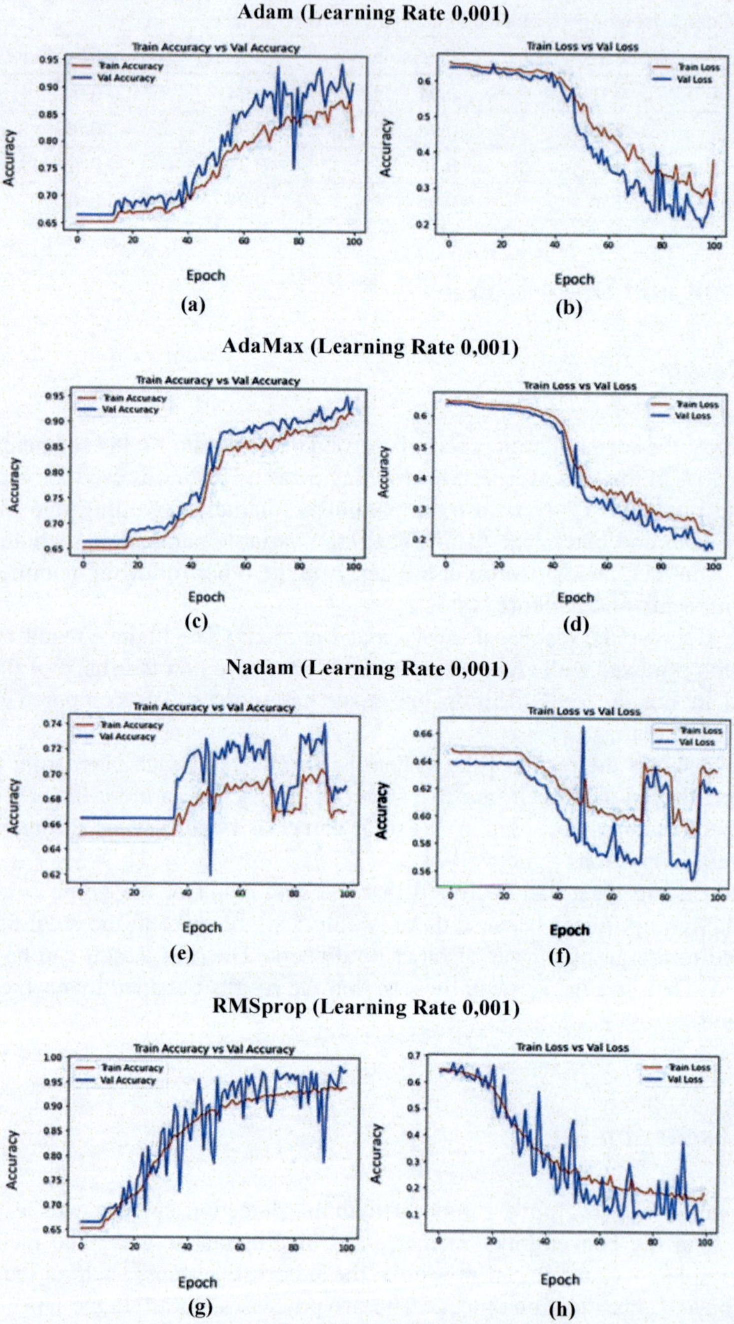

Fig. 6 Train accuracy and Train loss graph of the proposed model based on **(a)** and **(b)** Adam Optimizer; **(c)** and **(d)** AdaMax Optimizer; **(e)** and **(f)** Nadam Optimizer; **(g)** and **(h)**. RMSprop Optimizer

Table 2 System performance of each class from the best optimizer results

Class	Precision (%)	Recall (%)	F1-score (%)
Arrhythmia	0.96	0.98	0.97
Normal	0.95	0.93	0.94

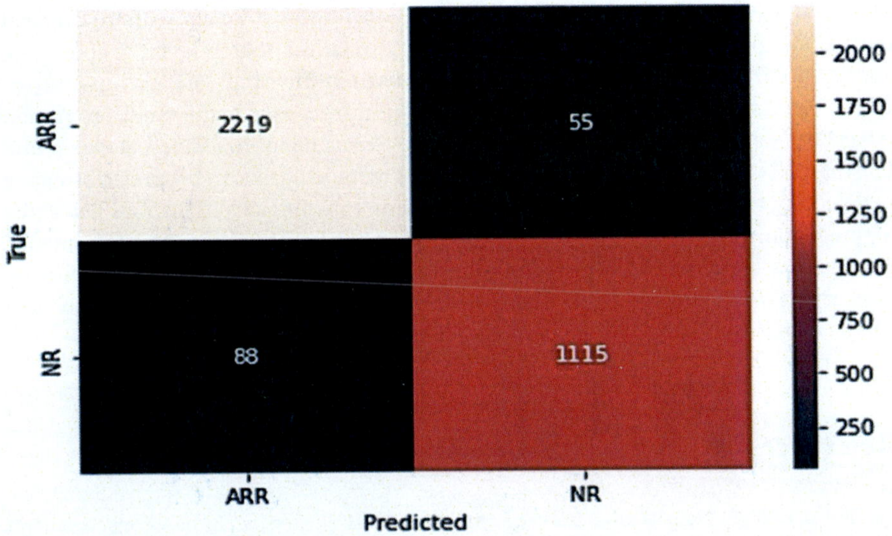

Fig. 7 Confusion matrix of validation data

is the AdaMax optimizer. The results of the performance accuracy of the test data obtained are 96% with a loss of 0.1602, the performance results obtained are quite good compared to several previous studies [17, 18]. The results of the accuracy of the training data are 91.42% with a loss of 0.2293 and the result of validation accuracy is 95.10%. The results of the accuracy are found in fold 3 of 5.

As shown in Fig. 6c, d, it can be seen that the research method with Adamax optimizer has a little bit of overfitting because it has a slight spike in the train accuracy and loss graphs and there is a distance between the curves of the train accuracy and validation accuracy. The distance between the train graph accuracy and validation is 3.68%. Overfitting that occurs in this model can be caused by noise contained in the dataset or the method used is still not appropriate. So, future experiment can use different datasets and use different methods. Figure 7 shows that this training model is quite promising to be used as a non-invasive tool for early detection of arrhythmia in the fetus so that it can be easier for medical personnel to provide appropriate treatment.

4 Conclusion

This study developed an automatic detection system to make it easier for a physician to detect arrhythmias in the fetus with two categories: Normal conditions and fetal arrhythmia conditions. This system is based on sound signal processing using a 1D CNN method. This method consists of 3 convolutional layers with 16 channel output, maxpooling with a length of 2, ReLU activation, flatten layer, dropout 0.5, and sigmoid activation. The fixed parameters used in this study are learning rate of 0.001, batch size of 64, and epoch of 100. The optimizers used in this study are Adam, AdaMax, Nadam, and RMSprop. Based on the experiments conducted, it was found that the CNN model with the AdaMax optimizer method produced better performance in detecting fetal arrhythmias with an accuracy of 96% and loss of 0.1602. The value of precision, recall, and F1-score is more than 90%. Based on the performance results, it is known that this system is promising to help physicians in diagnosing fetal arrhythmias and providing appropriate treatment. For future research, a system can be developed to classify the various types of fetal arrhythmias.

References

1. Behar J (2022) Non-Invasive fetal ecg arrhythmia database, https://physionet.org/content/nifeadb/1.0.0/, last accessed 2022/09/10. https://doi.org/10.13026/C2CT0S
2. Behar JA, Bonnemains L, Shulgin V, Oster J, Ostras O, Lakhno I (2019) Noninvasive fetal electrocardiography for the detection of fetal arrhythmias. Prenat Diagn 39:178–187. https://doi.org/10.1002/pd.5412
3. Balas VE, Kumar R, Srivastava R, Intelligent Systems Reference Library 172 Recent Trends and Advances in Artificial Intelligence and Internet of Things
4. Lecun Y, Bengio Y, Hinton G (2015). Deep learning. https://doi.org/10.1038/nature14539
5. Fu'adah YN, Pratiwi NC, Pramudito MA, Ibrahim N (2020) Convolutional neural network (CNN) for automatic skin cancer classification system. In: IOP Conference Series: Materials Science and Engineering. IOP Publishing Ltd. https://doi.org/10.1088/1757-899X/982/1/012005
6. Haryosuprobo IR, Sugiarto Y, Suryadi FX, Ekstraksi Ciri Sinyal EKG Aritmia Menggunakan Gelombang Singkat Diskrit
7. He R, Liu Y, Wang K, Zhao N, Yuan Y, Li Q, Zhang H (2019) Automatic cardiac arrhythmia classification using combination of deep residual network and bidirectional LSTM. IEEE Access. 7:102119–102135. https://doi.org/10.1109/ACCESS.2019.2931500
8. Institute of Electrical and Electronics Engineers (2018) In: 2018 4th International Conference on Frontiers of Signal Processing (ICFSP 2018) : September 24–27, Poitiers, France
9. Adnan Pramudito M, Nur Fu Y, Magdalena R, Rizal A, Frahma Taliningsih F, ECG signal processing using 1-D Convolutional Neural Network for Congestive Heart Failure Identification
10. Eren L, Ince T, Kiranyaz S (2019) A Generic intelligent bearing fault diagnosis system using compact adaptive 1D CNN classifier. J Signal Process Syst. 91:179–189. https://doi.org/10.1007/s11265-018-1378-3
11. Chen C, Hua Z, Zhang R, Liu G, Wen W (2020) Automated arrhythmia classification based on a combination network of CNN and LSTM. Biomed Signal Process Control. 57. https://doi.org/10.1016/j.bspc.2019.101819
12. Hanung T, Nugroho A, Rizal A, Caesarendra W, Lecture notes in electrical engineering 746.

13. Srivastava N, Hinton G, Krizhevsky A, Salakhutdinov R (2014) Dropout: a simple way to prevent neural networks from overfitting
14. Helen Josephine VL, Nirmala AP, Alluri VL (2021) Impact of hidden dense layers in convolutional neural network to enhance performance of classification model. IOP Conf Ser Mater Sci Eng. 1131:012007. https://doi.org/10.1088/1757-899x/1131/1/012007
15. Hamdi S, Abdallah A ben, Bedoui MH, Bedoui MH (2014) Grammar formalism for ECG signal interpretation and classification hardware architectures of reconfigurable neural networks using NoC view project shape analysis view project grammar formalism for ECG signal interpretation and classification
16. Bickel P, Diggle P, Fienberg S, Gather U, Olkin I, Zeger S, Springer series in statistics
17. IEEE Staff (2017) In: 2017 International Conference on Intelligent Computing, Instrumentation and Control Technologies (ICICICT). IEEE
18. Bangladesh University of Engineering and Technology. Department of electrical and electronic engineering, IEEE communications society. In: Bangladesh Chapter, Institute of Electrical and Electronics Engineers: 3rd IEEE International Conference on Telecommunications and Photonics (ICTP) : 28–30 December 2019, Dhaka, Bangladesh, Dept. of EEE, ECE Building, BUET, Dhaka, Bangladesh.

Diabetic Retinopathy Classification Based on Fundus Image Using Convolutional Neural Network (CNN) with MobilenetV2

Abel Bima Wiratama, Yunendah Fu'adah, Sofia Saidah, Rita Magdalena, Ibnu Da'wan Salim Ubaidah, and Richard Bina Jadi Simanjuntak

Abstract The amount of Diabetic Retinopathy (DR) patients is always increasing. There is a need to find a solution to prevent it, like regularly checking the eyes of patients to detect DR class. But the detection process also takes a long time and requires a large amount of money. So, this study proposed a deep learning method using CNN by implementing the MobilenetV2 architecture, which is a lightweight model and mobile-friendly architecture. In this study, we used the primary dataset from the APTOS 2019 dataset, which contains 3662 retinal fundus images. Diabetic retinopathy is divided into 5 classes, starting from No DR, Mild, Moderate, Severe, and Proliferative DR. To produce an optimal class classification in this study, first balance the dataset scheme to 800 in each class by using image augmentation and implementing circle cropping. So, the highest results are obtained with this method with the following parameters: batch size of 32, learning rate of 0.001, RMSProp optimizer, and epoch 100. Testing accuracy is 92.6% as a result of this parameter. The macro precision, recall, and f1-score are 92.8%, 92.6%, and 92.4%, respectively. Our results show that augmentation techniques and circle crop methods can make the MobileNetV2 architecture bring good performance results, and several parameters can bring significant system performance results. This research will provide information that MobileNetV2 has a good result on the parameters and this will be a lightweight model to classify DR into 5 classes.

Keywords Diabetic retinopathy · MobilenetV2 · Augmentation · Fundus image

1 Introduction

Diabetic Retinopathy (DR) is a chronic disease caused by complications of Diabetes Mellitus (DM) [1]. Based on data from the American Academy of Ophthalmology, DR is the leading cause of blindness in working-age adults worldwide. Published

A. B. Wiratama (✉) · Y. Fu'adah · S. Saidah · R. Magdalena · I. D. S. Ubaidah · R. B. J. Simanjuntak
School of Electrical Engineering, Telkom University, Bandung 40257, Indonesia
e-mail: abelwiratama@student.telkomuniversity.ac.id

T. Triwiyanto et al. (eds.), *Proceeding of the 3rd International Conference on Electronics, Biomedical Engineering, and Health Informatics*, Lecture Notes in Electrical Engineering 1008, https://doi.org/10.1007/978-981-99-0248-4_7

global data on DR includes: 387 million people with diabetes mellitus (DM) in the world in 2016 and is expected to increase to 592 million people by 2035, around 93 million people have DR in that year [2]. DR is estimated to threaten the eyesight of about 28 million people; the prevalence of DR worldwide in type 1 DM patients is 77.3%, and with type 2, it is 25.1%. According to data from the International Diabetes Management Practices Study, 8.8 million people in Indonesia are affected by DR, which is predicted to increase to 21.3 million in 2030 [3]. According to analysis of Indonesia's Basic Health in 2013 found that around 6.9% of the Indonesian population are affected by DR over 15 years old.

As this disease increases, it is necessary to properly prevent it by using existing technology such as conducting an early-scale examination. The manual technique used to diagnose DR today is that of ophthalmologists [4]. But unfortunately, the technology used today is not able to provide fast and precise results because the DR classification process takes a long time so automatic DR detection is needed [5].

In 2020, Shidqie Taufiqurrahman proposed research about Diabetic Retinopathy Classification Using A Hybrid and Efficient MobileNetV2-SVM Model [6]. An unbalanced dataset is the main problem that must be solved by converting the APTOS 2019 dataset into 700 fundus images for each image, with this research process, the model accuracy can be 85% and the model obtains a quadratic weighted kappa [7] value of 92.5%. A more compact model that makes the model lighter.

Also, in the same year, Sarah Sheikh proposed research Using MobileNetV2 to Classify the Severity of Diabetic Retinopathy [8]. In this research, he applied the MobileNetV2 model by preprocessing the EyePacs and APTOS 2019 datasets so as to obtain an accuracy of around 91.8%. Because the process of adding layers to the MobileNetV2 architecture is still not ideal, the research undertaken is still unable to offer improved accuracy.

In 2021, Wejdan L. Ayoubi proposed Diabetic Retinopathy Fundus Image Classification and Lesions Localization System Using Deep Learning to utilize some models like CNN299 and CNN512 for implementation in several datasets: DDR and APTOS 2019. As a result, the CNN512 model may achieve an accuracy rate of 88.6%. While CNN299 failed to detect the training process[4] but CNN512 use lot of time to train model.

In 2022, Yufiz Azhar et al. [9] conducted more investigation into the classification DR. The dataset used in this study is APTOS 2019 from the Kaggle website. In this study, the best accuracy is 89%. They also state that augmentation can reduce overfitting results and also test several pre-processing for the model. This study have limitations to increase the accuracy because the model needs improvement to do image enhancement.

The model provided has a large size, and the system to categorize diabetic retinopathy needs development, according to prior studies, which have various weaknesses. After learning that MobileNetV2 is one of the lightweight architectures and implements numerous approaches on datasets that we think can be deployed to mobile application, we proposed DR classification in this study that will be done using the Convolutional Neural Network (CNN) method. According to study, MobileNet and MobileNetV2 are two lightweight models that may be implemented on platforms like mobile, websites, and other prototypes [10, 11, 12, 13]. The contribution of this research is to check what parameters can bring good performance to MobileNetV2 and how to improve the accuracy of the model when classifying DR.

2 Material and System Design

2.1 Dataset

In this study, the dataset used came from the Kaggle website which was obtained from Aravind Eye Hospital, India, and was used for the competition at the Asia Pacific Tele-Opthalmology Society (APTOS) in 2019 [14]. The dataset was obtained using a fundus camera. The tool is used to retrieve retinal fundus images with a total of 3662 images consisting of 1805 No DR class images, 370 Mild class images, 990 Moderate class images, 193 Severe class images, and 295 Proliferate DR class images [15]. To make a balanced dataset, the augmentation process is implemented. In this study, the dataset will be augmented to become 800 images per class with a total of 4000 fundus images. According to research by Shidie that implemented 700 picture augmentation and resampling, the dataset's augmentation procedure will be resampled from No DR from 1805 class images to 800 [6]. Before the augmentation process, the image will be cropped with the circle cropping function and some method rescaling parameter of 1./255 [16]. The technique for augmentation is scikit random rotation and horizontal flip.

The diabetic retinopathy classes that we used in this study are shown in Fig. 1. No DR is a condition if the retina has no visible disease, Mild is localized swelling of the small blood vessels on the retina (microaneurysmis) [17], Moderate is mild class with minor bleeding (bleeding and spotting), leakage (hard discharge) or closure (cotton spots) of small blood vessels [18], Severe is moderate class plus further damage to blood vessels (interentinal hemorrhages, venous beading, intraretinal microvascular abnormalities) [1] and Proliferative DR is new vessels formation or vitreous/preretinal hemorrhages or tractional retinal detechment [19]. The results of certain resampling and augmentation processes are shown in Fig. 2.

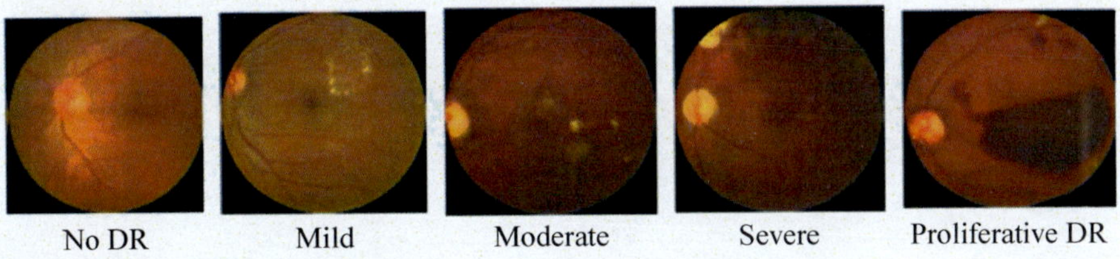

Fig. 1 Class of diabetic retinopathy

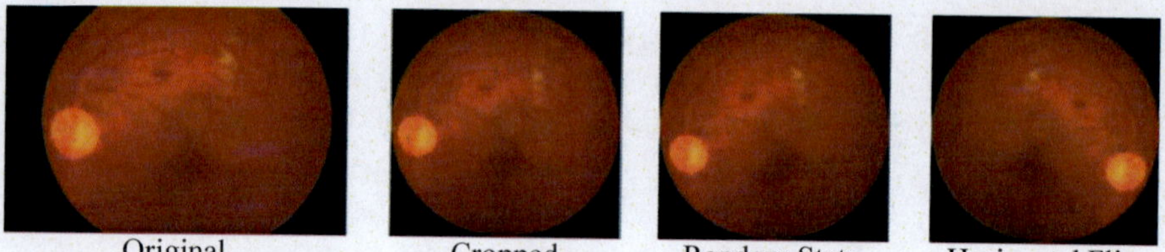

Fig. 2 Augmentation process

2.2 *Convolutional Neural Network*

Convolutional Neural Network (CNN) is a type of Neural Network that is used in digital image processing and RGB images [20], and a component of deep learning is capable of identifying and detecting some pictures [21]. CNN is the development of Multi-Layer Perception (MLP) [22] with the aim of processing data in two-dimensional form, while MLP still processes all data in one-dimensional fields.

In Fig. 3, there is an architecture of CNN, the CNN model includes a number of layers, including convolutional [23], pooling, fully connected, ReLU, and softmax activation. The main objective of this study is to analyze what scenarios bring good accuracy when classifying DR into 5 classes. This research paper proposes the implementation of the MobileNetV2 architecture which can provide a higher level of accuracy with several scenarios used. Before making the implementation, the paper will show the data augmentation and preprocessing steps that are used to improve the accuracy of the model.

Convolutional layer. The Convolutional Layer is one of the most basic layers in CNN [24], the function of this layer is to apply functions to the output of other functions repeatedly and to extract features from the input image. This process will produce a linear transformation of the data according to the spatial information of the data. This layer is composed of several neurons forming a filter that has length, height, and thickness. The calculation process of the convolutional layer can be seen in Fig. 4.

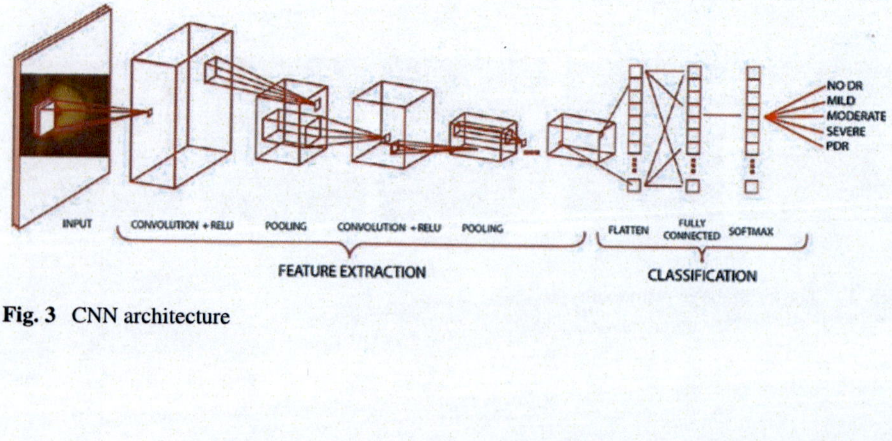

Fig. 3 CNN architecture

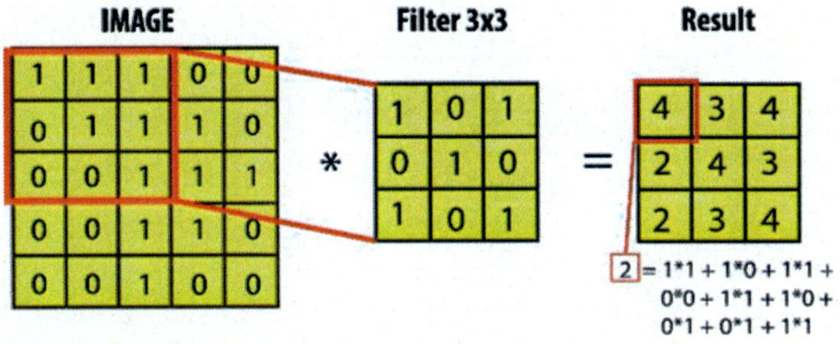

Fig. 4 Convolutional Layer

Pooling Layer. The pooling layer is very effective in reducing the dimensions of an image. This process aims to prevent overfitting of the model to be made. The most widely used pooling layer today is divided into 2, namely, max pooling and average pooling. Max pooling uses subregion mapping based on the maximum image value, while average pooling performs subregion mapping based on the average value of the image [25]. Implementation of the pooling layer can be seen in Fig. 5 provides a visualization of the average and maximum pooling layer usage calculation.

Rectified Linear Units (ReLU). The ReLU becomes a layer that will not change the size of the input image. ReLU has a function to increase the nonlinear transformation of the image and map the CNN input to the output which has a high nonlinear transformation [26]. ReLU also changes the value of feature maps, which was originally negative to 0, this is done to help the outline process of feature maps consisting of images. ReLU is also often referred to as the Activation function. The ReLU function is used to create the CNN model, the following functions Eq. (1):

$$f(x) = \begin{cases} x, x > 0 \\ 0, x \leq 0 \end{cases}, x = input\ value\ to\ neuron \tag{1}$$

Fig. 5 Pooling Layer

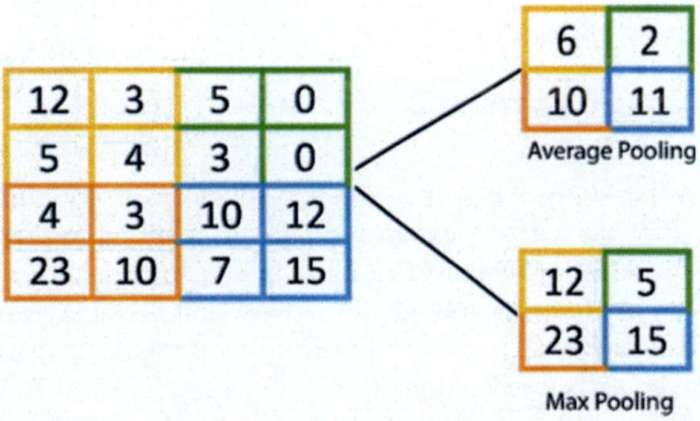

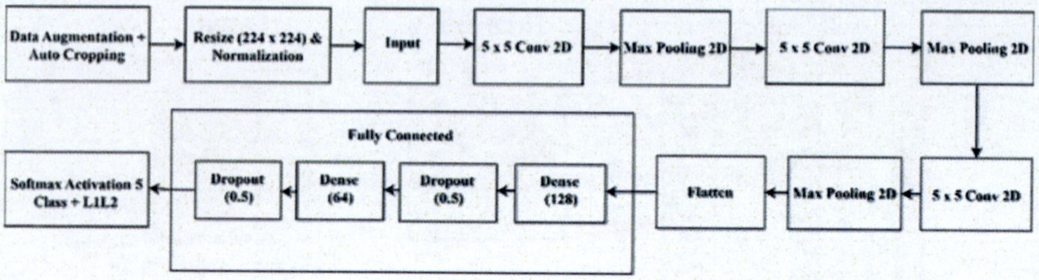

Fig. 6 Proposed CNN

In Eq. (1), when the value of f(x) is lower than 0 or negative, the result is 0. It is different if the input f(x) given is a value of 0 or above 0, then the result of the above equation is the number 0 and the value is positive.

2.3 Proposed CNN

In this study, the proposed CNN model is used to analyze how the results of the performance of the system designed with the CNN model. The architecture of the proposed CNN model consists of an input layer and 3 convolutional layers [24] that use the kernel, starting from 32, 64, and 128, respectively, which use ReLU in each layer [26]. Each convolutional layer is also accompanied by placing a pooling layer, the pooling layer used is Max Pooling 2D [25]. After the feature extraction has been completed, the next step will be to combine the layers using flatten [27]. In the FC layer there is a hidden layer with each layer size 128 plus dropout and hidden layer 64 and add dropout. In the last layer of architecture, it will be combined and classified into 5 classes using softmax activation [28] with regularization L1L2.

Figure 6 is a component of the proposed CNN that can be used to compare with MobileNetV2 architecture with several hyperparameters. This model has a total of 13,112,389 parameters that need to be trained when training the model.

2.4 MobileNetV2

In this study, we proposed a light model with MobileNetV2 architecture that each block has a 1×1 expansion layer in addition to the deep and dotted convolution layers [29]. MobileNetV2 has a residual connection that is useful for assisting the flow of gradients through the network and a total layer of MobilenetV2 17 bottleneck residual blocks in rows followed by 1×1 regular convolution, global average pooling layer, and classification layer.

Figure 7 show the proposed model of MobileNetV2 which is used in this study. The total parameter of this MobileNetV2 model is 2,340,293 which has many layers

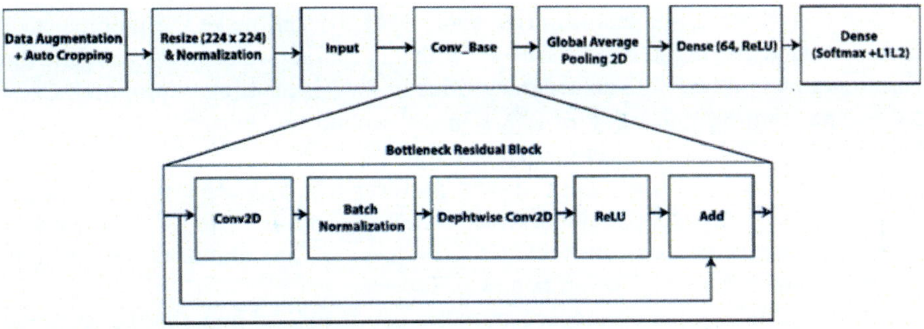

Fig. 7 Proposed MobileNetV2

build from MobileNet implementation of this Depthwise Separable [30] and pointwise convolutional [31] that improvement with bottleneck and residual block for MobileNetV2.

3 Results

In testing the scheme, it will use a dataset of 4000 retinal fundus images containing 5 classes with 800 fundus images in each class. Furthermore, it will be divided into 2, namely, 80% for training and 20% for testing. In this test, we will use cross validation with a fold size of 5 folds. For the first test, it focuses on the effect that the batch size parameter value can significantly increase or improve the accuracy value of the proposed MobileNetV2 and CNN models. The batch size values tested start from 16, 32, and 64.

Based on Table 1, the batch size value that can make a high accuracy value is the batch size 32 value with an accuracy value of 91.125%. The batch size 32 value will be tested in the second scenario.

In the second test, an analysis will be carried out on the effect of the learning rate parameter value in improving the performance of the system used. The proposed learning rates in this test are 0.1, 0.01, 0.001, 0.0001, and 0.00001.

Table 1 Comparison of performance in several batch size values

Model	Batch size	Acc (%)	Loss (%)	Precision (%)	Recall (%)	F1-Score (%)
MobileNetV2	16	88.500	0.495	88.60	89.00	88.40
	32	**91.125**	**0.445**	**91.20**	**91.00**	**91.00**
	64	88.125	0.558	88.40	88.1	88.00
Proposed CNN	16	50.125	1.191	49.60	50.00	48.20
	32	20.000	1.609	4.00	20.00	6.60
	64	78.500	0.949	78.80	78.60	79.00

Based on Table 2, the learning rate value of 0.001 can make the mobilenetV2 model produce good system performance with an accuracy value of 90%. While the learning rate of 0.0001 with an accuracy value of 80% is the highest proposed CNN value. The learning rate value of 0.001 in the second test becomes the reference parameter to be used in the third parameter test.

In the third test, an analysis of system performance will be carried out on the influence of the optimizer parameter which is able to increase system accuracy based on the reference of the previous parameter test results. The optimizers used include Adam, Nadam, Adamax, RMSprop, and SGD.

Based on Table 3, the optimizer parameter that is able to improve the accuracy and performance of the 2 models tested is the RMSprop optimizer, which gives an accuracy result of 91%. While the proposed CNN model has the most optimal results on the optimizer Adamax and SGD with an accuracy value of 77.625%. From the results of the third test, the most optimal optimizer used is RMSprop.

Table 2 Comparison of performance in several learning rate values

Model	Learning rate	Acc (%)	Loss (%)	Precision (%)	Recall (%)	F1-Score (%)
MobileNetV2	0.0001	82.375	0.799	82.40	82.40	82.40
	0.001	**90.000**	**0.506**	**90.40**	**90.00**	**90.00**
	0.01	78.625	0.717	78.80	78.60	78.60
	0.1	20.000	1.629	4.00	20.00	6.60
Proposed CNN	0.0001	80.000	0.876	79.80	79.80	79.80
	0.001	77.000	1.001	77.20	77.00	76.80
	0.01	20.000	2.983	4.00	20.00	6.60
	0.1	79.250	0.882	79.80	79.20	79.20

Table 3 Comparison of performance in several optimizers

Model	Optimizer	Acc (%)	Loss (%)	Precision (%)	Recall (%)	F1-Score (%)
MobileNetV2	Adam	90.000	0.506	90,40	90.00	90.00
	Nadam	89.375	0.560	89.60	89.20	89.20
	Adamax	88.500	0.581	88.60	88.40	88.40
	RMSprop	**91.000**	**0.421**	**91.60**	**91.00**	**91.00**
	SGD	62.000	1.312	51.60	61.80	61.40
Proposed CNN	Adam	77.000	1.001	77.20	77.00	76.80
	Nadam	76.750	0.757	77.00	76.80	76.80
	Adamax	77.625	0.978	78.00	77.40	77.80
	RMSprop	79.000	1.050	79.60	79.00	79.20
	SGD	77.625	0.978	78.00	77.40	77.80

Table 4 Comparison of performance in several epoch values

Model	Epoch	Acc (%)	Loss (%)	Precision (%)	Recall (%)	F1-Score (%)
MobileNetV2	10	77.625	0.770	79.80	77.60	77.60
	25	88.375	0.538	89.20	88.40	88.40
	50	90.500	0.468	90.80	90.80	90.60
	100	**92.625**	**0.382**	**92.80**	**92.60**	**92.40**
Proposed CNN	10	41.875	1.361	32.00	41.80	35.40
	25	70.350	0.908	71.00	70.40	70.20
	50	78.625	0.784	78.80	78.60	78.40
	100	20.000	1.609	4.00	20.00	6.60

In the last test, the system performance analysis will be carried out on the epoch parameters, which will use the previous parameters to find the most optimal results from the proposed system. The Epoch values used in this test are 10, 25, 50, and 100.

Based on table 4, the results of the analysis in the form of epoch values that can affect better system performance are obtained by epoch 100, which obtains an accuracy value of 92.625%.

4 Discussion

In this study, we developed a system that can assist in the process of classifying diabetic retinopathy. Several scenarios have been carried out, including testing the effect of batch size on the system, which obtained the best results using batch size 32. The second one tested the effect of the learning rate on the system and obtained the most optimal results for it, namely when the learning rate was 0.001. The third is to test the effect of which optimizer can give optimal results on the system, and it was found that the RMSprop optimizer can give the best results. The last one tests the effect of the epoch value that can give optimal results to the system. The best parameter results from several scenarios can be seen in Fig. 6., which presents the results of the confusion matrix and ROC curve, which are quite good compared to previous studies [8, 14] that have an accuracy lower than 92.625%. This model of MobileNetV2 has good accuracy but requires a technique to avoid overfitting, although in this study it was implemented cross-validation.

After implementation cross validation, the model has several best folds. Cross validation brings good information to know and easy detection which the fold that has minimum overfitting and has best accuracy. On this research the best performance system with several best parameter that give result that fold 3 is one best model that has train accuracy 99.4% with validation accuracy of 92.5%. From Fig. 8, the model has a small overfitting because the model has some noise on the dataset and maybe the model needs a dataset from another dataset like EyePACS, Messidor, DIABETIC0 and DIABETIC1.

The confusion matrix's output can be very good for system performance. The performance of the system utilizes an index prediction label and an actual label. The best model can predict every actual data point with a True Positive condition from Fig. 9. The system has a good result with a green image that is darker and the True Negative, False Positive, and False Negative darker. The system can predict every label from No DR/normal, mild, moderate, severe, and proliferative DR. To make sure that the model has good performance, we can see the result on the ROC curve.

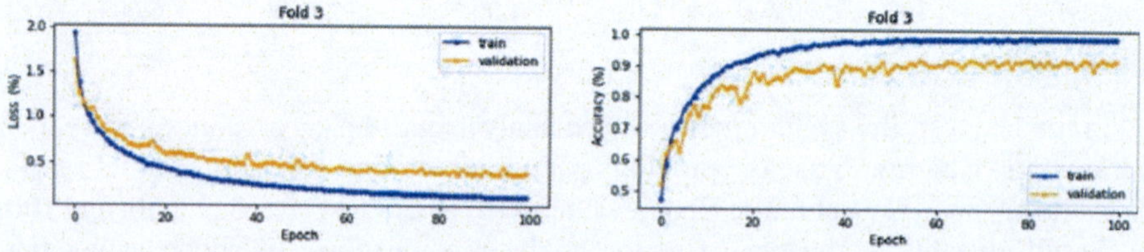

Fig. 8 Loss and Accuracy of the MobileNetV2 model

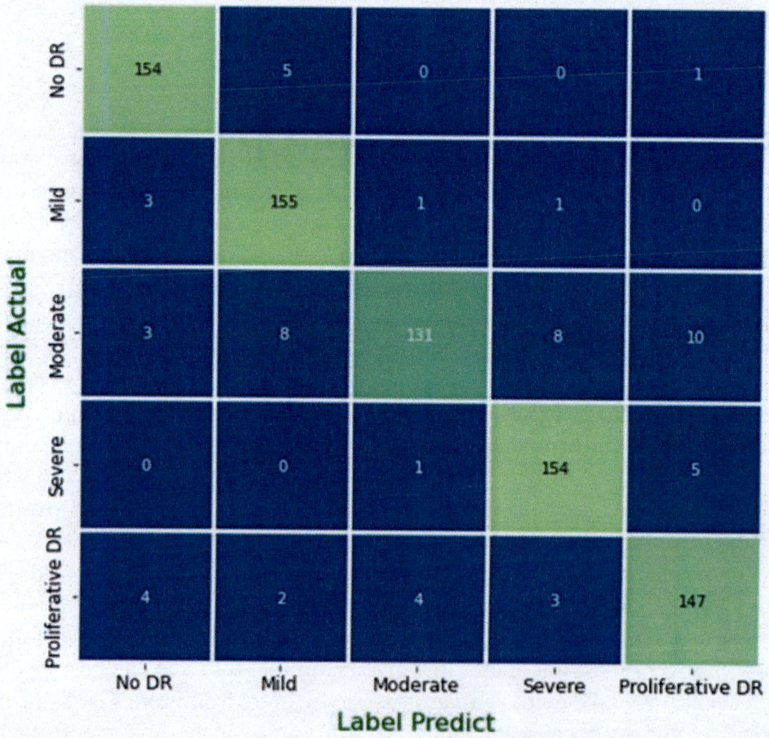

Fig. 9 Confusion Matrix Best Performance

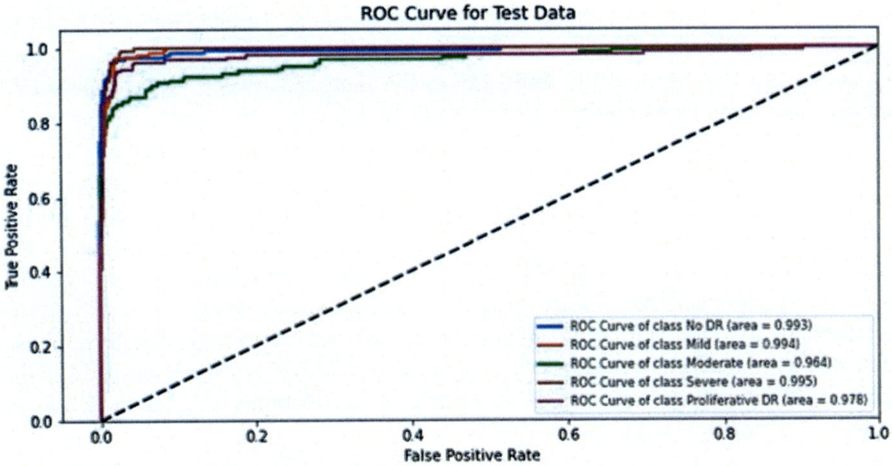

Fig. 10 ROC Curve of MobileNetV2 model

The ROC curve of the optimum MobileNetV2 is shown in Fig. 10. The result of every class from no DR/normal, mild, moderate, severe, and proliferative DR achieved the AUROC score of 0.993, 0.994, 0.964, 0.995, and 0.978, respectively.

The clinical approach to the diagnosis of DR disease is quite accurate, but they still have some limitations, such as the use of time on the detection and classification is still time- consuming and requires a high level of accuracy. As a result, computer-aided classifications in machine learning and deep learning are now being considered for the treatment of DR. In this study, we proposed a MobileNetV2 architectural model that has several adjustments to be able to classify diabetic retinopathy into several classes including No DR, Mild, Moderate, Severe, and Proliferative DR. However, in the research conducted, there are still some limitations such as limitations in using some existing datasets such as Messidor, EyePacs, and other datasets. As well as in the research we conduct, we always use the secondary dataset obtained from the Kaggle website.

In another study that was the same as ours, we sawthat our model gave promising results. In a related study by Sarah Sheikh [8], using datasets from APTOS 2019, EyePacs and Messidor. Techniques used in preprocessing is to change the luminous intensity of the image. previously obtained 91.68% accuracy results on a custom dataset and obtained a testing value of 50% with a dataset from Messidor dataset that was not used in the training process. Meanwhile, in the research that we conducted, we obtained a higher accuracy value than previous research with an accuracy value of 92.626% with some adjustments to the designed architecture such as implementing L2 regularization and changing the dataset only with auto cropping techniques on the APTOS 2019 dataset.

Another article provides [32] that research conducted mainly on image classification is divided into 2 classifications including DR and RDR (referable DR). In RDR, they use images with grade 0 and grade 1 for non-referable images, while grade 2 and grade 3 for RDR images. The model results obtained include the accuracy value at DR of 90.8%, while RDR of 92.3%. So this study provides a new technique for determining the threshold in the merger between the MobileNetV2 architecture with the MobileNet-Dense Bottleneck block and research conducted by Shidqie Taufiqurrahman [6]. The dataset used is APTOS 2019 by modifying the resolution range to 4288 × 2848 pixels. In their research, they use the QWK parameter to see the accuracy of the model and apply MobileNetV2-SVM to compare the results of the MobileNet2 values. The model used is able to get a QWK value of 92.5% and an accuracy value of 85%. And it is found that a small input image is able to promise a greater accuracy value. Based on this, the research we did got better results by implementing auto cropping, L2 regularization, and optimizing MobileNetV2 so that with our research, we got an accuracy result of 92.625% when compared to the proposed CNN which also uses the same settings as MobileNetV2 but does not get a higher accuracy value, that is, 78.625%.

As a result, we believe that a deep learning system can be used for computer-aided diagnosis to classify DR into the following categories: No DR, Mild, Moderate, Severe, and Proliferative DR. This addition in the approach can be potentially used as an assistant tool to help medical professionals make a more accurate diagnosis of DR. However, to confirm the clinical feasibility of our proposed approach, we should carry out further investigations using more datasets.

5 Conclusion

We have developed a system that can assist doctors in diagnosing and monitoring diabetic retinopathy patients automatically using the MobileNetV2 model, which can quickly classify DR levels. Based on the results of the experiment, the best parameters are batch size 32, learning rate 0.001, optimizer RMSprop, and epoch 100. This method can provide optimal results with an accuracy of 92.625%, and it can be considered a reference for future implementation. As a result of the research, it is necessary to increase the size of the dataset being used as well as to employ various techniques to reduce overfitting in the model. The implication of the proposed method is the existence of a system that is able to detect diabetic retinopathy with higher accuracy than previous studies with a simpler algorithm and faster computational time. In our research work, there are limitations in using secondary datasets in training the proposed model, so it is necessary to use primary dataset to get ready-to-go models direct.

References

1. Wang W, Lo ACY (2018) Diabetic retinopathy: pathophysiology and treatments. Int J Mol Sci 19. https://doi.org/10.3390/ijms19061816
2. Global Information (2016) Diabetic retinopathy—Asia 1–17
3. Prodi S, Telekomunikasi T, Elektro FT, Telkom U (2019) Klasifikasi diabetes retinopati menggunakan metode statistical region merging dan convolutional neural network classification of diabetic retinopathy using statistical region merging and convolutional neural. 6:4109–411
4. Alyoubi WL, Abulkhair MF, Shalash WM (2021) Diabetic retinopathy fundus image classification and lesions localization system using deep learning. Sensors 21:1–22. https://doi.org/10.3390/s21113704
5. Xu K, Feng D, Mi H (2017) Deep convolutional neural network-based early automated detection of diabetic retinopathy using fundus image. Molecules 22. https://doi.org/10.3390/molecules22122054
6. Taufiqurrahman S, Handayani A, Hermanto BR, Mengko TLER (2020) Diabetic retinopathy classification using a hybrid and efficient MobileNetV2-SVM Model. IEEE region 10's 9th annual international conference on proceedings/TENCON, 2020–November, pp 235–240. https://doi.org/10.1109/TENCON50793.2020.9293739
7. Vanbelle S (2016) A new interpretation of the weighted kappa coefficients. Psychometrika 81:399–410. https://doi.org/10.1007/s11336-014-9439-4
8. Sheikh S, Qidwai U (2020) Using MobileNetV2 to classify the severity of diabetic retinopathy. Int J Simul Syst Sci Technol 1–6. https://doi.org/10.5013/ijssst.a.21.02.16
9. Minarno AE, Mandiri MHC, Azhar Y, Bimantoro F, Nugroho HA, Ibrahim Z (2022) Classification of diabetic retinopathy disease using convolutional neural network. Int J Inf Vis 6:12–18. https://doi.org/10.30630/joiv.6.1.857
10. Cheng YJ, Lin W, Liu YZ, Sun L (2021) Classification of skin diseases based on improved MobileNetV2. In: 2021 33rd Chinese control and decision conference (CCDC), pp 598–603. IEEE. https://doi.org/10.1109/CCDC52312.2021.9602387
11. Kolonne S, Fernando C, Kumarasinghe H, Meedeniya D (2021) MobileNetV2 based chest X-rays classification. In: 2021 international conference on decision aid sciences and application DASA 2021, pp 57–61. https://doi.org/10.1109/DASA53625.2021.9682248
12. Shahi TB, Sitaula C, Neupane A, Guo W (2022) Fruit classification using attention-based MobileNetV2 for industrial applications. PLoS One 17:1–12. https://doi.org/10.1371/journal.pone.0264586
13. Dong K, Zhou C, Ruan Y, Li Y (2020) MobileNetV2 model for image classification. In: Proceedings of the 2020 2nd international conference on computer information science and application technology ITCA 2020, pp 476–480. https://doi.org/10.1109/ITCA52113.2020.00106
14. Sikder N, Masud M, Bairagi AK, Arif ASM, Nahid AAl, Alhumyani HA (2021) Severity classification of diabetic retinopathy using an ensemble learning algorithm through analyzing retinal images. Symmetry (Basel) 13. https://doi.org/10.3390/sym13040670
15. Asia Pacific Tele-Ophthalmology Society (APTOS): APTOS 2019 blindness detection
16. Adhinata FD, Tanjung NAF, Widayat W, Pasfica GR, Satura FR (2021) Comparative study of VGG16 and MobileNetV2 for masked face recognition. J Ilm Tek Elektro Komput dan Inform 7:230. https://doi.org/10.26555/jiteki.v7i2.20758
17. Azar AT, Balas VE (2013) Classification and detection of diabetic retinopathy. Stud Comput Intell 473:135–145. https://doi.org/10.1007/978-3-319-00029-9_12
18. Gupta A, Chhikara R (2018) Diabetic retinopathy: present and past. Procedia Comput Sci 132:1432–1440. https://doi.org/10.1016/j.procs.2018.05.074
19. Ayala A, Ortiz Figueroa T, Fernandes B, Cruz F (2021) Diabetic retinopathy improved detection using deep learning. Appl Sci 11. https://doi.org/10.3390/app112411970
20. Wahid FF, Raju G (2021) Diabetic retinopathy detection using convolutional neural network—a study. Lect Notes Netw Syst 132:127–133. https://doi.org/10.1007/978-981-15-5309-7_13

21. Saidah S, Fuadah YN, Alia F, Ibrahim N, Magdalena R, Rizal S (2021) Facial skin type classification based on microscopic images using convolutional neural network (CNN). Lect Notes Electr Eng LNEE 746:75–83. https://doi.org/10.1007/978-981-33-6926-9_7
22. Marius-Constantin P, Balas VE, Perescu-Popescu L, Mastorakis N (2009) Multilayer perceptron and neural networks. WSEAS Trans Circuits Syst 8:579–588
23. Wu J (2017) Introduction to convolutional neural networks 1–31
24. O'Shea K, Nash R (2015) An introduction to convolutional neural networks 1–11
25. Bodapati JD, Veeranjaneyulu N (2019) Feature extraction and classification using deep convolutional neural networks. J Cyber Secur Mobil 8:261–276. https://doi.org/10.13052/jcsm2245-1439.825
26. Agarap AF (2018) Deep learning using rectified linear units (ReLU) 2–8
27. Fu'adah YN, Sa'idah S, Wijayanto I, Ibrahim N, Rizal S, Magdalena R (2021) Computer aided diagnosis for early detection of glaucoma using convolutional neural network (CNN). Lect Notes Electr Eng LNEE 746:467–475. https://doi.org/10.1007/978-981-33-6926-9_40
28. Patel R, Chaware A (2020) Transfer learning with fine-tuned MobileNetV2 for diabetic retinopathy. 2020 International Conference for Emerging Technology, pp 6–9 (2020). https://doi.org/10.1109/INCET49848.2020.915401
29. Sandler M, Howard A, Zhu M, Zhmoginov A, Chen LC (2018) MobileNetV2: inverted residuals and linear bottlenecks. IEEE Conference on Computer Vision and Pattern Recognition, pp 4510–4520. https://doi.org/10.1109/CVPR.2018.00474
30. Chen H, Zeng X, Luo Y, Ye W (2019) Detection of diabetic retinopathy using deep neural network. Int Conf Digit Signal Process DSP, 2018–November. https://doi.org/10.1109/ICDSP.2018.8631882
31. Howard AG, Zhu M, Chen B, Kalenichenko D, Wang W, Weyand T, Andreetto M, Adam H (2017) MobileNets: efficient convolutional neural networks for mobile vision applications
32. Gao J, Leung C, Miao C (2019) Diabetic retinopathy classification using an efficient convolutional neural network. In: Proceedings of the 2019 IEEE International Conference on Agents, ICA 2019, pp 80–85. https://doi.org/10.1109/AGENTS.2019.8929191

Image Improvement and Dose Reduction on Computed Tomography Mastoid Using Interactive Reconstruction

Dwi Rochmayanti, Bagus Abimanyu, Ary Kurniawati, L. P. E. Santi, Betty Trimorti, Yeti Kartikasari, and Rini Indrati

Abstract Mastoid CT examination requires high detail and sharpness so that its iterative techniques can obtain optimal image quality along with the use of low exposure factors. The purpose of this study is to provide a profile of image quality and dose on various variations of ASIR by using varying tube voltages and currents as well. This research is a quantitative research study with a preexperimental approach. The phantom head was scanned with CT Mastoid protocol using varying tube currents of 100, 200, and 300 mA, and tube voltage of 80, 100, 120, and 140. Images are post-processed using iterative techniques on the CT Scan GE (ASIR) with variations of 30, 40, 50, 60, 70, and 80. The image was analyzed for anatomical clarity and the presence of artifacts/noise by a radiology specialist, especially in the area of Mastoid air cells. ROI is also carried out to get the pixel value of the image. Dosage information using CTDIvol and DAP. Results showed that the images of mastoid air cells in all mA and kVp areas had almost the same detail and sharpness. However, the highest assessment was the use of ASIR 50. At the use of 100 and 200 mA, noise and artifacts were still found, although not noticeable. The CTDI and DAP assessments showed linearity in the use of tube voltage and current, where the lowest doses were at 100 mA and 80 KVp with CTDI vol 9.53 mGy and DAP 225.54 mGy-cm, as well as the highest pixel values at 100 mA and 80 kVp at 463. For detailed and good images at lower doses, a combination exposure with tube voltage 100kVp and tube current 80 mA and setting ASIR 50 can be recommended. One can imply that the optimization of ASIR can be used to get a good image with the use of low exposure techniques.

D. Rochmayanti (✉) · L. P. E. Santi · B. Trimorti · Y. Kartikasari · R. Indrati
Department of Radiodiagnostic and Radiotherapy Engineering, Health Polytechnic, Ministry of Health, Semarang, Central Java, Indonesia
e-mail: dwirochmayanti@poltekkes-smg.ac.id

B. Abimanyu
Department Radiology of Regional General Hospital KRMT Wongsonegoro, Semarang, Indonesia

A. Kurniawati
Department Radiology of Regional General Hospital Sleman, Yogyakarta, Indonesia

T. Triwiyanto et al. (eds.), *Proceeding of the 3rd International Conference on Electronics, Biomedical Engineering, and Health Informatics*, Lecture Notes in Electrical Engineering 1008, https://doi.org/10.1007/978-981-99-0248-4_8

Keywords Image quality · Dose · ASIR · Tube voltage · Tube current · CT mastoid

1 Introduction

Over the last few decades, technological advances have markedly increased and expanded the computational reach in the clinical applications of tomography (CT). Computed Tomography has been chosen by many physicians as a modality in patient care innovation. The use of CT scanning has been widely documented, but along with this, increasing the radiation dose to the patient is also a concern. In response to this, the radiology community while carrying out the CT Scan examination procedure has used the ALARA (as low as reasonably achievable) principle [1]. This principle takes into account the principles of justification, optimization, and dose limitation. One of the optimization principles includes the selection of tools, techniques, tool operations, processing, and reading of radiographic images [2]. Taking clinical aspects into account, dose management is further developed by the latest CT Scan technology. Every imaging series, from tubes to detectors, has been developed with innovative imaging technology integrated with dose management and dose reporting systems. The algorithm makes it possible to manage doses while improving and maintaining image quality [1]. Basically, all MSCT has used a standard reconstruction, namely Filtered Back Projection (FBP). Although the overall performance is acceptable, the image reconstructed with FBP still produces high image noise, streak artifacts, and low contrast detectability in certain clinics [3]. As is the case in the acquisition examination of obese patients, situations that may occur with the use of low doses or limited tube strength will cause noise to appear in the image. Over time, the improvement of FBP continues to be improved to overcome these limitations, with advances in computing that makes it possible to explore with iterative reconstruction (IR) [1].

Iterative Reconstruction (IR) is present as a solution to overcome these biased artifacts and images. Actually, this IR has been developed for a long time but because of several shortcomings such as the difficulty of obtaining the accuracy of the number of rays due to quantum noise, patient movement, and long computation time. However, the present iterative reconstruction has been reused by using an adaptive linear filter to overcome the quantum mottle noise in the raw data. However, there are still drawbacks to this method, namely the decrease in spatial resolution and cannot reduce image noise [4].

Reconstruction algorithms in this case are mathematical equations that are convoluted to the measurement data in the form of software for each vendor. Reconstruction of this algorithm is very diverse and is always modified for better results. This is what makes the image results vary in several vendors [5]. Conventional FBP is based on the simple mathematical assumptions of the tomographic imaging system. The IR generates a series of projections that are synthesized by accurately modeling the data collection process in CT by incorporating statistical system information. The mathematically synthesized images are compared and corrected with actual measurements to adjust the object image estimation. This technique is then repeated until it is close to the actual size. This data processing can improve image quality, especially in noise and resolution, but the reconstruction process takes longer than FBP [6]. The existence of more computing capabilities on the workstation provides opportunities for the development of IR [7]. With better results, ASIR only requires a 30–50% process improvement from FBP [8].

All major CT Scan vendors now market some form of repetitive reconstruction. However, it has varying specifications. Among them is General Electrics (GE) which has introduced Adaptive Statistical Iterative Reconstruction (ASIR), which uses a mixture of FBP images filtered with repeated reconstructed images to reduce noise [9]. ASIR was developed as a corrective image processing application to improve image quality caused by noise. Noise will increase if the radiation dose is lowered. Low-dose CT scans combined with ASIR can reduce noise when compared to routine imaging (with FBP) [10]. Several studies related to the use of ASIR have been carried out for several examination objects such as applications to CT scans of the abdomen [11, 12], spine [13], head CT [14] and also implemented for pediatric examinations [15] the main focus is related to image quality and radiation dose [16, 17]. However, the existing research has not combined variations in the use of tubes and tube currents with variations in ASIR. There is also no research related to the use of ASIR in studies with mastoid examination.

Fulfilling the diagnostic value in imaging is very important. How an organ or object that has a small structure that requires good image detail must be able to be shown optimally. If the image is in a noisy condition, then the detail of the image that should be able to be shown will be reduced in quality. Included among the need for high-detail images is the examination of cases of mastoiditis.

Mastoiditis is the most common intratemporal complication of otitis media. This is confirmed in Lin YS's study, the most common complication of chronic suppurative otitis media is mastoiditis (14–74%). The diagnosis of otitis media is based on the results of clinical examinations (history and otologic examination) as well as to determine the presence or absence of complications through radiological examinations (plain photos, CT Scan, and MRI of the mastoid). The best imaging to assess the chronic disease of the middle ear and temporal bone (mastoid) including cholesteatoma is a CT scan because it can show bone destruction [18].

Because there are no similar studies related to the use of ASIR combined with variations in tube voltage and tube current in examinations that require high image detail such as mastoid CT examination, the researchers get this topic as a study. This study can provide a profile of image quality and dose with various variations of ASIR, tube voltage, and tube flow, and also a CT Scan examination protocol with mastoid with which this protocol is expected to reduce the dose received by the patient and also the resulting image still has good quality.

2 Data and Method

This research is a quantitative research study with a preexperimental approach. The phantom head was scanned with the CT Mastoid protocol using variations in tube currents of 100, 200, and 300 mA, at different tube voltages for each mA value. Variations in tube voltages are 80, 100, 120, and 140 kVp. Then the results of each image are post processed using iterative techniques on the CT Scan GE (ASIR) machine with variations of 30, 40, 50, 60, 70, and 80. The number of images assessed by respondents as many as 72 images. The results of the next image will be analyzed for anatomical clarity and the presence of artifacts/noise by a radiology specialist, especially in the area of Mastoid air cells. The concept framework of this research is shown in Fig. 1. On the resulting image, ROI is also carried out to get the pixel value of the image. Dosage information can be obtained by using CTDIvol and DAP (Dose Area Product). The data is then processed and analyzed descriptively to provide a profile of image quality and dose with various variations of ASIR, tube voltage, and tube current that produced good image quality and dose reduction. The parameters used for the head CT protocol are shown in Table 1.

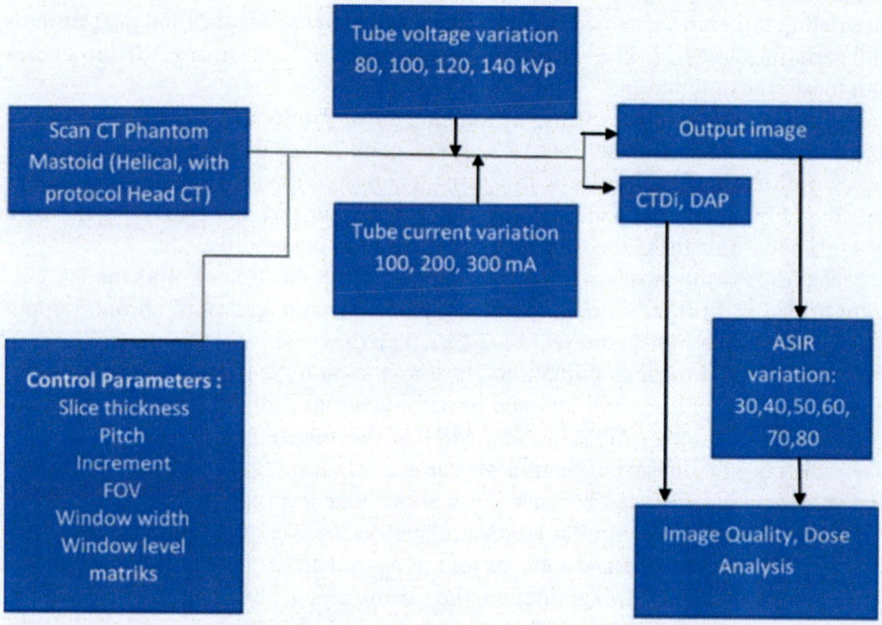

Fig. 1 Research concept framework

Table 1 Scan parameters for CT Mastoid examination (with the use of head CT protocol)

Parameters	Description
Tube voltage	80, 100, 120, and 140
Tube current	100, 200, and 300
Exposure time	12.51 s
Slice thickness	5 mm
Field of view (FOV)	25 cm
Image size	512 × 512
Window width	100
Window level	400
Scan technique	Helical
ASIR	30, 40, 50, 60, 70, and 80

3 Results

To assess image quality, two treatments were carried out. For the assessment of anatomical information, an assessment was carried out by 3 respondents (radiology specialists) which included the clarity of the Mastoid ais cells area and the external auditory canal as well as an assessment of the emergence of noise. Meanwhile, for measurements, use ROI in the mastoid air cell area with an ROI diameter of 0.5 cm, to get the pixel value which is a representation of the CT number. Windowing is adjusted to obtain information regarding the mastoid area with a window width of 2000 HU and a window level of 400 HU. Image results with variations in tube voltage and tube current, one of which is by using ASIR variations on tube voltage and tube current 300 mA, can be seen in Fig. 2.

From Fig. 2, subjectively, they look almost the same and don't look different, so it's bit difficult to distinguish clearly, therefore, apart from the respondents' assessments, pixel value measurements are also carried out with the image processing tool, to get a more objective image quality.

3.1 Image Information Quality Profile (Anatomy Assessment, Noise, and Pixel Value)

Profile of anatomical information of mastoid air cells with variations of tube current, tube voltage, and ASIR are shown in Fig. 3.

In Fig. 3a, the profile of the anatomical clarity assessment, especially on mastoid air cells where in the tube voltage range 80, 100 and 120 using ASIR variations of 30, 40, 60, 70 and 80 have the same clarity of mastoid air cells. At a tube voltage of 140 kVp, all variations of ASIR showed a maximum assessment where the mastoid air cell was the clearest and clearly demarcated. The interesting thing is that in ASIR 50, all variations of tube voltage show the maximum assessment, it can be

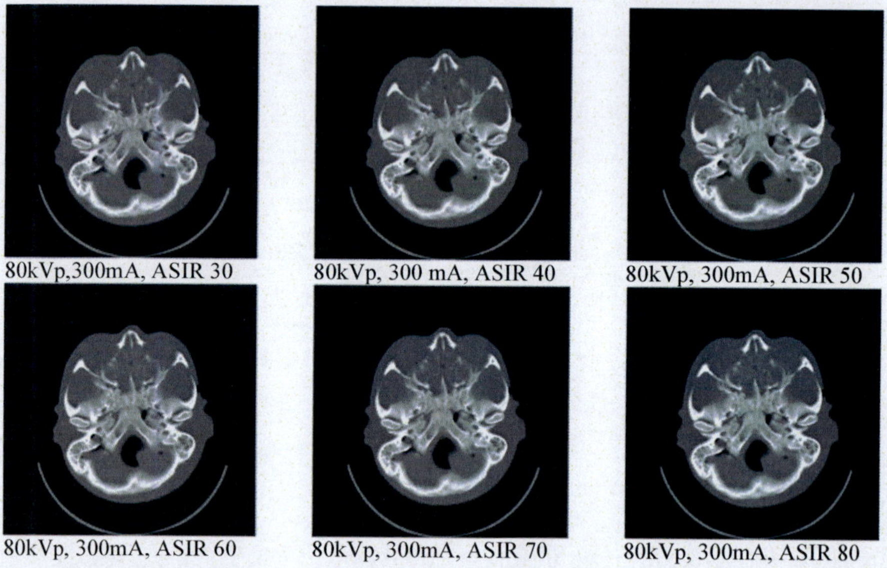

Fig. 2 Image with variations in tube voltage (80, 100, 120, and 140 kVp) and ASIR (30, 40, 50, 60, 70, and 80) with a fixed tube current (300 mA)

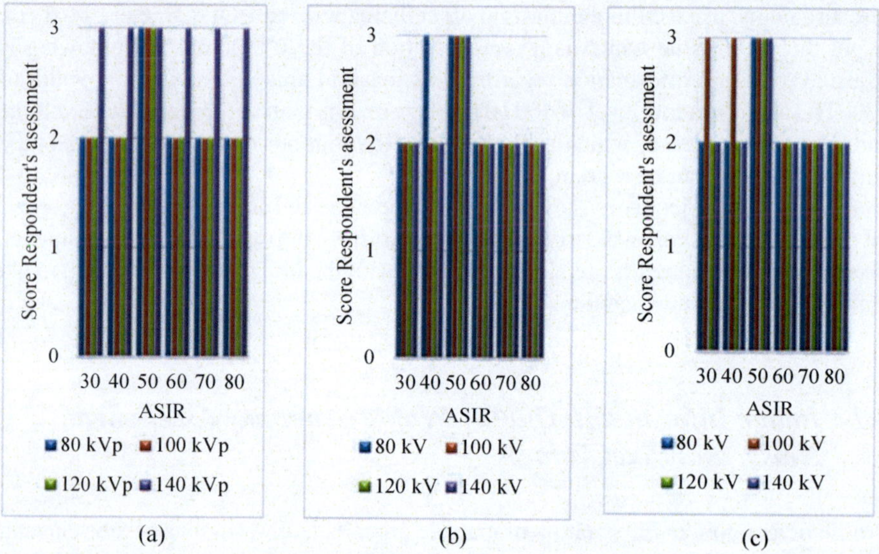

Fig. 3 Anatomical information of mastoid air cells with variations of tube current, tube voltage, and ASIR **a** 100 mA, **b** 300 mA, and **c** 300 mA

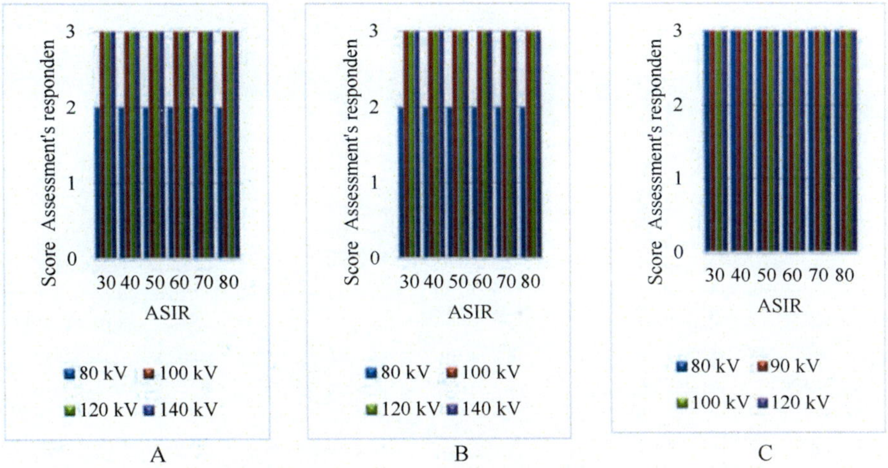

Fig. 4 Respondents' assessment presence of noise at various tube current with variations in tube voltage and ASIR. **a** 100 mA, **b** 200 mA, and **c** 300 mA

assumed that at ASIR 50 all voltages have the same anatomical quality. In Fig. 4b, the assessment looks more uniform in almost all tube current conditions of 200 mA with a tube voltage factor in almost all ASIR variations. A higher rating is shown at 80 kVp voltage on ASIR 40, and the highest rating is also ASIR 50 in all tube voltage variations. In Fig. 4c, it can be seen that at ASIR 60,70, and 80 in all tube voltages, there is a uniform assessment, meaning that there is no difference in that range. The various assessments for tube voltages of 100 on the use of ASIR 30 and 40 have the same assessment score, whereas the ASIR 30 and 40 have the same and no different ratings. The highest assessment score is also shown at ASIR 50, which has the highest assessment score, which means at a tube current of 300, at all tube voltages used, using ASIR 50, it will produce the clearest and most clearly defined mastoid air cell image.

In Fig. 4, it can be seen that based on the respondent's assessment, the use of tube voltages of 100, 120, and 140 kVp has the highest score for image quality, which means that noise is not found that interferes with the image in almost all ASIR variations. At a tube voltage of 80, in all ASIR noise is still visible even though it is not clearly visible and does not really interfere with the existing image. Meanwhile, the use of a 200 mA tube current has the same profile as the use of a 100 mA tube current. Different results are shown in the use of a tube current of 300 mA, a uniform assessment is found that there is no visible noise in all variations of the voltage and ASIR used.

In the image, ROI is given to the mastoid area with a diameter of ±0.5 cm to get the pixel value. This pixel value is a representation of the CT number. CT number is the value of the X-ray attenuation coefficient which is determined by the average energy of the X-rays and the atomic number of the absorber, this is expressed by the attenuation coefficient. In Fig. 5, it can be seen that at a tube current of 100 mA, the

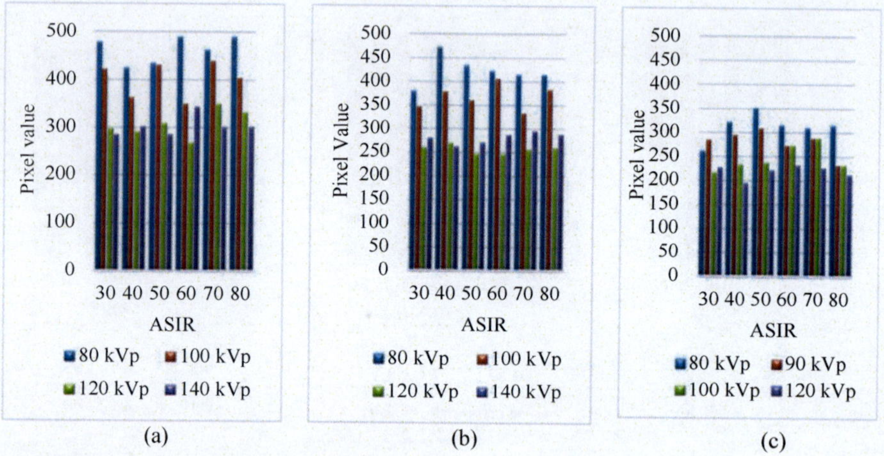

Fig. 5 Pixel value at various tube currents with variations in tube voltage and ASIR; **a** 100 mA, **b** 200 mA, and **c** 300 mA

higher the voltage factor used, the lower the pixel value. Almost all ASIR variations show a similar pattern at 120 kVp tube voltage there is the lowest pixel value at any ASIR value, while the highest pixel value at all ASIR values is at 80 kVp tube voltage. The assessment of the pixel value at a tube current of 300 mA has a smaller average value when compared to 100 and 200 mA.

3.2 *Dosage Profile on CT Mastoid*

In this study, measurements of radiation dose and image noise were carried out. For the measurement of radiation dose obtained from the value of CTDIvol and Dose length product (DLP) listed on the CT Scan computer monitor.

Figures 6 and 7 show that an increase in tube voltage and tube current will contribute to an increase in the value of CTDIvol and DAP so that it can be ascertained that the larger the tube current and the tube voltage used will give a large dose. From the data Fig. 6, it can be calculated the increase in CTDIvol value for every 20 increase in tube voltage at values of 100, 200 and 300 mA. The biggest percentage is when the tube voltage is changed from 80 to 100 k Vp, where there is an increase in CTDI vol and DAP values by 84% at 300 mA while at 100 and 200 mA values, there is an increase of 83%.

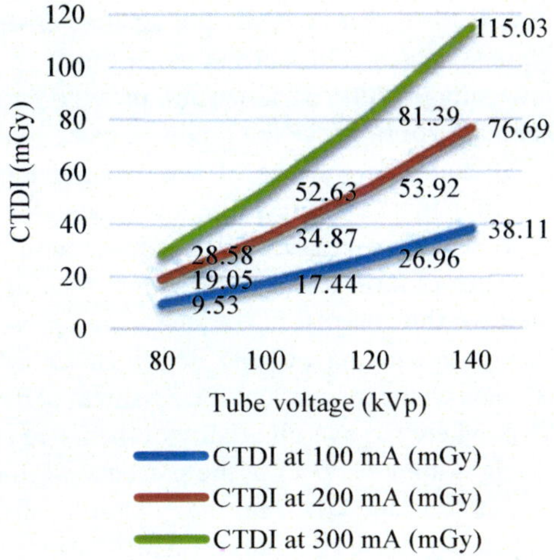

Fig. 6 Increasing trend CTDI vol (mGy) at different tube current and tube voltage

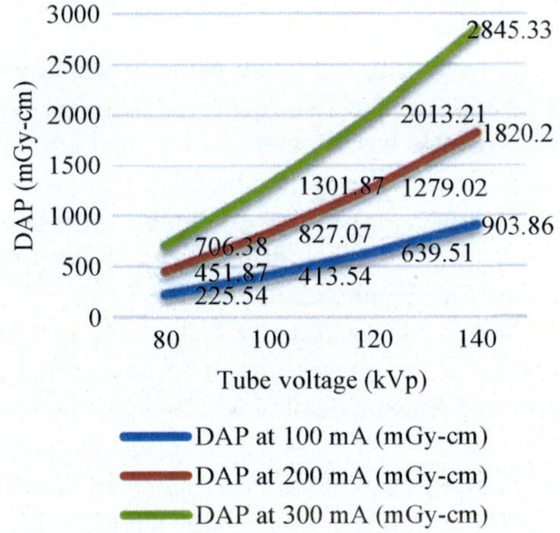

Fig. 7 Trend of increasing DAP (mGy-cm) at different tube current and tube voltage

4 Discussion

In the CT examination of the mastoid, efforts are needed to obtain good bone details, this must also be balanced with the acceptance of doses in patients that can be minimized, this is in accordance with Darmini et al. [19], which states that the application of CT scans for medical purposes must have good quality and relatively low dose, whereas CT scanning of the mastoid is usually preferred with high spatial resolution. CT Scan is an unquestionable modality to be able to provide high detail images of the temporal bone [20], including the mastoid.

The results showed that the assessment of the clarity of the mastoid air cell implemented using ASIR, at all tube voltage settings, gave almost the same assessment.

This is also seen in ASIR 50, all images on all variations of tube voltage have the highest scores. This means that even if the scanning technique is carried out at a low voltage (80kVp), it can still provide good anatomical clarity. So using ASIR has been able to improve the quality aspect even though using a low tube voltage.

Technically, the use of low technical factors (tube voltage and tube current), which in this case will cause low doses will also have an impact on noise generation [21], which of course will interfere with mastoid image needs that require high detail/resolution images. Although, technically, the use of a low tube voltage will increase the contrast of the image, the presence of noise with the use of a low tube voltage is also unavoidable. This is in accordance with the results of the study, which is based on the respondent's assessment of the presence of noise at a tube voltage of 80 kVp, where the overall quality of the noise can still be seen a little. In the use of tube voltages above 100 kVp, the presence of noise is almost invisible. The use of ASIR is able to reduce the presence of noise in the use of the low dose technique [22]. Regarding noise reduction, there is also a significant decrease, one study showed a noise reduction of up to 60% with the use of ASIR compared to FBP [23]. So this iterative technique is very useful for reducing noise due to the use of low dose techniques.

In measuring the pixel value, it was found that the largest pixel value was at 80 kVp tube voltage. This occurred in all variations of tube current. The use of 100 kVp tube voltage has a lower pixel value than 80 kVp, this is also supported by research [24]. The tube current value of 100 mA has a higher pixel value when compared to others. Each pixel of the CT image, represents a linear attenuation value of the x-rays interacting with each different tissue density, this attenuation value is called the CT number, or Hounsfield unit (HU) [25].

MSCT equipped with CT Dose Index (CTDI) measurement software, the CTDIw value and the Dose Length Product (DLP) value which can be observed on the operator console display which is obtained by mathematical calculations, which are automatically in the section computer data acquisition [26]. CTDI is a method of calculating the patient's average dose in one scan. The use of technical factors such as tube current and tube voltage has a significant role in contributing to the dose given to the patient. the largest dose at 300 mA and 140 kV was 115.03 mGy for CTDI vol, and DAP was 2845.33 mGy-cm. The lowest dose is shown at 80 kVp tube voltage and 100 mA tube arug usage. The results of the assessment show that in all variations of tube current, with increasing tube voltage, the dose increases. This shows the largest increase is from 80 to 100 kVp where there is an increase of 83–84%. In one study, it was stated that although the tube voltage did not linearly affect the dose, at 100 kVp, the X-ray output was 1.5 times greater than 80 kVp. In other words, reducing the tube voltage from 100 to 80 kVp will cause a dose reduction of 1.5 times. An increase in tube current will also lead to a linear increase in dose [22]. One study also mentioned a dose reduction in the range of 23–76% compared to FBP [27].

Decreasing dose does not necessary have to sacrifice image quality. Parameter optimization needs to be done to get optimal image quality with the lowest possible dose. In principle, the radiation dose depends on the tube current, slice scan time, and tube voltage. And during a CT scan, the patient gets radiation from all directions, causing the dose to be received largely [28]. Several studies have stated that reducing the tube voltage can significantly reduce the dose, but consequently lower the image quality factor. Because of this, several manufacturers, especially CT Scan modalities, have implemented automation of tube voltage selection in their equipment [29], clinical needs, and patient characteristics [22]. In recent decades, dose reduction can also be achieved with the use of mA modulation. Using the right mA modulation and ASIR is effective in reducing the dose and maintaining image quality [30]. using ASIR which is an iterative hybrid reconstruction technique can be used as a technique to reduce the dose compared to FBP [15].

Based on this discussion, the use of a tube current of 100 mA and a tube voltage of 80 kVp has an image quality in this case is the same good image resolution, with the highest pixel value. Although the use of low doses will produce noise, but the noise in the exposure factor is not too disturbing the image and can be minimized by using ASIR. ASIR with the highest quality is obtained at 50. The higher ASIR used, the resulting image looks less clear and sharp, of course, this will result in a reduction in the existing diagnostic value. This is also supported by setting the exposure factor (at 100 mA and 80 kVp), the lowest dose received (9.53 mGy) and decreasing the exposure to 80 kVp will reduce the dose received by the patient by almost 85%. This is supported by Prakash's study which stated that using ASIR there was a 25.1% reduction in CTDi compared to using the FBP technique on the use of ASIR 40% [12], The use of ASIR 40 is also recommended in abdominal examination with the most optimal image results [11].

Our research has weaknesses, where the assessment is still limited to the anatomy of the phantom study, in the future, it needs to be applied to pathology to see the suitability of the need for diagnostic identification according to medical needs. The object that is assessed also only focuses on mastoid air cells, further studies are needed regarding other anatomical assessments on CT mastoid. The iterative technique used is also still using statistical iterative techniques, there are still developments in other interactive techniques such as models based-IR [31]. The results of this study will provide experience in parameter optimization, especially in the CT scan of the mastoid to obtain optimum image details by using the right exposure technique so that the dose given to the patient can also be suppressed.

5 Conclusion

From the results of research on the topic of Image Improvement and Dose Reduction with Adaptive Statistical Interactive Reconstruction on the Mastoid, it can be concluded that on the CT Scan of the Mastoid using the CT head protocol using phantom, ASIR can be used to produce images with good quality, especially those that can display images with good detail across all mA variations. As for the mA values of 100 and 200, it is still found a little noise in the image at the use of 80 kVp tube voltage. The use of 80, 100, 120, and 140 tube voltages can also produce mastoid images with the same quality, but noise is still found at 80 kVp tube voltages with 100 and 200 mA, while the use of 300 tube currents shows the same results for all voltage variations and ASIR. The highest pixel value was obtained using a tube voltage of 80 kVp for all ASIR variations, where the highest was at 100 mA with an average pixel of 463. The best ASIR option for mastoid images to obtain detailed imagery was 50. The lowest dose value received by the object was on the use of 100 mA tube current and 80 kVp tube voltage CTDIvol 9.53 mGy and DAP 225.54 mGy-cm. To obtain an optimal mastoid image with a minimum dose, it is recommended to use a tube current of 100 mA and a tube voltage of 80 kVp with an ASIR 50. The future for the implementation of ASIR variations for clinical needs can use pathology in patients with post-traumatic conditions and reconstruction with more varied ASIR.

References

1. Mehta D, Thompson R, Morton T, Dhanantwari E, Shefer E (2013) Iterative model reconstruction simultaneously lowered computed tomography radiation dose and improved image quality
2. Woroprobosari NR (2016) Efek Stokastik Radiasi Sinar X Dental Pada Ibu Hamil dan Janin. ODONTO Dent J 3
3. Geyer LL, Schoepf UJ, Meinel FG, Nance JW, Bastarrika G, Leipsic JA, Paul NS, Rengo M, Laghi A, de Cecco CN (2015) State of the art: iterative CT reconstruction techniques. https://doi.org/10.1148/radiol.2015132766
4. Paper S, Ardley N, Buchan K, Lau K (2013) Efficacy of a liver detection algorithm for noise reduction in abdominal CT. 1–11
5. Bushberg JT, Seibert JA, Leidholdt EM, Boone JM (2003) The essential physics for medical imaging
6. Katsura M, Matsuda I, Akahane M, Sato J, Akai H, Yasaka K, Kunimatsu A, Ohtomo K (2012) Model-based iterative reconstruction technique for radiation dose reduction in chest CT: comparison with the adaptive statistical iterative reconstruction technique. Eur Radiol 22:1613–1623. https://doi.org/10.1007/s00330-012-2452-z
7. Beister M, Kolditz D, Kalender WA (2012) Iterative reconstruction methods in X-ray CT. Physica Med 28:94–108. https://doi.org/10.1016/J.EJMP.2012.01.003
8. Deák Z, Grimm JM, Treitl M, Geyer LL, Linsenmaier U, Körner M, Reiser MF, Wirth S (2013) Filtered back projection, adaptive statistical iterative reconstruction, and a model-based iterative reconstruction in abdominal CT: an experimental clinical study. Radiology 266:197–206. https://doi.org/10.1148/radiol.12112707
9. Leiner T, Velthuis B, Gietema H, de Jong PA, de Vries L, Hendrikse J (2011) Iterative reconstruction for reducing radiation dose at CT: review of technique and initial experience. https://doi.org/10.1594/ecr2011/C-2205
10. Hara AK, Paden RG, Silva AC, Kujak JL, Lawder HJ, Pavlicek W (2009) Iterative reconstruction technique for reducing body radiation dose at CT: feasibility study. AJR 193:764–771. https://doi.org/10.2214/AJR.09.2397
11. W LP, Indrati R, Biyono A (2020) Adaptive statistical iterative reconstruction for optimization image quality of Ct scan abdomen. Jurnal Riset Kesehatan 9:61–64. https://doi.org/10.31983/jrk.v9i1.5716
12. Prakash P, Kalra MK, Kambadakone AK, Pien H, Hsieh J, Blake MA, Sahani Dv (2010) Reducing abdominal CT radiation dose with adaptive statistical iterative reconstruction technique. Invest Radiol 45

13. Tsuda M, Yunaga H, Murakami A, Yata S (2021) Adaptive statistical iterative reconstruction for computed tomography of the spine. Radiography 27:768–772. https://doi.org/10.1016/j.radi.2020.12.002
14. Østerås BH, Heggen KL, Pedersen HK, Andersen HK, Martinsen ACT (2016) Can use of adaptive statistical iterative reconstruction reduce radiation dose in unenhanced head CT? An analysis of qualitative and quantitative image quality. Acta Radiol Open 5:205846011664583. https://doi.org/10.1177/2058460116645831
15. Westra SJ, Pavlicek W (2012) Radiation dose reduction with hybrid iterative reconstruction for pediatric CT related papers how I do it: managing radiat ion dose in CT. Radiol Soc N Am 263:537–546. https://doi.org/10.1148/radiol.12110268/-/DC1
16. Leng S, Dehn FE, Lane Jl, Keller KK, Witte RJ, Carter RE, McCollough CH (2015) Temporal bone CT: improved image quality and potential for decrease radiation dose using an ultra high resolution scan mode with an iterative reconstruction algorithm. Am J Neuroradiol 36:1599–1603. https://doi.org/10.3174/ajnr.A4338
17. Maxfield MW, Schuster KM, McGillicuddy EA, Young CJ, Ghita M, Jamal Bokhari S, Oliva IB, Brink JA, Davis KA (2012) Impact of adaptive statistical iterative reconstruction on radiation dose in evaluation of trauma patients. J Trauma Acute Care Surg 76. https://doi.org/10.1097/TA.0b013e318270d2fb
18. Oelan Sari R, Murtala B, Ilyas M, Liyadi F, Savitri E, Patellongi I, Ilmu Radiologi Fakultas Kedokteran B, Hasanuddin Makassar U (2013) Nilai Prediktif Radiografi Mastoid Dalam Mendeteksi Mastoiditis Pada Pasien Otitis Media Supuratif Kronik
19. Darmini, Ari Setiyono P, Rochmayanti D, Nino Kurniawan A, Nugroho Setiawan A (2020) The optimization of mastoid CT image using windows and kernel reconstructions. J Phys Conf Ser. Institute of Physics Publishing. https://doi.org/10.1088/1742-6596/1471/1/012015
20. Chatterjee P, Khanna S, Talukdar R (2015) Role of high resolution computed tomography of mastoids in planning surgery for chronic suppurative otitis media. Indian J Otolaryngol Head Neck Surg 67:275–280. https://doi.org/10.1007/s12070-015-0873-0
21. Silva AC, Lawder HJ, Hara A, Kujak J, Pavlicek W (2010) Innovations in CT dose reduction strategy: application of the adaptive statistical iterative reconstruction algorithm. AJR 194:191–199. https://doi.org/10.2214/AJR.09.2953
22. Lira D, Padole A, Kalra MK, Singh S (2015) Tube potential and CT radiation dose optimization. https://doi.org/10.2214/AJR.14.13281
23. Barca P, Marfisi D, Marzi C, Cozza S, Diciotti S, Traino AC, Giannelli M (2021) A voxel-based assessment of noise properties in computed tomography imaging with the asir-v and asir iterative reconstruction algorithms. Appl Sci (Switz) 11. https://doi.org/10.3390/app11146561
24. Chindasombatjaroen J, Kakimoto N, Shimamoto H, Murakami S, Furukawa S (2011) Correlation between pixel values in a cone-beam computed tomographic scanner and the computed tomographic values in a multidetector row computed tomographic scanner. J Comput Assist Tomogr 35:662–665. https://doi.org/10.1097/RCT.0b013e31822d9725
25. Afifi MB, Abdelrazek A, Deiab NA, Abd El-Hafez AI, El-Farrash AH (2020) The effects of CT X-ray tube voltage and current variations on the relative electron density (RED) and CT number conversion curves. J Radiat Res Appl Sci 13:1–11. https://doi.org/10.1080/16878507.2019.1693176
26. Kartikasari Y, Darmini, Masrochah S, Rochmayanti D (2021) Comparison of radiation dose and image noise in head computed tomography with sequence and spiral techniques. In: Lecture notes in electrical engineering. Springer Science and Business Media Deutschland GmbH, pp 557–566. https://doi.org/10.1007/978-981-33-6926-9_49
27. Willemink MJ, de Jong PA, Leiner T, de Heer LM, Nievelstein RAJ, Budde RPJ, Schilham AMR (2013) Iterative reconstruction techniques for computed tomography Part 1: technical principles. Eur Radiol 23:1623–1631. https://doi.org/10.1007/s00330-012-2765-y
28. Goldman LW (2007) Principles of CT: radiation dose and image quality. J Nucl Med Technol 35:213–225. https://doi.org/10.2967/jnmt.106.037846
29. Krazinski AW, Meinel FG, Joseph Schoepf U, Silverman JR, Canstein C, De Cecco CN, Geyer LL (2014) Reduced radiation dose and improved image quality at cardiovascular CT

angiography by automated attenuation-based tube voltage. Eur Soc Radiol 24:2677–2684. https://doi.org/10.1007/s00330-014-3312-9
30. Zhao Y, Xu Y, Bao Y, Geng X, Zhang T, Li D (2019) Comparative analysis of radiation dose and image quality between organ dose modulation and 3D smart mA modulation during head-neck CT angiography. Pub Med 27:97–100. https://doi.org/10.3233/XST-180443
31. Liu L (2014) Model-based iterative reconstruction—a promising algorithm for today's computed tomography imaging. J Med Imag Radiat Sci 45:131–136. https://doi.org/10.1016/j.jmir.2014.02.002

Classification of Pneumonia Based on X-Ray Images with ResNet-50 Architecture

Shafa Alifia Rachman, Dhimas Chandra Bagaskara, Rita Magdalena, and Sofia Sa'idah

Abstract Pneumonia is a disease that infects the lungs, it can be caused by a bacterial, viral, or fungal infection. A person can be known to have pneumonia or not by having a chest x-ray examination, meanwhile, it is difficult to identify the cause of pneumonia by just looking at the x-ray image results. This research was conducted to obtain a system that can classify the causes of pneumonia. This research can be used as a reference for development in further research. The classification system designed in this research was by using Convolutional Neural Network (CNN) method with ResNet-50 architecture. By using the proposed method, an analysis was carried out to obtain the best parameters for the system. CNN can imitate the image recognition system in the human visual cortex. By implementing a skip connection system, ResNet-50 is used to overcome the problem of declining system performance due to a high-depth architecture. The dataset used are secondary dataset x-ray images of the lungs, consisting of three classes, namely: bacterial pneumonia, viral pneumonia, and normal. This research produces the best accuracy of 88.88% and a loss of 0.4597. The precision, recall, and F1-Score parameters get a value of 83.34, 83.33, and 83.16%. The result shows that the pneumonia classification system designed using the CNN architecture ResNet-50 method is able to classify x-ray images of the lungs according to their respective classes. The classification system of pneumonia can be used to automate the identification of the cause of a pneumonia.

Keywords Pneumonia · Convolutional Neural Network · ResNet-50

1 Introduction

The lungs are important organs in human respiration. One of the diseases that attack the lungs is pneumonia. In the lungs of people with pneumonia, small pockets in the lungs, usually called alveoli, fill with pus and fluid. This will cause the patient's lungs to be limited in oxygen intake and have breathing difficulty [1]. The most common

S. A. Rachman · D. C. Bagaskara (✉) · R. Magdalena · S. Sa'idah
School of Electrical Engineering, Telkom University, Bandung, Indonesia
e-mail: dimascandrabagaskara@gmail.com

T. Triwiyanto et al. (eds.), *Proceeding of the 3rd International Conference on Electronics, Biomedical Engineering, and Health Informatics*, Lecture Notes in Electrical Engineering 1008, https://doi.org/10.1007/978-981-99-0248-4_9

causes of pneumonia are viral and bacterial infections. Pneumonia caused by a virus, called viral pneumonia, has more symptoms than bacterial pneumonia. However, when viewed clinically, the difference between viral pneumonia and bacterial pneumonia is difficult to find. Identification of x-ray images of the lungs just by looking at the x-ray images may cause misidentification because the eyes have a high level of subjectivity. With increasingly rapid technological advances, the identification of pneumonia can be done through x-ray image analysis. The use of Convolutional Neural Network (CNN) and Compressed Sensing (CS) on x-ray pictures of normal lungs and lung images of pneumonia patients showed a 97.34% accuracy rate [2]. The use of x-ray images with the Support Vector Machine (SVM) for image classification and the Linear Discriminate Analysis (LDA) method for feature extraction results in an accuracy of 92.775% [3]. Using a Computer Aided Diagnosis (CAD) system that is then segmented and extracted using Fully Convolutional Networks (FCN) and then the Deep Convolutional Neural Network (DCNN) model to classify viral or bacterial pneumonia based on x-ray images, researchers were able to achieve an accuracy of (0.80480.0202) [4]. Another study regarding the detection of pneumonia by utilizing the DCNN method and the use of augmentation strategies to improve model performance got an accuracy value of 83.38% [5]. Judging from these studies, the use of machine learning methods can be used to help classify pneumonia. However, the system that can classify the causes of pneumonia disease due to bacterial and viral is still lacking because there are similarities in the x-ray images of the two causes of pneumonia. In this proposed method, researchers used the CNN method and the ResNet-50 architecture to classify pneumonia. The CNN method was chosen because this method is known to have the most significant results in image recognition and can imitate the image recognition system in the human visual cortex so that it can process image information properly [6]. In addition, the CNN method was chosen because this method can train a large number of data so it corresponds to the data used in this research. The ResNet-50 architecture was chosen because the x-ray images of the lungs used in this research has a high level of similarity, so residual network was chosen because it can overcome complex image recognition problems by increasing the number of layers in deep learning without causing a decrease in system performance.

2 Basic Theory

2.1 The Lungs

In the human respiratory system, the lungs are vital organs. The right lung has three lobes, while the left lung has two lobes. The left lung has superior and inferior lobes. The right lung has three lobes: superior, medial, and inferior [7]. The exchange of oxygen and carbon dioxide in the blood is an important function of the lungs. The alveoli are where oxygen and carbon dioxide are exchanged. The carbon dioxide created by the body's cells will be carried through the bloodstream. When air is delivered, oxygen and carbon dioxide are exchanged in the alveoli [8].

2.2 Pneumonia

Pneumonia is a disease of the lungs in the form of parenchymal inflammation. Infection is caused by microorganisms such as bacteria, fungi, protozoa, and viruses, which produce inflammation [9]. Alveoli in normal lungs will be filled with air. However, in the lungs of people with pneumonia, the alveoli are filled with pus and fluid. Symptoms that commonly appear in patients with pneumonia are cough, sputum which has the medical term purulent sputum, fever, pleuritic pain, and shortness of breath [10]. There are two classifications of pneumonia based on the cause, namely bacterial pneumonia and viral pneumonia [11]. Bacterial pneumonia is caused by bacteria such as *Staphylococcus*, while viral pneumonia is caused by viruses such as RSV [12].

2.3 Digital Image Processing

Image can be interpreted as a two-dimensional function f(x, y) where x and y are coordinate pairs of a plane [13]. While the amplitude f is the gray intensity of an image at coordinates (x, y). Digital image processing is now widely used in imaging systems such as gamma rays, x-ray, ultraviolet, and so on. An x-ray is an electromagnetic wave with a wavelength ranging from 0.01 to 10 nm [14]. By focusing high-energy electrons onto tungsten, an x-ray can be produced. If the electrons have enough energy, the electrons in the tungsten atom's inner shell can be disabled. As a result, higher-energy electrons will replace the previously disabled electrons, allowing X-rays to be emitted [15].

2.4 Convolutional Neural Network

Convolutional Neural Network (CNN) is a deep learning method with linear operations in the form of convolution [16]. In general, the application of CNN has four stages of work. The first is to perform a convolution operation between the input image and the kernel. In the second process, the input of the convolution operation is changed using an activation function. Next, the third process is to do input pooling to minimize the feature map's dimension. In the fourth process, a classification operation is performed on the fully connected layer [17]. CNN architecture is divided into two parts: feature extraction layers and classification layers [18]. Figure 1 shows an overview of the CNN architecture.

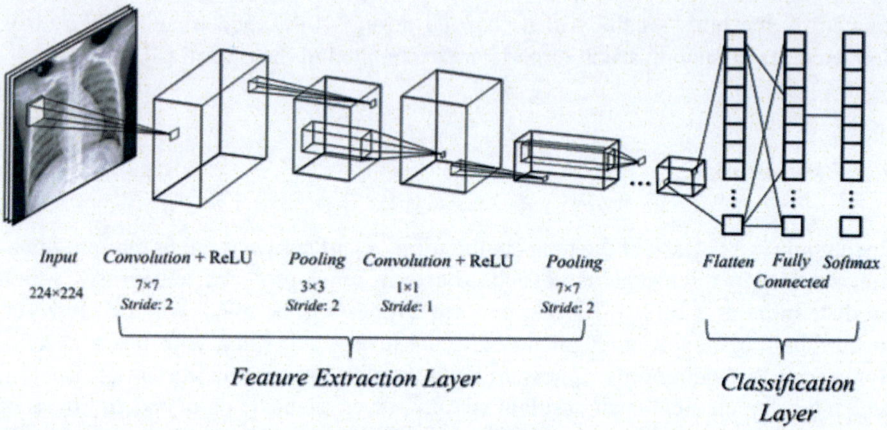

Fig. 1 Convolutional Neural Network (CNN) architecture [30]

Based on Fig. 1, the system is given input with x-ray images of the lungs. The input will be resized to 224 × 224 pixels and conducted with a convolution operation using kernel 7 × 7 and stride 2. The feature map from the convolution operation will pass the ReLU activation function. Furthermore, the pooling operation will be carried out on the feature map using kernel 3 × 3 and stride 2. The convolution operation will continue according to the number of layers used. When the feature extraction was completed, the system can recognize the characteristics of each image. Based on the output from feature extraction, image classification can be done on the classification layer.

Convolutional Layer. The main CNN processes take place in the convolutional layer [19]. In this layer, a convolution operation is performed to extract the input image features by using a kernel. The convolution operation is performed by multiplying the matrix between the input and kernel which produces an output in the form of a feature map, as shown in Fig. 2 [20]. There are several parameters in the convolutional layer, namely the kernel, stride, and padding. The kernel can be interpreted as a parameter in the form of a grid with weights that will be used to detect the input image pattern. Stride is a parameter used to determine the number of kernel shifts in the input image. Padding is a parameter used to minimize the amount of information lost from the input image by adding the number of zero pixels at each edge of the input image [21].

Pooling Layer. The pooling layer is the process of reducing the dimensions of the feature map by doing downsampling to overcome overfitting [22]. Average pooling and maximum pooling are the two types of pooling. The average value of the selected pixel region in the image is used in average pooling, while the maximum value of the selected pixel area in the image is used in max pooling [23]. Figure 3 is an illustration of max pooling and average pooling on feature map 4 × 4, kernel 2 × 2, and stride 2.

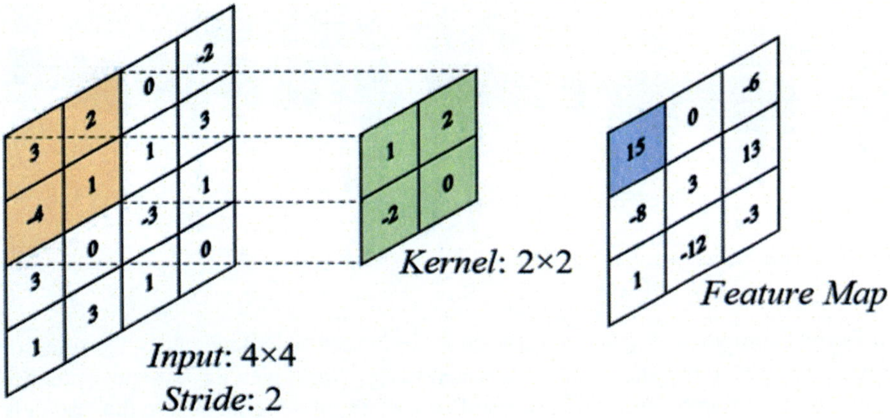

Fig. 2 Convolution process on the convolution layer [20]

Fig. 3 Pooling operation **a** Max pooling **b** Average pooling [20]

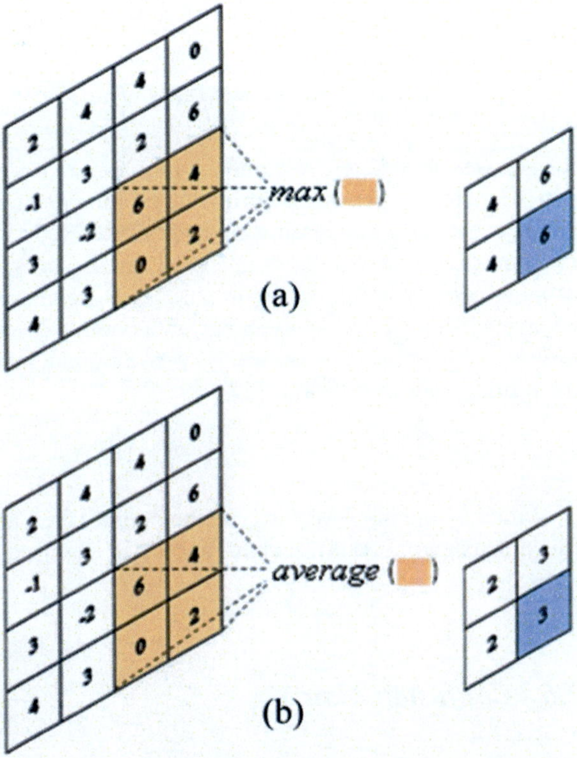

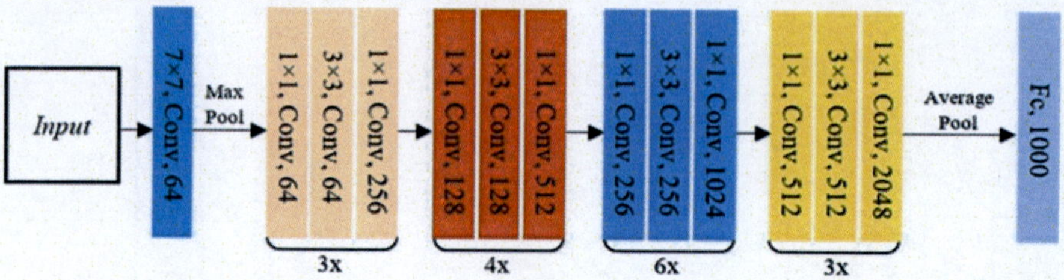

Fig. 4 ResNet-50 architecture [31]

Fully Connected Layer. A fully connected layer is a layer that functions to process images so that they can be classified [24]. In this layer, the flattening process on the feature map becomes a vector so that the output generated from the previous layer, which is still a multidimensional array, can be used as input to the fully connected layer [25].

2.5 *Residual Network (ResNet)*

ResNet was created to overcome the problem of decreasing system performance so that the error rate generated during the training and testing of data is high when the architecture has an increasing depth [20]. ResNet's way of dealing with this is by implementing a system skip connection, which works by way of input x will skip one or more layers without having to pass layer weights. ResNet is based on CNN, so its layers include a convolutional layer, a pooling layer, a fully connected layer, and a system skip connection on several convolutional layers [26]. Equation (1) depicts the residual block on ResNet [27].

$$y = F(x, \{W_i\}) + x \tag{1}$$

With x as the input vector, y as the output layer, and F as the residual mapping function to learn. In this research, ResNet-50 was used with an architecture as shown in Fig. 4.

2.6 *Confusion Matrix*

A confusion matrix is a matrix that is used to compare the predicted value to the actual value. The confusion matrix can be seen in Table 1 [28]. True Positive (TP), True Negative (TN), False Positive (FP), and False Negative (FN) are the four terms used in the confusion matrix. TP can be interpreted as a condition where the predicted value is the same as the actual value. An example of TP is Cell_1 in Table 1. TN is the

Table 1 Confusion matrix [28]

		Predicted Value		
Actual Value		Normal	Pneumonia *Viral*	Pneumonia *Bacterial*
	Normal	*Cell*$_1$	*Cell*$_2$	*Cell*$_3$
	Pneumonia *Viral*	*Cell*$_4$	*Cell*$_5$	*Cell*$_6$
	Pneumonia *Bacterial*	*Cell*$_7$	*Cell*$_8$	*Cell*$_9$

sum of all values other than the column and row values of the calculated class. For example, the sum of $Cell_5 + Cell_6 + Cell_8 + Cell_9$ is the TN value in the normal class. Furthermore, FP is the sum of the values of the column by class, without the TP value. For example, the sum of $Cell_4 + Cell_7$ is the FP value in the normal class. While FN can be interpreted as the number of values from the row based on its class, without the TP value. For example, the sum of $Cell_2 + Cell_3$ which is the FN value in the normal class [29].

3 System Design

There were several processes for the system to be able to classify x-ray images of the lungs into three classes. The processes of research are generally shown in Fig. 5.

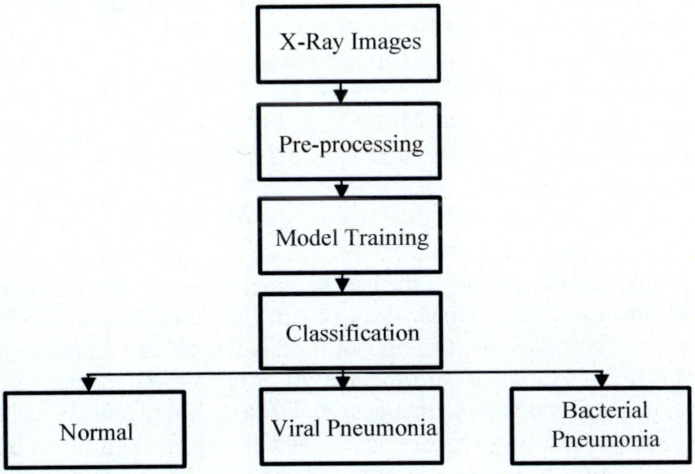

Fig. 5 The processes of research

The first stage was collecting data which was used as the system input. In this research, the data used is secondary data x-ray images of the lungs obtained from a dataset entitled "Chest X-Ray Images" on www.kaggle.com. At first, the data in the dataset were 5856 images with 1583 images in normal class, 2780 images in bacterial pneumonia, and 1493 images in viral pneumonia. There is an imbalance in the number of data, which can affect the performance of the designed system. To overcome that, the author generalizes the number of data in each class, so the distribution of data becomes balanced. The number of data used in this research was 4479 images consisting of 1493 images in each class. From 4479 images, 80% of the images were used as training data, 10% as validation data, and 10% as testing data. The second stage was pre-processing by resizing images to 224 × 224 for equalizing the size images. By using pre-processing images, a convolution operation was carried out which produces a feature map. As an activation function, if the feature map has a negative value index, ReLU will map the value into zero. In the pooling process, the dimensions of input are reduced with the max pooling method. The classification process is carried out on a fully connected layer using the softmax activation function. After the training stage was completed, a test was carried out aiming to determine the performance of the system in classifying x-ray images of the lungs. To check whether a system designed successfully classifies x-ray images, several performance parameters such as the value of accuracy, recall, precision, F1-Score, and loss were calculated.

4 Result and Discussion

The data ratio used in this research was split into three: 80% as training data, 10% as validation data, and 10% as test data. The testing phase consists of five test scenarios which included testing of the image size, the data ratio, the type of optimizer, the value of the learning rate, and the value of epoch. In the first test scenario, the image sizes used were 64 × 64, 128 × 128, and 224 × 224. In the second test scenario, the ratios used were 70:20:10, 75:15:10, and 80:20:20. In the third test scenario, the types of optimizers used were Adam, Nadam, SGD, and RMSprop. In the fourth scenario, learning rate values were 0.1, 0.01, 0.001, and 0.0001. In the last test scenario, the epoch values were 50, 60, 70, 80, 90, and 100. After the five test scenarios were completed, some of the best parameters were obtained to produce an optimal performance for the classification system. They are presented in Table 2.

The first test scenario aims to find out how is the effect of pre-processing in the form of resizing on system performance. After testing was carried out on three image sizes, it was found that the image size of 224 × 224 pixels obtained the best testing result and graph because each pixel contains information on an image. So, the larger the size of an image, the more detailed the information on the image. The second test scenario aims to find out how the ratio of training data, validation data, and testing data affects the system's performance. After testing was carried out on three data ratios, it was found that the data ratio of 80:10:10 obtained the best

Table 2 Best parameters

Parameter	Best result	
Size	224 × 224	
Ratio	Train	80
	Test	10
	Validation	10
Optimizer	SGD	
Learning rate	0.0001	
Epoch	100	
Batch size	64	

testing result and graph. It can produce the best test result because the number of images that can be learned by the system in the training process is increasing. This makes the characteristics of an image can continue to be studied and recognized by the system to improve the system's ability to classify x-ray images. The third test scenario aims to find out how the type of optimizer affects the system performance. The SGD optimizer was chosen to be the best optimizer because it can reduce the occurrence of overfitting on the testing graph and generate a smaller loss value than the other optimizers. This can happen because the optimizer SGD maximizes the optimum level of the designed system by updating the weights for each training data. The fourth test scenario aims to find out how the learning rate value affects the system performance. The learning rate value of 0.0001 was chosen to be the best learning rate value because it was able to reduce the occurrence of overfitting on the testing graph and produce a smaller loss value. This can happen because a small learning rate value affects the level of accuracy of the system in classifying so with learning rate value of 0.0001 the system can reach its optimum point. The last test scenario aims to find out how the epoch value affects the system performance. After testing was carried out on several epoch values, it was found that the greater the epoch value used, the more the resulting performance value increased. This happens because the system keeps repeating the training process as much as the epoch value used. So, the system becomes better at recognizing the characteristics of an image. The epoch value of 100 is chosen to be the best epoch because it obtains the highest testing result and graph. Testing results for accuracy value and loss value using the proposed method are shown in Fig. 6. Figure 6a, b show the result of the accuracy value and loss value for 100 epochs (iterations) of the training and the validation process. Based on Fig. 6a, b, it can be concluded that the designed system was not overfitting because there is no significant variation between the result of accuracy and the result of loss in the training and validation process. In this research, the best performance has reached the result of an accuracy value of 88.88%, precision of 83.34%, recall of 83.33%, F1-Score of 83.16%, and loss of 0.4597.

By using the confusion matrix, the test results of the system can be seen in Fig. 7. With a 10% data ratio of testing data, there are 450 images that were used as testing data consisting of 150 images in each class. From 150 images in normal class, 144

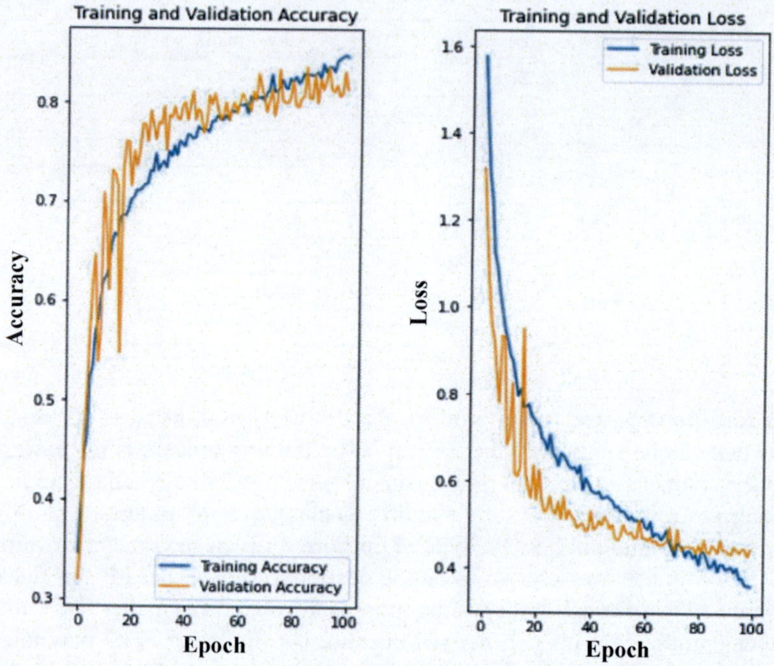

(a) (b)

Fig. 6 Testing results with best scenario **a** Accuracy **b** Loss

images can be classified appropriately, while 3 images are classified as bacterial pneumonia and 3 images are classified as viral pneumonia. Then from 150 images in the bacterial pneumonia class, 125 images can be classified appropriately, while 3 images are classified as normal, and 22 images are classified as viral pneumonia. Meanwhile, from viral pneumonia, 106 images are classified appropriately, while 8 images are classified as normal, and 36 images are classified as bacterial pneumonia.

From the confusion matrix, prediction errors most commonly occur in bacterial pneumonia and viral pneumonia. This is because the level of similarity between the image in bacterial pneumonia and viral pneumonia is high. The high degree of similarity makes the characteristics of images from bacterial pneumonia and viral pneumonia difficult to distinguish.

Based on Fig. 7, the system has successfully classified 375 images. This indicates the system designed using the CNN method with ResNet-50 architecture can be classified images appropriately. Although there are still images remaining, they are not classified appropriately because the degree of image similarity is complex. The result of the proposed method compared with previous results is shown in Table 3.

Systems using CNN with Compressed Sensing in research [2] and DCNN with augmentation in research [5] only detect whether a person has pneumonia or not, through x-ray images. While it is important to know the cause of pneumonia suffered

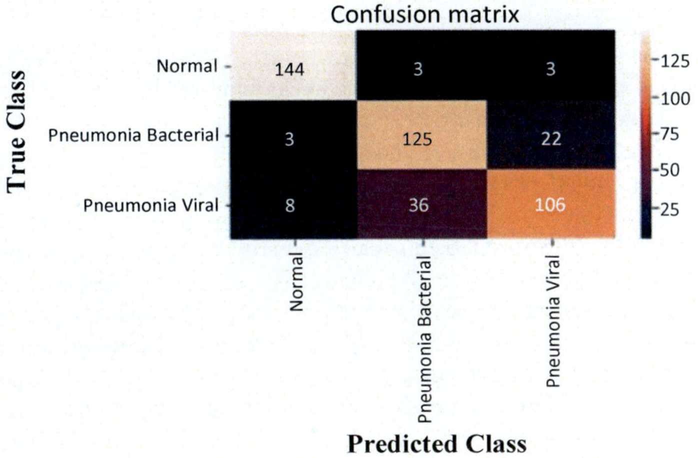

Fig. 7 Confusion matrix

Table 3 Comparison of accuracy results with different methods

Method	Accuracy (%)
CNN with compressed sensing [2]	97.34
LDA-SVM [3]	92.775
DCNN with transfer learning [4]	80.48
DCNN with augmentation [5]	83.38
CNN with ResNet-50 (proposed method)	88.88

by a person because each cause of pneumonia has a different way of treatment. In research [3], the system was designed to detect and classify pneumonia using one of the machine learning methods, namely LDA-SVM. Several weaknesses of this combination methods are the need for many iterations of training and too long computation time. When compared with research [2, 3], this research has a lower accuracy value which is because of the differences in the class of images used. In this research, the images of bacterial pneumonia and viral pneumonia classes have similarities, so this affects the accuracy value produced. Then when compared with research [4, 5], this research has a higher accuracy value in classifying x-ray images into three classes. This is because the method in this research is suitable for the characteristics of the x-ray image data used. With the classification system of pneumonia in this research, early detection can be carried out which is useful for recognizing symptoms and carrying out treatment in time to prevent conditions get worse.

5 Conclusion

Identifying the causes of pneumonia just by looking at the x-ray images of the lungs is difficult to do, not only because each x-ray images have a high degree of similarity, but also because eyes have a high level of subjectivity. As an early detection, a classification system for pneumonia is needed. The research aims to design a classification system of pneumonia based on x-ray images of the lungs using CNN ResNet-50 architecture which is carried out by analyzing the best parameters of the system. This research was also conducted because there is still a lack of a system that can classify the causes of pneumonia disease due to bacterial, viral and if looking from previous research, the accuracy value in classification system still can be improved. From the five test scenarios that have been carried out, the best parameters for the classification system are obtained. The best parameters for each scenario are an image size of 224 × 224 pixels, a data ratio of 80:10:10, an SGD optimizer, a learning rate of 0.0001, and an epoch of 100. The best performance values from the proposed method have reached an accuracy value of 88.88%, precision of 83.34%, recall of 83.33%, F1-Score of 83.16%, and loss of 0.4597. Based on the performance values obtained, it can be concluded that the classification system of pneumonia in this research can classify pneumonia based on x-ray images of the lungs into three classes, they are normal, bacterial pneumonia, and viral pneumonia. Images can be classified well because the proposed method is suitable for the characteristics of the x-ray images of the lungs used. There are several suggestions that can be given for further research to get a better performance value, which using primary data x-ray images of the lungs, using other pre-processing, and designing a classification system using a different architecture for comparison.

References

1. Divyashri S, Ganapathy D, Keerthisasanka L, Sivaswamy V (2022) Awareness on treatment protocols with pneumonia patients among the dental students. Int J Early Child Spec Educ (INT-JECS) 14. https://doi.org/10.9756/INT-JECSE/V14I3.994
2. Islam SR, Maity SP, Ray AK, Mandal M (2019) Automatic detection of pneumonia on compressed sensing images using deep learning. In: Canadian conference of electrical and computer engineering (CCECE)
3. Ling G, Cao C (2020) Atomatic detection and diagnosis of severe viral pneumonia CT images based on LDA-SVM. IEEE Sens J 20:11927–11934. https://doi.org/10.1109/JSEN.2019.2959617
4. Gu X, Pan L, Liang H, Yang R (2018) Classification of bacterial and viral childhood pneumonia using deep learning in chest radiography. In: ACM international conference proceeding series. Association for Computing Machinery. pp 88–93. https://doi.org/10.1145/3195588.3195597
5. Khoiriyah SA, Basofi A, Fariza A (2020) Convolutional neural network for automatic pneumonia detection in chest radiography. In: IES 2020—international electronics symposium: the role of autonomous and intelligent systems for human life and comfort. Institute of Electrical and Electronics Engineers Inc., pp 476–480. https://doi.org/10.1109/IES50839.2020.9231540
6. Clemson P, Lancaster G, Stefanovska A (2016). Reconstruct Time Depend Dyn. https://doi.org/10.1109/JPROC.2015.2491262

7. Kaminsky DA (2011) The netter collection of medical illustrations. Saunders Elsevier, Philadelphia
8. British lung foundation: how your lungs work. https://www.blf.org.uk/support-for-you/how-your-lungs-work/about-the-lungs
9. Khatiwada S, Subedi A (2020) Lung microbiome and coronavirus disease 2019 (COVID-19)-possible link and implications. Hum Microb J (2020) https://doi.org/10.1016/j.humic.2020.100073
10. Bourke SJ, Burns GP (2015) Lecture notes: respiratory medicine
11. Rahman T, Chowdhury MEH, Khandakar A, Islam KR, Islam KF, Mahbub ZB, Kadir MA, Kashem S (2020) Transfer learning with deep convolutional neural network (CNN) for pneumonia detection using chest X-ray. Appl Sci (Switzerland) 10. https://doi.org/10.3390/app10093233
12. Manohar P, Loh B, Nachimuthu R, Hua X, Welburn SC, Leptihn S (2020). Secondary Bact Infect Patients With Viral Pneumonia. https://doi.org/10.3389/fmed.2020.00420
13. Dwivedi RS (2017) Remote sensing of soils
14. Maier A, Steidl S, Christlein V, Hornegger J (2018) Medical imaging systems. Springer International Publishing, Cham (2018). https://doi.org/10.1007/978-3-319-96520-8
15. Clarke C, Dux A (2017) Chest X-rays for medical students. Wiley
16. Shyam R (2021) Convolutional neural network and its architectures. https://doi.org/10.37591/JoCTA
17. Agbinya JI (2019) Applied data analytics—principles and applications. River Publishers
18. Liu YH (2018) Feature extraction and image recognition with convolutional neural networks. In: Journal of physics: conference series. Institute of Physics Publishing. https://doi.org/10.1088/1742-6596/1087/6/062032
19. Mostafa S, Wu FX (2021) Diagnosis of autism spectrum disorder with convolutional autoencoder and structural MRI images. In: Neural engineering techniques for autism spectrum disorder: Volume 1: imaging and signal analysis. Elsevier, pp 23–38. https://doi.org/10.1016/B978-0-12-822822-7.00003-X
20. Khan S, Rahmani H, Afaq S, Shah A, Bennamoun M (2018) A guide to convolutional neural networks for computer vision. Morgan & Claypool. https://doi.org/10.2200/S00822ED1V01Y201712COV015
21. Albawi S, Mohammed TA, Al-Zawi S (2017) Understanding of a convolutional neural network. In: International conference on engineering and technology (ICET), pp 1–6
22. Djordjevic IB (2021) Quantum information processing, quantum computing, and quantum error correction: an engineering approach. Academic Press
23. Nurjannah AF, Kurniasari ASD, Sari Z, Azhar Y (2022) Pneumonia image classification using CNN with max pooling and average pooling 6:330–338. https://doi.org/10.29207/resti.v6i2.4001
24. Namatēvs I (2018) Deep convolutional neural networks: structure, feature extraction and training. Inf Technol Manage Sci 20. https://doi.org/10.1515/itms-2017-0007
25. Dai X, Spasić I, Meyer B, Chapman S, Andres F (2019) Machine learning on mobile: an on-device inference app for skin cancer detection. In: Fourth international conference on fog and mobile edge computing (FMEC), pp 301–305
26. Yamashita R, Nishio M, Do RKG, Togashi K (2018) Convolutional neural networks: an overview and application in radiology. Insights Imaging 9:611–629. https://doi.org/10.1007/s13244-018-0639-9
27. He K, Zhang X, Ren S, Sun J (2016) Deep residual learning for image recognition
28. Grandini M, Bagli E, Visani G (2020) Metrics for multi-class classification: an overview
29. Bharathi: Confusion Matrix for Multi-Class Classification. https://www.analyticsvidhya.com/blog/2021/06./confusion-matrix-for-multi-class-classification/

30. Singh I, Singh NP, Singh H, Bawankar S, Ngom A (2020) Blood cell types classification using CNN. In: Lecture notes in computer science (including subseries lecture notes in artificial intelligence and lecture notes in bioinformatics), pp 727–738. Springer. https://doi.org/10.1007/978-3-030-45385-5_65
31. Ali L, Alnajjar F, Jassmi H, Gochoo M, Khan W, Serhani MA (2021) Performance evaluation of deep CNN-based crack detection and localization techniques for concrete structures. Sensors 21:1–22. https://doi.org/10.3390/s21051688

A Model Convolutional Neural Network for Early Detection of Chili Plant Diseases in Small Datasets

Rifqi Akmal Saputra, Faisal Dharma Adhinata, Nur Ghaniaviyanto Ramadhan, and Rifqi Alfinnur Charisma

Abstract By the end of 2021 in Indonesia, there was an increase in the price of basic foodstuffs, including chili. This price increase was due to farmers' chili supply shortage because of disease that attacked chili plants in various areas. Early detection of chili plant diseases is essential to maintain the quality and productivity of crop yields. Research related to the detection of chili plant diseases has been developed by many researchers, for example, using machine learning techniques. Previous research used machine learning to classify three classes of chili diseases. The results of this research are not optimal because the amount of data used is small, so it only reaches 86% accuracy. Therefore, we propose using the Convolutional Neural Network (CNN) method, which is part of deep learning. This research contributes to building a CNN architectural model for processing small datasets. We developed the CNN architecture to process small amounts of data. The dataset consists of 5 classes: healthy, leaf curl, leaf spot, whitefly, and yellowish. The raw data obtained is pre-processed before going to the feature extraction stage. The reason for pre-processing is to homogenize the size and augment the data. The results of the pre-processing data will be used for feature extraction and classification using CNN. We also compare the results of using CNN with the DenseNet201 transfer learning model. The test results using the confusion matrix obtained an accuracy of 92% on the use of the DenseNet201 model, while on CNN, it produced an accuracy of 94%. Through these results, agricultural technology developers can use this method, especially for chili plants.

Keywords Chili plant · CNN · DenseNet201 · Disease · Transfer learning

R. A. Saputra · F. D. Adhinata (✉) · N. G. Ramadhan · R. A. Charisma
Faculty of Informatics, Institut Teknologi Telkom Purwokerto, Purwokerto, Indonesia
e-mail: faisal@ittelkom-pwt.ac.id

T. Triwiyanto et al. (eds.), *Proceeding of the 3rd International Conference on Electronics, Biomedical Engineering, and Health Informatics*, Lecture Notes in Electrical Engineering 1008, https://doi.org/10.1007/978-981-99-0248-4_10

1 Introduction

Chili plants are one of the vegetables that Indonesian people often consume as a spicy flavor in food. Many Indonesian people use chili as a cooking spice, so it is not surprising that it is easy to find chili in the market in various regions of Indonesia [1]. At the end of 2021, the price of chili tends to increase because the tourism sector has begun to open in this era of the COVID-19 pandemic. One of the causes of the increase in chili prices is farmers' shortage of chili supplies. The decline in chili production was due to erratic rainfall, and some areas were attacked by pests and diseases of chili plants [2]. The presence of these diseases and pests makes the chili yields not optimal. Several diseases and pests on chili plants include leaf curl, leaf spot, yellow virus, and white fly [3]. These diseases and pests need to be detected soon so that treatment can be carried out immediately. Disease detection in chili can be done through cross-sectional images of the leaves. This image can be processed using computer science, namely Artificial Intelligence for chili disease detection.

Recently, systems for the classification of various case studies have been developed. Researchers usually use machine learning or deep learning techniques to carry out the classification process. Several studies on plant disease classification, including the classification of corn plant diseases using machine learning techniques, namely Support Vector Machine (SVM), yielded an accuracy of 85% [4]. The data used are 50 in each class. Then in another research, the detection and classification of rice plant diseases using the K-Nearest Neighbor method resulted in an accuracy of 76.59% [5]. This research uses the amount of data 330 images. Rice disease classification was also carried out using the XGBoost method, which resulted in an accuracy of 86.58% [6]. The data used in this chili research is 100 data on each disease class, with the number of classes being three classes. Research with the same case research using a machine learning Decision tree also produces an accuracy of 86% [7]. The accuracy, which is still below 90%, is not yet optimal, so other methods are needed to process a small number of datasets. Based on several previous research descriptions, machine learning techniques' accuracy results are not optimal when later implemented for classifying chili plant diseases, mainly for using small datasets. Therefore, we propose the use of deep learning techniques. One of the deep learning methods to process image data is Convolutional Neural Network (CNN) [8, 9]. This research aims to create a CNN model to process a small number of datasets. In addition to traditional CNNs, transfer learning methods have been developed that are often used to process small datasets, for example, the transfer learning model DenseNet201 [10, 11].

Several studies that use DenseNet201 as a classification include the classification of diseases on corn leaves [12]. This research resulted in 93% accuracy in classifying four classes. Then, the pre-trained DenseNet201 model was also used to identify whether the patient is COVID-19 positive or not, which resulted in an accuracy of 97% [13]. The DenseNet201 model will be used to compare the CNN model created. We will evaluate the combination of epoch number and batch size parameters for optimal accuracy. The model's results with the best accuracy will be used for the testing process using a confusion matrix. The main contribution of this research is to create a CNN architecture for processing small datasets.

2 Materials and Method

The chili plant disease classification begins with inputting chili disease image data along with the identity of the disease, which is used as a label. The input data is divided into two parts: training data and validation data. All data is pre-processed in the form of resizing before being processed to the feature extraction stage using CNN or DenseNet201 models. The result of the feature extraction process using CNN or DenseNet201 is a model file with the extension.h5. The built model is evaluated using the best loss and accuracy values. The best modeling results will be used for evaluation using a confusion matrix. Figure 1 shows a flow diagram forming a chili plant disease classification.

2.1 Data Acquisition

This research used a dataset sourced from Kaggle [14]. This research uses a dataset in the form of chili diseases in Indonesia. The chili disease classification that we use consists of 5 classes: healthy, leaf curl, leaf spot, whitefly, and yellowish. Each class consists of 116 images. We divide the data into 70% training and 30% training data. Figure 2 shows an example of the data used in this research.

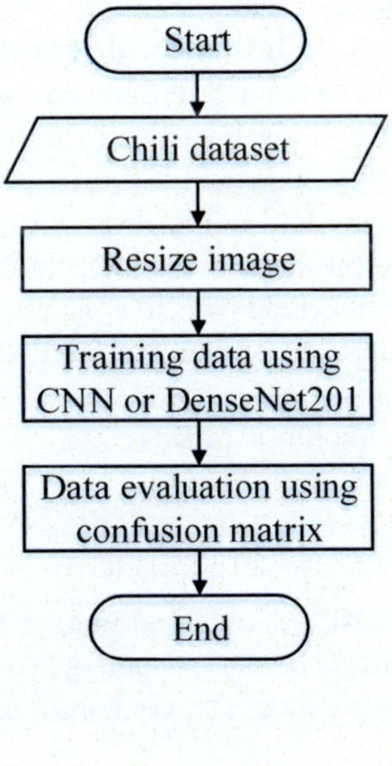

Fig. 1 Proposed system architecture

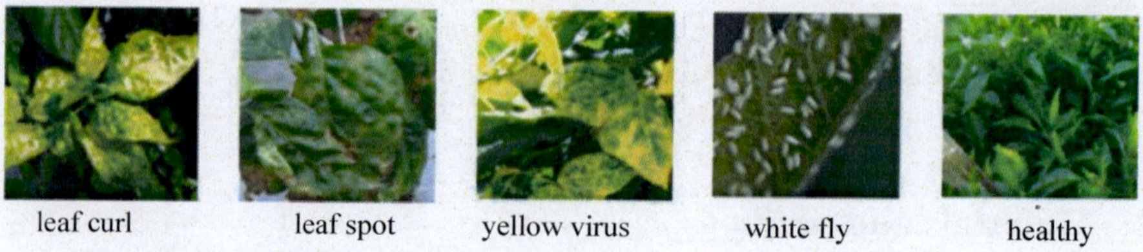

Fig. 2 Examples of data used in this research

2.2 Pre-Processing Data

The dataset being processed to the feature extraction stage using the CNN or transfer learning model is resized to a size of 150 × 150. The 150 × 150 size is used because, in previous research, it produced optimal accuracy with the CNN method [15]. This resizes operation uses the pre-processing library in the TensorFlow library [16]. This resizing is carried out in the preparation of both models so that the treatment is the same. The number of batch sizes used is 32 and uses categorical label mode because the number of data classes is more than two. The use of batch size is 32 because it produces optimal accuracy based on previous research [17, 18].

2.3 Convolutional Neural Network

Convolutional neural networks (ConvNets) are a type of Deep Learning algorithm [19] that can take in an input image, assign importance (learnable weights and biases), and distinguish between distinct aspects and objects in the image. When compared to other classification methods, ConvNet requires significantly less pre-processing work. While filters must be designed by hand for rudimentary approaches, ConvNets can be trained to develop such capabilities. The convolutional layer, the subsample or pooling layer, and the fully connected layer are the three layers that make up CNN in general [20, 21]. While the pooling layer performs a subsampling function to produce output from the convolutional layer and lower data rates from the layers below it, the convolutional layer shares a significant amount of weight. Several fully connected layers use the output from the pooling layer as their input. Convolutional filters or kernels are applied to the dataset to produce convolutional features, also known as feature maps [22, 23]. The following Eq. (1) can be used to represent the convolution process:

$$S(i, j) = (I * K)(i, j) = \sum_m \sum_n I(m, n) K(i - m, j - n) \tag{1}$$

where I is the input image, K is the convolution kernel or filter, m is a collection of images, and n is the image column. Reducing feature maps is done through subsample or pooling. The convolution filter applied to the input data is essentially the same idea behind the pooling process as it is behind the convolution process. However, in contrast to the convolution process, the pooling process in the shifting filter does not overlap in each filter [24].

The CNN architecture in this research is shown in Fig. 3. The CNN architecture used in this research consists of several layers, including an input layer with an input image size of 150 × 150 pixels and then passing through 5 convolutional layers, 5 batch normalization, five pooling layers (max pooling 2 × 2), five dropouts with a value of (0, 5), fully connected layer, and output layer. Furthermore, the architecture in DenseNet201 in this study consists of an input layer, convolution layer, poll layer, dense block 1, transition layer 1, dense block 2, transition layer 2, dense block 3, transition layer 3, dense block 4: global average polling layer, fully connected layer, activation layer, and classification layer. In the classification layer, the global average pooling operation of the DenseNet201 model is to determine the classification class.

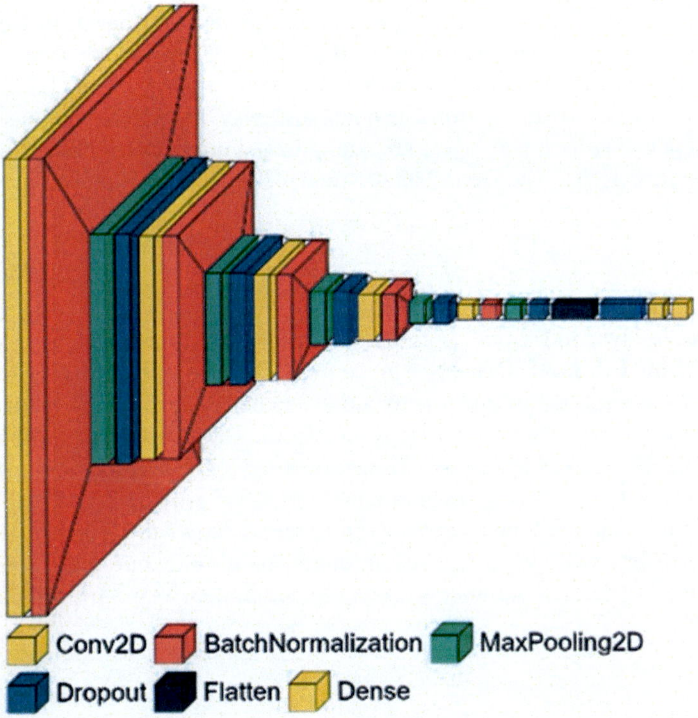

Fig. 3 CNN architecture in this research

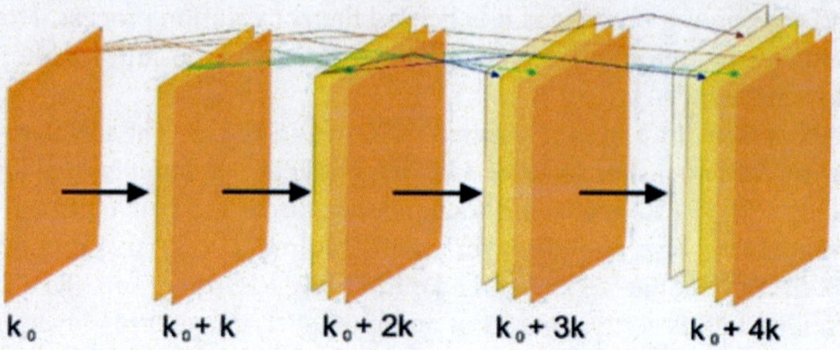

Fig. 4 DenseNet201 layer structure

2.4 DenseNet201

On multiple datasets, including ImageNet and CIFAR-100, the DenseNet201 has been shown to perform exceptionally well [25, 26]. The model's ability to reuse features across layers increases variety in subsequent layer input and boosts performance [27], so training the network is quick and easy. Direct connections between all preceding and subsequent layers are strengthened in the DenseNet201 model for increased connectivity. The DenseNet201 model's layers are displayed in Fig. 4.

$$x_l = H_l([x_0, x_1, x_2, \ldots, x_{l-1}]) \tag{2}$$

where l is the layer index and H is the nonlinear operation. Then, x_l is the characteristic of the l th layer. DenseNet made more changes to the model by concatenating all the output feature maps sequentially rather than summing them as it had in Eq. (2), which was the previous version's form. The concept of down-sampling on dense blocks was put forth [28]. To demonstrate a Dense Block case where the layer number is five and the growth rate is set to k, we provide Fig. 4. All previous layers' feature maps are sent to each layer. Figure 4 shows that H_l, k feature maps are produced for each operation. We can obtain $k_0 + 4k$ feature maps since Fig. 4 contains five layers. The number k_0 refers to the feature maps from the previous layer.

2.5 System Evaluation

In this research, the evaluation stage starts by evaluating the results of training validation loss between the two CNN and DenseNet201 models. The lowest validation loss value will be used for testing using the confusion matrix. In addition, we also provide graphs on the training process to determine whether the model made is overfitting or underfitting.

Table 1 Number of image data training and testing

Data	Healthy	Leaf curl	Leaf spot	White fly	Yellowish	Total
Training	80	80	80	80	80	400
Testing	36	36	36	36	36	180

3 Result and Discussion

In this section, we will discuss the results of the study. The discussion starts with the configuration of the dataset, the training results, the confusion matrix test results, and an example of the output of the detection results.

3.1 Dataset Configuration

The dataset used in this study uses data from Chile Plant Disease. The total image data collected is 580 image data. The data is divided into training and testing data consisting of 400 images as training data (70%) and 180 images as data testing (30%). Each training and testing data has five classes: healthy, leaf curl, leaf spot, whitefly, and yellowish. Table 1 shows an example of data sharing used in this research.

3.2 Training Result

The training results were obtained from experiments that have been carried out using 100 epochs, 32 batch sizes, loss functions using categorical cross entropy, and Adam's optimizer. Based on the Fig. 5, which shows the training results of the two graphs from the training process using CNN and DenseNet201, then for model.fit configuration, namely training data using train-ing_set and validation data using test_set there is no overfitting. The training process uses google collaborative using Google's GPU run time so that the CNN and DenseNet201 model training process can be done faster. Figure 5 shows the results of the training using the two models.

A comparison of the two models can be made by looking at the validation values of each of these models. The CNN model trained for 100 epochs results from the smallest validation loss value at the 90th epoch with a validation loss value of 0.2311. Then for the DenseNet201 model, which has the smallest process of 100 epochs, the results of the validation loss value are obtained at the 20 epochs with a loss validation value of 0.2507. The value of validation loss at the training stage is shown in Table 2.

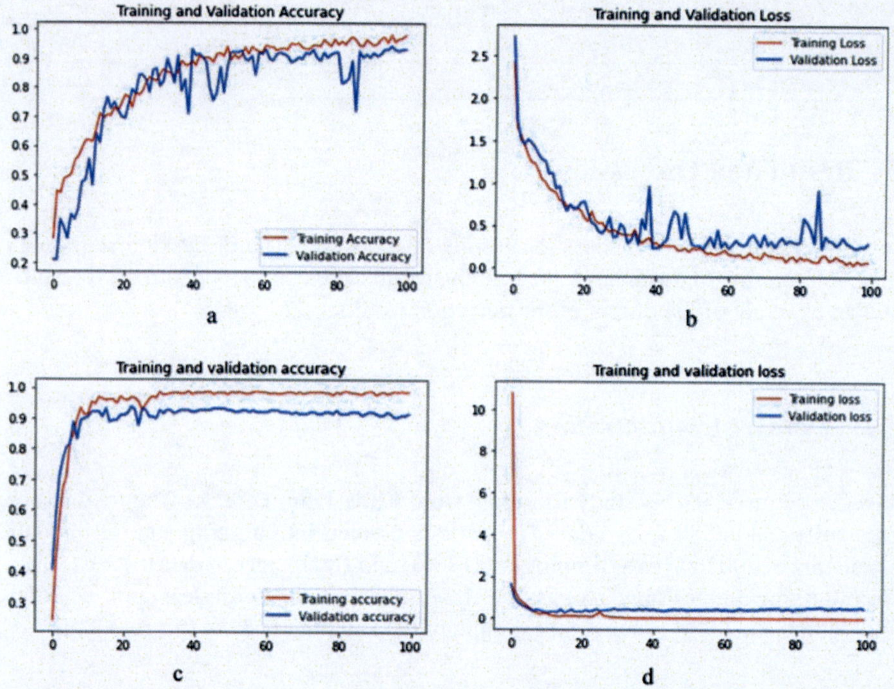

Fig. 5 Graphic of training results: **a** CNN training accuracy, **b** CNN training loss, **c**, DenseNet201 model accuracy, **d** DenseNet201 model loss

Table 2 Value validation loss from training results

Epoch	Validation loss	
	CNN	DenseNet201
10	1.2603	0.3247
20	0.7717	0.2507
30	0.3753	0.4712
40	0.2390	0.3998
50	0.4074	0.3934
60	0.3147	0.3948
70	0.2614	0.4244
80	0.3011	0.4141
90	0.2311	0.4568
100	0.2983	0.4874

3.3 Confusion Matrix Result

The evaluation of CNN and DenseNet201 models is using confusion matrix method, where testing it uses testing data consisting of 5 healthy classes, leaf curl, leaf spot, whitefly, and yellowish, where each class has 36 images. The confusion matrix results from the CNN and DenseNet201 models can be seen in the Table 3. In the CNN model, the results of image predictions were classified correctly; 33 out of 36 images were classified as "healthy", 36 out of 36 images were successfully classified as "leaf curl", 33 out of 36 images were successfully classified as "leaf spot", 35 out of 36 images were successfully classified "whitefly", and 32 out of the 36 images were successfully classified as "yellowish". Then for the DenseNet201 model, the results of the image prediction were classified correctly; 34 out of 36 images were classified as "healthy", 32 out of 36 images were successfully classified as "leaf curl", 32 out of 36 images were successfully classified as "leaf spot", 35 out of 36 images were successfully classified "whitefly", and 32 of the 36 images were successfully classified as "yellowish". Tables 3 and 4 show the confusion matrix results on the CNN and DenseNet201 models.

The confusion matrix can be used to calculate the precision, recall, f1-score, and accuracy value. Based on the confusion matrix table for the CNN and DenseNet201 models above, the calculation results for the precision, recall, f1-score, and accuracy values of the CNN and DenseNet201 models using the classification report function in the scikit learn library can be seen in Table 5. Based on these results, the CNN

Table 3 The result of confusion matrix from CNN model

		Prediction				
		Healthy	Leaf curl	Leaf spot	Whitefly	Yellowish
Actual	Healthy	33	2	0	1	0
	Leaf curl	0	36	0	0	0
	Leaf spot	1	1	33	1	0
	Whitefly	0	1	0	35	0
	Yellowish	0	4	0	0	32

Table 4 The result of confusion matrix from DenseNet201 model

		Prediction				
		Healthy	Leaf curl	Leaf cpot	Whitefly	Yellowish
Actual	Healthy	34	2	0	0	0
	Leaf curl	2	32	0	1	1
	Leaf cpot	0	1	32	2	1
	Whitefly	0	0	1	35	0
	Yellowish	0	2	2	0	32

Table 5 The result of precision, recall, F1-Score, and Accuracy

Model	Class	Precision (%)	Recall (%)	F1-score (%)	Accuracy (%)
Model CNN	0 (Healthy)	97	92	94	94
	1 (Leaf curl)	82	100	90	
	2 (Leaf spot)	100	92	96	
	3 (Whitefly)	95	97	96	
	4 (Yellowish)	100	89	94	
Model DenseNet201	0 (Healthy)	94	94	94	92
	1 (Leaf curl)	86	89	88	
	2 (Leaf spot)	91	89	90	
	3 (Whitefly)	92	97	95	
	4 (Yellowish)	94	89	91	

model has a better accuracy rate of 94%. Then the DenseNet201 model produces an accuracy rate of 92%.

3.4 *Testing Result*

The experiment uses random image data from the testing directory. The experimental and classification results using CNN can be seen in Fig. 6. The experimental results display 15 randomly selected test images and have two outputs: the actual image class and class classification carried out by the previously trained CNN and DenseNet201 models.

Experiments conducted using the DenseNet201 model resulted in 13 out of 15 images of chili plants being classified correctly according to their class, then 2 out of 15 images were still wrong in categorizing according to the actual class. Then for the experiment using the CNN model, 15 out of the 15 chili plant images were successfully classified according to their class. It can be concluded that the CNN model has 100% accuracy in classifying the 15 test images given.

3.5 *Analysis and Discussion*

In this research, deep learning algorithms are used to conduct training on images of chili plant diseases and classified using the CNN model. The results of this study show that the CNN model extracts important features in each image and has low efficiency in terms of memory and complexity. The accuracy results obtained in this research were excellent, reaching 94% using the CNN model. Table 6 compares the methods used in previous studies using standard feature-based and deep learning. The

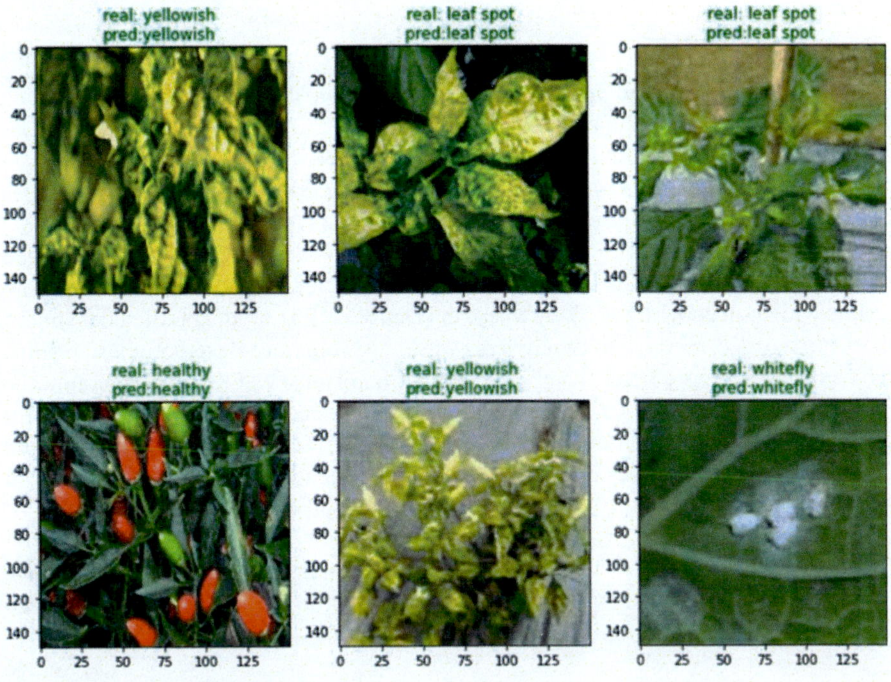

Fig. 6 Testing result using CNN model

results of the proposed research are still the greatest of previous studies. The accuracy results were not optimal in previous studies using deep learning and machine learning approaches. However, the proposed method also has a weakness in using deep learning, namely the long training time. The training process is also very dependent on the computer device used. So that future research can use other models whose training process is not too long. Then, this research is expected to help farmers detect diseases in chili plants so they can carry out countermeasures quickly and precisely according to the detected disease.

Table 6 Comparison of the proposed method with previous studies

Classification model	Accuracy (%)
Color, size, and texture features [29]	80
Faster R-CNN + DNN [30]	65
GLCM + KNN [31]	93
InceptionV3, DenseNet201 + SVM [32]	90.76
Proposed Method (CNN)	94

4 Conclusion

Chili farmers can carry out proper handling according to diseases and pests that attack chili plants. This research provides solutions to chili farmers in identifying diseases and problems in chili plants. This study uses a deep learning approach by comparing two models, namely CNN and DenseNet201, which can be used to classify the types of diseases in chili plants correctly. The experimental results of the CNN model obtained testing results with a success rate of 100%, where the CNN model managed to predict 15 out of the 15 images. Then the DenseNet201 model obtained testing results with a success rate of 87%, where the DenseNet201 model predicted 13 out of the 15 images correctly, and two images were mispredicted. Based on these results, the CNN model has a better level of accuracy than DenseNet201 in conducting the disease classification process in chili plants. It is hoped that further research will apply other models or combine them with the CNN model and can be implemented in the form of an application or mobile so that chili can be used to detect pests on chili plants.

Acknowledgements The author would like to thank the Lembaga Penelitian dan Pengabdian Masyarakat (LPPM) Institut Teknologi Telkom Purwokerto, which has provided funds to develop this research.

References

1. Surya R, Tedjakusuma F (2022) Diversity of sambals, traditional Indonesian chili pastes. J Ethnic Foods 9(1):1–19
2. Islam AHMS, Schreinemachers P, Kumar S (2020) Farmers' knowledge, perceptions and management of chili pepper anthracnose disease in Bangladesh. Crop Prot 133:1–7
3. Das Chagas Silva Araujo S, Malemath VS, Sundaram KM (2021) Symptom-based identification of G-4 chili leaf diseases based on rotation invariant. Front Robot AI 8:1–8
4. Setiawan W, Syarief M, Prastiti N (2019) Maize leaf disease image classification using bag of features. Jurnal Infotel 11(2):48–54
5. Suresha M, Shreekanth KN, Thirumalesh BV (2017) Recognition of diseases in paddy leaves using knn classifier. In: 2017 2nd international conference for convergence in technology, vol 2017, pp 663–666
6. Azim MA, Islam MK, Rahman MM, Jahan F (2021) An effective feature extraction method for rice leaf disease classification. Telkomnika (Telecommun Comput Electron Control) 19(2):463–470
7. Zuain SS, Fitriyah H, Maulana R (2021) Disease detection in chili leaves based on HSV and GLCM features using the C4.5 algorithm based on Raspberry Pi. Jurnal Pengembangan Teknologi Informasi dan Ilmu Komputer 5(9):3934–3940
8. Alzubaidi L et al (2021) Review of deep learning: concepts, CNN architectures, challenges, applications, future directions. J Big Data 8(1):1–74
9. Wahyono, Harjoko A, Dharmawan A, Adhinata FD, Kosala G, Jo KH (2021) Real-time forest fire detection framework based on artificial intelligence using color probability model and motion feature analysis. Fire 5(1):1–15

10. Junaidi A, Adhinata FD, Iskandar AR, Lasama J (2022) Image classification for egg incubator using transfer learning VGG16 and inceptionV3. In: Proceedings of the 2nd international conference on electronics, biomedical engineering, and health informatics, pp 85–95
11. Adhinata FD, Rakhmadani DP, Wibowo M, Jayadi A (2021) A deep learning using densenet201 to detect masked or non-masked face. JUITA: Jurnal Informatika 9(1):115–121
12. Adhinata FD, Fitriana GF, Wijayanto A, Pajar M, Putra K (2021) Corn disease classification using transfer learning and convolutional neural network. JUITA: Jurnal Informatika 9(2):1–7
13. Jaiswal A, Gianchandani N, Singh D, Kumar V, Kaur M (2021) Classification of the COVID-19 infected patients using DenseNet201 based deep transfer learning. J Biomol Struct Dyn 39(15):5682–5689
14. Prakoso DD (2021) Chili plant disease. Kaggle, Kaggle.com
15. Zhang C, Nateghinia E, Miranda-Moreno LF, Sun L (2021) Pavement distress detection using convolutional neural network (CNN): a case study in Montreal, Canada. Int J Transp Sci Technol 11(2):298–309
16. Ruvinga C, Malathi D, Dorathi Jayaseeli JD (2020) Human concentration level recognition based on vgg16 cnn architecture. Int J Adv Sci Technol 29(6):1364–1373
17. Bengio Y (2012) Practical recommendations for gradient-based training of deep architectures BT—neural networks: tricks of the trade, 2nd edn. Springer, Heidelberg, pp 437–478
18. Kandel I, Castelli M (2020) The effect of batch size on the generalizability of the convolutional neural networks on a histopathology dataset. ICT Express 6(4):312–315
19. Abdusalomov A, Baratov N, Kutlimuratov A, Whangbo TK (2021) An improvement of the fire detection and classification method using YOLOv3 for surveillance systems. Sensors 21(19):1–18
20. Li H, Huang J, Ji S (2019) Bearing fault diagnosis with a feature fusion method based on an ensemble convolutional neural network and deep neural network. Sensors 19(9):1–18
21. Patil A, Rane M (2021) Convolutional neural networks: an overview and its applications in pattern recognition. Smart Innov Syst Technol 195:21–30
22. Zhou Y, Liao L, Gao Y, Huang H (2021) Extracting salient features from convolutional discriminative filters. Inf Sci 558:265–279
23. Zou J, Rui T, Zhou Y, Yang C, Zhang S (2018) Convolutional neural network simplification via feature map pruning. Comput Electr Eng 70:950–958
24. Anton A, Nissa NF, Janiati A, Cahya N, Astuti P (2021) Application of deep learning using convolutional neural network (CNN) method for women's skin classification. Sci J Inform 8(1):144–153
25. Mahanty C, Kumar R, Patro SGK (2022) Internet of medical things-based COVID-19 detection in CT images fused with fuzzy ensemble and transfer learning models. New Gener Comput
26. Sharma A, Mishra PK (2022) Image enhancement techniques on deep learning approaches for automated diagnosis of COVID-19 features using CXR images. Multimedia Tools Appl
27. Huang G, Liu Z, Van Der Maaten L, Weinberger KQ (2017) Densely connected convolutional networks. In: Proceedings—30th IEEE conference on computer vision and pattern recognition. CVPR 2017, pp 2261–2269
28. Wang S-H, Zhang Y-D (2020) DenseNet-201-based deep neural network with composite learning factor and precomputation for multiple sclerosis classification. ACM Trans Multimedia Comput Commun Appl 16(2):1–19
29. Patil DP, Kurkute SR, Sonar PS (2017) An advanced method for chilli plant disease detection using image processing. In: Proceedings of the 2nd international conference on education, science, and technology, pp 309–313
30. Saad WHM, Karim SAA, Razak MSJA, Radzi SA, Yussof ZM (2020) Classification and detection of chili and its flower using deep learning approach. J Phys Conf Ser 1502(1):0–7
31. Patil A, Lad K (2021) Chili plant leaf disease detection using SVM and KNN classification. Adv Intell Syst Comput 1187:223–231
32. Ahmad Loti NN, Mohd Noor MR, Chang SW (2021) Integrated analysis of machine learning and deep learning in chili pest and disease identification. J Sci Food Agric 101(9):3582–3594

Early Risk Pregnancy Prediction Based on Machine Learning Built on Intelligent Application Using Primary Health Care Cohort Data

Eka Miranda, Meyske Kumbangsila, Mediana Aryuni, Richard, Alfi Yusrotis Zakiyyah, and Albert Verasius Dian Sano

Abstract Early detection has already reduced pregnancy risk, complications, emergency situations, and also maternal mortality cases. Our study's goal was to build on the intelligent application for early risk pregnancy prediction based on machine learning. We examined 997 patient data and 114 attributes from the electronic medical records on primary health care cohort data from the ENA System of the Sawah Besar Primary Health Care. Subsequently, eight attributes were chosen based on the Indonesian Ministry of Health, Maternal and Child Health Handbook, and medical doctor-supervised as classifier attributes. Machine learning and Knowledge Discovery from Data (KDD) technique was also applied to build an intelligent prediction in this work. In addition, we investigated the decision tree C4.5, random forest, and naive bayes algorithms for seeing which one was the right match for our application. The accuracy values for decision tree C4.5, random forest, and naive bayes were 98.01, 98.51, and 68.81%, respectively. On most accuracy measures, the random forest algorithm exceeded the decision tree C4.5 and the naive bayes algorithm. As a consequence, we employed random forest to build the web-based application. Additionally, all three algorithms obtained AUCs ranging from 0.95 to 0.99, indicating perfect prediction accuracy. Our study's contribution was to pave the way for machine learning potential in intelligent applications for early risk pregnancy prediction. In conclusion, we successfully developed an intelligent application for risk pregnancy prediction based

E. Miranda (✉) · M. Aryuni · Richard
Information Systems Department, School of Information Systems, Bina Nusantara University, Jakarta 11480, Indonesia
e-mail: ekamiranda@binus.ac.id

M. Kumbangsila
Sawah Besar Community Health Service, Jakarta, Indonesia

A. Y. Zakiyyah
Mathematics Department, School of Computer Science, Bina Nusantara University, Jakarta 11480, Indonesia

A. V. D. Sano
Computer Science Department, School of Computer Science, Bina Nusantara University, Jakarta 11480, Indonesia

T. Triwiyanto et al. (eds.), *Proceeding of the 3rd International Conference on Electronics, Biomedical Engineering, and Health Informatics*, Lecture Notes in Electrical Engineering 1008, https://doi.org/10.1007/978-981-99-0248-4_11

on machine learning and revealed potential implications in providing self-checking and early detection of pregnancy risk based on machine learning.

Keywords Decision tree C4.5 · Random forest · Naïve Bayes · Knowledge discovery from data · Risk of pregnancy

1 Introduction

In 2017, the WHO reported an unacceptably high maternal mortality rate, with approximately 295,000 women dying after or during pregnancy, including during childbirth. Every day in 2017, approximately 810 women died due to preventable causes related to pregnancy and childbirth [1]. Maternal death is defined as a woman dying during pregnancy or death within 42 days of giving childbirth as just a consequence of the pregnancy or treatment, not as a result of an accident or injury [2]. The maternal mortality rate in Indonesia reached 359 per 100,000 live births in 2012, according to the Indonesian Demographic and Health Survey (IDHS) [3].

Based on the 2018 Sampling Registration System (SRS) data, the Ministry of Health of the Republic of Indonesia reported nearly 76% of maternal mortality occurred during and after pregnancy and childbirth, 24% occurred during pregnancy, 36% occurred during childbirth, and 40% occurred after childbirth [4]. Maternal mortality was caused by some combination of factors during the pre-pregnancy phase, namely anemic condition, obesity, syphilis, hepatitis B, and HIV. During pregnancy, the mother may experience various complications, such as hypertension, hemorrhage, anemia, diabetes, infections, heart disease, and other causes. Additionally, during the Covid-19 pandemic, the maternal mortality rate increased [4]. Early detection has already reduced pregnancy risk, complications, emergency situations, and also maternal mortality cases. Antenatal Care (ANC) examinations and medical testing for blood sugar, hemoglobin, weight, height, and urine protein can be used to monitor pregnancy health [5]. Self-checking tool is possible action by using intelligent tools as a couple of medical checking by a doctor. An intelligent prediction model has already been constructed based on a machine learning approach. This model was trained and tested using electronic medical records in this way. For many cases, an intelligent prediction model such as random forest, decision tree C4.5, naïve bayes, AdaBoost, and KNN in the medical field has already been developed [6–10]. Research by Kim [6] has already developed a machine learning approach for active vaccine safety monitoring, but only the model and not the application. Uddin [7] has already performed a comparative performance analysis of the KNN algorithm and its various variations for disease prediction. They revealed the potential use of KNN and its variants for disease prediction but did not develop a model or application for a specific purpose. Machine learning has already been employed to predict the risk of stillbirth and preterm pregnancy by Koivu [8]. The model was constructed using algorithms such as logistic regression, an artificial neural network, and a gradient boosting decision tree. However, they merely created the model and did not develop the application. Another research has already been reported by Amit [9]. Using machine learning, they estimated the risk of postpartum depression from electronic health records. They constructed the machine learning model but not the application. Barbounaki [10] has already revealed intelligent systems in obstetrics and midwifery based on machine learning. However, they did not conclude the research with application development.

Further research must be conducted to fully leverage machine learning's viable solution. There was a research gap found in the previous research. Previous research mostly focused on machine learning experiments but only a few explained machine learning as an intelligent application. Therefore, our study filled the gap. Our study goal was to build on an intelligent application based on machine learning for early risk pregnancy prediction. The intelligent application paved the way for potential implications in providing self-checking and early detection of pregnancy risk based on machine learning. Pregnant women can use our application to check their own pregnancy and avoid serious risks. In this study, three machine learning algorithms have been observed: decision tree C4.5, random forest classification, and naive bayes. Afterward, the prominent algorithm in the form of accuracy measures was used in the application, and it was embedded into the website of Sawah Besar's primary health care. To complete this study, we proposed the research questions:

R1: For prediction, we employed eight classifier attributes. Which attributes were the most important for prediction?

R2: Which algorithm was the most prominent in terms of accuracy measures for predicting the risk of pregnancy?

R3: How was a prediction model employed in the development of an intelligent application for predicting pregnancy risk?

2 Methodology

2.1 Data

During 2020 and 2021, dataset was collected from the cohort of pregnant women in the electronic medical record on primary health care cohort data from the ENA System (Primary Health Care Hospital Information System) of the Sawah Besar Primary Health Care. The dataset consists of 997 patient data and 114 attributes. Subsequently, the primary attributes were evaluated based on medical doctor-supervised and standards for predicting pregnancy risk. The attributes were (eight attributes): Parity (number of previous pregnancy), LILA (upper arm circle) (cm), Hb (gr/dl), Urine Protein (+/−), Blood Sugar, Syphilis (+/−), Hepatitis B (+/−), and VCT for HIV status (+/−). Afterward, the intelligent application in this study investigated and predicted the patient risk prediction classes, namely: Pregnancy with risk or Pregnancy without risk class.

2.2 Study Design

Machine learning and Knowledge Discovery from Data (KDD) steps were also used to develop the intelligent prediction. Data cleaning and integration, data selection and transformation, data mining, evaluation, and presentation all were steps inside the KDD process [11].

This research method involved six steps: (1) Problem definition. This study developed an intelligent prediction model for predicting pregnancy risk using a machine learning approach. This model and application could also be used to perform self-detection as the first step toward further medical intervention, (2) Literature study. This step involved examining medical documents and also machine learning algorithms, (3) Data collection. Data was gathered from the pregnant women cohort data in the ENA System of the Sawah Besar Primary Health Care, (4) Data pre-processing. Data cleaning and pre-processing were part of this step. The data was cleaned by examining duplicate and incomplete data, (5) Development of prediction model. The prediction model was built using machine learning algorithms such as decision tree C4.5, random forest classification, and naive bayes, (6) Implementation of the prediction model in the application. The accuracy value for each algorithm was examined using the confusion matrix, and the application was constructed using the algorithm with the highest accuracy value. Figure 1 illustrates the research method.

2.3 Feature Variables

Feature variables were selected based on medical doctor-supervised and The Ministry of Health the Republic of Indonesia, Maternal and Child Health Handbook [12]. Table 1 displays an explanation of the variables and the threshold value.

2.4 Machine Learning Algorithm

We investigated machine learning algorithms such as decision tree C4.5, random forest classification, and naive bayes in order to construct an intelligent prediction model.

C4.5 Decision Tree. C4.5 is a decision tree generating algorithm. C4.5's decision trees can be used for classification. The C4.5 decision tree step covered several tasks [11]: (1) Generate a decision tree by using the data partition's training tuples, (2) Partition. Data partition D is a set of training tuples and the class labels that go along with them, (3) describe the attribute. The set of candidate attributes is denoted by the attribute list, and (4) the attribute selection technique is a method for finding the splitting criterion that best splits data tuples into individual classes. The prediction model was evaluated by counting the number of correct predictions and the number

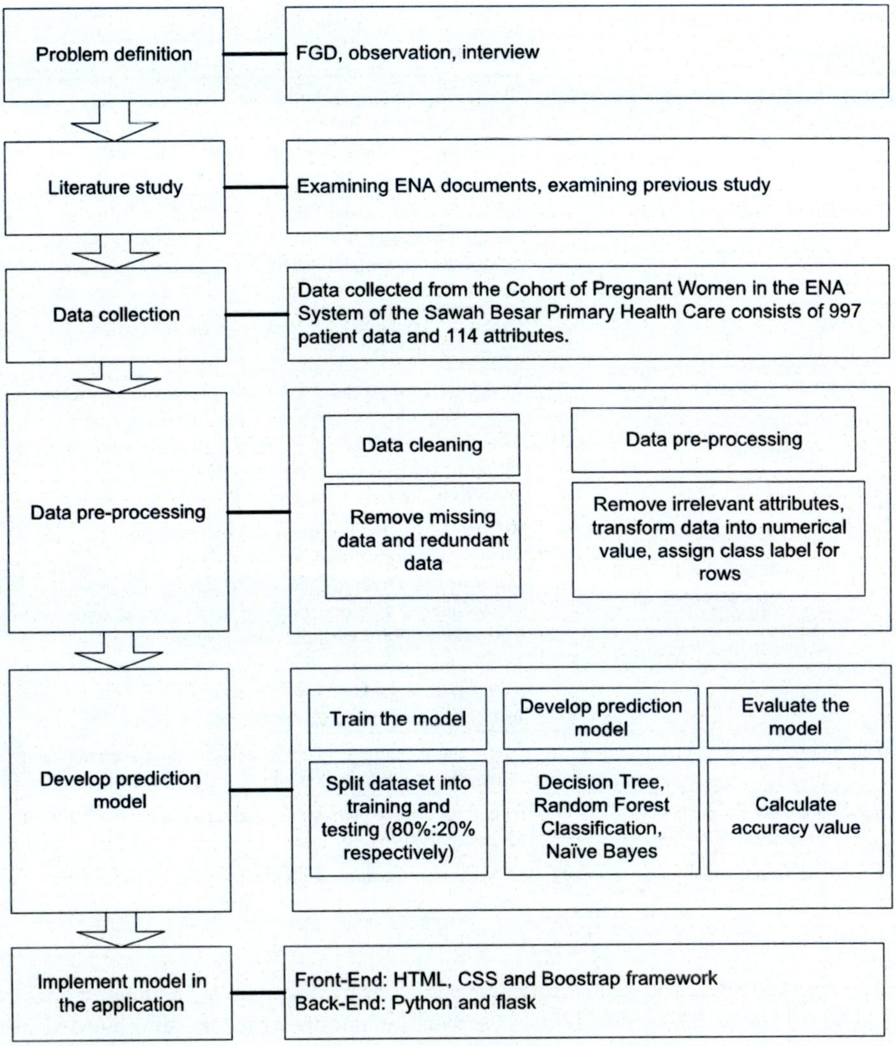

Fig. 1 Research method

of incorrect predictions for each class [13]. The splitting rules were established by attribute selection measures. Let node N represents or hold the partition D tuple. As the splitting attribute for node N, the attribute with the highest information gain is chosen. Entropy is the expected info needed to classify a tuple in D [11] based on Eq. (1).

$$\text{Gain}(D, A) = \sum_{i=1}^{n} (-p_i) * \log_2 p_i - \sum_{i=1}^{n} \frac{(D_i)}{|D|} * \text{Entropy}(D_i) \quad (1)$$

Table 1 Data explanatory [12]

Attribute	Explanation
Parity (number of previous pregnancy)	Pregnant women who give birth frequently, more than 4 times, get a higher chance of experiencing a high-risk pregnancy. During pregnancy, childbirth, and postpartum, the risk was found
LILA (upper arm circle) (cm)	LILA has a standard value = 23.5 cm. A pregnant woman with LILA less than 23.5 appears to indicate malnutrition, which also has a negative impact on either the mother or the fetus
Hb (gr/dl)	Anemia is diagnosed in pregnant women when the hemoglobin level is less than 11 gr/dl
Urine protein (+/−)	Pregnant women that have urine protein levels of far more than 300 mg every 24 h have an abnormal condition. A high level of protein in urine could lead to complications in a pregnant woman, such as preeclampsia
Blood sugar (mg/dl)	Diabetes-affected pregnant women experienced chronically high blood sugar levels during pregnancy (Gestational Diabetes Mellitus (GDM)). Diabetes is characterized as blood glucose levels greater than 200 mg/dl (along with classic hyperglycemia symptoms) or fasting blood glucose levels greater than 126 mg/dl or glucose levels greater than 200 mg/dl 2 h after OGTT or HbA1C values greater than 6.5%
Syphilis (+/−)	In pregnant women, syphilis can cause miscarriage, stillbirth, or the baby's death shortly after birth
Hepatitis B (+/−)	The detection of HBsAg (+) indicated the possibility of Hepatitis B transmission
VCT for HIV status (+/−)	HIV (human immunodeficiency virus) is a virus that attacks the body's immune system

where P_i represents the probability that an arbitrary tuple in D belongs to class C_i. The entropy of D, or info (D), is the average amount of information needed to identify the class label of a tuple in D. Based on the class label attribute, expected information subsequently classifies a tuple from D [14] Gain (A) (Eq. 1) in denotes that we want to split the attribute A that would produce the best classification [11]. Several previous studies have revealed the decision tree's accomplishment in the medical field [15, 16].

Random Forest. The random forest is composed of several individual decision trees and operates like an ensemble. Moreover, this algorithm outperforms the decision tree algorithm [17]. Previous researchers in the medical field have already investigated random forest machine learning [18, 19].

Naive Bayes. The naive bayes classifier works on Bayes Theorem Eq. (2).

$$Pr(G = G_i|X) = \frac{Pr(X|G = G_i).Pr(G = G_i)}{Pr(X)} \quad (2)$$

where $G = G_i$ denotes the classes that could be attributed to a data point X. Or put this another way, we compute the posterior probability $Pr(G = G_i|X)$ using prior knowledge with observed data.20. The researchers have been attracted to a machine learning classifier naive bayes for the construction of a health prediction model [20, 21]. Table 2 displays a list of machine learning in pregnancy and childbirth application.

3 Results

3.1 Data Pre-processing

Data pre-processing involved both data cleaning and data pre-processing. Data cleaning was initiated by checking empty data and redundant data. The rows which contained empty data for one or more attributes would be deleted. As a result, we removed only one row and found no redundant data. Data pre-processing was initiated by identifying the data; only numerical data can be processed by a machine learning algorithm. Consequently, we converted categorical data to numerical data. We converted Urine Protein (+/−), Syphilis (+/−), Hepatitis B (+/−), and VCT for HIV status (+/−) into positive integer value (1) or negative integer value (−1). Finally, we converted class prediction to predict patient data into integer values, namely: Pregnancy with risk converted into (−1) and Pregnancy without risk converted into (1).

3.2 Model Prediction

Decision Tree C4.5 Classifier. The entropy for the prospective split was utilized to evaluate attribute selection for the decision tree. The R1 focused on the most important attributes for prediction. The best split was a significant attribute with the highest entropy, namely Hb (gr/dl), LILA, and urine protein. Figure 2 displays the important attributes based on entropy.

A summary of the prediction results was shown in the form of a confusion matrix. The number of correct and incorrect predictions was summarized with count values and grouped by class. Furthermore, classification performance measures were calculated based on a confusion matrix. Accuracy, Precision, F-score, and Recall were the measures. In Eqs. (3), (4), (5), and (6), the formula for each accuracy value was presented [7]. Accuracy is defined as the ratio of True (positive and negative) predictions to overall data. Precision is defined as the percentage of truly positive predictions

Table 2 Compilation of machine learning techniques in pregnancy and childbirth application

Health application	Machine learning technique	Result and limitation
Preterm pregnancies	Ensemble learning [8]	Robustness in the repeatable performance of the models The information spanned multiple years, locations, and hospitals. In addition, the amount of inaccurate data entries should be decreased to negligible proportions
Early pregnancy loss	Logistic regression (LR), support vector machine (SVM), decision tree (DT), back propagation neural network (BNN), XGBoost and random forest (RF) [22]	Random forest attained a higher prediction accuracy rate Only one medical center provided data. To boost performance and dependability, multicenter datasets and external verification are being investigated
Covid-19 infected pregnant	Random forest, C5.0, and deep neural networks [23]	The classification accuracy range from 64.86 to 97.3%
Macrosomia	Random forest, logistic regression [24]	The sensitivity, specificity, and area under the curve for the random forest model were 91.7, 91.7, and 95.3%, accordingly, and 56.2, 82.6, and 72.0% for the logistic regression model The ultrasound has a sensitivity and specificity of 29.6 and 97.5%, correspondingly
Cardiovascular in women with preeclampsia	Logistic regression, SVM, Naïve Bayes, XGBoost, random forest [25]	The random forest algorithm showed the best performance. Systolic blood pressure, urea nitrogen, neutrophil count, glucose, and D-Dimer were the most important variables in the random forest algorithm. The study was performed in a single place, and the missing data were estimated in this study. The study did a good job of excluding negative patients but accomplished a slightly poor job of distinguishing positive patients

(continued)

Table 2 (continued)

Health application	Machine learning technique	Result and limitation
Postpartum depression	Support vector machine (SVM) and random forest [26]	The model based on SVM and RF performed the best in terms of prediction (sensitivity = 0.69, area under the curve = 0.78) The model's applicability may have been impacted by the 50% loss of data and the small sample size. A larger number of possible classifiers would have been helpful
Fetal birth weight	Convolutional neuron networks (CNN), random forest (RF), linear-regression, support vector regression (SVR), back propagation neural Network (BPNN), and the hybrid-LSTM [27]	Most of the machine learning models beat the empirical formula
Pregnant women with congenital heart disease	Support vector machine, random forest, AdaBoost, decision tree, k-nearest neighbor, Naïve Bayes, and multilayer perceptron [28]	The maternal model had an accuracy of 0.76–0.86 in the development cohort and 0.72–0.86 in the validation cohort, according to the algorithms Two reliable predictive accuracy prenatal assessment models for mothers and offspring were successfully established A potential bias in the development cohort due to the small sample size
Biopsychosocial factors and type of childbirth	C4.5 decision tree [29]	High accuracy 8% sample loss was found. To solve this problem, we had to call the mothers on the phone to gather information about the childbirth process, which impacted the accuracy of the information
Uterine activity outside pregnancy	Support vector machine (SVM), K-nearest neighbors (KNN), Gaussian mixture model (GMM), and Naive Bayes [30]	The SVM classifier performed best on accuracy The small dataset includes only 7 patients and 24 viable data

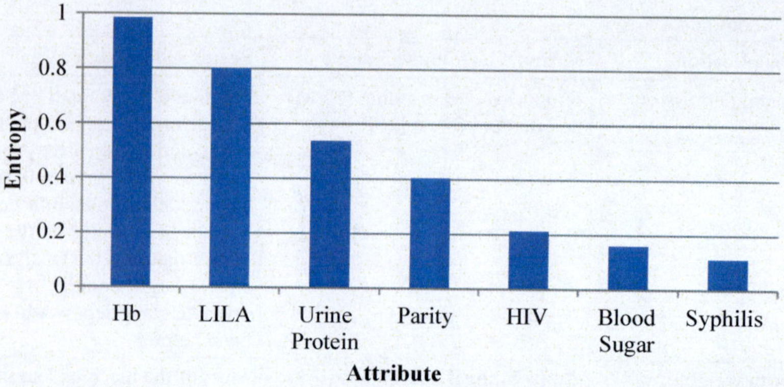

Fig. 2 Important attributes based on entropy. The y-axis shows entropy value for each attribute

to overall positive expected results. Recall is defined as the percentage of totally positive predictions to totally positive overall data. The F1-Score is a weighted average of precision and recall [7]. True Positive (TP) is the number of positive data correctly classified by the model. True Negative (TN) is the number of negative data classified correctly by the model. False Negative (FN) is the negative outcome of data that the model incorrectly classified. False Positive (FP) is the number of positive data that the model incorrectly classified [7]. Based on Eqs. (3), (4), (5), and (6) accuracy, precision, and recall are calculated.

$$\text{Accuracy} = \frac{(TP + TN)}{(TP + TN + FP + FN)} \tag{3}$$

$$\text{Precision} = \frac{(TP)}{(FP + TP)} \tag{4}$$

$$\text{Recall} = \frac{(TP)}{(FN + TP)} \tag{5}$$

$$F1 - \text{Score} = 2 \times \frac{(\text{precision} \times \text{recall})}{(\text{precision} + \text{recall})} \tag{6}$$

Table 3 represents the confusion matrix for both the training and testing data for decision tree C4.5, random forest, and naïve bayes. The confusion matrix displays and compares the actual or predicted model value to generate evaluation metrics such as Accuracy (accuracy), Precision, Recall, and F1-Score or F-Measure. Since pregnancy without risk indicated a positive condition and pregnancy with risk indicated a negative condition, we classified the pregnancy without risk class label as true positive and the pregnancy with risk class label as true negative for the confusion matrix. The testing data matrix revealed 84 data that actually belonged to the Pregnancy with risk class, and the C4.5 classifier model in our study predicted the data as Pregnancy with risk class as well. The matrix revealed 114 testing data that actually belong to the Pregnancy without risk class, and the C4.5 classifier model in our study predicted the data as Pregnancy with risk class for testing data as well. Table 4 presents the classification performance measures for the decision tree C4.5, random forest, and naïve bayes. The precision achieved the highest result among other measures for testing data in the performance measure for C4.5. Precision helped to visualize the machine learning model's reliability in classifying the model.

Decision Tree C4.5 Classifier. Random forests generate decision trees from randomly selected data samples, generated predictions from each tree, and then vote on the best solution. Among other measures for testing data, the performance measure for random forest demonstrated precision and achieved the highest result.

Naïve Bayes Classifier. The naive bayes classifier calculates the probability of an event in the following steps: Calculate the prior probability for the given class labels and Compute the likelihood probability for each attribute for each class. Put these numbers into the bayes formula and compute the posterior probability. Consider whether the input belongs to the higher probability class, and determine which class has a higher probability. Among other measures for testing data, the performance measure for naive bayes revealed recall achieved the highest result. The recall measure assesses the model's ability to identify positive samples. Considering the

Table 3 Confusion metric for training dataset and testing dataset: decision tree C4.5, random forest, Naïve Bayes. The numbers in the confusion matrix show the amount of data used

		Predicted pregnancy with risk		Predicted pregnancy without risk	
		Predicted pregnancy with risk	Predicted pregnancy without risk	Predicted pregnancy with risk	Predicted pregnancy without risk
Decision tree	Actual pregnancy with risk	346 (TN)	0 (FP)	84 (TN)	1 (FP)
	Actual pregnancy without risk	0 (FN)	458 (TP)	3 (FN)	114 (TP)
Random forest	Actual pregnancy with risk	84 (TN)	1 (FP)	84 (TN)	1 (FP)
	Actual pregnancy without risk	2 (FN)	115 (TP)	2 (FN)	115 (TP)
Naive Bayes	Actual pregnancy with risk	80 (TN)	266 (FP)	23 (TN)	62 (FP)
	Actual pregnancy without risk	0 (FN)	458 (TP)	1 (FN)	116 (TP)

Table 4 Accuracy, precision, f-score, and recall for decision tree C4.5, random forest, and Naïve Bayes

		Training dataset	Testing dataset
Decision tree	Accuracy (%)	100.00	98.01
	Precision (%)	100.00	99.13
	F-score (%)	100.00	98.27
	Recall (%)	100.00	97.43
Random forest	Accuracy (%)	100.00	98.51
	Precision (%)	100.00	99.13
	F-score (%)	100.00	98.71
	Recall (%)	100.00	98.29
Naïve Bayes	Accuracy (%)	66.92	68.81
	Precision (%)	63.26	65.16
	F-score (%)	77.50	78.64
	Recall (%)	100.00	99.14

high recall value, achieving more positive samples was detected. The higher the recall, the more positive samples were identified.

4 Discussion

We developed a model by working with three machine learning algorithms: decision tree C4.5, random forest, and naive bayes. The R2 was obtained using the empirical results of the three algorithms: decision tree C4.5, random forest classification, and naive bayes. Our experiment revealed that random forest gained the highest accuracy value for the testing dataset (see Table 3). Therefore, we employed random forest to build the web-based application. In some cases, accuracy was insufficient to determine a model's performance (the case of imbalanced data for example). On our classification result for decision tree C4.5, random forest, and naive bayes, we found imbalanced data (the number of TN and TP were not balanced). Therefore, we calculated another performance measure, namely AUC. When working with unbalanced data, the property was highly appealing. AUC is a useful method to summarize the test's overall diagnostic accuracy. It accepts values ranging between 0 to 1, with 0 representing a perfectly inaccurate test and 1 representing a perfectly accurate test [31]. The AUC for the three algorithms ranged from 0.95 to 0.99, indicating accurate prediction.

Following that, we developed an intelligent application on a random forest and integrated it into Sawah Besar's primary healthcare website. The R3 focused on how to implement an algorithm into an intelligent prediction model for predicting the risk of pregnancy built on an intelligent application. Python programming language was used for back end construction, and it was supported by flask, which took action to manage data flow. Furthermore, as part of the website's UI/UX, the front end was constructed with HTML, CSS, and the Bootstrap framework. The application also displayed the prediction result as well as the classifier attributes. An intelligent model was developed to predict the risk of pregnancy into two classes: pregnancy with risk and pregnancy without risk. Classifier attributes were chosen based on medical doctor-supervised and the Maternal and Child Health Handbook published by the Ministry of Health of the Republic of Indonesia [12]. Parity (number of previous pregnancies), LILA (upper arm circle) (cm), Hb (gr/dl), Urine Protein (+/−), Blood Sugar, Syphilis (+/−), Hepatitis B (+/−), and VCT for HIV status (+/−) were chosen as compulsory predictor attributes, while body weight and body height were optional attributes. If all compulsory attributes met the threshold value, then the prediction result returned to Pregnancy without Risk; on the other hand, if one of the compulsory attributes did not meet the threshold value, then the prediction result returned to Pregnancy with Risk. The red color on the classifier attributes indicated a value that exceeded the threshold. Figure 3 demonstrates the application's visualization.

In comparison to Koivu's [8] previous study, we successfully developed not only the machine learning model prediction, but also the intelligent application for risk pregnancy prediction based on the model. The proposed study was novel in that it used machine learning to construct an intelligent model as a non-invasive approach by analyzing electronic medical record data to design an intelligent model and subsequently used the model in a web-based application to predict the risk of pregnancy. Our study revealed the novelty, namely the theoretical and clinical significance accrued across these aims, which included (1) The data based on electronic medical records on the ENA System of the Sawah Besar Primary Health Care, (2) The development and testing of an intelligent prediction model based on machine learning, KDD, medical doctor-supervised and Maternal and Child Health Handbook Ministry of Health The Republic of Indonesia, (3) Evaluation of each algorithm for prediction model calculated based on confusion matrix to determine prominent algorithm, and (4) Prediction application for predicting risk of pregnancy built on the basis of the prominent algorithm. Although this study did not investigate all prediction attributes based on WHO criteria, the model and application would be important because they have been constructed using actual data and supervised by a medical doctor. As a result, the practical contribution of this research on how to develop an intelligent model and integrate it into an intelligent application based on actual data has been presented. We enhanced scientific knowledge in the field of pregnancy risk prediction through the use of machine learning for pregnancy risk prediction. Furthermore, the social implication of the study was promising since it offered self-checking and early detection for pregnant women as couples for medical tests. Since primary health care has played an important role in providing the best maternal and child health care, it must be supported by e-health technology to ensure data accuracy [32]. In contrast to the previous study by [26, 30], which used a small number of predictive factors and a small sample size, our study used a large number of predictive factors (114 candidates' predictive attributes and 8 predictive attributes selected) and a large sample size (997 patient data). Beyond the positive impact, we found limitations in our research for attribute classifiers used. We only examined 8 mandatory attributes (see

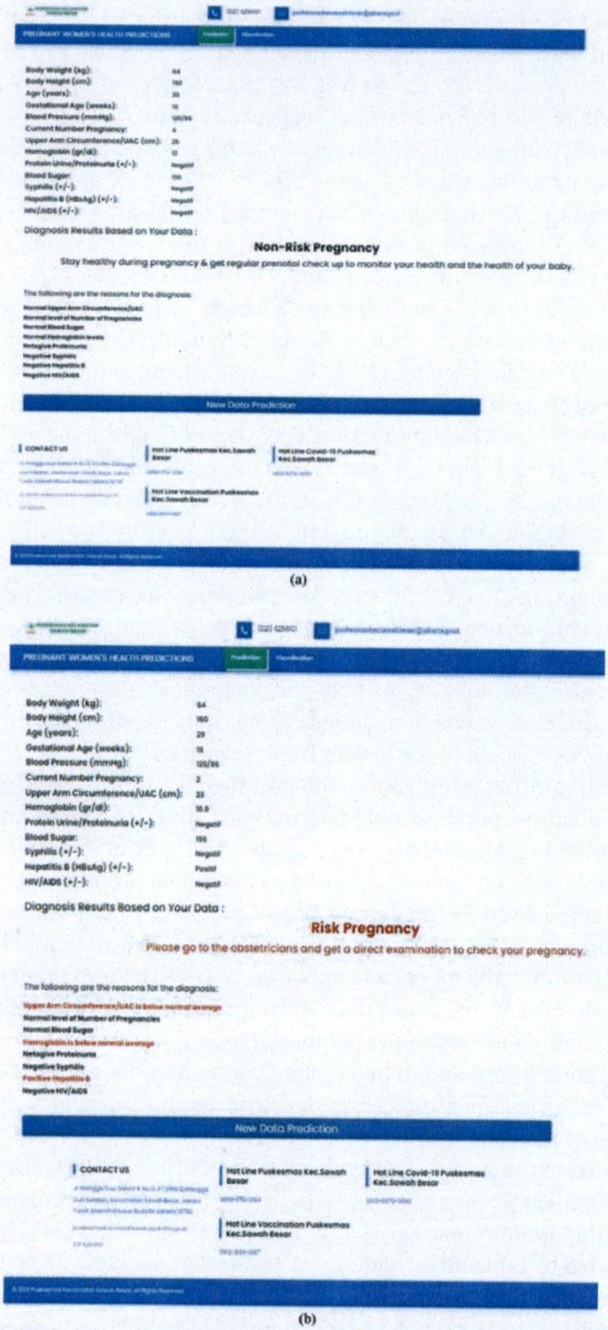

Fig. 3 Visualization of the application intelligent prediction model for predicting risk level of pregnancy **a** No-risk pregnancy prediction, **b** Risk pregnancy prediction

Table 1) and did not look at all of the WHO criteria for antenatal care for a positive pregnancy experience; also, data were collected from only one primary health care.

5 Conclusion

The study goal was to build on an intelligent application based on machine learning for early risk pregnancy prediction. Our study, being of a revealing nature, raises a number of opportunities for future research both in terms of machine learning techniques and healthcare application development for pregnancy risk prediction. Hb (gr/dl), LILA, and urine protein were the most important attributes for prediction based on entropy value. The accuracy was 98.01, 98.51, and 68.81%, respectively, for decision tree, random forest, and naïve bayes. Our experiment revealed that random forest gained the highest accuracy value for the testing dataset. More research will be necessary to refine our findings. Collecting data from multi-center datasets, completing prediction attributes based on WHO criteria for prediction [33], and investigating other machine learning techniques to increase performance and reliability are some of the challenges for future work.

Acknowledgements This work is supported by Research and Technology Transfer Office, Bina Nusantara University as a part of BINUS Research Untuk Nusantara (BRUN) Research Grant entitled "Web-Based Application for Predicting the Health of Pregnant Women and Toddler Nutrition Using a Data Mining Approach" with contract number: No: 064/VR.RTT/IV/2022 and contract date: 8 April 2022. We also appreciate the support provided by Puskesmas Kecamatan Sawah Besar, Jakarta Pusat, who helped our students (Ivan Wijaya, Caroline Losari, and Gloriana Chalsy Roman) in the research process.

References

1. World Health Organization (WHO) https://www.who.int/news-room/fact-sheets/detail/maternal-mortality. Accessed 2022/4/26
2. Data and information Center the Ministry of Health the Republic of Indonesia. https://www.kemkes.go.id/article/view/15021800009/situasi-kesehatan-ibu.html. Accessed 2022/4/26
3. Data and information Center The Ministry of Health the Republic of Indonesia. https://pusdatin.kemkes.go.id/resources/download/pusdatin/profil-kesehatanindonesia/PROFIL_KESEHATAN_2018_1.pdf. Accessed 2022/4/26
4. The Ministry of Health the Republic of Indonesia https://sehatnegeriku.kemkes.go.id/baca/umum/20210914/3738491/kemenkes-perkuat-upaya-penyelamatan-ibu-dan-bayi/. Accessed 2022/4/26
5. The United Nations Children's Fund (UNICEF) https://data.unicef.org/topic/maternal-health/antenatal-care/. Accessed 2022/4/26
6. Kim Y, Jang JH, Park N, Jeong NY, Lim E, Kim S et al (2021) Machine learning approach for active vaccine safety monitoring. J Korean Med Sci 36(31):1–13
7. Uddin S, Haque I, Lu H, Moni MA, Gide E (2021) Comparative performance analysis of K-Nearest Neighbour (KNN) algorithm and its different variants for disease prediction. Sci Rep 12:1–11

8. Koivu A, Sairanen M (2020) Predicting risk of stillbirth and preterm pregnancies with machine learning. Health Inform Sci Syst 8(1):1–12
9. Amit G, Girshovitz I, Marcus K, Zhang Y, Pathak J, Bar V et al (2021) Estimation of postpartum depression risk from electronic health records using machine learning. BMC Pregnancy Childbirth 21:1–10
10. Barbounaki S, Vivilaki VG (2021) Intelligent systems in obstetrics and midwifery: applications of machine learning. Eur J Midwifery 5:1–12
11. Han J, Kamber M, Pei Y Data mining: concepts and technique, 3rd edn. Morgan Kaufman, San Francisco (2012)
12. The Ministry of Health the Republic of Indonesia. https://kesga.kemkes.go.id/assets/file/pedoman/BUKU%20KIA%20REVISI%202021%20LENGKAP.pdf. Accessed 2016/11/21
13. Chern CC, Chen YJ, Hsiao B (2019) Decision tree-based classifier in providing telehealth service. BMC Med Inform Decis Mak 19:1–15
14. He Q, Xu Z, Li S, Li R, Zhang S, Wang N (2019) Novel entropy and rotation forest-based credal decision tree classifier for landslide susceptibility modeling. Entropy 21(2):1–24
15. Wiharto W, Kusnanto H, Herianto H (2016) Interpretation of clinical data based on C4.5 algorithm for the diagnosis of coronary heart disease. Healthc Inform Res 22(3):186–195
16. Ryu KJ, Yi KW, Kim YJ, Shin JH, Hur JY, Kim T et al (2021) Machine learning approaches to identify factors associated with women's vasomotor symptoms using general hospital data. J Korean Med Sci 36(17):1–11
17. Han S, Kim H (2019) On the optimal size of candidate feature set in random forest. Appl Sci 9(5):1–13
18. Byeon H (2020) Is the random forest algorithm suitable for predicting Parkinson's disease with mild cognitive impairment out of Parkinson's disease with normal cognition? Int J Environ Res Public Health 17(7):1–14
19. Lee J (2017) Patient-specific predictive modeling using random forests: an observational study for the critically Ill. JMIR Med Inform 5(1):1–12
20. Wood A, Shpilrain V, Najarian K, Kahrobaei D (2019) Private naive bayes classification of personal biomedical data: application in cancer data analysis. Comput Biol Med 105:144–150
21. Gibbons KS, Chang AMZ, Ma RCW, Tam WH, Catalano PM, Sacks DA et al (2021) Prediction of large for gestational age infants in relation to hyperglycemia in pregnancy—a comparison of statistical models. Diabetes Res Clin Pract 78:1–8
22. Liu L, Jiao Y, Li X, Ouyang Y, Shi D (2020) Machine learning algorithms to predict early pregnancy loss after in vitro fertilization-embryo transfer with fetal heart rate as a strong predictor. Comput Methods Programs Biomed 196:1–8
23. Guleken Z, Jakubczyk P, Wiesław P, Krzysztof P, Bulut H, Öten E et al (2022) Characterization of covid-19 infected pregnant women sera using laboratory indexes, vibrational spectroscopy, and machine learning classifications. Talata 237:1–10
24. Wang F, Wang Y, Ji X, Wang Z (2022) Effective macrosomia prediction using random forest algorithm. Int J Environ Res Public Health 19(6):1–10
25. Salhi DE, Tari A, Kechadi MT (2021) Using machine learning for heart disease prediction. In: Senouci MR, Boudaren MEY, Sebbak F, Mataoui M (eds) Conference 2020, LNNS, vol 199. Springer, Heidelberg, pp 70–81
26. Zhang W, Liu H, Silenvio VMB, Qiu P, Gong W (2020) Machine learning models for the prediction of postpartum depression: application and comparison based on a cohort study. JMIR Med Inform 8(4):1–13
27. Tao J, Yuan Z, Sun L, Yui K, Zhang Z (2021) Fetal birth weight prediction with measured data by a temporal machine learning method. BMC Med Inform Decis Mak 21:1–10
28. Chu R, Chen W, Song G, Yao S, Xie L, Song L et al (2020) Predicting the risk of adverse events in pregnant women with congenital heart disease. J Am Heart Assoc 9(14):1–23
29. Hajimirzaie SS, Tehranian N, Mousavi SA, Golabpour A, Mirzaii M, Keramat A et al (2021) Predicting the relation between biopsychosocial factors and type of childbirth using the decision tree method: a cohort study. Iran J Med Sci 46(6):437–443

30. Raisa JF, Kaiser MS, Mahmud M (2022) A machine learning approach for early detection of postpartum depression in Bangladesh. In: Mahmud M, He J, Vassanelli S, van Zundert A, Zhong N (eds) Conference 2022, LNAI, vol 13406. Springer, Heidelberg, pp 241–252
31. Verbakel JY, Steyerberg EW, Uno H, Cock BD, Wynantys L, Collin GS et al (2020) ROC curves for clinical prediction models part 1. ROC plots showed no added value above the AUC when evaluating the performance of clinical prediction models. J Clin Epidemiol 126:207–216
32. Ansariadi A, Manderson L (2015) Antenatal care and women's birthing decisions in an Indonesian setting: does location matter? Rural Remote Health 15(2):1–17
33. World Health Organization (WHO) https://www.who.int/publications/i/item/9789241549912. Accessed 2016/11/21

Uretery Stone Detection with CT Scan Image Contrast Analysis

Nanang Sulaksono, Kusworo Adi, Rizal Isnanto, and Budi Warsito

Abstract Kidney disease is one of the vital organs that prevent the buildup of waste and control the fluid balance in the body in order to maintain the composition of the blood. In terms of public health, chronic kidney disease (CKD) is a big problem. One method for determining kidney function is the CT scan, the need for proper stone assessment to assist doctors in diagnosing. This study's goal was to evaluate the effectiveness of stone contrast in aiding the accurate diagnosis of urinary tract stones. This research method uses experiments using CT scan images of the urinary tract with various thicknesses of 1–3 slices, and the images used are primary data taken directly at the hospital as many as 21 images. The study was conducted by assessing the area of stones and ureters using the MATLAB program to perform a contrast analysis to determine the optimal image and detect the presence of stones in the ureter. There was a noticeable difference in the histogram results after utilizing the MATLAB application to perform gram historical analysis on CT scan pictures of stones and ureters, which was dominated by the gray level of the ureteral organ, which was 29.298 and dominated by perfect white color in the ureter organ stone, which is 65,535. The outcomes of the substantial difference in the contrast value show this, which is 36,237. The use of analysis of the contrast value of ureteral stone images using MATLAB can help in diagnosing the urinary tract.

Keywords CT scan · Stones · Ureter · MATLAB · Contrast analysis

N. Sulaksono (✉)
Doctoral Program of Information System, School of Postgraduate Studies, Diponegoro University, Semarang, Indonesia
e-mail: nanangsulaksono@poltekkes-smg.ac.id

Poltekkes Kemenkes Semarang, Semarang, Indonesia

K. Adi · R. Isnanto · B. Warsito
School of Postgraduate Studies, Diponegoro University, Semarang, Indonesia

T. Triwiyanto et al. (eds.), *Proceeding of the 3rd International Conference on Electronics, Biomedical Engineering, and Health Informatics*, Lecture Notes in Electrical Engineering 1008, https://doi.org/10.1007/978-981-99-0248-4_12

1 Introduction

The kidneys are crucial organs that prevent waste from building up and regulate the body's fluid balance in order to maintain blood composition [5, 11, 13]. The artificial intelligence (AI)-based systems are now starting to be used in medical imaging to assist wizard assessments for diagnostic information [8, 9], such as assessing urinary tract lesions [26, 28], developing medical image segmentation [8], detecting COVID-19 with Non-CT Scan Contrast [17], abdominal abnormalities [21], liver tumors [10], malignancy of musculoskeletal disease [12], and coronary artery abnormalities in detecting calcium score [25], and CCTA interpretation can assess the presence of stenosis [6].

One of the medical imaging currently using AI is in establishing abnormalities in the urinary tract. Kidney disease occurs in anyone, regardless of age and gender, the significance of renal illness early diagnosis. A person's death may result from untreated chronic renal disease. Artificial intelligence models can be applied in various fields using medical images [24] and can be applied to evaluate abnormalities in CT Scan modalities and greatly assist radiology doctors in confirming the diagnosis of abnormalities, the use of artificial intelligence in detecting kidney stones and normal conditions [2, 7, 27], and assess the composition of the type of kidney stone [3, 29], described in Table 1.

Selection of the right examination modality can detect the presence of stones in the urinary tract (Urolithiasis) [4]. Non-Contrast Computed Tomography (NCCT) is used to detect diseases of the urinary tract. The NCCT has emerged as the go-to imaging technique for identifying sudden onset low back pain. Sensitivity and specificity of low-dose NCCT were 93.1 and 96.6%, respectively, for detection. NCCT is the gold standard for detecting and characterizing urolithiasis with sensitivity and specification close to 100% because urolithiasis has sufficient density to describe [22].

Table 1 Research in detecting stones in the urinary tract

Researcher name and year	Method	Detection
Yildrim et al., 2021 [27]	XResNet-50	Stone, normal
Baygin M et al., 2022 [2]	ExDark19	Stone, normal
Fitri LA et al., 2020 [7]	Convolutional neural network (CNN)	Stone type
Black KM et al., 2020 [3]	Convolutional neural network (CNN), ResNet-101 (ResNet, Microsoft)	Stone composition
Shkolyar et al., 2019 [23]	CystoNet	Bladder cancer
Ke Yan et al., 2018 [26]	CADe/CADx	Assessing lesions of the urinary tract
Alnazer Israa et al., 2021[1]	Deep learning	Detect chronic kidney
Rice Patrick et al., 2021 [20]	Neural networks (ANN)	Shockwave lithotripsy (SWL)

Currently, in the field of radiology, there are still problems faced in establishing a diagnosis, including the following. It takes time to perform image processing in reconstructing the CT Scan modality and a long time to determine stones in the ureter, so a MATLAB device is needed to analyze images to help accurately assess abnormalities in the diagnosis [22]. This study aims to prove that the use of urinary tract image contrast analysis can produce optimal images and detect stones in the ureters.

2 Materials and Methods

It is possible to obtain answers to research questions and tools for researchers to control or control numerous influential variables in a study via the use of research design. The type of research used is an experimental research design with Pretest–Posttest Control Design. The treatment group consisted of three treatment groups with the use of tracking reconstruction with variations in slice thickness 1, 2, 3, and Window abdomen.

This study uses experiments using CT scan images of the urinary tract with various thicknesses of 1, 2, 3, and Window abdomen, the images used are primary data taken directly at the hospital as many as 21 images. The study was conducted with image contrast values using the MATLAB program to perform Contrast analysis in the ureter and stone area to determine the best image and determine whether there are stones in the ureter.

Data analysis was done to look for variations between each group's MSCT pictures of the urinary tract. Prior to testing, the Shapiro–Wilk test ($n = 50$) was used to check the normality of the data. The One-Way Anova test is run followed by the Post Hoc Tukey test if the data is normally distributed ($p > 0.05$), and the Kruskal–Wallis test is run afterward followed by the Mann–Whitney test if the data is not normally distributed ($p < 0.05$). To determine the optimal image, after obtaining the best image in multivariate analysis, a contrast analysis was performed on the ureter and stone area using MATLAB programming.

3 Results and Discussion

The urinary tract tracking CT scan images used were from patients who underwent the most abdominal MSCT examinations; for most CT scan images were obtained from patients with an average age of 40 years and over [16]. Here are some images of the urinary tract's MSCT examination results with various slice thicknesses, shown in Figs. 1, 2 and 3.

The Shapiro–Wilk test was run on the results of pictures with different slice thicknesses, including 1 mm for the abdomen, 2 mm for the abdomen, and 3 mm for the abdomen, to assess the data's normalcy, showed in Table 2.

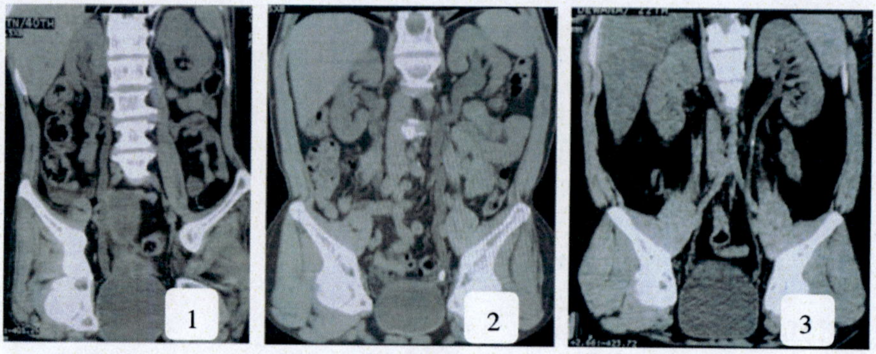

Fig. 1 (1), (2), and (3) urinary tract images with a slice thickness of 1 mm abdomen

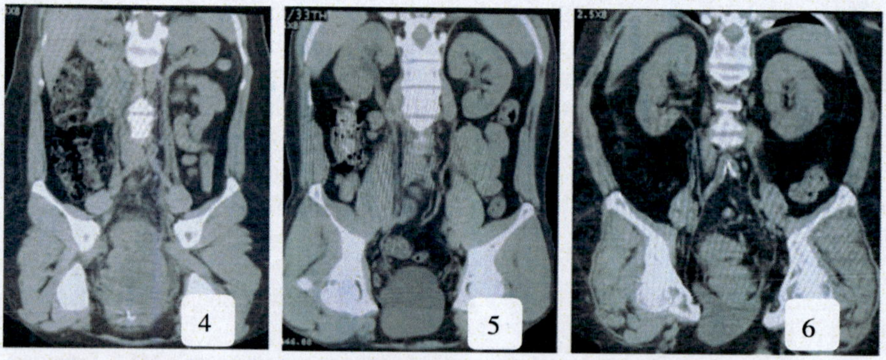

Fig. 2 (4), (5), and (6) urinary tract images with a slice thickness of 2 mm abdomen

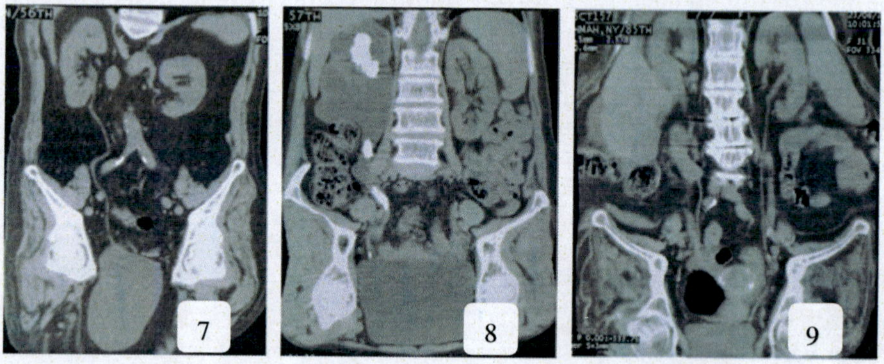

Fig. 3 (7), (8), and (9) urinary tract images with a slice thickness of 3 mm abdomen

Table 2 Results of the Shapiro–Wilk test to check the data's normality

Variable	P	Information
Pre	0,000	Not normally
Post	0,000	Not normally

Table 3 Results of the CT scan slice thickness test

Variable	Mean rank	Mean ± SD	*P*
Slice thickness 1, abdomen	9.33	16.22 ± 1.093	
Slice thickness 2, abdomen	8.33	15.67 ± 0.866	0.006
Slice thickness 3, abdomen	5.33	16.00 ± 0.707	

Table 4 Shows the analysis of the Mann–Whitney test results

Variable	X2	X3
X1	0.297	0.730
X2		0.387

Following the Shapiro–Wilk normality test, which revealed that the data acquired before and after treatment were not normally distributed ($p < 0.05$), the Kruskal–Wallis test was conducted, and Mann–Whitney analysis was then carried out. Table 3 displays the outcomes of the Kruskal–Wallis test before employing tracking.

To determine whether groups had significant differences, Table 3 shows that the findings of the MSCT image analysis of the urinary tract showed a significant difference with a *p*-value of 0.006 ($p < 0.05$) based on the Mann–Whitney test. Table 4 displays the Mann–Whitney test findings.

Table 4 shows the outcomes of the MSCT image analysis of the urinary tract following the use of tracking, showing that there is no significant difference between X1/slice thickness of 1 mm abdomen, with X2/slice thickness of 2 mm abdomen (*p*-value 0.297), X3/slice thickness 3 mm abdomen (*p*-value 0.730), and X2/slice thickness 2 mm abdomen with X3/slice thickness 3 mm abdomen (*p*-value 0.387).

Following modifications in slice thickness, the findings of the CT Scan image analysis of ureteral stones were obtained, the highest value was 16.22 which occurred in the 1 mm abdominal slice thickness. CT Scan image analysis of ureteral stones was performed using MATLAB to perform contrast on the stone and ureter area. Analyze the contrast value between the stone and the ureter to get the optimal image. In this study, the assessment of image analysis was carried out by cropping the area of the stone and ureter to obtain different contrast values. The following is an overview of the best images analyzed using the MATLAB program with a slice thickness of 1 mm abdomen. This is shown in Fig. 4.

The first cropped CT scan image is displayed in Fig. 4, and Figs. 5, 6, and 7 display the outcomes of the CT scan contrast analysis of ureteral stones using MATLAB.

A substantial difference in the histogram results, which were dominated by the gray level of the ureter organs, was found after histogram analysis of CT scan pictures of stones and ureters using the MATLAB program, which was 29.298 and dominated by perfect white color in the ureter organs stone which is 65,535. This can be seen in the results of the significant difference in contrast values, which is 36,237.

The optimal contrast value in the urinary tract between the stone and the ureter can show a significant difference in the picture [23]. This can be seen from the results of the density between the stone and the ureter so that the quality of the

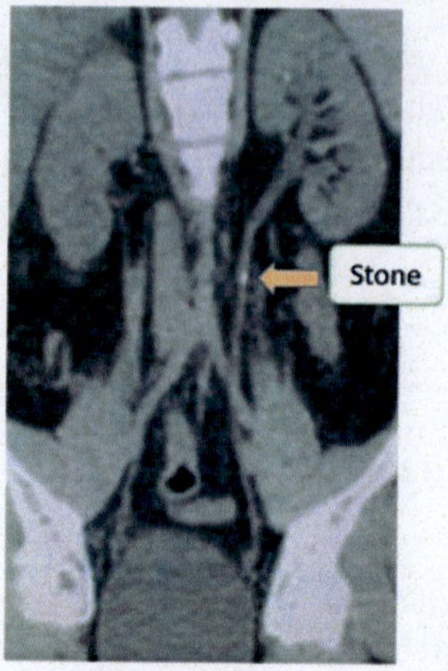

Fig. 4 The best urinary tract image with a slice thickness of 1 mm and abdomen

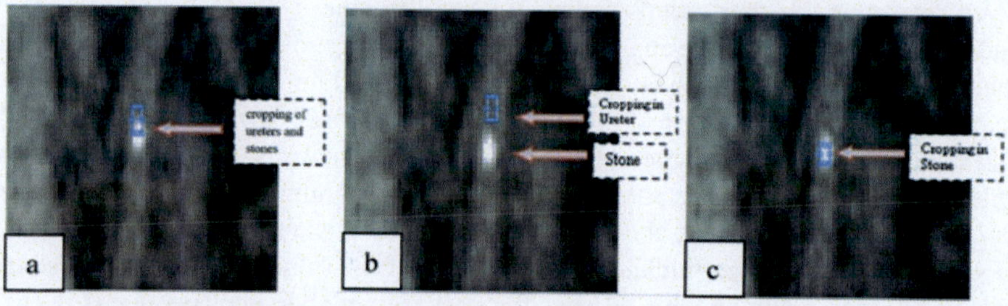

Fig. 5 The cropped MATLAB image. **a** Image cropping the ureter and stone, **b** image cropped in the ureter area, and **c** image cropped in the stone area MATLAB on the ureter

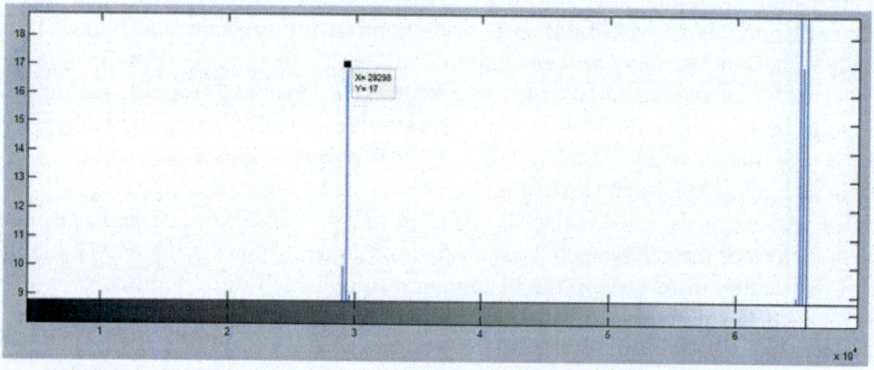

Fig. 6 Histogram of urinary tract image contrast analysis using MATLAB on the ureter

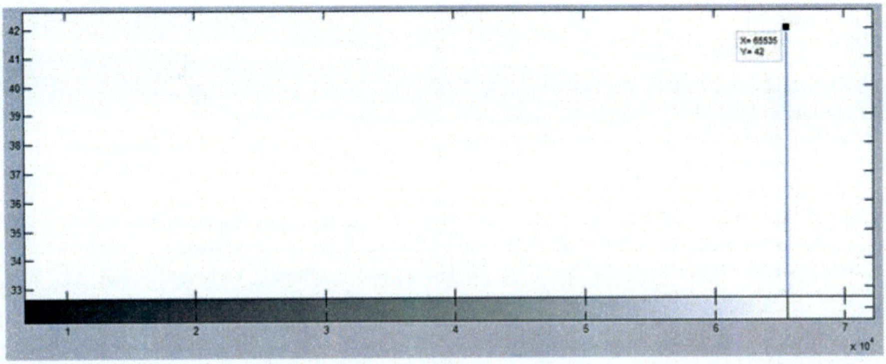

Fig. 7 The histogram of the contrast analysis result of urinary tract image using MATLAB on stone

channel can detect the presence of stones in the ureter. In addition, it can support a diagnosis by improving the quality of CT Scan images for urinary tract examination. So that it can detect kidney disease and prevent kidney failure, reduce severe pain, and decrease human quality of life [15, 18, 19]. Developments in analyzing and detecting abnormalities in establishing medical imaging diagnoses need to be further developed with artificial intelligence (AI)-based systems so that they can provide accurate diagnostic information [6, 14, 21, 25, 26].

4 Conclusion

Utilizing a 1 mm slice thickness reconstruction with an abdominal window improves the quality of a CT scan of the urinary system performed without the use of a contrast agent. Identification of CT scan of the urinary tract in the area of stones and ureters using MATLAB can analyze images in assessing stones well, with a contrast value of 36,237. In this study, there are still shortcomings because it cannot automatically detect stones in the urinary tract, and the need for further development in detecting stones or diseases in the urinary tract area, especially the kidney and ureter. To swiftly and accurately detect, developers can utilize artificial intelligence, machine learning, and deep learning, so that it can assist radiology doctors in assessing abnormalities in the kidneys or ureters.

References

1. Alnazer I et al (2021) Recent advances in medical image processing for the evaluation of chronic kidney disease. https://doi.org/10.1016/j.media.2021.101960
2. Baygin M et al (2022) Exemplar Darknet19 feature generation technique for automated kidney stone detection with coronal CT images. Artif Intell Med 127. https://doi.org/10.1016/j.artmed.2022.102274
3. Black KM et al (2020) Deep learning computer vision algorithm for detecting kidney stone composition. BJU Int 125(6):920–924. https://doi.org/10.1111/bju.15035
4. Brisbane W et al (2016) An overview of kidney stone imaging techniques. Nat Rev Urol 13(11):654–662. https://doi.org/10.1038/nrurol.2016.154
5. Chewcharat A, Curhan G (2021) Trends in the prevalence of kidney stones in the United States from 2007 to 2016. Urolithiasis 49(1):27–39. https://doi.org/10.1007/s00240-020-01210-w
6. Choi AD et al (2021) CT evaluation by artificial intelligence for atherosclerosis, stenosis and vascular morphology (CLARIFY): a multi-center, international study. J Cardiovasc Comput Tomogr 15(6):470–476. https://doi.org/10.1016/j.jcct.2021.05.004
7. Fitri LA et al (2020) Automated classification of urinary stones based on micro-computed tomography images using convolutional neural network. Physica Med 78:201–208. https://doi.org/10.1016/j.ejmp.2020.09.007
8. Hesamian MH et al (2019) Deep learning techniques for medical image segmentation: achievements and challenges. J Digit Imaging 32(4):582–596. https://doi.org/10.1007/s10278-019-00227-x
9. Homepage J et al (2019) Pemanfaatan Machine Learning dalam Berbagai Bidang: review paper. IJCIT (Indones J Comput Inf Technol)
10. Hsu TMH et al (2021) Artificial intelligence to assess body composition on routine abdominal CT scans and predict mortality in pancreatic cancer—a recipe for your local application. Eur J Radiol 142. https://doi.org/10.1016/j.ejrad.2021.109834
11. James SL et al (2018) Global, regional, and national incidence, prevalence, and years lived with disability for 354 diseases and injuries for 195 countries and territories, 1990–2017: a systematic analysis for the Global Burden of Disease Study 2017. The Lancet 392(10159):1789–1858. https://doi.org/10.1016/S0140-6736(18)32279-7
12. Kijowski R et al (2020) Deep learning for lesion detection, progression, and prediction of musculoskeletal disease. J Magn Reson Imaging 52(6):1607–1619. https://doi.org/10.1002/jmri.27001
13. Lampignano et al. Bontrager's textbook of radiographic positioning and related anatomy
14. Luckin R et al. Intelligence unleashed an argument for AI in education
15. New F, Somani BK (2016) A complete world literature review of quality of life (QOL) in patients with kidney stone disease (KSD). Curr Urol Rep 17(12):88. https://doi.org/10.1007/s11934-016-0647-6
16. O'Connor A (2007) Pathology. Mosby
17. Ozturk T et al (2020) Automated detection of COVID-19 cases using deep neural networks with X-ray images. Comput Biol Med 121. https://doi.org/10.1016/j.compbiomed.2020.103792
18. Penniston KL, Nakada SY (2013) Development of an instrument to assess the health related quality of life of kidney stone formers. J Urol 189(3):921–930. https://doi.org/10.1016/j.juro.2012.08.247
19. Purnomo B (2015) Dasar Dasar Urologi
20. Rice P et al (2021)Machine learning models for predicting stone-free status after shockwave lithotripsy: a systematic review and meta-analysis. https://doi.org/10.1016/j.urology.2021.04.006
21. Roth HR et al (2018) Deep learning and its application to medical image segmentation. https://doi.org/10.11409/mit.36.63
22. Shaaban MS, Kotb AF (2016) Value of non-contrast CT examination of the urinary tract (stone protocol) in the detection of incidental findings and its impact upon the management. Alex J Med 52(3):209–217. https://doi.org/10.1016/j.ajme.2015.08.001

23. Shkolyar E et al (2019) augmented bladder tumor detection using deep learning. Eur Urol 76(6):714–718. https://doi.org/10.1016/j.eururo.2019.08.032
24. Türk C et al (2016) EAU guidelines on diagnosis and conservative management of urolithiasis. Eur Urol 69(3):468–474. https://doi.org/10.1016/j.eururo.2015.07.040
25. Xu J et al (2021) Performance of artificial intelligence-based coronary artery calcium scoring in non-gated chest CT. Eur J Radiol 145:110034. https://doi.org/10.1016/j.ejrad.2021.110034
26. Yan K et al (2018) DeepLesion: automated mining of large-scale lesion annotations and universal lesion detection with deep learning. J Med Imaging 5(03):1. https://doi.org/10.1117/1.jmi.5.3.036501
27. Yildirim K et al (2021) Deep learning model for automated kidney stone detection using coronal CT images. Comput Biol Med 135:104569. https://doi.org/10.1016/j.compbiomed.2021.104569
28. Zhang X, Dahu W (2019) Application of artificial intelligence algorithms in image processing. J Vis Commun Image Represent 61:42–49. https://doi.org/10.1016/j.jvcir.2019.03.004
29. Zhou SK et al (2021) Deep reinforcement learning in medical imaging: a literature review. https://doi.org/10.1016/j.media.2021.102193

Accuration of Classification of Covid with Convolutional Neural Network-Based Image Chest X-ray with Variations in Image Size and Batch Size

Dwi Rochmayanti, Kusworo Adi, Catur Edi Widodo, Budi Warsito, Adi Wibowo, W. Andi Nur Intan, and Aris Kiswanto

Abstract The use of convolutional neural networks in Covid classification has a positive impact on the speed of justification and can provide high accuracy. But on the one hand, the many parameters on CNN will also have an impact on the resulting accuracy. CNN requires time and a heavy level of computation. Setting the right parameters will provide high accuracy. This study examines the performance of CNN with variations in image size and minibatch. Parameter settings used are max epoch values of 100, minibatch variations of 32, 64, and 128, and learning rate of 0.1 with image size inputs of 50,100, and 150 variations on the level of accuracy. The dataset consists of training data and test data, 200 images, which are divided into two categories of normal and abnormal images (Covid). The results showed an accuracy with the use of minibatch 128 with the highest level of accuracy at image size 150 × 150 on test data of 99,08%. The size of the input matrix does not always have an impact on increasing the level of accuracy, especially on the minibatch 32.

D. Rochmayanti (✉)
Department of Radiodiagnostic and Radiotherapy Engineering, Health Polytechnic, Ministry of Health, Semarang, Central Java, Indonesia
e-mail: dwirochmayanti@poltekkes-smg.ac.id

K. Adi · C. E. Widodo
Department of Physics, Faculty of Science and Mathematics, Diponegoro University, Semarang, Indonesia

B. Warsito
Department of Statistics, Faculty of Science and Mathematics, Diponegoro University, Semarang, Indonesia

A. Wibowo
Department of Informatics, Faculty of Science and Mathematics, Diponegoro University, Semarang, Indonesia

W. Andi Nur Intan
Muhammadiyah Makassar Health Polytechnic, Makassar, Indonesia

A. Kiswanto
Department of Electrical Engineering, University of Muhammadiyah Semarang, Semarang, Indonesia

T. Triwiyanto et al. (eds.), *Proceeding of the 3rd International Conference on Electronics, Biomedical Engineering, and Health Informatics*, Lecture Notes in Electrical Engineering 1008, https://doi.org/10.1007/978-981-99-0248-4_13

The parameter setting on CNN was dependent on the CNN architecture, the dataset used, and the size of the dataset. One can imply that optimization parameter in CNN can approve good accuration.

Keywords CNN · Acurration · Covid · Image size · Minibatch

1 Introduction

Since it was announced by the World Health Organization (WHO), which declared COVID-19 as a global disease in March 2020, after two years there has been a downward trend. On the official Covid site (https://covid19.go.id/), there is a map of the distribution and trends in Indonesia as of May 28, 2022, which were confirmed positive in Indonesia for as many as 279 people. Where the highest peak in the range of the first trimester of 2022 occurred in February which experienced a peak, 63,596 people were confirmed positive [1], and worldwide resulting in more than 6,529,331 deaths [2].

To detect Covid, Reverse Transcription Polymerase Chain Reaction (RT-PCR) and CT Scan have good sensitivity [3], but this method is expensive and time-consuming [4]. In addition to this, imaging modalities such as chest radiography have an important role in providing information related to Covid [5, 6]. Radiographic diagnostic accuracy generally refers to how well the examination can predict the presence of a disease or condition. Technology plays an important role in increasing diagnostic accuracy by providing diagnostic images [7]. The increasing number of medical images and the rapidly increasing development of modalities must take into account the possible risks of error and delayed diagnosis. The current answer to these problems was in computer-aided detection (CADe) and diagnosis (CADx) systems [8]. Machine learning has the potential to improve and support clinical decisions regarding the interpretation of results [9]. Many of research has been done regarding the detection and classification of Covid, using a deep learning approach with a convolutional neural network (CNN) [10–16]. Confirmation of the presence of Covid with several graded tests will take longer, and delaying the results will also have fatal consequences. Therefore, trusted with CNN can be used for classification and faster decisions [17]. CNN has the advantage of being able to learn directly from data classification features [18].

Medical images have a unique character compared to ordinary images [8]. The need for diagnostic value from medical images has its own advantages, so standardized image quality is needed. High resolution is an important requirement to ensure the image does not lose detail so that the level of diagnostic accuracy can be achieved. The standard format for medical images is Digital Imaging and Communications in Medicine (DICOM). A DICOM image file consists of a header containing metadata and raw data. DICOM image matrix size is 512×512 for CT Scan and 2048×2048 for Computed Radiography and Digital Radiography [19]. Digital medical images have a very large number of features. One digital chest X-ray image in DICOM format generated by computer radiography has dimensions of $1024 \times 1024 = 1{,}048{,}576$ features [20]. The addition of X-ray images as training data and the number of iterations will increase the accuracy of the Deep Convolution Neural Network model [21].

In one study it was stated that the image dimensions of 256 and 512 pixels provide optimal accuracy, after which the accuracy decreases [22]. Therefore, research related to image size is carried out below this range, with image size inputs of 50,100, and 150. In this study, the image will be downscaled. This is because the image in DICOM format has a large enough memory, so the number of features that must be recognized by the CNN algorithm in the image processing process is very large, which can cause computer equipment to be heavier in the processing process. The amount of training data is large so that it is more burdensome and the image processing process will take longer, while the purpose of artificial intelligence applied in this research is to recognize images quickly and accurately. Minibatch variations are also carried out to find the highest accuracy. The purpose of this study was to compare the matrix and minibatch size parameters on CNN to see the accuracy.

2 Data and Method

This research is a quantitative descriptive study by varying the size of the input image on the performance and accuracy of the CNN concept framework as shown in (see Fig. 1). From the two variations that are carried out and cross each other, the best parameters will be determined in the training data class and test data.

2.1 Identification of Covid with Chest X-ray Image

Chest imaging is less sensitive in justifying Covid and often shows a normal picture early in the course of the disease. Bilateral/multilobular distribution is common in COVID-19 patients [23]. Interpreting normal and abnormal chest radiographs requires instructions and an understanding of the anatomy and physiology of the chest X-ray organs and their limitations. To make it easier, use the help method ABCDEFGHI [24], (A) Assessment of quality, ensuring that the identity listed on the chest X-ray image matches the patient being examined and ensures the appropriateness of the image quality. Next (B) Bones and soft tissue, (C) Cardiac, (D) Diaphragm, (E) Effusion, (F) Field, fissures, and foreign bodies, (G) Great vessel and gastric bubble, (H) Hilla and mediastinum, and (I) Impressions. The image is indicated for Covid, there are typical Covid lesions, ground-glass opacity, and a picture of spots [25].

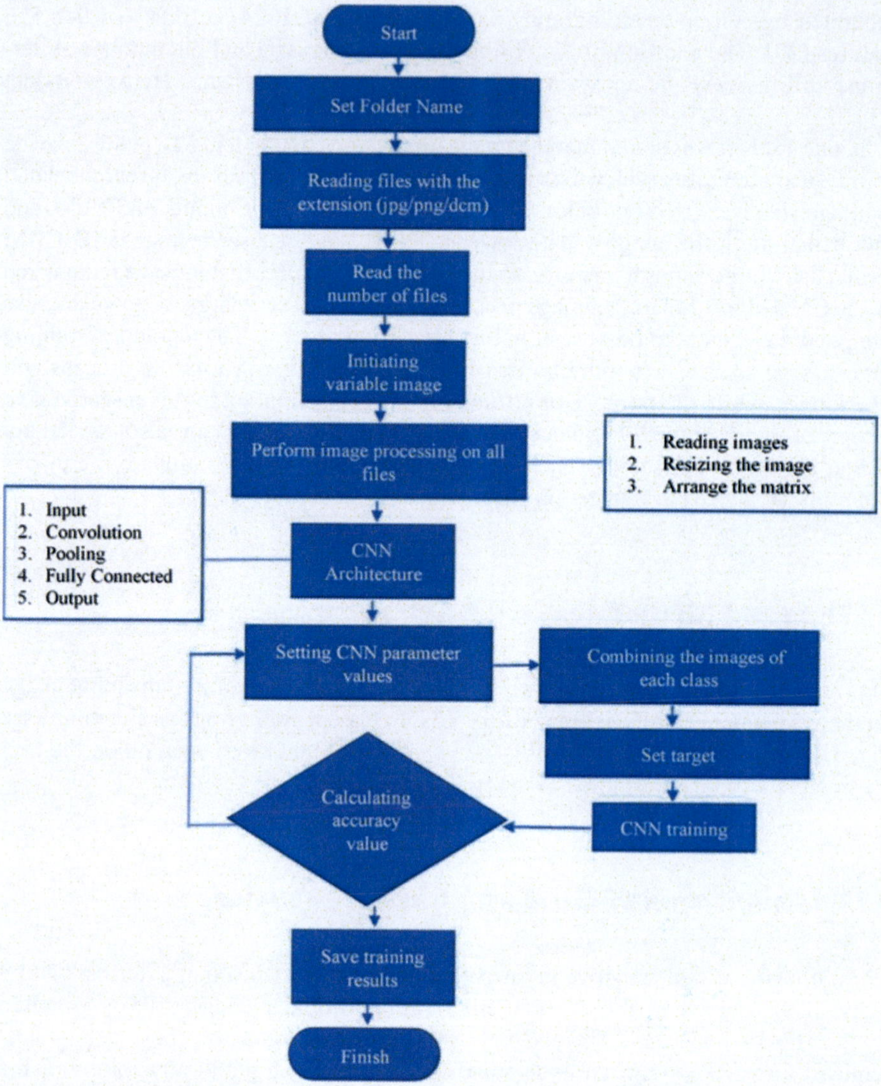

Fig. 1 Research concept framework of CNN

2.2 Collecting Data

Data were extracted from modality computed radiography in dicom format. The sample image is the result of an adult chest radiograph that has obtained the readings of a radiologist with more than 5 years of experience. Image collection consists of two categories, both normal and confirmed images of Covid. Images that are categorized as Covid are identified by cross-checking the results of the RT-PCR test. Data retrieval

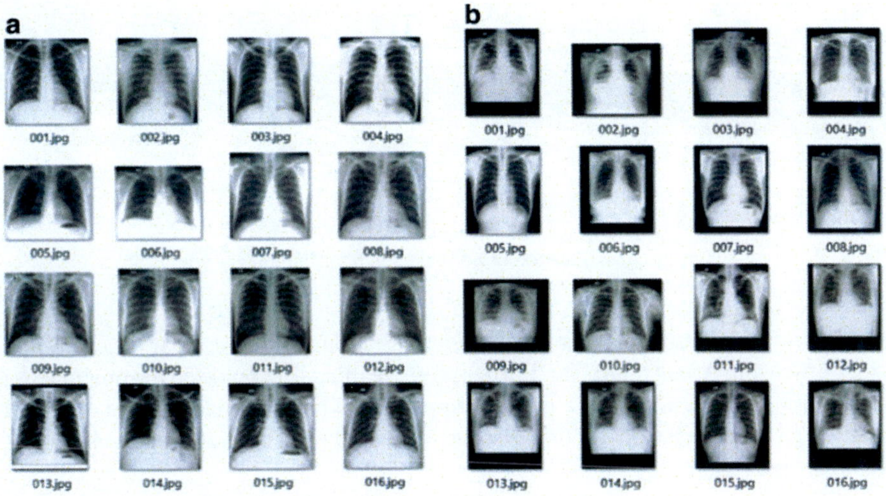

Fig. 2 Dataset for normal (**a**) and abnormal (**b**) training categories

using purposive sampling method is by considering the established criteria, namely the established category, namely the thoracic image of adults normal and covid image categories were confirmed by RT-PCR results. The image is also conditioned with the entire lung field in collimation/irradiation, where the apex area and costophrenic sinus are not cut, and in a symmetrical condition, the heart and diaphragm are clear. Furthermore, the image data is stored in a DVD-RW and organized into two categories as training data and test data, where each category consists of two folders which are classified as normal image data and abnormal images (confirmed by Covid). The group of images (Fig. 2). The number of images for training data is 200 images with 100 images per category each. As for the test data used as many as 23 abnormal images and 196 normal images. The file name is adjusted to the normal or COVID-19 category. To facilitate the image processing, the data is converted into JPG format. The image has been freed from the patient's data and identity. Training data is prepared and used as input in training programming during the CNN algorithm development process. The image obtained from the dataset with a size of 1024 × 1024 pixels is then downscaled with variations of 50 × 50, 100 × 100, and 150 × 150 with minibatch variations of 32, 64, and 128 to find the highest training data accuracy.

2.3 CNN Architecture

The CNN algorithm is built based on several convolution layers including Image Input Layer, Convolution 2D layer, ReLU layer, Fully Connected Layer three times, Softmax Layer, and Classification Output Layer. Next, parameter settings are set, max epoch at 100 and learning rate at 0.1 with minibatch variations of 32, 64, and

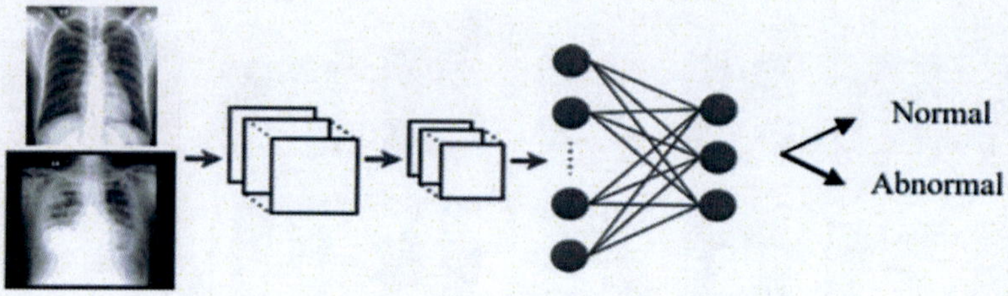

Fig. 3 Illustration Concept Classification of normal and abnormal images with CNN

100. Previously, the image was resized with variations of 50 × 50, 100 × 100, and 150 × 150 using Adam optimizer. Furthermore, readings are made on the output class by looking at the results of the input training data whether it has met the expected criteria and calculating the accuracy of the training data. The tool used is MATLAB R2022a, (see Fig. 3).

3 Results and Discussion

The CNN model uses the Convnet architecture. The output image results are in the form of a classification between COVID-19 which is called abnormal and normal. In training, the image size is varied from 50 × 50, 100 × 100, and 150 × 150. The parameter settings used are max epoch values of 100, minibatch variations of 32, 64, and 128, and learning rate of 0.1. The parameters used are used to control the running of the CNN that is made so that it can produce classification predictions correctly.

In the architectural preparation process, each convolution layer is carried out as much as 1 × 1 per layer until the last hidden layer (see Fig. 2). The convolution layer plays a role in detecting edges, lines, and visual elements as well as typical local areas in the chest X-ray image. One of the architectures used is to use a 150 × 150 input image, (see Fig. 4) and detail architecture in Table 1.

The CNN training data was carried out with three variations of image resize at 50 × 50, 100 × 100, and 150 × 150 with minibatch variations of 32, 64, and 128. The training algorithm performance data can be shown in Table 2.

Furthermore, Classification is carried out with test data. The test data are 196 normal images and 23 abnormal images. From the classification results, the accuracy level is obtained as shown in Table 3.

From Table 2, with the input image of 50 × 50, the use of minibatch 32 and 64 has the same accuracy, while at 100 × 100 it produces erratic accuracy, while for the input image of 150 × 150, the accuracy decreases with increasing use of minibatch. Meanwhile, the accuracy of the test data has different characteristics from the accuracy results of the training data. In the 50 × 50 input image, the accuracy increases with the addition of minibatches with the same number on the 64 and 128 minibatches. In the 100 × 100 image, very different results are produced with

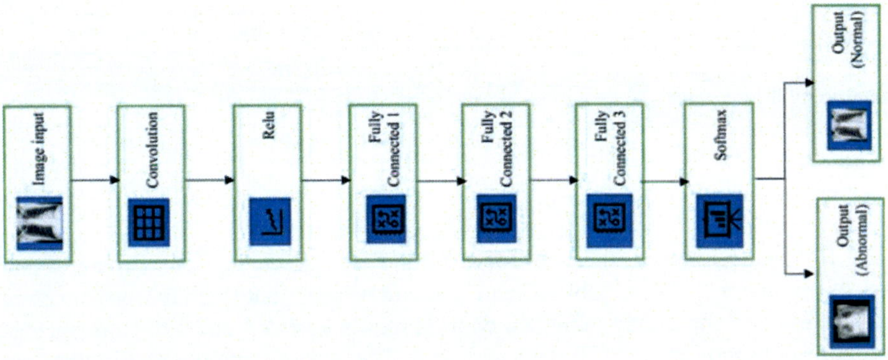

Fig. 4 CNN architecture

Table 1 Detailed architecture of CNN of image input 150 × 150

Type	Activations	Learnable properties
Image input	150(s) × 150(s) × 1(C) × 1(B)	–
Convolution	150(s) × 150(s) × 16(C) × 1(B)	Weight 3 × 3x1 × 16 Bias 1 × 1x16
ReLu	150(s) × 150(s) × 16(C) × 1(B)	
Fully connected (fc_1)	1(s) × 1(s) × 384(C) × 1(B)	Weight 384 × 360x1 Bias 384 × 1x16
Fully connected (fc_2)	1(s) × 1(s) × 384(C) × 1(B)	Weight 384 × 384x1 Bias 384 × 1
Fully connected (fc_3)	1(s) × 1(s) × 2(C) × 1(B)	Weight 2 × 384 Bias 2 × 1
Softmax	1(s) × 1(s) × 2(C) × 1(B)	-
Classoutput ("0" and "1")	1(s) × 1(s) × 2(C) × 1(B)	-

Table 2 Accuracy of training data on variations in the size of the image matrix and minibatch (in percentage)

	50 × 50	100 × 100	150 × 150
32	100	50	100
64	100	100	99.5
128	98.5	97	98

Table 3 Accuracy of test data on variations in the size of the image matrix and minibatch (in percentage)

	50 × 50	100 × 100	150 × 150
32	97,26	10,50	73,97
64	98,63	97,26	98,17
128	98,63	98,80	99,08

the 32 minibatch where the accuracy has a significantly different number, which is only 10.50%. While at 150 × 150 for test data, accuracy increases with increasing use of minibatches. From Tables 2 and 3, it can be seen that there is consistency in the accuracy of the training and test data on minibatches 64 and 128 from various variations of input images (50, 100, and 150). The size of the input matrix does not always have an impact on increasing the level of accuracy, this can be seen in the use of minibatch 32, and there are irregular fluctuations in the level of accuracy resulting from various variations of the input image. More stable results were obtained with the minibatch parameter of 128. Even though the 32 and 64 batch size settings did not provide linear information. From these results, it can be seen that parameter determination is important to maximize performance in reading existing data.

Characteristics of the data are important, so as not to bias the performance of the algorithm used. This is supported by the research of Uyar (2021) which stated that the parameter setting on CNN is very dependent on the CNN architecture, the dataset used, and the size of the dataset [26]. The size of the input image needs to be considered so as not to lose the input data resolution; image quality is also important to get better accuracy. Classification depends on visual information and image resolution, if the resolution is reduced, the missing image information will increase so that it will reduce the ability to detect edges and textures in the image and increase blurring [22, 27]. High accuracy can be obtained by using a large image size [28].

The use of minibatch is also an important parameter for optimization so that the correct value will be obtained to be applied to all types of data. In general, if you use a large minibatch, the resulting accuracy will be smaller and it will require faster computations. A small minibatch will consume computational time but the results are more optimal when compared to a large minibatch [29]. So, it is also necessary to experiment with the use of a small minibatch [26].

From the results of this study, it is important to note that all aspects must be considered in building an architecture in CNN. In addition to the architecture in which there are parameters that can be set for optimization, input data and the amount are also things that need to be considered. Another thing that also needs to be fulfilled is that more training data and the quality of the training data will increase the accuracy performance [8]. The classification of image networks is strongly influenced by the network architecture and dataset, and it is even mentioned that the dataset has a significant impact on the accuracy of the test [30].

The limitation of this research is the result of only an accuration between a training and data test, not including F1 score and confusion matrix and that the dataset used does not take into account the proportional training and test data. Because we use training data and custom test with a proportional 1:1. The number of training datasets also only amounts to 200 with 100 images each in the image group.

4 Conclusion

From the results of the study, it was found that the image input matrix did not have a specific impact on the accuracy of the training data and test data, as well as the variation of the minibatch used. The accuracy results appear stable when using minibatch 128 in all variations of the image matrix (50,100, and 150). Efforts need to be made to improve the training data for research and the quality of the resulting data. In future work, more analysis includes the f1 score and confusion matrix and more dataset.

References

1. Satuan Tugas Penanganan COVID-19: Perkembangan Kasus Terkonfirmasi Positif Covid-19. https://covid19.go.id/. Last accessed 11 May 2022
2. Wordometers. Coronavirus death toll and trends—worldomet. https://www.worldometers.info/coronavirus/coronavirus-death-toll/. Last accessed 17 September 2022
3. He JL, Luo L, Luo ZD, Lyu JX, Ng MY, Shen XP, Wen Z (2020) Diagnostic performance between CT and initial real-time RT-PCR for clinically suspected 2019 coronavirus disease (COVID-19) patients outside Wuhan, China. Respir Med 168. https://doi.org/10.1016/j.rmed.2020.105980
4. Hassantabar S, Ahmadi M, Sharifi A (2020) Diagnosis and detection of infected tissue of COVID-19 patients based on lung X-ray image using convolutional neural network approaches. Chaos Solitons Fractals 140:110170. https://doi.org/10.1016/j.chaos.2020.110170
5. Irmak E (2021) COVID-19 disease severity assessment using CNN model. IET Image Process 15:1814–1824. https://doi.org/10.1049/ipr2.12153
6. Singh KK, Siddhartha M, Singh A (2020) Diagnosis of coronavirus disease (COVID-19) from chest X-ray images using modified XceptionNet
7. Tafti A, Byerly DW (2022) X-ray radiographic patient positioning. StatPearls Publishing LLC
8. Cho J, Lee K, Shin E, Choy G, Do S (2016) How much data is needed to train a medical image deep learning system to achieve necessary high accuracy? ICLR
9. Choy G, Khalilzadeh O, Michalski M, Do S, Samir AE, Pianykh OS, Raymond Geis J, Pandharipande PV, Brink JA, Dreye KJ (2018) Current applications and future impact of machine learning in radiology. RSNA 2:318–328. https://doi.org/10.1148/radiol.2018171820
10. Nigam B, Nigam A, Jain R, Dodia S, Arora N, Annappa B (2021) COVID-19: automatic detection from X-ray images by utilizing deep learning methods. Expert Syst Appl 176. https://doi.org/10.1016/j.eswa.2021.114883
11. Tahir AM, Chowdhury MEH, Khandakar A, Rahman T, Qiblawey Y, Khurshid U, Kiranyaz S, Ibtehaz N, Rahman MS, Al-Maadeed S, Mahmud S, Ezeddin M, Hameed K, Hamid T (2021) COVID-19 infection localization and severity grading from chest X-ray images. Comput Biol Med 139. https://doi.org/10.1016/j.compbiomed.2021.105002
12. Padmakala S, Revathy S, Vijayalakshmi K, Mathankumar M (2022) CNN supported automated recognition of Covid-19 infection in chest X-ray images. Mater Today Proc. https://doi.org/10.1016/j.matpr.2022.05.003

13. Jain G, Mittal D, Thakur D, Mittal MK (2020) A deep learning approach to detect Covid-19 coronavirus with X-Ray images. Biocybern Biomed Eng. 40:1391–1405. https://doi.org/10.1016/j.bbe.2020.08.008
14. Sekeroglu B, Ozsahin I (2020) Detection of COVID-19 from chest X-ray images using convolutional neural networks. SLAS Technol 25:553–565. https://doi.org/10.1177/2472630320958376
15. Ibrahim AU, Ozsoz M, Serte S, Al-Turjman F, Yakoi PS (2021) Pneumonia classification using deep learning from chest X-ray images during COVID-19. Cognit Comput. https://doi.org/10.1007/S12559-020-09787-5
16. Hertel R, Benlamri R (2022) A deep learning segmentation-classification pipeline for X-ray-based COVID-19 diagnosis. Biomed Eng Adv 100041. https://doi.org/10.1016/j.bea.2022.100041
17. Shambhu S, Koundal D, Das P, Sharma C (2022) Binary classification of COVID-19 CT images using CNN: COVID diagnosis using CT. Int J E-Health Med Commun 13. https://doi.org/10.4018/IJEHMC.20220701.oa4
18. Ahmed WS, Karim A, Amir A (2020) The impact of filter size and number of filters on classification accuracy in CNN. In: 2020 international conference on computer science and software engineering (CSASE). IEEE, pp 88–93. https://doi.org/10.1109/CSASE48920.2020.9142089
19. Mishra VK, Kumar S, Shukla N (2017) Image acquisition and techniques to perform image acquisition. SAMRIDDHI: A J Phys Sci Eng Technol 9:21–24. https://doi.org/10.18090/samriddhi.v9i01.8333
20. Bushong S (2012) Radiologic science for technologists. Elsevier Mosby, St. Louis
21. Thirukrishna JT, Reddy S, Krishna S, Shashank P, Srikanth S, Raghu V, Srikanth S, Raghu V (2022) Survey on diagnosing CORONA VIRUS from radiography chest X-ray images using convolutional neural networks 124:2261–2270. https://doi.org/10.1007/s11277-022-09463-x
22. Philips MB, Luke JJ, Joseph R, Balaji M (2019) Impact of image size on accuracy and generalization of convolutional neural networks. IJRAR19SP012 Int J Res Anal Rev
23. Salehi S, Abedi A, Balakrishnan S, Gholamrezanezhad A (2020) Coronavirus disease 2019 (COVID-19): a systematic review of imaging findings in 919 patients. https://doi.org/10.2214/AJR.20.23034
24. American College of Radiology (2017) ACR–SPR–STR: practise parameter chest radiography
25. Colman J, Zamfir G, Sheehan F, Berrill M, Saikia S, Saltissi F (2021) Chest radiograph characteristics in COVID-19 infection and their association with survival. Eur J Radiol Open. 8:100360. https://doi.org/10.1016/j.ejro.2021.100360
26. Uyar K, Taşdemir Ş, Özkan Ilker A (2021) The analysis and optimization of CNN hyperparameters with fuzzy tree model for image classification. Turk J Electr Eng Comput Sci. https://doi.org/10.3906/elk-2107-130
27. Thambawita V, Strümke I, Hicks SA, Halvorsen P, Parasa S, Riegler MA (2021) Impact of image resolution on deep learning performance in endoscopy image classification: an experimental study using a large dataset of endoscopic images. Diagnostics 11. https://doi.org/10.3390/diagnostics11122183
28. Rukundo O (2022) Effects of image size on deep learning. https://doi.org/10.48550/arXiv.2101.11508
29. Rochmawati N, Hidayati HB, Yamasari Y, Tjahyaningtijas HPA, Yustati W, Prihanto A (2021) Analysis of learning rate and batch size on covid classification using deep learning with Adam's optimizer. J Inf Eng Educ Technol 5:44–48
30. Luo C, Li X, Wang L, He J, Li D, Zhou J (2018) How does the data set affect CNN-based image classification performance? In: 2018 5th international conference on systems and informatics (ICSAI). IEEE, pp 361–366 (2018). https://doi.org/10.1109/ICSAI.2018.8599448

Automatic Water Monitoring and Draining System Manufacturing for Aquascape Based on Water Quality Using Fuzzy Logic Method

Namira Ainannisa, Desri Kristina Silalahi, and Porman Pangaribuan

Abstract In order to maintain the survival of those aquatic vegetation, aquariums need to be treated with several treatments, such as feeding routines for fish and environmental maintenance (temperature, water turbidity, humidity, and pH). Those mentioned treatments will be more efficient and optimal if it is carried out with technology, such as aquascape with automatic draining and monitoring system in real time and remotely. The system that will be built in this research is a system that can monitor water humidity, turbidity, temperature, and pH in real time and remotely for aquascapes as well as design an algorithm for the automatic draining system based on pH and water turbidity using Fuzzy Logic method. The system uses DFRobot pH sensor with a pH range of 6.5–8.5 and a turbidity sensor SHT11 with a turbidity range of 5–25 NTU, which is then processed using NodeMCU8266 and continued with fuzzy logic programming. The monitoring process of water condition is carried out using the Blynk application that is installed on android smartphones. The result of the monitoring system design is functioning well, as indicated by the reading of the aquascape water environmental condition values with a distance of 5–20 m between the Wi-Fi router and the system successfully displaying data with 100% accuracy through the Blynk application. Also, the result of the algorithm design in the automatic draining system is functioning well, indicated by the result of the entire system test where the automatic draining output given goes according to the conditions of the aquascape.

Keywords Automatic drainage system · Aquascape · Water quality

N. Ainannisa (✉) · D. K. Silalahi · P. Pangaribuan
Bachelor of Electrical Engineering, School of Electrical Engineering, Telkom University, Bandung, Indonesia
e-mail: namiraainannisa@student.telkomuniversity.ac.id

T. Triwiyanto et al. (eds.), *Proceeding of the 3rd International Conference on Electronics, Biomedical Engineering, and Health Informatics*, Lecture Notes in Electrical Engineering 1008, https://doi.org/10.1007/978-981-99-0248-4_14

1 Introduction

Aquascape is an art that uses techniques by combining plants, fish, wood, stones, and other components to make it pleasing to the eye [1]. Basically, aquascape is a water garden, because one of the components in an aquascape are fish and aquatic plants. Currently, the aquascape manufacturing industry is very busy among the people, both small, medium, and large-scale industries. So, the aquascape industry is an industry engaged in ornamental fish and ornamental plants [2].

Aquascape is the art of arranging an aquarium, in which there are usually living creatures, both fish and aquatic plants [3]. The growth of fish and plants in the aquarium is affected by the quality of the water. Water quality parameters are seen based on temperature, power of Hydrogen or abbreviated as pH, and water turbidity. Good water conditions for fish and plants, in aquascapes have a temperature of 20–28 °C [4] with a pH of 6.0–8.0 [5]. If the temperature is below the standard interval, the fish's body temperature will decrease, suppressing the fish's immune response, reducing appetite, and activity, and resulting in decreased growth [6]. Likewise in plants will result in a slowdown in plant growth. Conversely, if the temperature exceeds the upper limit of the standard interval, what happens is that the fish's body temperature rises and the metabolism in the fish's body will increase so that it requires more oxygen levels which makes the fish easy to stress. Likewise with plants, high water temperatures can cause plants to wither quickly because they require high levels of carbon dioxide.

Humidity conditions also affect the room and plant growth in the aquascape [7]. High humidity can cause mold growth in the aquascape [8]. The low pH value of the water will cause imperfect growth in fish, as well as in aquatic plants [9]. If the pH is too high it can cause incompatibility with the characteristics of the fish [10]. This is because in general aquascapes use freshwater fish.

The turbidity of the water in the aquascape also needs to be controlled, because this parameter is used to be able to take action to drain the water in the aquascape by replacing the new water [11]. Thus, in order for each parameter to meet good aquascape conditions, a device is needed that can monitor humidity, temperature, water pH, and turbidity in real time and the results of temperature and pH measurements can be seen directly on the installed device or remotely.

Research on aquascape design already exists. One of them is an IoT-based aquascape that has a remote monitoring and control system for ornamental fish-rearing aquariums using Arduino mega 2560 as a microcontroller [12]. The research focused on monitoring temperature, pH, and turbidity using ThingSpeak as a cloud for IoT. However, this research can be developed by adding a test parameter, namely the humidity value. The research is monitoring environmental parameters using Blynk in the monitoring and control system of mushroom plants. The environmental parameters that were controlled in this research were temperature and humidity, as well as giving orders to control the watering of the mushroom plants using the fuzzy logic method [13].

Thus, in this research, the development of previous research was carried out. This study designed a system that can monitor the conditions of humidity, turbidity, temperature, and pH of the water using sensors which then the measurement results are processed using the Fuzzy logic method to determine the process of draining water automatically. Aquascape water draining is automatically carried out if the water quality, which includes pH and turbidity, does not meet the requirements set by the user. The pH range used in this study was 6.5–8.5 [5], while the turbidity range used in this research was 5–25 NTU (Nephelometric Turbidity Unit) [14]. The monitoring process is carried out through the display of data on the LCD and the Blynk application on the android smartphone.

2 Literature Review

2.1 Aquascape Industry

In general, aquariums are divided into two types, those are seawater and fresh-water aquarium. Seawater aquarium is also called oceanarium or the popular term is reefarium. Aquariums require maintenance to maintain the survival of fish and aquatic vegetation contained in them. Aquascape is the art of arranging aquatic plants and rocks, coral, coral, or driftwood, naturally and beautifully in an aquarium so that it gives an effect like gardening under water [15]. Treatments such as feeding routines for fish, and maintenance of environmental parameters (temperature, water turbidity, humidity, and pH) are things that must be maintained regularly in an aquarium, especially aquascape-type aquariums [12].

2.2 Temperature

Temperature plays an important role in Aquascape, especially the influence on plants. A temperature of 26–28 °C is the ideal temperature, which can be said to be true, because apart from plants being able to grow optimally, the whole ecosystem is not disturbed [16]. Temperature affects the biota in the Aquascape which can affect the fish's immune response, appetite, activity, and growth of fish. Temperature is also one of the factors that affect the rate of plant growth. In this study, the DS18B20 temperature sensor is used to detect the air temperature in a room digitally and uses a single wire.

2.3 Humidity

Humidity is the amount of water contained in the air, usually expressed as a percentage. This humidity is related or influenced by air temperature and jointly between temperature. The relatively low humidity of less than 20% can cause dryness of the mucous membranes, while high humidity will increase the growth of micro-organisms such as mold growth in the environment. In this study, the SHT11 sensor is used which can detect air humidity. This sensor has an output in the form of a calibrated digital signal.

2.4 Turbidity

A water environment can be said to be cloudy if there are particles that are not dissolved by water in it, for example, such as sand, soil, mud, and organic and inorganic chemicals. Particles that are not dissolved by the water form a suspension in the water, causing the water to become turbid [11]. Turbidity is closely related to dissolved oxygen levels in the water. The value of turbidity is written in units of measurement NTU or Nephelometric Turbidity Units. The standard of clean water is indicated by a turbidity value of <25 NTU [17]. The relationship between turbidity and dissolved oxygen levels is inversely proportional [18], namely the higher the turbidity value, the smaller the dissolved oxygen content in the water. On the other hand, if the turbidity value is low, the dissolved oxygen content in the water will increase [19]. In this study, the SKU SEN0819 turbidity sensor was used to measure the level of turbidity in the water.

2.5 Power of Hydrogen

Power of hydrogen (pH) is the degree or measure of the strength of an acid solution [20]. pH has a scale of acidity (acid) and alkalinity (base) which is worth 0–14. A solution or water environment can be said to be acidic if the pH value is 0–7, then it can be said to be alkaline if the pH value is 7–14 [18]. The optimum pH value varies in the species of fish found in the aquarium, for most species of seawater fish can live and thrive at a pH of ±8.2 [21]. Based on the test of measuring the pH quality of betta fish [22], the optimal pH obtained was in the range of 6.7–7.4. These results are evidenced by the growth of betta fish which is quite good in water conditions with a pH value that is neither acidic nor alkaline (neutral). This study uses a pH sensor DFRobot.

2.6 Blynk

Blynk is a platform in the form of a server service that is commonly used to assist the work process of the Internet of Things system [23]. This platform supports the iOS operating system version 9+ and Android OS version 4.2+ and can even be downloaded using an Android emulator on a laptop or computer device. There are more than 400 hardware that can be used with Blynk, including ESP8266, ESP32, NodeMCU, Arduino, and Raspberry Pi. The provision of the Blynk platform aims to monitor and control hardware remotely using the Internet or intranet network in the form of visual data display using numbers, graphics, or colors.

2.7 Fuzzy Logic

Developments in the field of informatics make it easier for researchers to make decisions using the desired method or algorithm. One of them is the use of fuzzy methods in making decisions in a system [24]. The word fuzzy comes from an English word which means unclear (indistinct) or the same (vague). This fuzzy theory was first introduced in 1965 by an engineer in the field of machinery as well as an informatics scientist named Lotfi Asker Zadeh [25].

The fuzzy logic method in this study is the method used to determine water drainage by processing the humidity, temperature, and pH values of the water in the aquascape. Draining is carried out if the parameters including humidity, temperature, and pH of the water do not match the settings specified by the User. Fuzzy logic systems are used because they are able to adapt to problems or data that are uncertain or vague. Fuzzy logic has a logical value of 0 to 1, while strict logic or conventional logic has absolute values of 0 and 1 so that it can be concluded with the terms little, fair, and very [26]. The stages of fuzzy logic used in this study are as follows:

(1) Fuzzification

Fuzzification is the first step to determine the sensor membership set [27]. Each water environment parameter has a different membership value. In the turbidity parameter section, the membership values include limpid, normal, and turbid. Meanwhile, in the pH parameter section, the membership values include acid, neutral, and base. Drain speed in minutes with membership values including fast, medium, and slow. The values are depicted (see Fig. 1).

(2) Inference

The inference stage is the stage of determining the fuzzy rules [28]. The determination of these rules is based on the set value of the water environment parameters that have been determined in the fuzzification process. In Table 1, the following are fuzzy logic rules for each parameter of temperature, humidity, turbidity, and pH level.

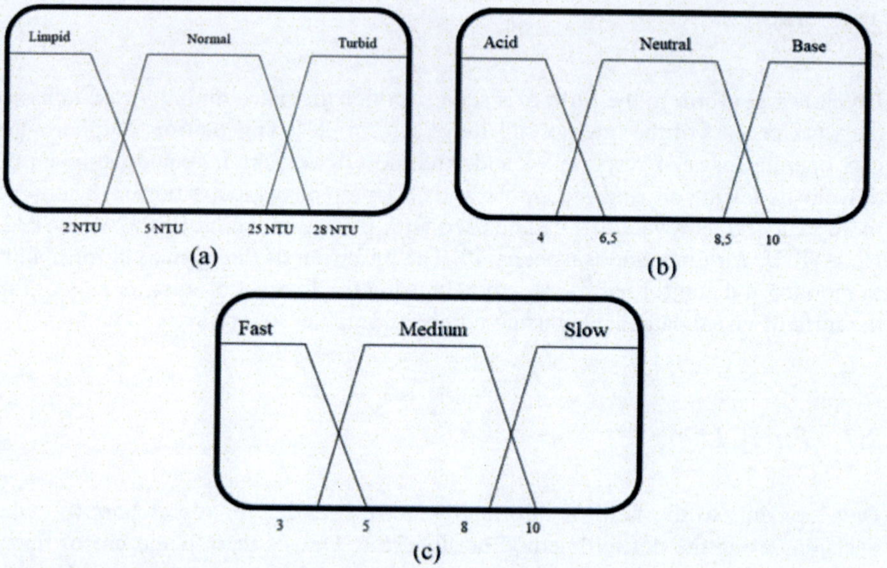

Fig. 1 Membership function: **a** turbidity; **b** pH; and **c** drain speed

(3) Defuzzification

The defuzzification stage is the last stage that functions as a mapping of a fuzzy space value into a crisp value [29]. The resulting crisp values will then be used in the implementation and final analysis. In this study, the defuzzification process of Mamdani's rules was used with the discrete COA (Center of Area) method which can be formulated as follows [30]:

$$z = \frac{\sum_{j=1}^{n} Z_j \mu(z_j)}{\sum_{j=1}^{n} \mu(z_j)} \quad (1)$$

Table 1 Fuzzy logic rules

No	Rules
1	**IF** turbidity (limpid) **AND** pH (acid) **THEN** Water Pump (active, fast)
2	**IF** turbidity (limpid) **AND** pH (neutral) **THEN** Water Pump (active, slow)
3	**IF** turbidity (limpid) **AND** pH (base) **THEN** Water Pump (active, fast)
4	**IF** turbidity (normal) **AND** pH (acid) **THEN** Water Pump (active, medium)
5	**IF** turbidity (normal) **AND** pH (neutral) **THEN** Water Pump (non-active)
6	**IF** turbidity (normal) **AND** pH (base) **THEN** Water Pump (active, medium)
7	**IF** turbidity (turbid) **AND** pH (acid) **THEN** Water Pump (active, slow)
8	**IF** turbidity (turbid) **AND** pH (neutral) **THEN** Water Pump (non-active)
9	**IF** turbidity (turbid) **AND** pH (base) **THEN** Water Pump (active, slow)

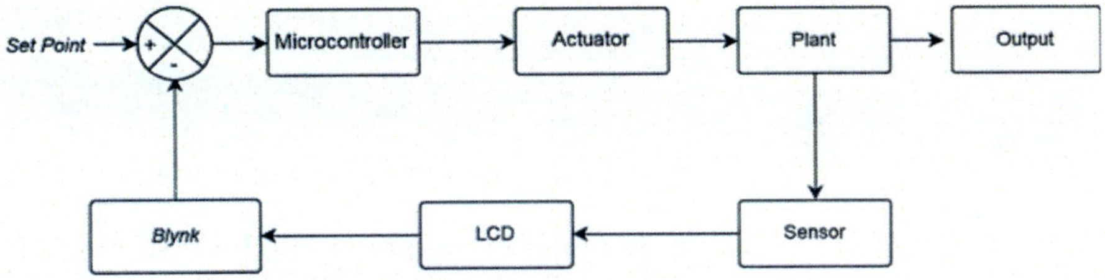

Fig. 2 Monitoring and controlling block diagram system

where z is defined as the crisp value and $\mu(z_j)$ is the membership value of the crisp.

3 System Designing

3.1 System Design

According to (see Fig. 2), the monitoring system begins with a set point in the form of water parameter values, namely temperature (24–28 °C) and humidity (40–60%) in the aquascape. After that, the water environmental parameter values will be processed by the NodeMCU8266 microcontroller. If the temperature value does not match the set point, then the temperature adjustment is carried out by the heater and fan as actuators in the aquascape. The environmental parameter values were read by the DS18B20 temperature sensor and the SHT11 humidity sensor. Then, the processed data will be displayed on the LCD (Liquid Crystal Display) and the Blynk application via the WI-FI network.

According to (see Fig. 3), the automatic draining system begins with a set point in the form of water parameter values, namely pH (6.5–8.5) and turbidity (5 NTU–25 NTU) in the aquascape. After that, the water environmental parameter values will be processed by the NodeMCU 8266 microcontroller. If the pH and turbidity values do not match the set point, then the automatic draining is carried out by the in and out pumps as actuators in the aquascape. The environmental parameter values were read by the DFRobot pH sensor and SKU SEN0819 turbidity sensor. Then, the processed data will be displayed in the Blynk application installed on the smartphone via the WI-FI network.

3.2 Hardware Design

The aquascape used is 60 cm × 30 cm × 30 cm which contains betta fish and ornamental plants that do not use O¬2 elements. The aquascape can accommodate a water capacity of approximately 52 L (52 cm^3). In this aquascape design, researchers

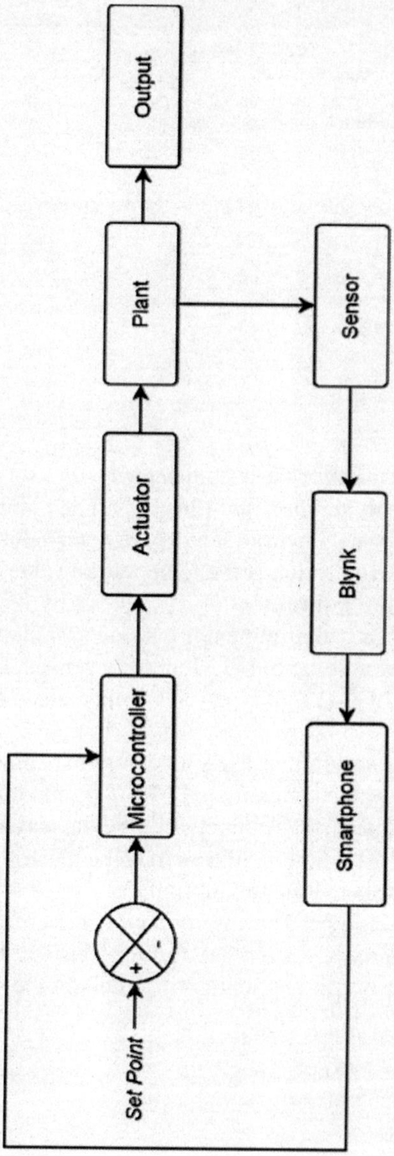

Fig. 3 Drain system block diagram

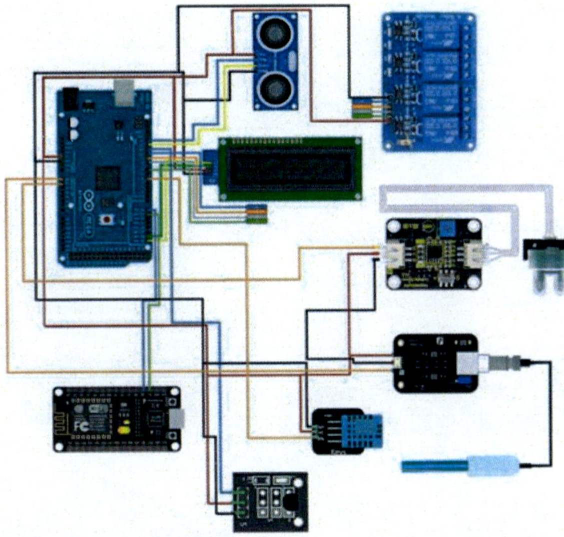

Fig. 4 Wiring diagram

use three types of sensors to determine the water quality in the aquascape, namely temperature sensors, humidity sensors, and pH sensors. Each water environment parameter uses a different sensor, the DS18B20 sensor to measure temperature, the SKU SEN0819 sensor to measure the turbidity of the water, the SHT11 sensor to measure humidity, and the DFRobot sensor to measure the degree of acidity in the aquascape.

This Research also used ultrasonic sensors to measure the water level. This aquascape design also has an LCD (Liquid Crystal Display) installed as a medium for displaying water quality data. As for the use of a water pump for drainage and filling of water, and an electromechanical relay that functions to provide mechanical movement of the water pump when it receives a signal from the microcontroller. The system hardware design is as shown (see Fig. 4). This system integrates pH, turbidity, temperature, and humidity sensors which are controlled by the controller and then displays the output using the Blynk application.

3.3 System Work Flowchart

Based on the system flowchart depicted (see Fig. 5), the stages of the system begin with filling water along with freshwater biota which includes fish and plants. The water in the aquascape is a compound whose quality will be measured by the sensor according to the specified parameters, namely the degree of acidity (pH), temperature, level of turbidity, and humidity.

Next, the sensors installed in the aquascape begin to detect the water parameter values. The sensor then transmits the water parameter value in the form of an analog

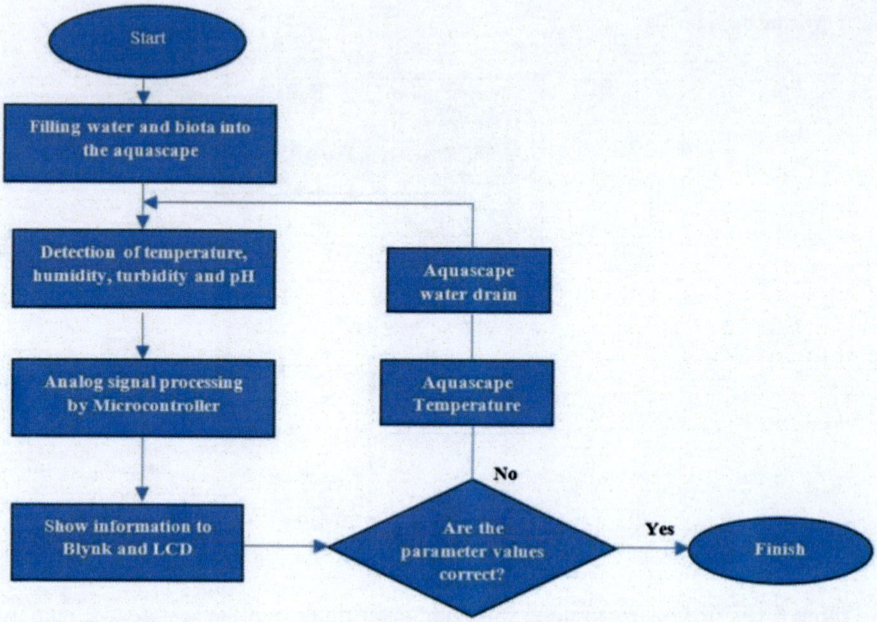

Fig. 5 System work flowchart

signal to the microcontroller to be processed into a digital signal. This digital signal will be displayed on the LCD and the Blynk application that is already installed on the Smartphone via the WI-FI network. The information displayed is a number that shows the water parameter values in the aquascape. If the water parameter values (turbidity and pH) are not in accordance with the provisions set by the user, then the draining process is carried out using the fuzzy logic method. Meanwhile, if the water in the aquascape is in accordance with the provisions, the draining process is not carried out. Then, if the temperature value on the Aquascape does not match the provisions set by the user, then the temperature setting is carried out by the heater or cooling fan. The workings of draining water are described in the following flowchart:

In (see Fig. 6), this automatic draining stage begins with reading the parameter values of the water environment which are read by the sensor, then forwarded to the microcontroller for fuzzy logic testing. The suitability of the values that have been determined in the fuzzy logic program will determine the presence or absence of the drain command. If the turbidity and pH values do not match the set that has been set by the user, then water pump 1 will be active for draining water, otherwise if the water environmental parameter values are appropriate, then water pump 1 will stop. The method of draining water is based on the water level in the aquascape. Water pump 1 will continue to drain water until 1/3 of the aquascape's capacity has been drained. If the water level detected by the ultrasonic beam reaches 1/3 of the aquascape capacity, then water pump 1 will stop, and water pump 2 will be active

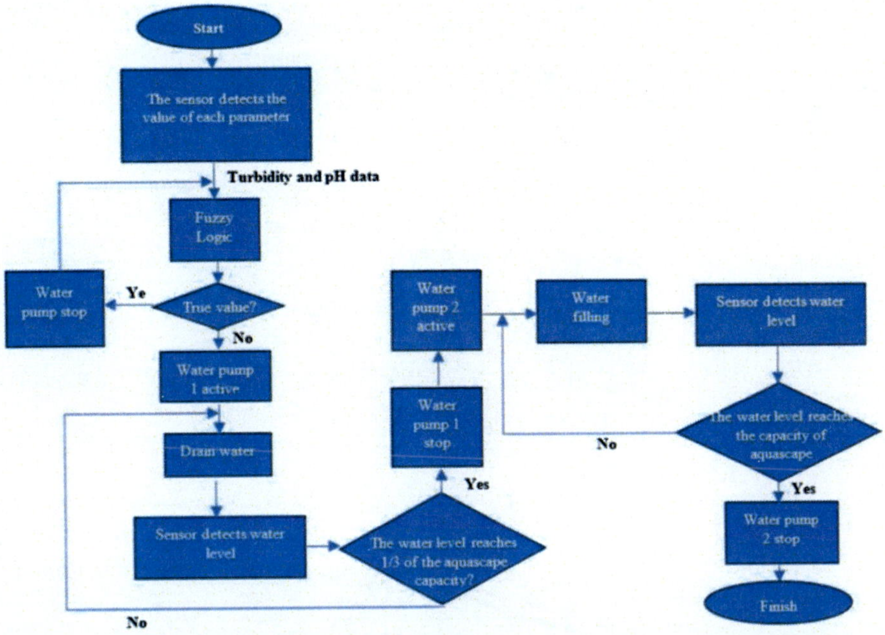

Fig. 6 Automatic water drain flowchart in aquascape

for water filling. The water filling process stops when the water pump 2 has filled the water according to the capacity of the aquascape.

4 Results

4.1 Sensor Accuracy Test

Smart aquascape system designed using supporting sensors. To get a value that is close to the measuring instrument, it is necessary to test the accuracy of the sensor.

Testing the accuracy of the DS18B20 sensor is done by comparing the results of digital thermometer measurements. Water samples used various types to obtain varying temperature values. This test was carried out 20 times. The test results are depicted (see Fig. 8). Based on (see Fig. 7), an error of 3.09% is obtained, which means that the accuracy of the DS18B20 sensor test is 97.91%, stating that the sensor used is feasible.

Testing the accuracy of the SHT11 sensor is done by comparing the results of the comparison sensor measurements. The tests were carried out in different types of rooms to obtain varying humidity values. The test was carried out 10 times. The test results are depicted (see Fig. 8). Based on (see Fig. 8), an error of 7.47% is obtained,

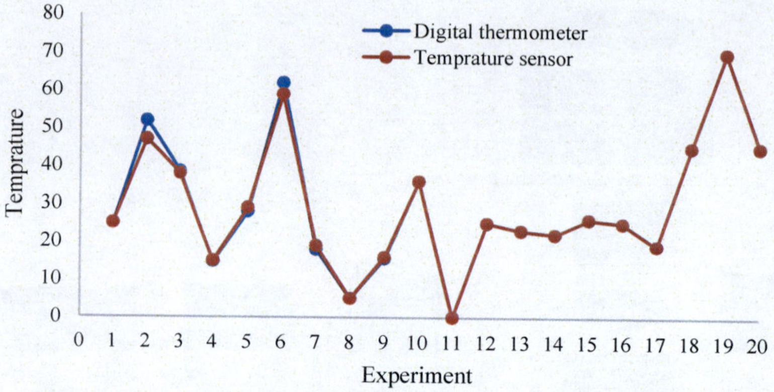

Fig. 7 Accuracy testing of the DS18B20 sensor

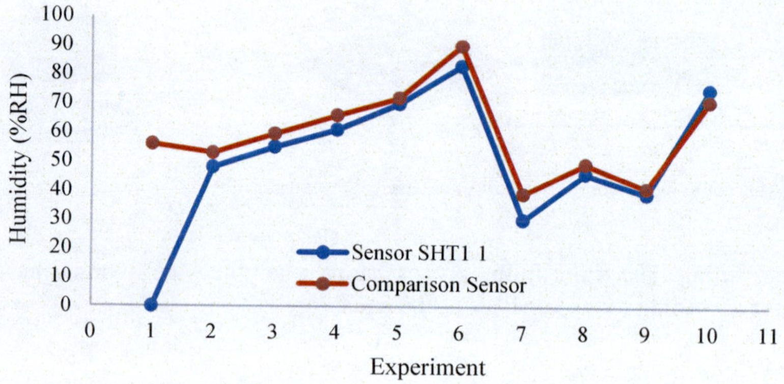

Fig. 8 Accuracy testing of the SHT11 sensor

which means that the accuracy of the SHT11 sensor test is 92.53%, stating that the sensor used is feasible. Testing the accuracy of the SKU SEN0189 sensor is done by comparing the measurement results of the comparison sensor. Tests were carried out on different types of solutions to obtain varying turbidity values. The test was carried out 5 times. The test results are depicted (see Fig. 9). Based on (see Fig. 10), an error of 5.19% is obtained, which means that the accuracy of the SKU SEN0189 sensor test is 94.81%, stating that the sensor used is feasible.

Testing the accuracy of the pH sensor is done by comparing the measurement results of the ATC pH meter sensor. To get a varying pH value, pH up and pH down were used to give different pH conditions. In addition, this test was carried out 30 times, with 15 experiments using acidic liquids and 15 more experiments using alkaline liquids. Based on the results of the sensor accuracy test, an error of 5.09% is obtained, which means that the accuracy of testing the DFRobot pH sensor is 94.91%, stating that the sensor used is feasible (see Figs. 10 and 11).

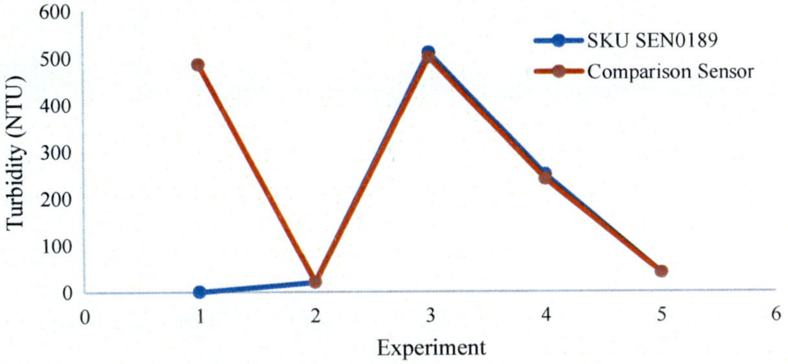

Fig. 9 Accuracy testing of the SKU SEN0189 sensor

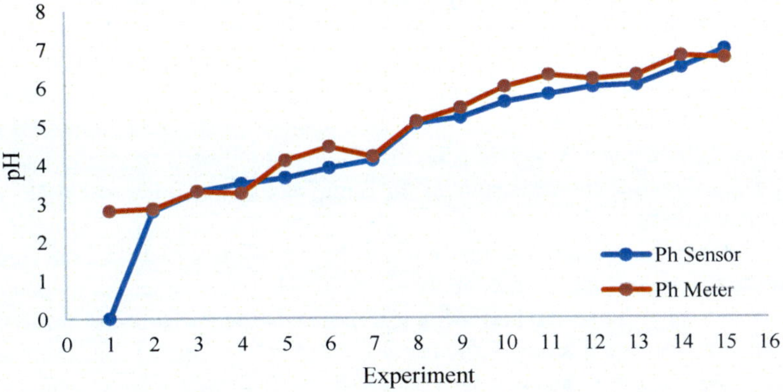

Fig. 10 Testing the accuracy of the DFRobot pH sensor in acid liquids

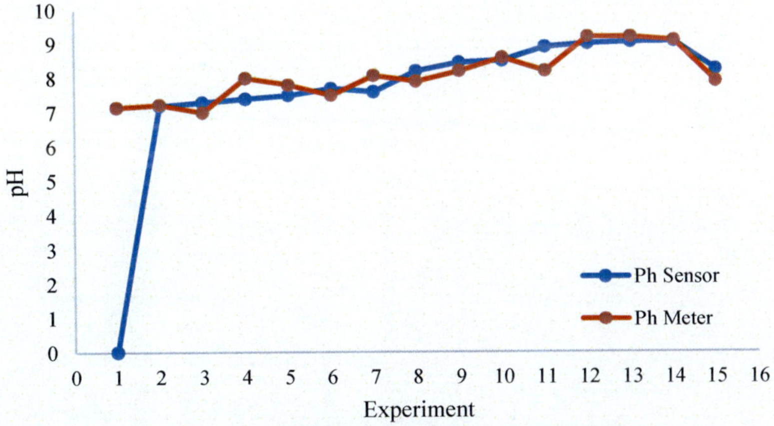

Fig. 11 Testing the accuracy of the DFRobot pH sensor in base liquids

4.2 System Drainage Test

Testing the aquascape drain system consists of several tests, namely testing the heater and fan, testing the pump, and testing the drain. The heater and fan tests are carried out to determine the fan speed in lowering the water temperature and determine the heater speed in increasing the water temperature in the aquascape. Heater testing is done by turning on the heater for 20 min. Aquascape temperature recording is done every 2 min with an initial temperature of 21 °C. Fan testing is done by turning on the fan for 20 min. Then the aquascape temperature was recorded every 2 min with an initial temperature of 29 °C. The following are the results of the heater and fan testing data (see Fig. 12).

Furthermore, pump testing is carried out to determine the timing of the pump in and pump out speeds used for draining. The testing step begins with fully filling the aquascape with water. Then, drain the aquascape by pumping out in one condition, then the aquascape begins to refill with the pump under one condition. Draining with a pump out was carried out with the initial distance condition of 27 cm then every 1 cm decrease was recorded until the final distance of 12 cm was recorded. Meanwhile, the pump is carried out with the opposite condition, namely the initial distance of 12 cm, then every 1 cm increase is recorded until the final distance is 27 cm. The following are the results of the pump test by recording the time, which is illustrated (see Fig. 13).

Drain testing is carried out to find out whether the system work is in accordance with the fuzzy logic system that has been designed. In addition, it can determine the effect of the pH sensor and turbidity (turbidity) on the flame of the pump in and pump out in aquascape drainage. The test is carried out by making the conditions of the aquascape into five types, namely alkaline-normal; normal-cloudy; acid-normal; sour-turbid; and muddy. The following results of the draining test are described in Table 2.

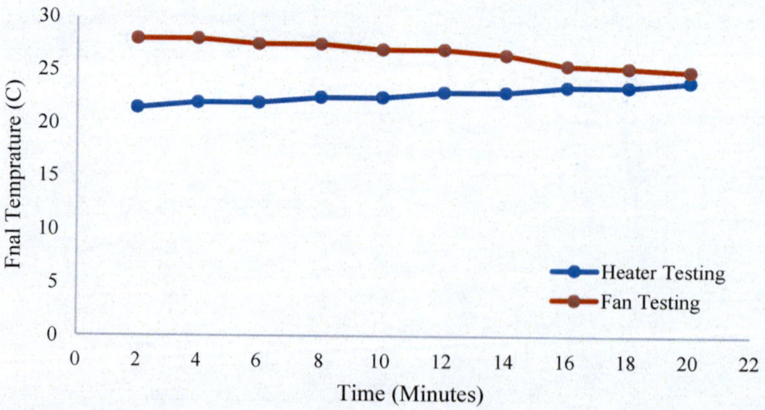

Fig. 12 Heater and fan test

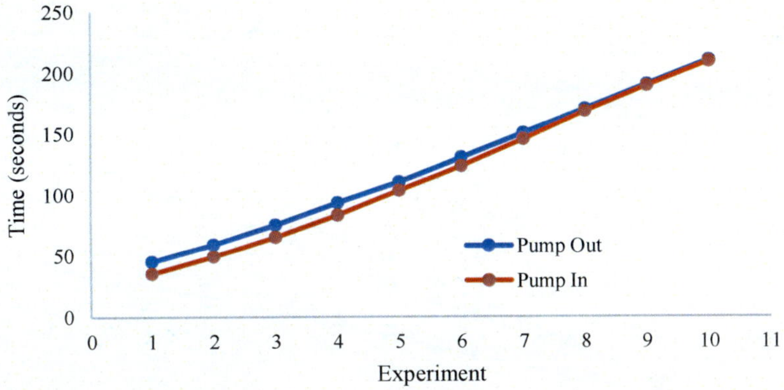

Fig. 13 Pump out and pump in test

Table 2 Drain test results

No	Type	pH sensor	Turbidity sensor (NTU)	COA value (minutes)	Drain speed
1	Base-normal	8.71	10.16	6.85	Medium
2	Normal-turbid	7.79	27.02	8.08	Slow
3	Acid-normal	5.57	10.72	6.97	Medium
4	Acid-turbid	4.48	27.72	3.78	Fast
5	Base-turbid	9.92	27.72	4.43	Fast

Based on Table 1, it can be stated that the drain system automatically runs according to the provisions of Fuzzy Logic. Under normal conditions—cloudy and acid—clean, the draining speed runs slowly according to the conditions set by the user. Under conditions of clear-base, the rate of draining is moderate, while under conditions of acid-turbid and alkaline-cloudy, the rate of draining is fast. Then a drain test is carried out at the specified distance. The test results are depicted (see Fig. 12).

In (see Fig. 14), the average draining time required in acid-turbid conditions from a distance of 26–12 cm is 227 s, then the average draining time required for alkaline-turbid conditions from a distance of 26–12 cm is equal to 265 s, then the average draining time required under base-normal conditions from a distance of 26–12 cm is 411 s, while the average draining time required under normal-turbid conditions from a distance of 26–12 cm is equal to 480 s, and the average draining time required under acid-normal conditions from 26 to 12 cm is 418 s.

4.3 *Notification Testing System*

Notification testing aims to find out that there are no obstacles that occur to the system in hardware. The system constraints in question are in the design of hardware

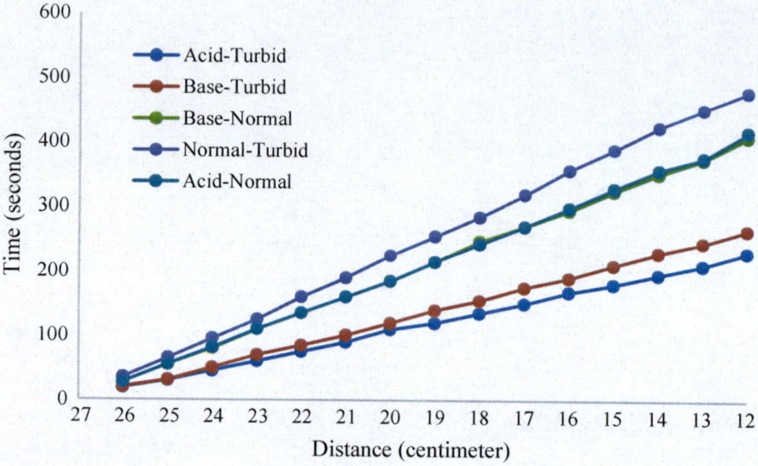

Fig. 14 Drain test results in various conditions

and component wiring. The test was carried out by making the conditions of the aquascape into five types, namely base-limpid; neutral-turbid; acid-limpid; acid-turbid; and base-turbid. When the drain occurs, the Blynk will display the state that the aquascape is being drained.

According to Table 3, it can be stated that there are no problems in the system which include hardware design and component wiring. The system is able to display drain notifications on the Blynk app.

Based on Table 4, it can be stated that from a distance of 2 m to 25 m, the notification test with a distance of 2–20 m shows a percentage of 100%, while the notification test with a distance of 22 m begins to decrease, which is 60%. The signal can no longer be received by the Smartphone when testing a distance of 25 m.

Table 3 Drainage system notification test result without IoT

No	Type	pH sensor	Turbidity sensor (NTU)	Pump out	Pump in	LCD display
1	Base-limpid	>8.5	5–25	On	On	Active drain
2	Normal-turbid	6–8.5	>25	On	On	Active drain
3	Acid-limpid	<6	5–25	On	On	Active drain
4	Acid-turbid	<6	>25	On	On	Active drain
5	Base-turbid	>8.5	>25	On	On	Active drain

Table 4 Drainage system notification test result with IoT

No	Testing distance (meters)	Successful notification frequency (time)	Notification frequency failed (time)	Success percentage (%)
1	2	10 time	–	100
2	5	10 time	–	100
3	10	10 time	–	100
4	15	10 time	–	100
5	20	10 time	–	100
6	22	6 time	4 time	60
7	25	–	10 time	0

5 Conclusion

Based on the research results, then the conclusion obtained is the test of reading the value of the water environment with the distance of the WI-FI router and the system as far as 5–20 m successfully displays data with 100% accuracy through the Blynk application. The monitoring system displayed by the monitor also works well. If the Wi-Fi router is between 5 and 20 m and the Internet network is available, then the control of water quality in the form of pH and turbidity can work 100%. The design of the algorithm in the automatic control system begins with determining the turbidity value of 5–25 NTU and pH of 6.5–8.5 for the aquascape which is then processed using fuzzy logic. Fuzzy Logic is applied in an automatic drain system by comparing the measurement of the turbidity and pH values by the sensor with the crisp values obtained from the fuzzy logic processing results. The design of the algorithm in the automatic draining system is functioning well, as shown by testing the whole system, where the output of the automatic draining is given according to the conditions of the aquascape.

References

1. Azri Bin Mohammad M, Norisikin Abas S, Ihwan Zakariah M, Sheriff SM (2021) Aquascape ornamental industry in Malaysia: a perspective review. In: IOP conference series: earth and environmental science. https://doi.org/10.1088/1755-1315/860/1/012044
2. Anjur N, Sabran SF, Daud HM, Othman NZ (2021) An update on the ornamental fish industry in Malaysia: aeromonas hydrophila-associated disease and its treatment control. Vet World 14. https://doi.org/10.14202/vetworld.2021.1143-1152
3. Meena Kumari K, Varun Kumar N, Kumari Scholar C, Kumari C (2021) Art and science of aquascaping. ~ 240 ~Pharma Innov J
4. Encinas C, Ruiz E, Cortez J, Espinoza A (2017) Design and implementation of a distributed IoT system for the monitoring of water quality in aquaculture. In: Wireless telecommunications symposium. https://doi.org/10.1109/WTS.2017.7943540

5. Emerenciano MGC, Martínez-Córdova LR, Martínez-Porchas M, Miranda-Baeza A (2017) Biofloc Technology (BFT): a tool for water quality management in aquaculture. In: Water Qual. https://doi.org/10.5772/66416
6. Volkoff H, Rønnestad I (2020). Effects of temperature on feeding and digestive processes in fish. https://doi.org/10.1080/23328940.2020.1765950
7. Lee JM, Ban H, Lee Y, Cho K-C, Koh H-B, Lee K (2017) Impact of aquariums on indoor environmental quality. Korean J Environ Heal Sci 43. https://doi.org/10.5668/jehs.2017.43.1.87
8. Hardyanto RH, Ciptadi PW, Asmara A (2019) Smart aquarium based on internet of things. J Bus Inf Syst (e-ISSN 2685–2543) 1. https://doi.org/10.36067/jbis.v1i1.12
9. Devi PA, Padmavathy P, Aanand S, Aruljothi K (2017) Review on water quality parameters in freshwater cage fish culture. Int J Appl Res 3
10. Boyd CE (2017) General relationship between water quality and aquaculture performance in ponds. In: Fish diseases: prevention and control strategies. https://doi.org/10.1016/B978-0-12-804564-0.00006-5
11. Quality W (2008) Turbidity: description, impact on water quality, sources, measures. Water Qual 3
12. Ertyan PV, Pangaribuan P, Wibowo AS (2019) System monitoring and controlling the aquarium in the maintenance fish from a distance. e-Proceeding Eng 6:3102–3108
13. Handi FH, Setyawan GE (2019) Sistem Pemantauan Menggunakan Blynk dan Pengendalian Penyiraman Tanaman Jamur Dengan Metode Logika Fuzzy. J Pengemb Teknol Inf dan Ilmu Komput 3
14. Adityas Y, Ahmad M, Khamim M, Sofi K, Riady SR (2021) Water quality monitoring system with parameter of pH, temperature, turbidity, and salinity based on internet of things. JISA(Jurnal Inform. dan Sains) 4 https://doi.org/10.31326/jisa.v4i2.965
15. Akshitha S (2020) Girwani: aquascaping: an incredible art under water. Vigyan Varta 1:59–62
16. Mishra BK, Khalid MA, Narayan SL (2019) Assessment of the effect of water temperature on length gain, feed conversion ratio (FCR) and protein profile in brain of Labeo rohita (Hamilton 1822) fed Nigella sativa incorporated diets. Int J Fish Aquat Stud 7:6–13
17. Adiyaksa IP (2022) Water quality assessment at Tanggulangin cultural park. J Sumberd Alam dan Lingkung 8:33–37
18. Yehia HMA-S, Said SM (2021) Drinking water treatment: pH adjustment using natural physical field. J Biosci Med 09. https://doi.org/10.4236/jbm.2021.96005
19. Cantera-Cantera LA, Calvillo-Téllez A, Lozano-Hernández Y (2020) Turbidity, dissolved oxygen and pH measurement system for grey water treatment process by electrocoagulation. Rev del Desarro Tecnol. https://doi.org/10.35429/jtd.2020.14.4.20.27
20. Kahlert H, Leito I (2019) Generalization of acid-base diagrams based on the unified pH-Scale. Chem Phys Chem 20. https://doi.org/10.1002/cphc.201900388
21. Kleinhappel TK, Burman OHP, John EA, Wilkinson A, Pike TW (2019) The impact of water pH on association preferences in fish. Ethology 125. https://doi.org/10.1111/eth.12843
22. Spence R, Gerlach G, Lawrence C, Smith C (2008) The behaviour and ecology of the zebrafish. Danio Rerio. https://doi.org/10.1111/j.1469-185X.2007.00030.x
23. Rif'an M (2019) Internet of Things (IoT): BLYNK framework for smart home KnE Soc Sci 3. https://doi.org/10.18502/kss.v3i12.4128
24. Kahraman C, Onar SC, Oztaysi B (2015) Fuzzy multicriteria decis making. Lit Rev. https://doi.org/10.1080/18756891.2015.1046325
25. Hardyanto RH, Wahyu P (2019) Konsep "AQU PINTAR" aquarium pintar 4.0 berbasis IoT. In: Seri prosiding seminar nasional dinamika informatika, pp 81–83
26. Tadeus DY, Azazi K, Ariwibowo D (2019) Model sistem monitoring pH dan kekeruhan pada akuarium air tawar berbasis internet of things. METANA 15. https://doi.org/10.14710/metana.v15i2.26046
27. Siahaan APU (2017) Fuzzification of college adviser proficiency based on specific knowledge. Adv Res Comput Sci Softw Eng 6

28. Agusta A, Arini FY, Arifudin R (2020) Implementation of fuzzy logic method and certainty factor for diagnosis expert system of chronic kidney disease. J Adv Inf Syst Technol 2
29. Thaker S, Nagori V (2018) Analysis of fuzzification process in fuzzy expert system. in: procedia computer science. https://doi.org/10.1016/j.procs.2018.05.047
30. Rajagiri AK, Mn SR, Nawaz SS, Suresh Kumar T (2019) Speed control of DC motor using fuzzy logic controller by PCI 6221 with MATLAB. In: E3S web of conferences. https://doi.org/10.1051/e3sconf/20198701004

Comparison of Principal Component Analysis and Recursive Feature Elimination with Cross-Validation Feature Selection Algorithms for Customer Churn Prediction

Muhammad Afif Afdholul Matin, Agung Triayudi, and Rima Tamara Aldisa

Abstract Customers choose services from telecommunication companies which are usually based on service quality, price, to security issues. If the customer is not satisfied with the services provided, the customer tends to churn or switch to another company. Churn prediction using data mining techniques is necessary because getting new customers is taking a higher cost than retaining customers that already subscribed. Many previous studies have discussed customer churn and used various classification algorithms. However, the research that focuses on comparing algorithms for feature selection to predict customer churn is still few. This study aims to find the impact of Principal Component Analysis (PCA) and Recursive Feature Elimination with Cross-Validation (RFECV) feature selection algorithms on the eXtreme Gradient Boost (XGBoost) classifier. This study aims to obtain more optimal classification results with fewer predictor attributes. This study was conducted to perform feature selection using PCA and RFECV on the available datasets, then build customer churn prediction models using the XGBoost algorithm, and the quality of each model is measured using accuracy, precision, sensitivity, f1-score, and Area Under the Curved (AUC) score. The results showed that the use of RFECV-XGBoost resulted in higher accuracy and f1-score and the XGBoost model without feature selection resulted in a higher AUC than the classification model using feature selection. The results of the modeling after RFECV feature selection, the accuracy reaches 0.96, the precision reaches 0.859, the sensitivity reaches 0.83, the f1-score reaches 0.844, and the AUC reaches 0.904. The use of RFECV feature selection can exceed XGBoost classification results without feature selection.

Keywords Customer churn · Classification · PCA · RFECV · XGBoost

M. A. A. Matin · A. Triayudi (✉) · R. T. Aldisa
Universitas Nasional, Jl. Sawo Manila, Pasar Minggu, Pejaten 12520, Indonesia
e-mail: agungtriayudi@civitas.unas.ac.id

T. Triwiyanto et al. (eds.), *Proceeding of the 3rd International Conference on Electronics, Biomedical Engineering, and Health Informatics*, Lecture Notes in Electrical Engineering 1008, https://doi.org/10.1007/978-981-99-0248-4_15

1 Introduction

Customers are an important element in business that makes a company survive in market competition. In a competitive market, customers make their own choices to choose the services offered [1]. These decisions are usually based on price, quality of customer service, to the reliability of features [2]. If the service provided is unsatisfactory, the customer inevitably decides to churn or move from one service to another company [3].

The big challenge of a service company or service is when customers decide to unsubscribe or churn. Because this can have an impact on decreasing the company's income. The average percentage of churn rates in the telecommunications industry sector is around 1.9–2.1% per month, and per year it can reach 10–67% [4]. In addition to decreasing company revenues, churn by customers can incur additional costs to acquire new customers [5]. This is because old customers already recognize the previous service. Meanwhile, to find new customers, companies must introduce their products again because new potential customers do not necessarily recognize what is offered and what are the advantages of the services provided by the company. Therefore, many companies are switching strategies from finding new customers to focusing on retaining existing ones, especially for companies that prioritize a high return on investment (ROI) [6]. As for how companies can improve service quality, seek to find out customer complaints, seek predictions of customers who tend to churn using machine learning techniques [7].

Churn prediction uses a supervised learning classification technique which means that modeling requires training data and test data that uses predictor attributes or features and target attributes that determine data into a class [8]. Generally, in the case of churn prediction, the target attribute output consists of two classes: churn and non-churn [9]. Therefore, churn prediction is also referred to as binary classification [10].

Previously, many studies discussed churn prediction, especially in the telecommunications industry. Research [1] proposes an experiment using the most effective classification algorithm in recent years, namely eXtreme Gradient Boosting (XGBoost). The performance of XGBoost is tested after being combined with the oversampling method to overcome class imbalances in the dataset. The model is compared with other classification algorithms and the results show that the performance of XGBoost and the random forest is better than other classification algorithms and the resampling method does not improve the f1 measurement results and accuracy.

Research [3] analyzed the best classification algorithm. Classifier performance is measured by accuracy and f-measure. The correlation of the predictor with the target is used to select features. The dataset is modeled using KNN, random forest, and XGBoost. The results show that the XGBoost algorithm produces the best performance.

Research [5] proposes a model that applies feature selection to select relevant features and improves the churn prediction model. The selected feature selection method is the Sequential Forward Selection (SFS) wrapper technique, Sequential

Backward Selection (SBS), Sequential Forward Floating Selection (SFFS), and Sequential Backward Floating Selection (SBFS). Modeling using the Naive Bayes algorithm. The dataset was tested by applying tenfold cross-validation. The results show that the selection of the four algorithms produces the same accuracy value but is better than not using feature selection.

Research [11] compares the heuristic feature selection methods Ant Search Method (ASM), Cuckoo Search Method (CSM), Particle Swarm Optimization (PSO), Linear Forward Selection (LFS), and Principal Component Analysis (PCA). After feature selection, the dataset is modeled using a decision tree and evaluated using the specified metrics. As a result, the ASM algorithm showed better performance with an accuracy of 94.2% and a ROC of 0.78.

Research [10] proposed the use of PCA for feature reduction. The dataset used is a dataset of telecommunications companies in the United States consisting of 100,000 data, 171 predictor attributes, and one target attribute. The dataset was successfully reduced to 55 features from 90% variation. The proposed model yields an accuracy of 92% and an AUC of 0.67 which is better than other classification algorithms.

Research [12] proposed the use of Recursive Feature Elimination with Cross-Validation (RFECV) to reduce features in the employee reduction dataset. The results showed that the use of RFECV with the Random Forest and AdaBoost classification algorithms resulted in a good performance with an accuracy of 98.63 and 95.83% with f1-scores of 0.96 and 0.91, respectively.

But as far as the literature that has been found, there are still few who propose the effect of feature selection on the customer churn dataset of telecommunications companies and use RFECV as feature selection and XGBoost as a modeling algorithm for customer churn prediction [5, 11].

This study proposes a comparison of PCA and RFECV algorithms as feature selection and uses XGBoost for modeling customer churn classification on public datasets of the telecommunications industry. The effect of the feature selection algorithm is then compared to the results of the accuracy, precision, sensitivity, f1-score, and AUC metrics from the modeling.

2 Methods

2.1 Research Framework

The framework for this research is summarized in Fig. 1. This study uses three datasets described in Table 1. Based on the research framework in Fig. 1, the experiment begins by importing each dataset into a program using the Python programming language using the Jupyter Notebook platform. After the dataset is imported, the next step is the data preprocessing stage. Data preprocessing is the process of cleaning data so that it can be classified. Data cleaning can be in the form of overcoming empty data, normalizing data into a numeric form, to feature selection. In this study, the feature selection process is separated into two different methods which will be evaluated at the end of the experiment.

The process of cleaning data of categorical type is converted into a numeric value, and this technique can also use normalization for each category in the attribute into binary data. If the categorical data type has only two labels, then the sample data is replaced with binary data. Examples of target attribute data "Churn" in the form of "TRUE" and "FALSE" changed to 1 and 0. The empty data cleaning process is

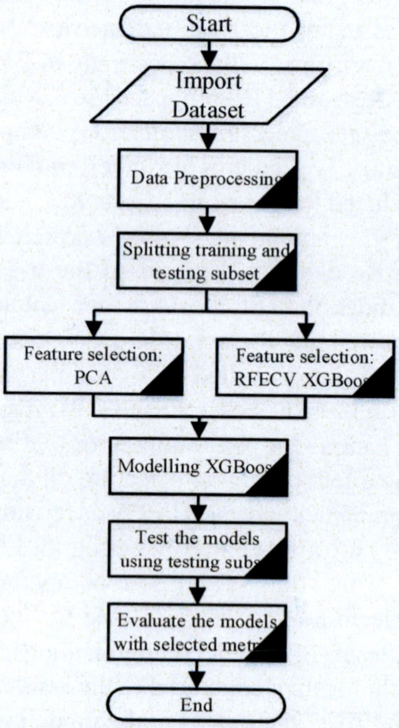

Fig. 1 Research framework

Table 1 Description of the dataset used in this study

Description	Dataset 1	Dataset 2	Dataset 3
Number of records	72,274	3333	3333
Number of attributes	11	21	11
Number of classes	2	2	2
Positive class percentage (%)	55.4	14.5	14.5
Negative class percentage (%)	44.6	85.5	85.5
Dataset sources	Kaggle [13]	Kaggle [14]	Kaggle [15]

done by filling the data with the average of the existing data. If the empty data on the attribute is below 1% of the total sample data, then the sample data is deleted because it does not have a major effect on the classification process [16]. The data preprocessing process also includes deleting attributes or features that are not related to the classification process, for example, telephone numbers and state codes, because if normalized it will make the dimensions of the dataset very large.

After going through the data preprocessing stage, the next step is to separate the dataset into training data, namely data that will be used as modeling with a ratio of 80% and test data for testing models that have been trained with a ratio of 20%.

The next stage is feature selection which is further described in Sects. 2.2 and 2.3. The purpose of feature selection is to be able to select attributes that a contribution to classification. Feature selection is also used to eliminate features that can interfere with the performance of the classification or also known as noise [17]. With this application, it is expected that the performance of the classification model with feature selection can approach or exceed the performance of the model that does not use feature selection.

After the feature selection process, the data is modeled using the XGBoost algorithm which is described further in Sect. 2.4 and measured by the metrics of accuracy, precision, sensitivity, f1-score, and Area Under the Curve (AUC). The sensitivity or recall metric was chosen because in predicting customer churn, the prediction is prioritized to find customers who are likely to churn to prioritize customers who want to switch in retention efforts. The f1-score metric was chosen to determine the feasibility of the modeling which cannot rely solely on accuracy metrics. Since the dataset in churn prediction is highly unbalanced, performance cannot be measured solely with accuracy. The accuracy value is usually large because the correct non-churn prediction or false negative (FN) is greater than the true positive (TP) which indicates the churn class is very small.

2.2 *Principal Component Analysis (PCA)*

PCA is a linear combination of initial variables which geometrically obtains the coordinates of this new linear combination obtained from the original rotation. PCA is used for data that has a large number of variables and has a correlation between variables. The purpose of PCA is to select variables without losing important information contained in the initial dataset [8, 18–20]. The stages in finding the PCA value are as follows:

Calculating the covariance matrix from the dataset. The covariance matrix is a matrix of covariance values in each cell obtained from sample data. The formula for finding the covariance matrix is as follows [8].

$$\mathrm{Cov}(x, y) = \frac{1}{n-1}\sum_{i=1}^{n}(x_i - \mu_x)(y_i - \mu_y) \quad (1)$$

where x and y are the selected features to calculate the covariance. μ_x and μ_y are the averages of the sample features x and y. x_i and y_i are i-th sample data with x and y features. The n is the number of sample data. The results of the covariance calculation are arranged in the form of a matrix that has a size of $m \times m$, where m is the number of features.

Finding the eigenvalues and eigenvectors of the covariance matrix. Eigenvalues (λ) are scalar numbers and A is a matrix with a size of $m \times m$. The equation to obtain the m eigenvalues ($\lambda_1, \lambda_2, \ldots, \lambda_m$) is as follows.

$$|A - \lambda I| = 0 \tag{2}$$

A is the covariance matrix $m \times m$, λ is the eigenvalue, and I is the identity matrix. The equation to get the eigenvector is

$$\begin{aligned} Ax &= \lambda x \\ Ax - \lambda x &= 0 \\ (A - \lambda)x &= 0 \\ (A - \lambda I)x &= 0, x \neq 0 \end{aligned} \tag{3}$$

where A is an $m \times m$ matrix that has the m number of the eigenvalue (λ_m). x is a non-zero matrix and I is an identity matrix.

Selecting several Principal Components (PCs). The main component or principal component chosen is the component that has a maximum contribution of 99% of the variance threshold. This value was chosen because it is considered to meet the total covariance variance of the original attribute [8]. The value of the proportion of variance is calculated by the following equation:

$$\text{PC}(\%) = \frac{\text{eigen value}}{\text{covariance variance}} \times 100\% \tag{4}$$

which is the covariance variance obtained from the sum of the diagonal values of the covariance matrix.

1. Calculating attribute weights with eigenvector values

The PC that has been selected is calculated in its cumulative value until it meets the predetermined threshold. The weight of the attributes is determined by the eigenvector matrix and the highest absolute value is selected in the matrix in each PC.

2. Selecting the original attribute using the eigenvector weight

Selected features that have met the threshold are used to create a prediction model.

2.3 Recursive Feature Elimination with Cross-Validation (RFECV)

RFECV is an improvement of Recursive Feature Elimination (RFE), and the difference is that RFE must determine how many features will be used and RFECV does not need to specify the number of attributes desired [21]. RFECV removes attributes that are repetitive and have a weak effect on the classifier. This algorithm uses an iterative procedure to compare attributes. This algorithm first builds a model of all the attributes in the dataset. Then the attributes are ranked for their effect on the classifier. RFECV removes the attribute that has the lowest correlation and repeats it to recalculate the rank of the attribute. The main purpose of RFECV is to select the best number of attributes through automatic cross-validation [22–24].

RFE is a feature selection wrapper that uses a machine learning model, calculates the importance of features, then eliminates features with the lowest ranking until they meet the specified number of features [25].

The purpose of using cross-validation is to overcome the previous weakness of the RFE algorithm which is less stable in determining the training data. By using cross-validation, RFE is more stable and more reliable in ranking attributes. This study uses a fivefold cross-validation.

2.4 eXtreme Gradient Boosting (XGBoost)

XGBoost is an implementation of a gradient-boosted decision tree designed for speed and performance. This algorithm is a supervised learning and ensemble learning algorithm that combines trees to further generalize machine learning models that are built from a large number of trees and average the prediction results for better predictions. Decision trees are built from one to another where the faults of the previous tree can be corrected and focus on increasing accuracy in the next tree. Due to good optimization, XGBoost produces good results but takes longer to iterate [3].

2.5 Evaluation Metrics

The classification results are placed in the confusion matrix. The confusion matrix places the correct prediction data with positive data or churn is declared true positive (TP), correct prediction data with negative or non-churn data is declared true negative (TN), and non-churn prediction data while the reality of churn is declared false negative (FN), and churn prediction data but non-churn reality data were declared false positive (FP) [26].

The placement of predictions in the confusion matrix is then calculated as metrics of accuracy, precision, sensitivity, f1-score, and Area Under the Curve (AUC). Accuracy is the proportion of correct predictions, which is calculated by Eq. (5) where the number of correct predictions is divided by the number of test samples. Precision is the proportion of prediction with churn class and true churn. Equation (6) is a precision calculation where the correct churn prediction (TP) is divided by the number of predicted churn classes [27–29].

$$\text{Accuracy} = \frac{\text{TP} + \text{TN}}{\text{TP} + \text{TN} + \text{FP} + \text{FN}} \tag{5}$$

$$\text{Precision} = \frac{\text{TP}}{\text{TP} + \text{FP}} \tag{6}$$

Sensitivity or recall or TP-rate is the proportion of churn class that is classified correctly. Equation (7) describes a sensitivity calculation in which the number of correct churn predictions is divided by all samples of the churn class [26].

$$\text{Sensitivity} = \frac{\text{TP}}{\text{TP} + \text{FN}} \tag{7}$$

F1-score is the average of precision and sensitivity which is used as a performance measurement of the classification results [3]. The f1-score calculation is described in Eq. (8).

$$\text{F1 score} = \frac{2 \times \text{precison} \times \text{sensitivity}}{\text{precision} + \text{sensitivity}} \tag{8}$$

AUC is the area under the Receiver Operating Characteristic (ROC) curve on a two-dimensional graph where the Y-axis is the TP level, and the X-axis is the FP level. ROC shows the exchange between TP and FP. The closer the curve to the point (0, 1), the better the model. Diagnostic testing of a classification algorithm is measured using the AUC value. The calculation of the AUC value is shown in Eq. (9).

$$\text{AUC} = \frac{1 + \text{TP}_{\text{rate}} + \text{FP}_{\text{rate}}}{2}, \text{ where } \text{FP}_{\text{rate}} = \frac{\text{FP}}{\text{TN} + \text{FP}} \tag{9}$$

3 Results and Discussion

3.1 Results

The research started by importing the dataset. Datasets that have been imported are preprocessed for data. Irrelevant variables are eliminated so that the remaining attributes can be classified. One of the attributes in dataset 1 [13] with the name "remaining_contract" has a very large number of empty values, namely 29.8%. However, according to the source of the dataset, an empty value in the attribute concerned has meaning, if the attribute is empty, it means the customer has not entered into a term contract, while if it is filled then the data is the remaining time of the contract [13]. Therefore, feature engineering is carried out by changing the perception of these features. If the attribute value is empty then it is replaced with 0 while the non-empty value is filled with 1. The result of the feature engineering is then saved to the new attribute "is_time_range_contract" and the old attribute "remaining_contract" is deleted. Dataset 2 [14] and dataset 3 [15] have no empty values in all of their attributes so they can proceed to the next stage, namely splitting or separating the dataset into training and testing subsets with a ratio of 80:20.

The selection of PCA features is carried out by calculating the covariance matrix to find correlations between attributes [8, 30, 31]. Then calculate the covariance variance by adding up the diagonal cells of the covariance matrix. Search for eigenvalues and eigenvectors for calculating the proportion of principal components (PC). The PC proportion is calculated using Eq. (4) whose results are shown in Tables 2, 3, and 4.

Based on Table 2, the cumulative threshold of 99% variance proportion is met in PC 3 in dataset 1 which means there will be three selected attributes. In Table 3, the cumulative threshold of dataset 2 is met in PC 9 which means there are 9 selected attributes. In Table 4, the cumulative threshold of dataset 3 is met in PC 4 which means there are four selected attributes.

After the number of PCs on each dataset is determined, the predetermined attribute is selected through the highest absolute value in the eigenvector matrix. After the attributes are selected, modeling is done using XGBoost.

Table 2 The proportion of PCs in dataset 1

Principal component	Eigenvalues	Variance proportion	Cumulative
PC 1	3733.915	94.7416%	94.7416%
PC 2	140.258	3.5588%	98.3%
PC 3	**60.681**	**1.5397%**	**99.84%**
PC 4	4.146	0.1052%	99.95%
...	⋮	⋮	⋮
PC 9	0.1053	0.0027%	100.0%

Table 3 The proportion of PCs in dataset 2

Principal component	Eigenvalues	Variance proportion	Cumulative
PC 1	3029.344	23.279%	23.28%
PC 2	2652.471	20.383%	43.66%
PC 3	2541.777	19.5323%	63.19%
PC 4	1808.55	13.8978%	77.09%
PC 5	1585.09	12.1807%	89.27%
PC 6	407.471	3.1312%	92.4%
PC 7	404.812	3.1108%	95.51%
PC 8	383.482	2.9469%	98.46%
PC 9	**183.924**	**1.4134%**	**99.88%**
PC 10	8.504	0.0653%	99.94%
…	⋮	⋮	⋮
PC 18	7.621	0.0%	100.0%

Table 4 The proportion of PCs in dataset 3

Principal component	Eigenvalues	Variance proportion	Cumulative
PC 1	3030.984	58.0283%	58.03%
PC 2	1592.588	30.4902%	88.52%
PC 3	403.896	7.7326%	96.25%
PC 4	**180.34**	**3.4526%**	**99.7%**
PC 5	7.857	0.1504%	99.85%
…	⋮	⋮	⋮
PC 9	0.0007	0.0%	100.0%

In the selection of RFECV features, each dataset is selected with a fivefold cross-validation using the f1-score metric. The classification algorithm used in the feature selection is the same as the main classification algorithm in this study, namely XGBoost. The results of the RFECV feature selection are shown in Table 5. The results of feature selection in each dataset are shown in Table 6. After the features are selected, modeling is carried out with training data using the XGBoost algorithm. The results of the modeling were tested using test data. The results of the modeling test are summarized in Table 7.

Based on the results of the study which are summarized in Table 7, the use of RFECV feature selection with the XGBoost classification algorithm (RFECV-XGBoost) produces very good performance when compared to PCA with XGBoost (PCA-XGBoost). RFECV-XGBoost's accuracy performance in dataset 1 can match the accuracy of the XGBoost model without feature selection, and in datasets 2 and 3, RFECV-XGBoost's accuracy outperforms PCA-XGBoost and XGBoost without

Table 5 RFECV feature selection result

Datasets	Number of selected attributes
Dataset 1	8
Dataset 2	8
Dataset 3	9

feature selection. Likewise, with precision, RFECV-XGBoost is only 0.001 below XGBoost's performance in dataset 1 and can outperform the other two methods in datasets 2 and 3.

In the sensitivity measurement, the performance of RFECV-XGBoost outperformed XGBoost in dataset 1, the same score in dataset 2, and only a 0.011 difference under dataset 3. For the f1-score measurement, the performance of RFECV-XGBoost could match XGBoost in dataset 1 and outperformed both other methods in datasets 2 and 3. In AUC measurements, XGBoost's performance outperformed both feature selections in datasets 1 and 3 and was comparable to RFECV-XGBoost in dataset 2.

The visualization of the metric comparison results from the applied method is shown in Figs. 2, 3 and 4.

All of the metrics shown in Figs. 2 through 4 show that PCA-XGBoost's performance cannot match the performance of RFECV-XGBoost and XGBoost without feature selection. This can happen because the number of selected features is different from the results obtained by the RFECV selection and the features selected by PCA are different from RFECV. The number of attributes in the datasets used in this study is still relatively small compared to previous studies. Also, this study does not use time metrics on modeling and feature selection to be considered with the proposed methods.

3.2 *Discussion*

From the results above, it can be shown that the performance of PCA feature selection cannot match the results of RFECV feature selection performance or XGBoost modeling without feature selection in the three datasets. Although the use of PCA succeeded in reducing the number of features significantly, the metric results did not show the maximum performance of the model. RFECV does not reduce features significantly but shows a model performance that can balance modeling without feature selection except in dataset 2.

This result is not in line with the results of research [10] which did succeed in significantly reducing features, but the performance produced in this study is not so good. In addition, it is also constrained by the number of features, which is that study uses 171 features meanwhile this study has less than 30 features.

The use of RFECV proved to exceed the performance of the sequential feature selection wrapper technique used in the study [5]. This result is also influenced by the modeling algorithm used to eliminate features, namely XGBoost, while in this

Table 6 The results after the feature selection process

Datasets	Methods	Number of features	Selected features
Dataset 1	PCA–XGBoost	3	'bill_avg', 'download_avg', 'upload_avg'
	RFECV–XGBoost	8	'is_tv_subscriber', 'is_movie_package_subscriber', 'subscription_age', 'bill_avg', 'download_avg', 'upload_avg', 'download_over_limit', 'is_time_range_contract'
	XGBoost	9	'is_tv_subscriber', 'is_movie_package_subscriber', 'subscription_age', 'bill_avg', 'service_failure_count', 'download_avg', 'upload_avg', 'download_over_limit', 'is_time_range_contract'
Dataset 2	PCA–XGBoost	9	'account length', 'area code', 'number vmail messages', 'total day minutes', 'total day calls', 'total eve minutes', 'total eve calls', 'total night minutes', 'total night calls'
	RFECV–XGBoost	8	'international plan', 'voice mail plan', 'total day minutes', 'total eve minutes', 'total night minutes', 'total intl minutes', 'total intl calls', 'customer service calls'
	XGBoost	18	'account length', 'area code', 'international plan', 'voice mail plan', 'number vmail messages', 'total day minutes', 'total day calls', 'total day charge', 'total eve minutes', 'total eve calls', 'total eve charge', 'total night minutes', 'total night calls', 'total night charge', 'total intl minutes', 'total intl calls', 'total intl charge', 'customer service calls'
Dataset 3	PCA–XGBoost	4	'AccountWeeks', 'DayMins', 'DayCalls', 'MonthlyCharge'
	RFECV–XGBoost	9	'ContractRenewal', 'DataPlan', 'DataUsage', 'CustServCalls', 'DayMins', 'DayCalls', 'MonthlyCharge', 'OverageFee', 'RoamMins'
	XGBoost	10	'AccountWeeks', 'ContractRenewal', 'DataPlan', 'DataUsage', 'CustServCalls', 'DayMins', 'DayCalls', 'MonthlyCharge', 'OverageFee', 'RoamMins'

Table 7 The results of the evaluation of feature selection with the XGBoost algorithm

Datasets	Methods	Accuracy	Precision	Sensitivity	F1-score	AUC score
Dataset 1	PCA–XGBoost	0.751	0.805	0.725	0.763	0.754
	RFECV–XGBoost	**0.858**	0.905	**0.831**	**0.866**	0.861
	XGBoost	**0.858**	**0.906**	0.83	**0.866**	**0.862**
Dataset 2	PCA–XGBoost	0.897	0.744	0.33	0.467	0.656
	RFECV–XGBoost	**0.96**	**0.859**	**0.83**	**0.844**	**0.904**
	XGBoost	0.958	0.849	**0.83**	0.839	**0.904**
Dataset 3	PCA–XGBoost	0.874	0.534	0.352	0.425	0.653
	RFECV–XGBoost	**0.939**	**0.805**	0.705	**0.752**	0.839
	XGBoost	0.936	0.778	**0.716**	0.746	**0.842**

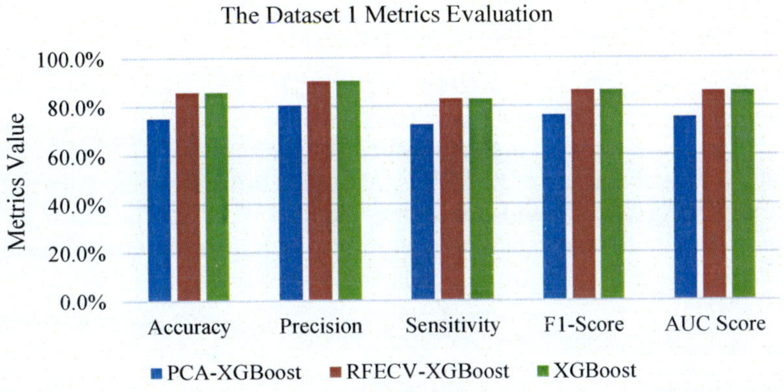

Fig. 2 The metrics result and methods comparison of dataset 1

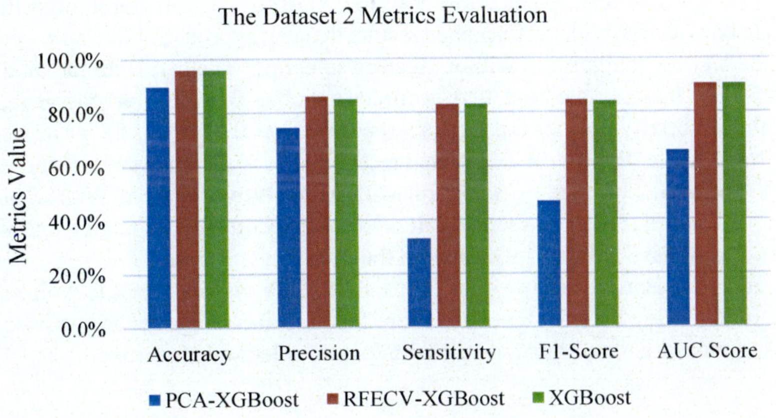

Fig. 3 The metrics result and methods comparison of dataset 2

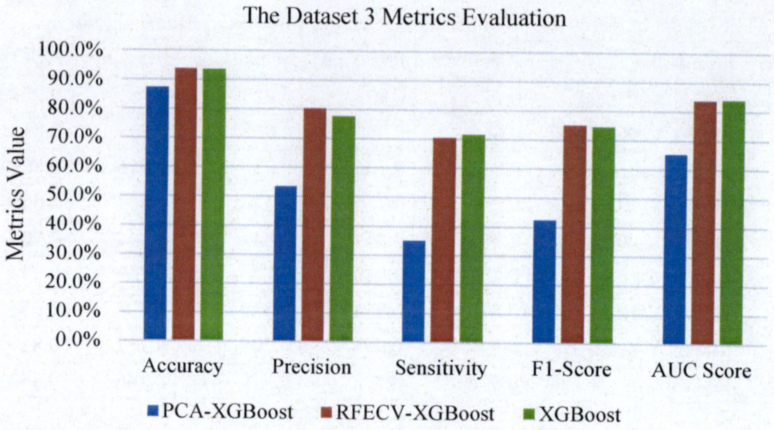

Fig. 4 The metrics result and methods comparison dataset 3

study using Naïve Bayes. However, what needs to be considered in RFECV is a very long time that is not included in the measurement metric.

In future research, the use of RFECV can be tested further by using a dataset with a larger number of features and considering the time variable. The use of RFECV has proven to be able to maintain optimal results with fewer features in predicting customer churn.

4 Conclusion

The use of RFECV feature selection with the XGBoost classification algorithm is proven to be effective with performance results that can approach and even exceed the use of the XGBoost algorithm without feature selection. The results of the modeling after RFECV feature selection, the accuracy reaches 0.96, the precision reaches 0.859, the sensitivity reaches 0.83, the f1-score reaches 0.844, and the AUC reaches 0.904. Meanwhile, the use of PCA has not been able to compensate for the use of RFECV and XGBoost feature selection without feature selection. With a smaller number of features, it can be seen which features affect the classification and which features do not have a major influence on the modeling process.

For future research, the use of PCA and RFECV as feature selection can be considered by using datasets that have more features and research can consider time metrics to measure the performance of the feature selection algorithm.

References

1. AL-Shatnwai AM, Faris M (2020) Predicting customer retention using XGBoost and balancing methods. Int J Adv Comput Sci Appl 11. https://doi.org/10.14569/IJACSA.2020.0110785
2. Senthan P, Rathnayaka R, Kuhaneswaran B, Kumara B (2021) Development of churn prediction model using XGBoost—telecommunication industry in Sri Lanka. In: 2021 IEEE International IOT, electronics and mechatronics conference (IEMTRONICS). IEEE, pp 1–7. https://doi.org/10.1109/IEMTRONICS52119.2021.9422657
3. Raja JB, Pandian SC (2020) An optimal ensemble classification for predicting churn in telecommunication. J Eng Sci Technol Rev 13:44–49. https://doi.org/10.25103/jestr.132.07
4. Hughes A. Churn reduction in the telecom industry. http://www.dbmarketing.com/2010/03/churn-reduction-in-the-telecom-industry/. Last accessed 22 Nov 2021
5. Yulianti Y, Saifudin A (2020) Sequential feature selection in customer churn prediction based on Naive Bayes. IOP Conf Ser Mater Sci Eng 879:012090. https://doi.org/10.1088/1757-899X/879/1/012090
6. García DL, Nebot À, Vellido A (2017) Intelligent data analysis approaches to churn as a business problem: a survey. Knowl Inf Syst 51:719–774. https://doi.org/10.1007/s10115-016-0995-z
7. Dhini A, Fauzan M (2021) Predicting customer churn using ensemble learning: case study of a fixed broadband company. Int J Technol 12:1030–1037. https://doi.org/10.14716/ijtech.v12i5.5223
8. Dewi C, Arisoesilaningsih E, Mahmudy WF (2022) Solimun: performance of information gain and PCA feature selection for determining ripen susu banana fruits. In: 2022 IEEE International conference on cybernetics and computational intelligence (CyberneticsCom), pp 323–328. https://doi.org/10.1109/CyberneticsCom55287.2022.9865623
9. Parmar P, Serasiya S (2021) Telecom churn prediction model using XgBoost classifier and logistic regression algorithm. Int Res J Eng Technol (IRJET) 8:1100–1105
10. Jamalian E, Foukerdi R (2018) A hybrid data mining method for customer churn prediction. Eng Technol Appl Sci Res 8:2991–2997. https://doi.org/10.48084/etasr.2108
11. Raja JB, Sandhya G, Peter SS, Karthik R, Femila F (2020) Exploring effective feature selection methods for telecom churn prediction. Int J Innov Technol Explor Eng 9:632–635. https://doi.org/10.35940/ijitee.C8121.019320
12. Yadav S, Jain A, Singh D (2018) Early prediction of employee attrition using data mining techniques. In: 2018 IEEE 8th International advance computing conference (IACC). IEEE, pp 349–354. https://doi.org/10.1109/IADCC.2018.8692137
13. Kunt MS. Internet service provider customer churn. https://www.kaggle.com/datasets/mehmetsabrikunt/internet-service-churn. Last accessed 27 May 2022
14. Mnassri B. Telecom churn dataset. https://www.kaggle.com/datasets/mnassrib/telecom-churn-datasets. Last accessed 27 May 2022
15. Kumar B. Customer churn. https://www.kaggle.com/datasets/barun2104/telecom-churn. Last accessed 27 May 2022
16. Elhassan A, Abu-Soud SM, Alghanim F, Salameh W (2021) ILA4: overcoming missing values in machine learning datasets—an inductive learning approach. J King Saud Univ Comput Inf Sci. https://doi.org/10.1016/j.jksuci.2021.02.011
17. Mustaqim AZ, Adi S, Pristyanto Y, Astuti Y (2021) The effect of recursive feature elimination with cross-validation (RFECV) feature selection algorithm toward classifier performance on credit card fraud detection. In: 2021 International conference on artificial intelligence and computer science technology (ICAICST), pp 270–275. https://doi.org/10.1109/ICAICST53116.2021.9497842
18. Liu B, Li X, Li J, Li Y, Lang J, Gu R, Wang F (2018) Comparison of machine learning classifiers for breast cancer diagnosis based on feature selection. In: 2018 IEEE International conference on systems, man, and cybernetics (SMC), pp 4399–4404. https://doi.org/10.1109/SMC.2018.00743

19. Lu P, Zhuo Z, Zhang W, Tang J, Wang Y, Zhou H, Huang X, Sun T, Lu J (2021) A hybrid feature selection combining wavelet transform for quantitative analysis of heat value of coal using laser-induced breakdown spectroscopy. Appl Phys B 127:19. https://doi.org/10.1007/s00340-020-07556-8
20. Sanchez A, Raya L, Mohedano-Munoz MA, Rubio-Sánchez M (2021) Feature selection based on star coordinates plots associated with eigenvalue prob-lems. Vis Comput 37:203–216. https://doi.org/10.1007/s00371-020-01793-w
21. Kim Y-E, Kim Y-S, Kim H (2022) Effective feature selection methods to detect IoT DDoS attack in 5G core network. Sensors 22:3819. https://doi.org/10.3390/s22103819
22. Mustaqim AZ, Adi S, Pristyanto Y, Astuti Y (2021) The effect of recursive feature elimination with cross-validation (RFECV) feature selection algorithm toward classifier performance on credit card fraud detection. In: 2021 International conference on artificial intelligence and computer science technology (ICAICST). IEEE, pp 270–275. https://doi.org/10.1109/ICAICST53116.2021.9497842
23. Duan X, Li Y, Liu C, Li X, Liu W, Li G (2022) Research on the method of selecting the optimal feature subset in big data for energy analysis attack. In: Gladyshev P, Goel S, James J, Markowsky G, Johnson D (eds) Digital forensics and cyber crime. Springer International Publishing, Cham, pp 109–126
24. Shoumo SZH, Dhruba MIM, Hossain S, Ghani NH, Arif H, Islam S (2019) Application of machine learning in credit risk assessment: a prelude to smart banking. In: TENCON 2019—2019 IEEE region 10 conference (TENCON), pp 2023–2028. https://doi.org/10.1109/TENCON.2019.8929527
25. Priscilla CV, Prabha DP (2021) A two-phase feature selection technique using mutual information and XGB-RFE for credit card fraud detection. Int J Adv Technol Eng Explor 8:1656–1668. https://doi.org/10.19101/IJATEE.2021.874615
26. Mohammad NI, Ismail SA, Kama MN, Yusop OM, Azmi A (2019) Customer churn prediction in telecommunication industry using machine learning classifiers. In: Proceedings of the 3rd international conference on vision, image and signal processing. ACM, New York, NY, pp 1–7. https://doi.org/10.1145/3387168.3387219
27. Pathy A, Meher S, Balasubramanian P (2020) Predicting algal biochar yield using eXtreme Gradient Boosting (XGB) algorithm of machine learning methods. Algal Res 50:102006. https://doi.org/10.1016/j.algal.2020.102006
28. Wang H, Liu C, Deng L (2018) Enhanced prediction of hot spots at protein-protein interfaces using extreme gradient boosting. Sci Rep 8:14285. https://doi.org/10.1038/s41598-018-32511-1
29. Hanif I (2020) Implementing extreme gradient boosting (XGBoost) classifier to improve customer churn prediction. In: Proceedings of the 1st international conference on statistics and analytics, ICSA 2019, 2–3 August 2019, Bogor, Indonesia. EAI (2020). https://doi.org/10.4108/eai.2-8-2019.2290338
30. Yu B, Qiu W, Chen C, Ma A, Jiang J, Zhou H, Ma Q (2020) SubMito-XGBoost: predicting protein submitochondrial localization by fusing multiple feature information and eXtreme gradient boosting. Bioinformatics 36:1074–1081. https://doi.org/10.1093/bioinformatics/btz734
31. Ni L, Wang D, Wu J, Wang Y, Tao Y, Zhang J, Liu J (2020) Streamflow forecasting using extreme gradient boosting model coupled with Gaussian mixture model. J Hydrol (Amst) 586:124901. https://doi.org/10.1016/j.jhydrol.2020.124901

Implementation and Evaluation of Prototype Photoplethysmography for Healthy Person-Based Internet of Things

Sevia Indah Purnama, Mas Aly Afandi, Raditya Artha Rochmanto, and Dwi Prasetyo

Abstract A decrease in the oxygen rate of blood flow will lead a human to death because it affects the oxygen supplied to the heart and its pumping. A normal heart rate ranges from 60 to 100 BPM and a normal oxygen saturation ranges from 95 to 100%. This study aimed to develop a heart rate and oxygen saturation monitoring device with non-invasive method and linear regression modeling. Photoplethysmography is developed using the MAX30100 sensor. The NodeMCU ESP8266 V3 acts as a microcontroller with a Wi-Fi module to transmit data. Firebase is used as a web server, and MIT App Inventor is used to create a monitoring application. Some features are embedded in the monitoring application and sent heart rate and oxygen saturation data to Firebase. After several tests, it was found that linear regression improves heart rate reading from 95.06 to 96.30% and oxygen saturation reading from 95.74 to 96.81%. Data are sent to the database through the Internet connection. After retrieval of 20 data, the connection (network) test obtained an average throughput of 108.157, an average delay of 96.168 ms, and an average packet loss of 0.44%. Finally, it is concluded that the proposed device can be used to monitor heart rate and oxygen saturation for a healthy person.

Keywords Heart rate · Oxygen saturation · Photoplethysmography · Sensors

1 Introduction

Heart rate is one of the vital signs of humans [1]. Measurement of heart rate can be done by using non-invasive method [2]. This measurement method utilizes the effect of light reflection. Light wavelength and light receiver are keys for measuring heart rate. This method has been proven and used to make Heart Rate Monitoring

S. I. Purnama (✉) · M. A. Afandi · D. Prasetyo
Institut Teknologi Telkom Purwokerto, Jl. DI Panjaitan No.128, Purwokerto, Indonesia
e-mail: sevia@ittelkom-pwt.ac.id

R. A. Rochmanto
Politeknik Negeri Semarang, Jl. Prof. Sudarto, Semarang, Indonesia

T. Triwiyanto et al. (eds.), *Proceeding of the 3rd International Conference on Electronics, Biomedical Engineering, and Health Informatics*, Lecture Notes in Electrical Engineering 1008, https://doi.org/10.1007/978-981-99-0248-4_16

Pulse Oximetry. This Pulse Oximetry has been used by nurses to monitor patients' heart rates [3]. This Pulse Oximetry can be used not only for sick people, but also for normal people (healthy people) [4–6]. Normal people usually use Pulse Oximetry after doing some sport, like jogging, cardio exercise, and athletic activities [7]. Heart rate monitoring device is also commonly used by athletes to measure heart conditions [8].

The Internet of Things (IoT) is a technology for developing measuring devices anytime and anywhere [9]. IoT has been used in many cases such as smart classrooms [10–12], smart warehouses [13–15], and smart agricultures [16–18]. IoT has also been used for developing medical devices, such as electrocardiographs [19], electromyographs [20], and electroencephalographs [21]. IoT technology also drives the improvement of Pulse Oximetry. Many studies have been done to develop heart rate monitoring device in several decades.

Studies on Oximetry using the photoplethysmography (PPG) method have been developed in many aspects. A study on sensor using LED and photodiode to capture PPG signal has been done [22]. The study has proven that the configuration can be used to capture PPG signal. Although, LED and photodiode is not a robust system. Therefore, improvements are still needed to make a robust system for PPG signal reading. Another study has used a built-in sensor in a module [23]. A built-in sensor in a module is more robust than the previous configuration but it is more complex too. It uses two minimum systems, the first one is Arduino Uno and the second one is Raspberry Pi. The system may be robust but it still can be improved. Another study to improve the development of Oximetry using the PPG method in a simpler system has been done [24]. The system also uses a built-in sensor with one minimum system and sends the data to a smartphone. Data are sent to a smartphone using Bluetooth. This system is good but it still can be improved. Another study on the improvement to developing Oximetry has been done by adding human temperature measurements. The system uses a built-in sensor to measure SPO2 and a temperature sensor to measure temperature in one device. The system is good but lacks accuracy in SPO2 reading.

This study aimed to develop a simpler device to measure both heart rate and SPO2 with high accuracy. Output data from the device are sent to an Internet server and can be seen in a smartphone application.

2 Method

The system configuration of the proposed device is shown in Fig. 1. The Device development consists of hardware and software. Hardware is devices used, consisting of a MAX30100 sensor, NODEMCU ESP8266 microcontroller, and LED indicator. Software is a smartphone application for the output data reading. The MAX30100 is a built-in sensor for heart rate reading using the photoplethysmography concept. The concept is heart rate reading by maintaining the stroke volume of blood by reading

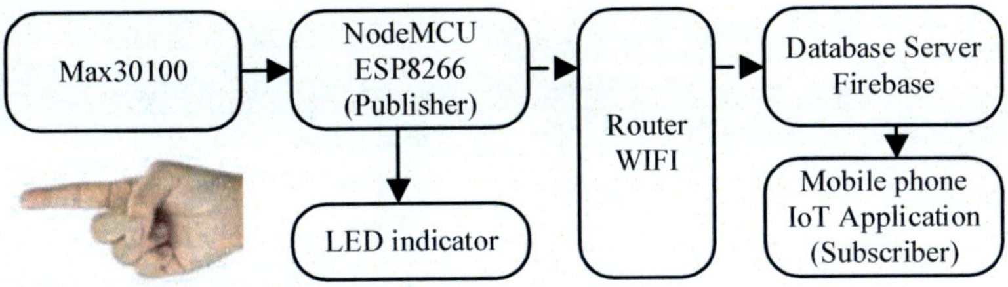

Fig. 1 System configuration of the proposed device

the amount of blood pumped by the ventricle [25]. The mathematical modeling of the photoplethysmography concept obtained from [26] is shown in Eq. (1).

$$v_0(t) = k * \left(\frac{\sin\omega t}{c_1} + \frac{\sin 2\omega t}{c_2} \right) \quad (1)$$

where $v_0(t)$ is the voltage output in volts, k is the constant, c_1 is the capacitance offered by the epidermis layer, and c_2 is the capacitance offered by the dermis layer of both pF. As for $\omega = \sqrt{(LC)}$ since the photoplethysmography signal is periodic. The MAX30100 sensor will read the heart rate and SPO2 from the finger and send it to the NODEMCU ESP8266. The NODEMCU ESP8266 is a microcontroller with embedded Wi-Fi. It will process the data and send it to Google Firebase through the Wi-Fi connection. A smartphone application will grab the data from Google Firebase and display it.

The hardware configuration pin from the component to the microcontroller is shown in Table 1. The MAX30100 sensor is communicated through the inter-integrated circuit (I2C) protocol. It needs serial data (SDA) and serial clock (SCL) pins in the microcontroller. The SDA pin is D2 and the SCL pin is D1 in the microcontroller. The LED indicator can use any microcontroller pin with D6 and D7 pins. The power supply output is 3.3 V because both the sensor and NODEMCU ESP8266 need a supply output of 3.3 V. The smartphone application design is shown in Fig. 2. The application is built using the MIT APP Inventor. The application will get the data from Google Firebase and show it to the application. First, users need to pick the data measurement. It can be heart rate or SPO2 data. Second, users need to pick a condition. It can be a relaxed condition or after doing exercises. After that, the application will get the data from Google Firebase and show it. The final device development is shown in Fig. 3. Figure 3 shows how the prototype works. The hardware system will measure heart rate or SPO2. After that, it will send the data to the database through Wi-Fi (Internet connection). Data from the cloud will be captured and shown in the application. Users can see the result of measurement through the application. Measurement data will be saved in the database. Data saving is needed for assessing and measuring system performance. The system performance in this study consists of calculating accuracy and error. The system data will be compared with

Table 1 Hardware configuration pin

Component part	NODEMCU ESP8266 pin
MAX30100	D1, D2, 3.3 V, GND
LED indicator	D6, D7, GND
Power supply	Vin, GND

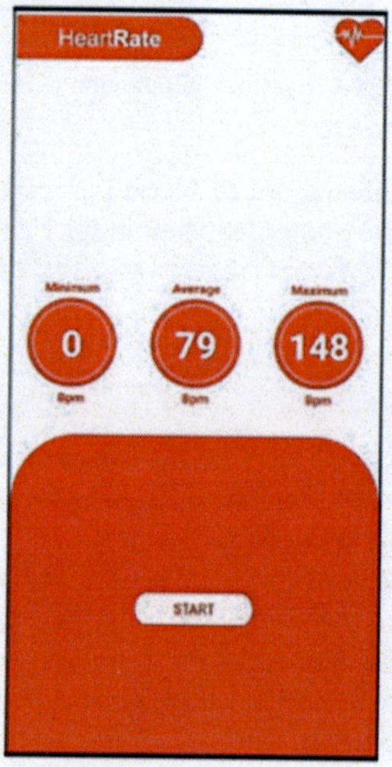

Fig. 2 Design of the smartphone application

the standard oxygen saturation and heart rate. The system also uses linear regression to model sensor output [27–29]. Linear regression is proven to give more accurate data through many applications [30–32]. This study also improves data reading from the sensor using linear regression. Linear regression is chosen because from the datasheet information, the sensor characteristic is linear Eq. (2).

$$y = ax + c \tag{2}$$

$$a = \frac{n\left(\sum xz\right) - \left(\sum x\right)\left(\sum z\right)}{n\left(\sum x^2\right) - \left(\sum x\right)^2} \tag{3}$$

$$c = \frac{\left(\sum z\right)\left(\sum x^2\right) - \left(\sum x\right)\left(\sum xz\right)}{n\left(\sum x^2\right) - \left(\sum x\right)^2} \tag{4}$$

The linear regression model is shown in Eq. (2) where y in formula 1 is the output linear regression model, x is the data reading from the sensor, a is the slope from

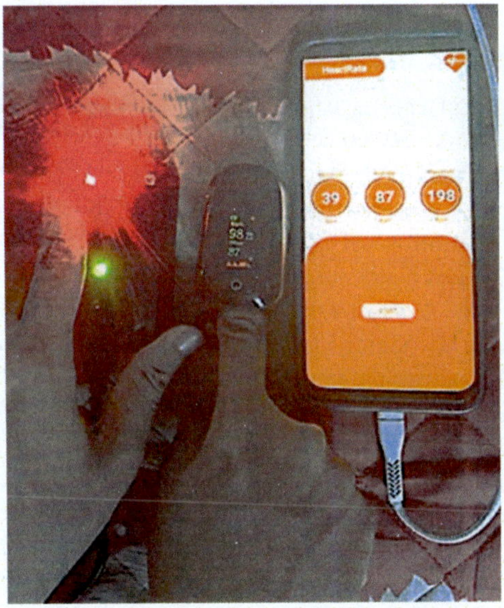

Fig. 3 Hardware and software development

the line, and c is the intercept. To calculate a and b uses formulas (2) and (3), where n in formula (2) and (3) is the total data retrieval and z is the data from the standard device. This modeling will be used in both oxygen saturation and heart rate.

$$\text{error} = \left| \frac{\text{sensor value} - \text{oximetry value}}{\text{oximetry value}} \right| \times 100 \tag{5}$$

$$\text{accuracy} = 100 - \text{error} \tag{6}$$

The error value is calculated using Eq. (5) and accuracy is calculated using Eq. (6). Both error and accuracy need to be calculated for the device's validation. Sensor value is obtained from the MAX30100 sensor and oximetry value is obtained from common oximetry. Another test parameter is the calculation of the T-Test between the sensor and oximetry (Eq. 7).

$$t = \frac{\bar{x}_1 - \bar{x}_2}{\sqrt{\frac{s_1^2}{n_1} + \frac{s_2^2}{n_2} - 2r\left(\frac{s_1}{\sqrt{n_1}}\right)\left(\frac{s_2}{\sqrt{n_2}}\right)}} \tag{7}$$

3 Results

Several tests have been done after designing a prototype photoplethysmography using the MAX30100 Sensor. Data testing was done by comparing the prototype with a common pulse oximetry. Data testing was done with 4 respondents, 2 conditions, and 2 parameters. Every respondent did 4× tests, so the total number of tests in every condition was 16 for each parameter. Therefore, the total number of tests was 32. The parameters used were without and with modeling.

The first test was done 4× by the four respondents, so the total number of tests was 16 in the condition after jogging. The expected output is an accelerated heartbeat. The output data are shown in Table 2, and the comparison of data taken using the prototype and oximetry device is shown in Fig. 4. The T value from this data is −0.69.

The second test was done 4× by the four respondents, so the total number of tests was 16 in the condition after jogging. The expected output is an accelerated SPO2. The output data are shown in Table 3, and the comparison of data taken using the prototype and oximetry device is shown in Fig. 5. The T value from this data is −3.89.

The condition in this study refers to the respondents' conditions after jogging and while relaxing. The parameters in this study refer to the heart rate and SPO2 parameters. The comparison of data for the heart rate parameter of respondents in

Table 2 Comparison of heart rate data after jogging condition without modeling

Number of respondents	Prototype output (bpm)	Oximetry output (bpm)	Error (%)	Accuracy (%)	Diff (bpm)
1	90	91	1.10	98.90	1
	83	83	0.00	100.00	0
	93	96	3.13	96.88	3
	95	98	3.06	96.94	3
2	109	109	0.00	100.00	0
	109	111	1.80	98.20	2
	94	96	2.08	97.92	2
	99	101	1.98	98.02	2
3	94	95	1.05	98.95	1
	95	96	1.04	98.96	1
	87	88	1.14	98.86	1
	93	95	2.11	97.89	2
4	93	95	2.11	97.89	2
	95	96	1.04	98.96	1
	93	95	2.11	97.89	2
	93	96	3.13	96.88	3

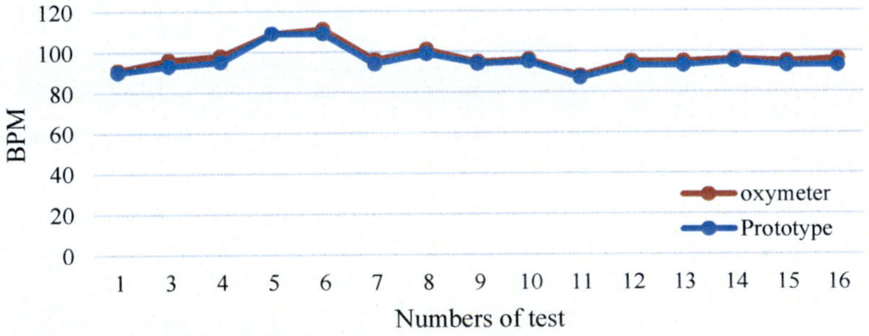

Fig. 4 Graph of comparison of heart rate data after jogging condition without modeling

Table 3 Comparison of SPO2 data after jogging condition without modeling

Number of respondents	Prototype output (%)	Oximetry output (%)	Error (%)	Accuracy (%)	Diff (%)
1	94	94	0.00	100.00	0
	90	91	1.10	98.90	1
	93	95	2.11	97.89	2
	90	94	4.26	95.74	4
2	95	97	2.06	97.94	2
	95	98	3.06	96.94	3
	95	98	3.06	96.94	3
	95	98	3.06	96.94	3
3	96	98	2.04	97.96	2
	95	98	3.06	96.94	3
	94	98	4.08	95.92	4
	93	95	2.11	97.89	2
4	94	97	3.09	96.91	3
	94	97	3.09	96.91	3
	94	97	3.09	96.91	3
	94	97	3.09	96.91	3

the condition after jogging is shown in Table 2, and the SPO2 parameter of the respondents in the condition after jogging is shown in Table 3. Data from Tables 2 and 3 were obtained from the respondents after jogging, with an average of 10 data with 5 min of reading, respectively. The age of respondents 1, 2, 3, and 4 is 16, 18, 21, and 24 years old with a normal heart condition. From the comparison of heart rate data in Table 2, it can be seen that the prototype has different values of heart rate measurement. The minimum difference is 0 at respondent 1 in the second data. The maximum difference is 3 at respondent 1 in the third and fourth data, and at respondent 4 in the fourth data. According to data retrieval, the maximum accuracy

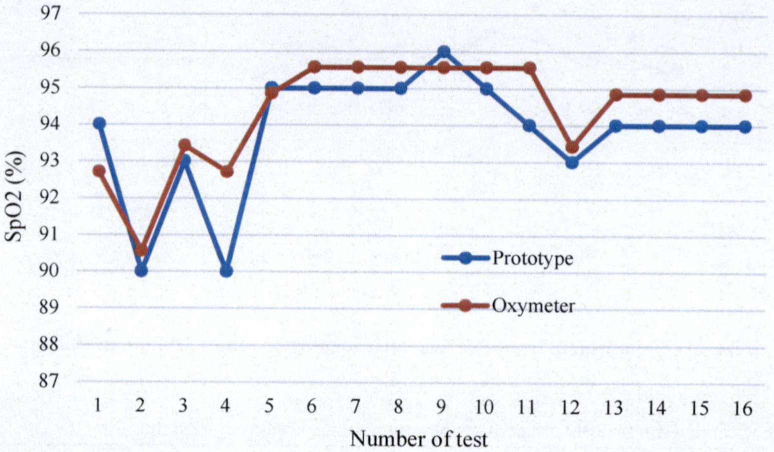

Fig. 5 Graph of comparison of SPO2 data after jogging condition without modeling

is 100% and the minimum accuracy is 96.88%. From the SPO2 measurement in Table 3, it can be seen that the prototype also has different values of measurement. The minimum difference is 0 at respondent 1 in the first data. The maximum difference is 4 at respondent 1 in the fourth data, and at respondent 3 in the third data. According to data retrieval, the maximum accuracy is 100% and the minimum accuracy is 95.74%. Different measurement reading values in heart rate and SPO2 occurred because of the different timings in the measurement.

The first measurement was done using Oximetry, after that the second measurement was done using the prototype. The different timings were approximately 5 min, and it is suspected as the cause of the error in data reading from the proposed prototype and Oximetry. Nevertheless, the difference value is quite small. Accuracy of above 95% with 3 error values in heart rate and 4 error values in SPO2 is acceptable if it is used by healthy people. However, this error is not acceptable if it is used by people with pneumonia disease. After this experiment, it can be specified that the proposed prototype is valid for measuring heart rate and SPO2 for healthy people. The advantage of the proposed prototype with Oximetry is the implementation of IoT. The third test was done 4× by the four respondents, so the total number of tests was 16 in the condition after jogging with modeling. The expected output is a similar value of the prototype and oximetry pulse. The output data are shown in Table 4, and the comparison of data taken using the prototype and oximetry device shown is shown in Fig. 6. The T value from this data is 0.16. The fourth test was done 4× by the four respondents, so the total number of tests was 16 in the condition after jogging with modeling.

The expected output is an accelerated SPO2 which is similar to the prototype and oximetry. The output data are shown in Table 5, and the comparison of data taken using the prototype and oximetry device is shown in Fig. 7. The T value from this data is 0.44.

Table 4 Comparison of heart rate data after jogging condition with modeling $y = 1.006x + 1.2$

Number of respondents	Prototype output (bpm)	Oximetry output (bpm)	Error (%)	Accuracy (%)	Diff (bpm)
1	92	91	1.10	98.90	1
	85	83	2.41	97.59	2
	95	96	1.04	98.96	1
	97	98	1.02	98.98	1
2	111	109	1.83	98.17	2
	111	111	0.00	100.00	0
	96	96	0.00	100.00	0
	101	101	0.00	100.00	0
3	96	95	1.05	98.95	1
	97	96	1.04	98.96	1
	89	88	1.14	98.86	1
	95	95	0.00	100.00	0
4	95	95	0.00	100.00	0
	97	96	1.04	98.96	1
	95	95	0.00	100.00	0
	95	96	1.04	98.96	1

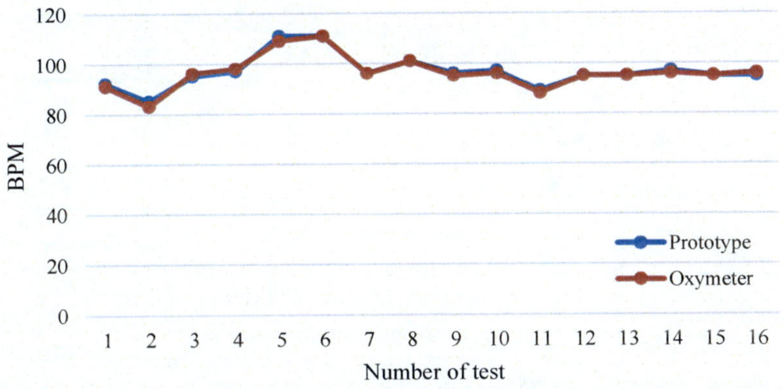

Fig. 6 Graph of comparison of heart rate data after jogging condition with modeling $y = 1.006x + 1.2$

Heart rate and SPO2 data after modeling are shown in Tables 4 and 5. It can be seen that modeling with linear regression improves the data measurement using sensors. The minimum accuracy in heart rate data without modeling is 96.88% and with modeling is 97.59%. The minimum accuracy in SPO2 data without modeling is 95.74% and with modeling is 96.81%. Linear regression improves the accuracy of both heart rate and SPO2 in jogging conditions.

Table 5 Comparison of SPO2 data after jogging condition with modeling $y = 1.04x - 1.17$

Number of respondents	Prototype output (%)	Oximetry output (%)	Error (%)	Accuracy (%)	Diff (%)
1	97	94	3.19	96.81	3
	92	91	1.10	98.90	1
	96	95	1.05	98.95	1
	92	94	2.13	97.87	2
2	98	97	1.03	98.97	1
	98	98	0.00	100.00	0
	98	98	0.00	100.00	0
	98	98	0.00	100.00	0
3	99	98	1.02	98.98	1
	98	98	0.00	100.00	0
	97	98	1.02	98.98	1
	96	95	1.05	98.95	1
4	97	97	0.00	100.00	0
	97	97	0.00	100.00	0
	97	97	0.00	100.00	0
	97	97	0.00	100.00	0

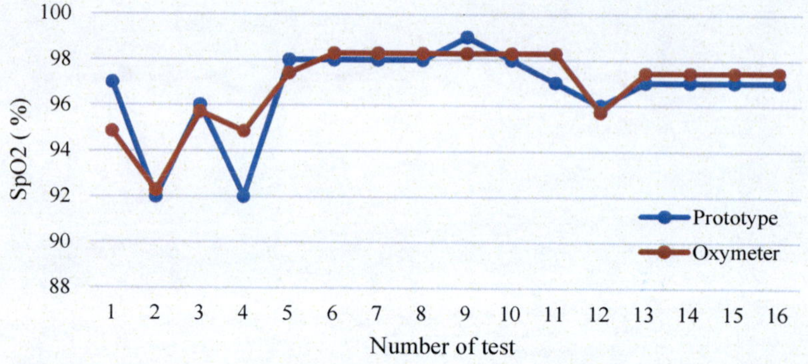

Fig. 7 Graph of comparison of SPO2 data after jogging condition with modeling $y = 1.04x - 1.17$

The fifth test was done 4× by the four respondents, so the total number of tests was 16 in relaxing condition without modeling. The expected output is a similar heart rate value of the prototype and oximetry. The output data are shown in Table 6, and the comparison of data taken using the prototype and oximetry device is shown in Fig. 8. The T value from this data is −0.39.

The sixth test was done 4× by the four respondents, so the total number of tests was 16 relaxing conditions without modeling. The expected output is a similar SPO2

Table 6 Comparison of heart rate data in relaxing conditions without modeling

Number of respondents	Prototype output (bpm)	Oximetry output (bpm)	Error (%)	Accuracy (%)	Diff (bpm)
1	87	88	1.14	98.86	1
	81	83	2.41	97.59	2
	77	77	0.00	100.00	0
	77	81	4.94	95.06	4
2	83	83	0.00	100.00	0
	82	83	1.20	98.80	1
	82	85	3.53	96.47	3
	72	73	1.37	98.63	1
3	95	96	1.04	98.96	1
	78	79	1.27	98.73	1
	69	69	0.00	100.00	0
	68	68	0.00	100.00	0
4	82	83	1.20	98.80	1
	82	83	1.20	98.80	1
	71	71	0.00	100.00	0
	69	70	1.43	98.57	1

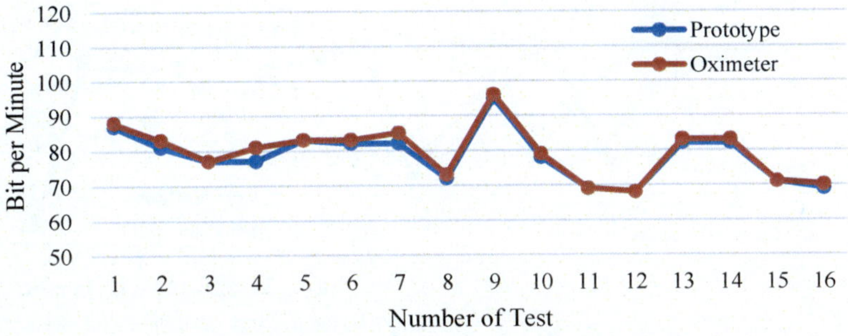

Fig. 8 Graph of comparison of heart rate data in relaxing condition without modeling

value of the prototype and oximetry. The output data are shown in Table 7, and the comparison of data taken using the prototype and oximetry device is shown in Fig. 9. The T value from this data is −0.62.

From the comparison of heart rate data in Table 6, it can be seen that the prototype has different values of heart rate measurement. The minimum difference is 0 at respondent 1 in the third data, while the maximum difference is 4 at respondent 1 in the fourth data. The maximum accuracy is 100% and the minimum accuracy is 95.06% in heart rate data. Meanwhile, from the comparison of SPO2 in Table 7, it can be seen that the prototype also has different values of measurement. The minimum

Table 7 Comparison of SPO2 data in relaxing condition without modeling

Number of respondents	Prototype output (%)	Oximetry output (%)	Error (%)	Accuracy (%)	Diff (%)
1	95	98	3.06	96.94	3
	93	96	3.13	96.88	3
	90	91	1.10	98.90	1
	83	83	0.00	100.00	0
2	94	95	1.05	98.95	1
	91	94	3.19	96.81	3
	88	88	0.00	100.00	0
	80	81	1.23	98.77	1
3	95	96	1.04	98.96	1
	94	95	1.05	98.95	1
	93	92	1.09	98.91	1
	87	88	1.14	98.86	1
4	93	96	3.13	96.88	3
	93	96	3.13	96.88	3
	93	95	2.11	97.89	2
	75	75	0.00	100.00	0

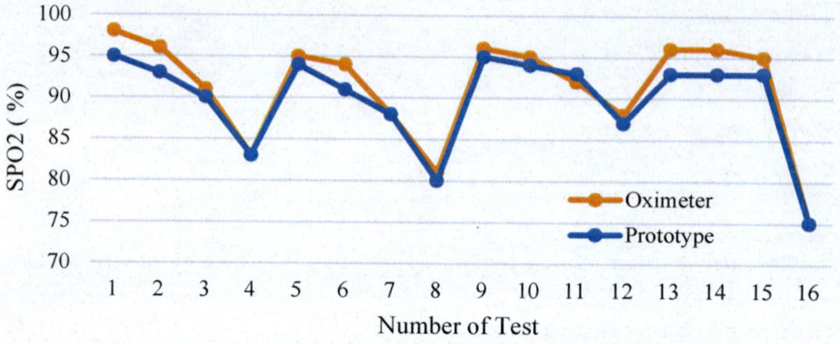

Fig. 9 Graph of SPO2 data comparison in relaxing condition without modeling

difference is 0 and the maximum difference is 3. The maximum accuracy is 100% and the minimum accuracy is 96.81%.

The seventh test was done 4× by the four respondents, so the total number of tests was 16 in relaxing condition with modeling. The expected output is a similar heart rate value of the prototype and oximetry. The output data are shown in Table 8 and the comparison of data taken using the prototype and oximetry device is shown in Fig. 10. The T value from this data is −0.02. The eighth test was done 4× by the four respondents, so the total number of test was 16 in relaxing condition with modeling. The expected output is a similar value of the prototype and oximetry. The output

Table 8 Heart rate data comparison in relaxing condition with modeling $y = x + 1$

Number of respondents	Prototype output (bpm)	Oximetry output (bpm)	Error (%)	Accuracy (%)	Diff (bpm)
1	88	88	0.00	100.00	0
	82	83	1.20	98.80	1
	78	77	1.30	98.70	1
	78	81	3.70	96.30	3
2	84	83	1.20	98.80	1
	83	83	0.00	100.00	0
	83	85	2.35	97.65	2
	73	73	0.00	100.00	0
3	96	96	0.00	100.00	0
	79	79	0.00	100.00	0
	70	69	1.45	98.55	1
	69	68	1.47	98.53	1
4	83	83	0.00	100.00	0
	83	83	0.00	100.00	0
	72	71	1.41	98.59	1
	70	70	0.00	100.00	0

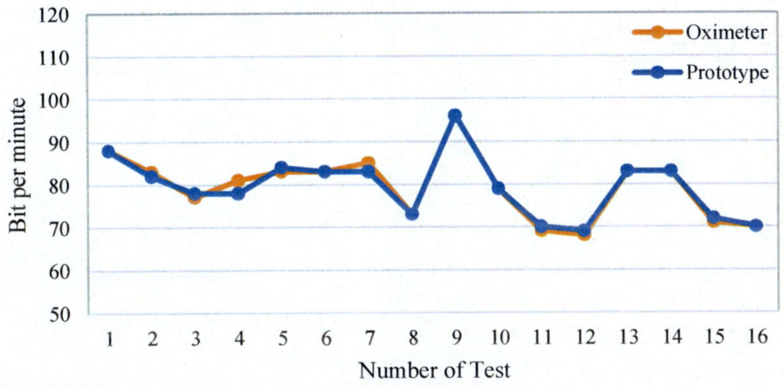

Fig. 10 Graph of comparison of heart rate data in relaxing condition with modeling $y = x + 1$

data are shown in Table 9, and the comparison of data taken using the prototype and oximetry device is shown in Fig. 11. The T value from this data is −0.25.

Heart rate and SPO2 data after modeling are shown in Tables 8 and 9. Modeling with linear regression improves the accuracy of measurement using sensors. The minimum accuracy in heart rate data without modeling is 95.06% and with modeling is 96.30%. The minimum accuracy in SPO2 data without modeling is 96.81% and

Table 9 Comparison of SPO2 data in relaxing condition with modeling $y = 1.02 - 1.17$

Number of respondents	Prototype output (%)	Oximetry output (%)	Error (%)	Accuracy (%)	Diff (%)
1	96	98	2.04	97.96	2
	94	96	2.08	97.92	2
	91	91	0.00	100.00	0
	83	83	0.00	100.00	0
2	95	95	0.00	100.00	0
	92	94	2.13	97.87	2
	89	88	1.14	98.86	1
	80	81	1.23	98.77	1
3	96	96	0.00	100.00	0
	95	95	0.00	100.00	0
	94	92	2.17	97.83	2
	88	88	0.00	100.00	0
4	94	96	2.08	97.92	2
	94	96	2.08	97.92	2
	94	95	1.05	98.95	1
	75	75	0.00	100.00	0

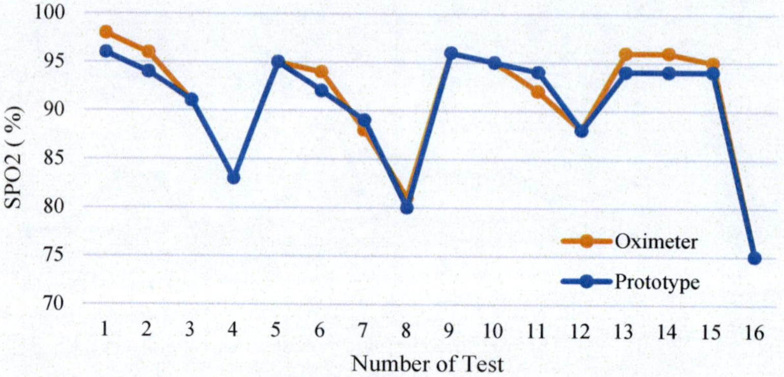

Fig. 11 Graph of comparison of SPO2 data in relaxing condition with modeling $y = 1.02 - 1.17$

with modeling is 97.83%. Linear regression improves the accuracy of both heart rate and SPO2 in relaxing conditions.

Network testing also has been done in this study. Network testing parameters retrieved in this study are throughput, packet loss, and delay. According to the test, the prototype has an average throughput of 108.157, 480 from 20 data. This parameter is bad according to the TIPHON standard. The prototype has an average delay of 96.168 ms from 20 data. This parameter is excellent according to the TIPHON

Table 10 Comparison of feature

System feature	Proposed system	Previous system 1 [23]	Previous system 2 [24]
Heart rate accuracy	Max accuracy 100% Min accuracy 96.30%	Doesn't have	Average Accuracy 93.8%
SPO2 accuracy	Max accuracy 100% Min accuracy 96.81%	Max accuracy 98.86% Min accuracy 95.2%	Average Accuracy 95.2%
Can be seen anywhere and anytime	Yes	No	No
Complexity system	Simple	Complex	Simple

standard. The prototype also has an average packet loss of 0.44% from 20 data. This parameter is good according to the TIPHON standard. According to parameters testing, the prototype can send data with good delay and packet loss but with bad throughput. This condition means that the prototype can send data in good condition.

4 Discussion

After doing several tests and obtaining data research, the device's performance was compared to another device. Comparison consists of device feature, system accuracy, and the complexity.

The comparison between the proposed system with another system is presented in Table 10. Heart rate accuracy from the proposed system is better compared to the previous system. SPO2 accuracy from the proposed system is also better compared to the previous system. This comparison proves that linear regression gives improvements in heart rate and SPO2 measurement. The system also uses the IoT concept that makes users can see heart rate and SPO2 measurements anytime and anywhere through a smartphone application. The limitation of this prototype is that it can only be used by healthy people, while the implication is that it can be used anywhere and anytime.

5 Conclusion

Based on the results and discussion of this study, it can be concluded that the proposed system can be used to measure the heart rate and SPO2 of healthy people. The comparison run has proven that the system is better than another system. The development of the system was done using an IoT system which is simpler and uses a connection feature. The IoT system makes output data that can be seen anytime and anywhere. The system is also simpler and can be used by people without specific requirements like nurses or doctors. Heart rate measurement maximum accuracy is 100% and minimum accuracy is 95.06%. SPO2 measurement maximum accuracy is 100% and minimum accuracy is 95.74%. Each of these measurements was done before the use of the linear regression model. Linear regression improves the minimum accuracy from 95.06 to 96.30% for heart rate measurement and from 95.74 to 96.81% for SPO2 measurement. The IoT connection (network) testing also gave good results. After retrieval of 20 data, the connection test obtained an average throughput of 108.157, an average delay of 96.168 ms, and an average packet loss of 0.44%. Although the results are good, this device still needs improvement in many aspects such as data security, data management, and digital filtering.

References

1. Brekke IJ, Puntervoll LH, Pedersen PB, Kellett J, Brabrand M (2019) The value of vital sign trends in predicting and monitoring clinical deterioration: A systematic review. PLoS One 14:e0210875. https://doi.org/10.1371/journal.pone.0210875
2. Abdulhay WE, Oweis JR, Alhaddad MA, Sublaban NF, Radwan AM, Almasaeed MH (2014) Review article: non-invasive fetal heart rate monitoring techniques. Biomed Sci Eng 2:53–67
3. Enoch AJ, English M, Shepperd S (2016) Does pulse oximetry use impact health outcomes? A systematic review. Arch Dis Child 101:694–700. https://doi.org/10.1136/archdischild-2015-309638
4. Ajrina A (2021) Pulse oximetry usage in patient COVID-19 treatment: at a glance. J Vocat Heal Stud 5:53–57. https://doi.org/10.20473/jvhs.V5.I1.2021.53-57
5. Alboksmaty A, Beaney T, Elkin S, Clarke JM, Darzi A, Aylin P, Neves A-L (2022) Effectiveness and safety of pulse oximetry in remote patient monitoring of patients with COVID-19: a systematic review. Lancet Digit Heal 4:e279–e289. https://doi.org/10.1016/S2589-7500(21)00276-4
6. Gaskin L, Thomas J (1995) Pulse oximetry and exercise. Physiotherapy 81:254–261. https://doi.org/10.1016/S0031-9406(05)66819-8
7. Mengelkoch LJ, Martin D, Lawler J (1994) A review of the principles of pulse oximetry and accuracy of pulse oximetry estimates during exercise. Phys Ther 74:40–49. https://doi.org/10.1093/ptj/74.1.40
8. Martín-Escudero P, Cabanas AM, Fuentes-Ferrer M, Galindo-Canales M (2021) Oxygen saturation behavior by pulse oximetry in female athletes: breaking myths. Biosensors 11. https://doi.org/10.3390/bios11100391
9. Kumar S, Tiwari P, Zymbler M (2019) Internet of Things is a revolutionary approach for future technology enhancement: a review. J Big Data 6:111. https://doi.org/10.1186/s40537-019-0268-2
10. Afandi MA, Nurandi S, Enriko IKA (2021) Automated air conditioner controler and monitoring based on internet of things. IJEIS Indonesian J Electron Instrum Syst 11:83. https://doi.org/10.22146/ijeis.64563
11. Pacheco A, Cano P, Flores E, Trujillo E, Marquez P (2018) A smart classroom based on deep learning and osmotic IoT computing. In: 2018 Congreso Internacional de Innovación y Tendencias en Ingeniería (CONIITI), pp 1–5. https://doi.org/10.1109/CONIITI.2018.8587095
12. Inayathulla ZM, Shyamala C (2021) IoT based Cloud integrated smart classroom for smart and a sustainable campus 9:91–95
13. Putri AK, Prakasa A, Afandi MA (2021) Sistem Pemantau Densitas Debu Gudang Elektronik: Perancangan dan Analisanya. J Telecommun Electron Control Eng 3:81–86. https://doi.org/10.20895/jtece.v3i2.367

14. Kim JA, Jeong J (2018) Smart warehouse management system utilizing IoT-based autonomous mobile robot for SME manufacturing factory. J Inst Internet 0238:237–244
15. Sung W-T, Lu C-Y (2018) Smart warehouse management based on IoT architecture. In: 2018 international symposium on computer, consumer and control (IS3C), pp 169–172. https://doi.org/10.1109/IS3C.2018.00050
16. Saha S, Halder S, Paul S, Majumder K (2017) Smart agricultural system: better accuracy and productivity. In: 2017 devices for integrated circuit (DevIC), pp 316–320. https://doi.org/10.1109/DEVIC.2017.8073960
17. Afandi MA, Fadhlan F, Rochmanto RA, Widyantara H (2022) Perangkat Budidaya Microgreen berbasis Internet of Things. ELKOMIKA J Tek Energi Elektr Tek Telekomun Tek Elektron 10:581. https://doi.org/10.26760/elkomika.v10i3.581
18. Prathibha SR, Hongal A, Jyothi (2017) MP IOT based monitoring system in smart agriculture. In: 2017 international conference on recent advances in electronics and communication technology (ICRAECT), pp 81–84. https://doi.org/10.1109/ICRAECT.2017.52
19. Mahdy LN, Ezzat KA, Tan Q (2018) Smart ECG holter monitoring system using smartphone. In: 2018 IEEE international conference on internet of things and intelligence system (IOTAIS), pp 80–84. https://doi.org/10.1109/IOTAIS.2018.8600891
20. Nguyen M, Gia TN, Westerlund T (2021) EMG-based IoT system using hand gestures for remote control applications. In: 2021 IEEE 7th world forum on internet of things (WF-IoT), pp 911–912. https://doi.org/10.1109/WF-IoT51360.2021.9595957
21. Laport F, Dapena A, Castro PM, Vazquez-Araujo FJ, Iglesia D (2020) A prototype of EEG system for IoT. Int J Neural Syst 30:2050018. https://doi.org/10.1142/S0129065720500185
22. Madona P (2016) Akuisisi Data Sinyal Photoplethysmograph (PPG) Menggunakan Photodioda. J Elektro dan Mesin Terap 2:32–41. https://doi.org/10.35143/elementer.v2i2.187
23. Bakhri S, Rosiana E, Saputra RC (2020) Design of low cost pulse oximetry based on Raspberry Pi. J Phys Conf Ser 1501. https://doi.org/10.1088/1742-6596/1501/1/012003
24. Nugroho CR, Yuniarti E, Hartono A (2020) Alat Pengukur Saturasi Oksigen Dalam Darah Menggunakan Metode Photoplethysmograph Reflectance. Al-Fiziya J Mater Sci Geophys Instrum Theor Phys 3:84–93. https://doi.org/10.15408/fiziya.v3i2.17721
25. Suprayitno EA, Marlianto MR, Mauliana MI (2019) Measurement device for detecting oxygen saturation in blood, heart rate, and temperature of human body. J Phys Conf Ser 1402:033110. https://doi.org/10.1088/1742-6596/1402/3/033110
26. Adhikari L, Pahuja SK (2020) Mathematical modeling and simulation of photoplethysmography. In: Proceedings of 2020 IEEE international conference on communication and signal processing ICCSP 2020, pp 1307–1311. https://doi.org/10.1109/ICCSP48568.2020.9182070
27. Su X, Yan X, Tsai C-L (2012) Linear regression. Wiley Interdiscip Rev Comput Stat 4:275–294. https://doi.org/10.1002/wics.1198
28. Aalen OO (1989) A linear regression model for the analysis of life times. Stat Med 8:907–925. https://doi.org/10.1002/sim.4780080803
29. Maulud D, Abdulazeez AM (2020) A review on linear regression comprehensive in machine learning. J Appl Sci Technol Trends 1:140–147. https://doi.org/10.38094/jastt1457
30. Lesch SM, Corwin DL (2008) Prediction of spatial soil property information from ancillary sensor data using ordinary linear regression: model derivations, residual assumptions and model validation tests. Geoderma. 148:130–140. https://doi.org/10.1016/j.geoderma.2008.09.014
31. Ma L, Zhu H, Nallamothu G, Ryu B, Zhang Z (2008) Impact of linear regression on time synchronization accuracy and energy consumption for Wireless Sensor Networks. In: MILCOM 2008—2008 IEEE military communications conference, pp 1–7 (2008). https://doi.org/10.1109/MILCOM.2008.4753563
32. AlMallahi AA, Kataoka T (2013) Estimation of mass flow of seeds using fibre sensor and multiple linear regression modelling. Comput Electron Agric 99:116–122. https://doi.org/10.1016/j.compag.2013.09.005

Enhancing Temperature Control in a Miniature Green House for Corn Plantation System Using Model Predictive Controller

Yulian Zetta Maulana, Aji Pangestu, and Sigit Pramono

Abstract In order to grow normally, Corn plantation required a temperature between 28 °C and 32 °C, and it can give problems if we want to grow it in a cold area. It is possible to put that plant inside a miniature Green House with sufficient temperature. Temperature controller in the Corn Plantation Green House for this research used a NI DAQ device as an interface between Personal Computer, where the controller is created using LabVIEW software, and a heater. The control process is carried out using Model Predictive Controller (MPC). The purpose is to obtain a sufficient temperature value in the Corn Green House system. The output is in a duty cycle percentage that is connected to driver L298N which is also connected to the heater. This research uses DAQ LabVIEW. The temperature is measured by LM35 Sensor. Various Prediction Horizon (Np), Control horizon (Nc), and static Gain are used to find the most suitable parameter to control the temperature using Model predictive controller. Using a sufficient tuning, the right value for temperature to grow Corn plantation can be obtained. Results show that the best parameter can be reached by using MPC at Np = 30, Nc = 2, Static Gain = 3, and Delay = 5. This setting can achieve a stable temperature of 30,8 °C faster than other settings. But for different parameters, it can reach a stable temperature albeit at different set points. It can be concluded that Different parameters in Prediction Horizon and Control horizon give significant effect to the performance. This research can obtain the right adjustment to get sufficient temperature using Model Predictive Control for Miniature Green House. This can be used for Corn farmers who want to control the temperature inside the Green House.

Keywords First keyword · Temperature · Model predictive controller · Miniature green house · LabVIEW

Y. Z. Maulana (✉) · A. Pangestu · S. Pramono
Institut Teknologi Telkom Purwokerto, Purwokerto, Indonesia
e-mail: yulian@ittelkom-pwt.ac.id

T. Triwiyanto et al. (eds.), *Proceeding of the 3rd International Conference on Electronics, Biomedical Engineering, and Health Informatics*, Lecture Notes in Electrical Engineering 1008, https://doi.org/10.1007/978-981-99-0248-4_17

1 Introduction

1.1 Background

Corn Green House is a place for plant cultivation with some variable arrangements within to meet the needs of the growth and development of corns that are being cultivated inside it. The problems occurred when we want to grow corn in a cold area, especially indoor. These variables that need to be regulated in the Green House system are temperature, air humidity, and light intensity [1, 2]. With the development of technology in the field of electronics, it is possible to control these variables automatically and continuously [3]. The results of the trial showed that the tool is able to control the desired parameters in accordance with the program on a controller device and is able to reduce the effects of weather conditions outside the Green House [4]. This study used the method of designing a model of the Green House temperature regulation system using predictive control model which then tested each subsystem of the model. At the end after subsystem testing, an overall system model test is performed to see the success rate of the Green House temperature setting system model using the designed Predictive Control Model.

Sufficient temperature is needed in order to grow corn Plantation in a Green House. Usually, the temperature is around 30 °C [5]. It can be conducted by applying intelligent control for dynamical physiological system [6]. Research was conducted in a system that has unsteady temperature in [7], and Model Predictive Controller can overcome that problem. In [8], it was also shown that MPC can control Batch Temperature with large time delays. Based on research in [9], it is strongly recommended to use an optimal control to increase profit in cultivating plant inside Green House. In [10] MPC is compared with other types of controllers, such as PI controller and Stochastic Model Predictive Controller (SMPC), and the result shows that MPC and SMPC controllers have similar results. There are many devices that can be used to apply Model predictive Controller, and RS-485 bus can be used. However, in [11], the results of using that device even though can be considered reliable, but needed further researches. Other types of controller used MATLAB software in temperature control in [12]. It meets satisfying result, but it is only a simulation.

Further research about non-linearity in system is conducted in [13], but it is applied in HVAC system. In order to have a great MPC controller, a great and sufficient model is required, but in [14], the research that is conducted shows that model-free control approach can also be applied. In saturated control input, a robust model is required. The research in [15] creates a robust MPC system to improve controller performance. MPC can also be applied to reduce energy needed, but at the same time still meet the temperature required in [16]. The research in Green House using other types of controller was used in [17] that using feedback-forward optimization in Proportional Integral Controller. In [18] and [19], the performance of conventional controller and MPC Controller was being compared, and the result shows that MPC controller outperformed conventional Controller, albeit not significant. Two advanced controllers also being compared in [20], which are Generalized predictive auto-tuning controller and Generalized Minimum Variance. It shows that GPC adaptive controller has better stability and robustness compared to the GMV adaptive.

Multivariable control using MPC is conducted in [21], and the result shows that two points control structure which is multivariable MPC attained better performance for the system, compared to the single-point control structure. In [22], there is comparison between normal MPC and feedforward MPC, there are no big differences in term of performance between two types of controllers. Other advanced controllers are applied in [23], which is GA-based adaptive Neuro-fuzzy Controller. It can be concluded this controller gives significant improvement in the system response, but it is still in simulation. Based on the research that is conducted in [24], environment controller is something that can be considered very important in the future, and the problems within this scope are enormous. It can be very complex, and in [25], the complex situation is solved using Complex Event Processing, so basically the research here aims to use the data gathered from many parameters. But, the downside of this research is that it seems too complicated. The complex situation has also become the theme of the research in [26]. The research here uses Fuzzy logic controller, that has advantages of creating something complicated to be simplifier. But the disadvantage of using this method is that it can oversimplify many parameters.

In order to control humidity in green house, then a model predictive controller is applied in [27], but this time, using a constrained version. It can be concluded based on this research that the constrained model predictive control that can achieve high performance is Single Input Single Output Situation. System using Multiple Input and Output parameters is conducted in [28]. It integrates parameters such as PH and Turbidity. It uses fuzzy logic controller. Other software and devices are used to control temperature of heat exchanger using model predictive control in [29]. It also used constrained model, and the result was compared with PID Control. The result shows that a state observer can improve control performance when there was inaccuracy in the model created before. Further research using LabVIEW is needed. Comparison using distributed and Centralized Model Predictive control is shown in [30]. This research aims to investigate the energy required to achieve the temperature set point in energy building. The research shows that using a distributed MPC is effective to reduce energy that is required to control the temperature inside the building.

The previous research that is conducted covers many areas of research using Model Predictive Controller to control the temperature. The research can be used using different types of Hardware and algorithm. This research gap here is that there is no particular research related to Model Predictive Control that aims to know the different effects of difference Prediction Horizon, Control Horizon, with various Gain and Time delay.

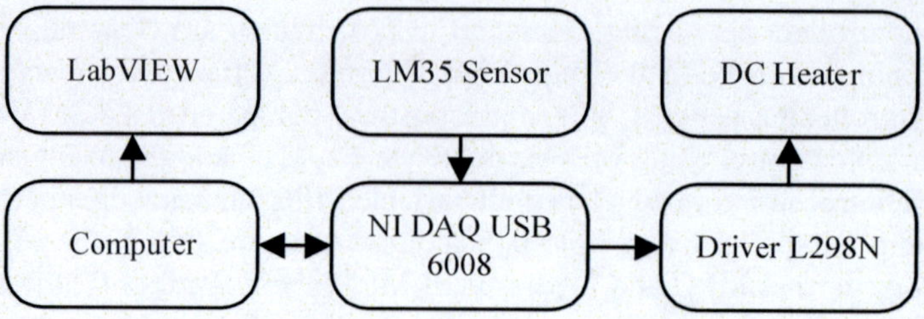

Fig. 1 Hardware system diagram block

2 Materials and Methods

2.1 Hardware Configuration

NI DAQ is one of LabVIEW components with low-cost portable devices and one of the digital to analog and analog to digital data processing devices. NI DAQ USB 6008 is used in this research as interface to PC. The MPC program is created in LabVIEW software that is installed on the PC. This temperature control and monitoring system is a prototype that controls the temperature of Green House using LM 35 as temperature sensor. The block diagram can be seen in Fig. 1.

From the picture of the block diagram above, it can be explained about each block. It starts with the MPC that has been programmed in LabVIEW, and has set point for the Green House system. NI DAQ USB 6008 is an interface between the heater and the MPC program on LabVIEW. The LM35 Sensor detects the environment temperature and retrieves data, after which the LabVIEW software display the set point value that has been set. The heater gets the voltage from the NI DAQ output and is connected to the L298N driver. The voltage obtained will vary depending on the output of MPC and NI DAQ adjusted the condition of the Green House system. The Component that is used is temperature sensor in the form of LM35 that has resolution of 0,1 °C, DC Power Supply with 12 V output voltage [31]. Heater is with 5–12 input voltage and 120 W output [32]. Driver L298N to adjust the current, and NI DAQ USB 6008 as an interface between hardware and LabVIEW Software.

2.2 Model Predictive Controller

MPC is s a discrete-time control methodology, that only produces control actions at a certain discrete time range. Additionally, it requires a particular system model that has the ability to predict behavior of the system within a number of time steps from this time periods into the future. This time period is named the prediction horizon. An MPC controller aims to find the optimum control input sequence inside the prediction horizon that can reduce cost function. The prediction is based on the system model.

In Model Predictive Control, the equation for variable horizon can be obtained in Eq. (1) and Eq. (2).[33]

$$J^*(x(k) = \min_{u(k)N(k)} \sum_{j=0}^{N(k)-1} l(x(k+j|k), u((k+j|k) \tag{1}$$

That can be applied within time constraints:

$$u((k + j \geq |k) \in U) \tag{2}$$

$$x((k + j \geq |k) \in X) \tag{3}$$

$$x((k + N(k)|k) \in T) \tag{4}$$

The horizon length N(k) in Eq. (3) and Eq. (4) is a variable in the constrained optimization problem that is solved at each k. Naturally, N(k) means the first time step when the set T is entered. The corresponding optimal horizon length is defined by N ∗ (k). Additionally, with varied prediction Horizon, the input sequence can be defined using this equation [34].

$$\hat{u}(k+1) \in \left\{u^*((k+1|k),\ u^*((k+2|k), \ldots, u^*(k+N^*(k)-1|k\right\} \tag{5}$$

Equation (5) gives a sufficient solution to solve the problem at time k + 1, the horizon length that used is N ∗ (k) − 1. The state of the system is carried into the final set T in N(k) steps. The control action is switched once the output set is stable. Completion is obtained within time limit. So, it ensures that for all j < N ∗ (k), the constant can be defined as c ∈ R + , such that

$$l(x(k+j|k), u(k+j|k)) \geq c \tag{6}$$

By looking at Eq. (6), it can be seen that because the state prediction x(k + j|k) is not inside the terminal set. It must be shifted using correct input at time k + 1 inside horizon length N ∗ (k) − 1, which is shown in Eq. (7).

$$J^*(x(k+1)) - J^*(x(k)) \leq \widehat{J}(x(k+1) - J^*(x(k)) = -l(x(k), u^*(k|k)) = -c \tag{7}$$

Because the horizon length is, a simple minimum-time value function with the form as shown in Eq. (8).

$$J^*(x(k) = \min_{N(k)} N(k) \tag{8}$$

It can be defined, which will adjust the time needed. The value function then takes the form

$$J^*(x(k) = \min_{u(k)N(k)} \sum_{j=0}^{N(k)-1} 1 + \gamma||u(k + j(k)||_p \tag{9}$$

for some p-norm of the inputs weighted by $\gamma > 0$. It can be seen based on Eq. (9), that the proposed predictive control has a cost function: Where e(k) is the kth error signal which is the difference between the temperature measured at k in the system and the kth target [35]:

$$(k) = (k) - y(k) \tag{10}$$

From Eq. (10), it can be seen that u(k) is the kth control signal and (k) is the rate of change of the kth control signal. The value of u(k) is limited to the range 0–5. The variable is the prediction horizon which is used to determine the extent to which the system prediction must be made if given input from the optimization results. The result of the equation is a control signal that minimizes the cost function with the following arrangement in Eq. (11):

$$\mathrm{u}(k+1)\,, u(k+2),\ \ldots\ , u(k+Nc). \tag{11}$$

2.3 Software System Design

This system uses LabVIEW to adjust the model predictive Controller. There are Predictive Control Model diagram blocks, PWM program block diagrams, and other hardware components. The process model runs from the beginning until the specified time stops. From the Flowchart diagram in Fig. 2, it can be explained that the use of the MPC process model can predict the upcoming output within a certain time span and minimize a criterion function in the controller circuit [36]. Additionally, MPC systems have the ability of feedforwarding controllers to compensate interference and can take into account limitations or constraints in designing controllers. The control signal is sent to the process, while the next predictable control signal is discarded. Then the first step is repeated with the output value of the new process. In order to get the best parameter for model predictive control, predictable output values must be calculated using the best estimation of the current state variable [37]. The parameters are prediction horizon, control horizon, gain, and delay time. Gain and delay time are related to the model transfer function proposed.

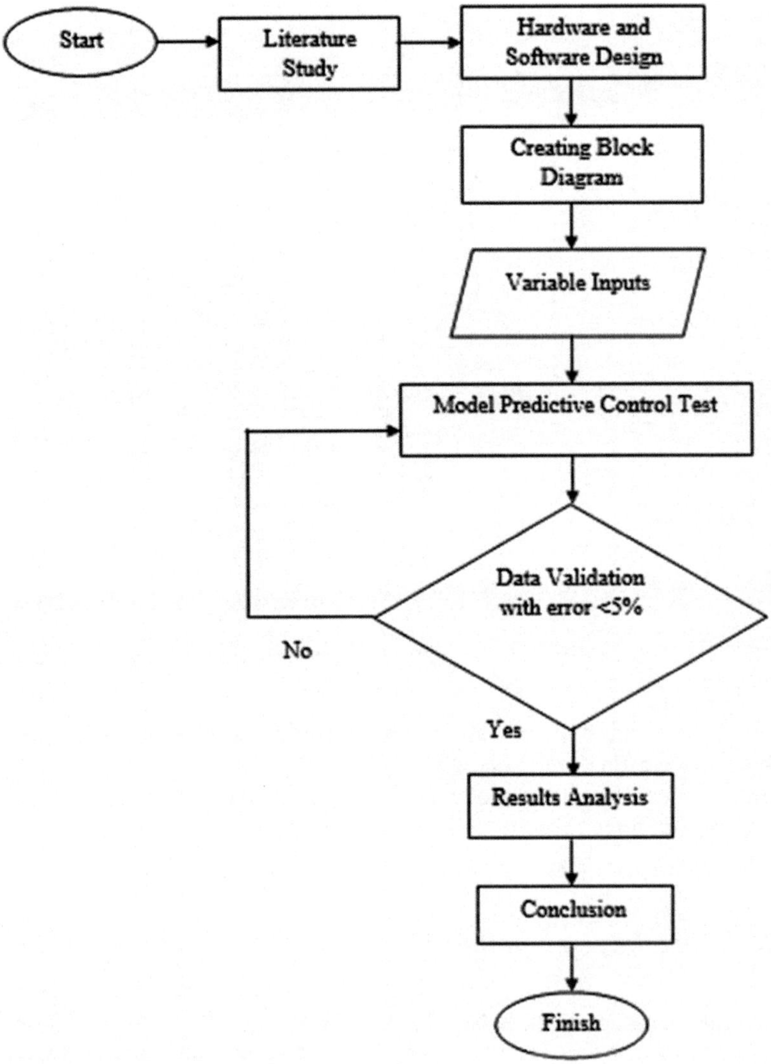

Fig. 2 System flowchart

3 Result

3.1 Hardware Device Implementation

The implementation of Corn Green House control is carried out using NI DAQ USB 6008 with component such as LM35 Sensors, L298N Drivers, and Heaters.

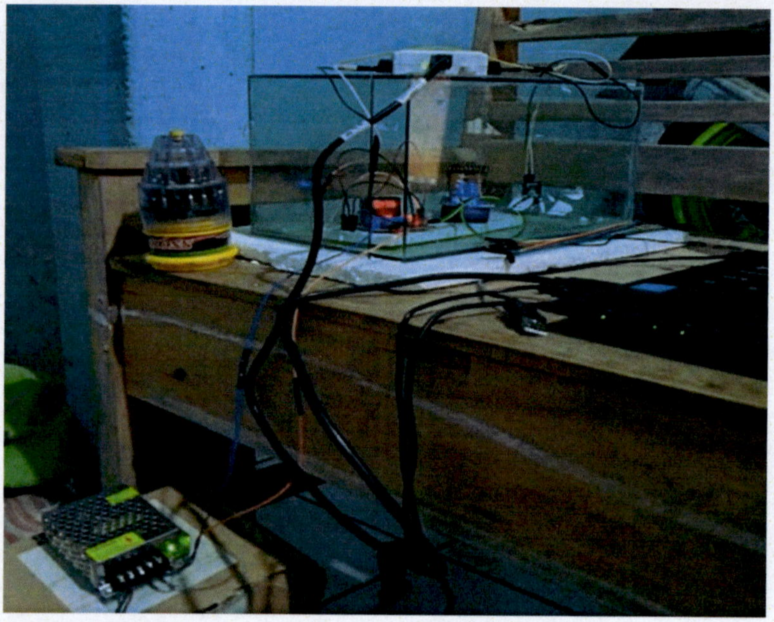

Fig. 3 Hardware implementation

Figure 3 shows an implementation of hardware design that has been assembled and arranged according to the hardware system diagram block. Once the hardware has been arranged, then it is connected to NI DAQ USB 6008 which is located on top of a miniature Green House.

3.2 *Software Implementation*

Final program is used to activate the hardware systems, so it can be used to regulate the temperature of corn Green House systems. The diagram can be seen in Fig. 4. This test program with MPC controllers can be explained when the program is running, and the sensor will detect the temperature of the Green House. The LM35 temperature sensor gets voltage from NI DAQ USB 6008 so that it can detect heat in the form of voltage at the Green House.

After being converted and created a subsystem program, the voltage is obtained by the sensor and passed to the MPC Controller input subsystem. It will be processed to be displayed on the front panel shown in Fig. 5. Additionally, the MPC Controller Input subsystem program will also provide data in the form of voltage to the PWM program which is used to turn on the heater. Then, the temperature in the Green House will rise. DAQ Assistant is used to acquire sensor signal data and L298N

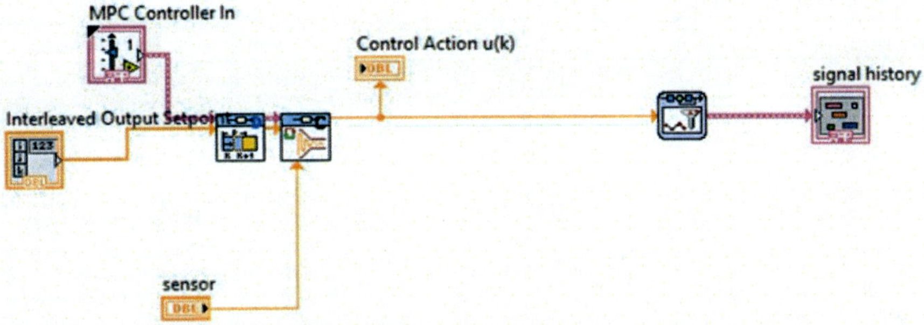

Fig. 4 Testing program with MPC controller

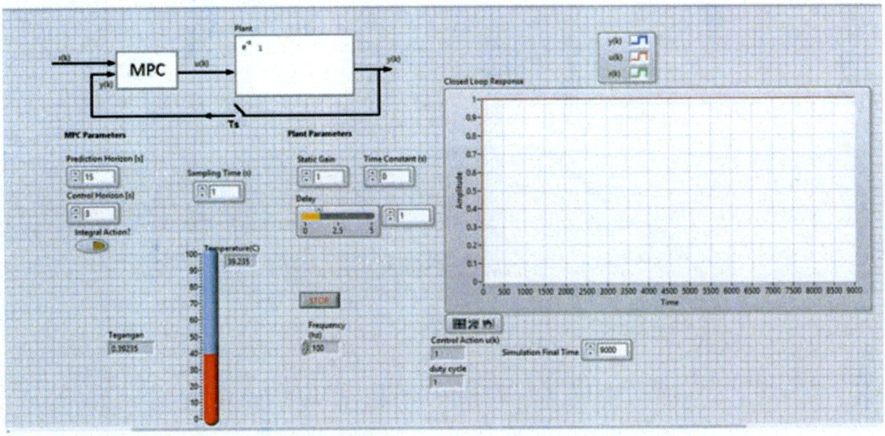

Fig. 5 Test panel front with MPC controller

drivers, which are usually analog signals, convert them into digital signals and then forward the data to the MPC Controller.

4 Analysis and Discussion

At this stage of testing the overall system, several test experiments were conducted from the Green House system temperature setting by using the Predictive Controller Model to get a stable temperature according to the desired set point and for the data retrieval is taken once every 5 min until it gets a stable value. The following is a table of the results of the data collection. The data is based on the parameter such as prediction Horizon, Control Horizon, Gain, and Time Delay. The parameter setting can be seen in Table 1, and the results can be seen in Fig. 6.

Table 1 Parameter setting

Setting	Prediction horizon	Control horizon	Gain	Time delay
1	9	3	4	1.5
2	15	3	1	1
3	12	6	0.5	2.5
4	20	10	0.4	1.5
5	30	10	3	5
6	12	6	1	1.5
7	15	3	0.9	1
8	8	4	0.5	2.5
9	10	5	0.5	1.5
10	30	10	0.2	5

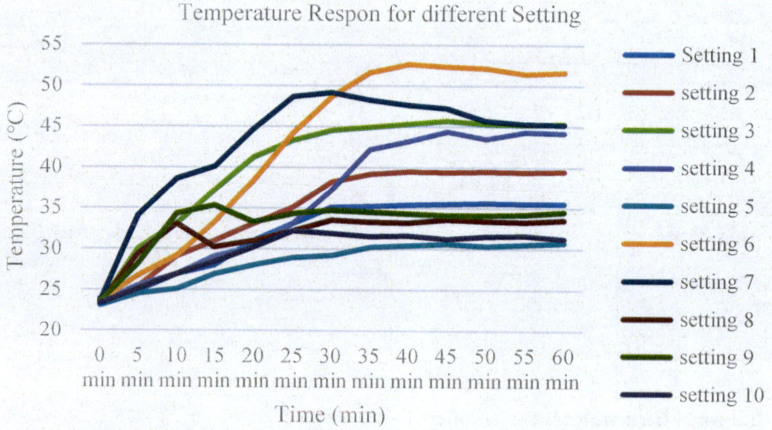

Fig. 6 Temperature response for different settings

In the overall system testing that is conducted, each of them is carried out as many as 10 tests for various prediction Horizon (Np) and Control Horizon (Nc) parameter value with different Gain and Time Delay. The overall result can be seen in Fig. 6. The results are obtained by counting the time that is needed for the temperature to reach the set point. It can be seen that different settings have different outcomes. The first setting obtained a stable value in the 30th minute which is 35.1 °C, which is not suitable for Corn Green House. For the second setting, a stable value was obtained in the 35th minute of 39.2 °C and the value did not change until the 45th minute. The same thing also occurred in other various settings, when the output temperature did not meet the set point. From the data obtained, it can be concluded that prediction horizon and control horizon value gave significant effect on output. It can be interpreted that using different sets of parameters, the output is very varied.

The set point can only be achieved for a specific parameter that is used. The study before shows that Prediction Horizon and Control Horizon did not affect the output that much, but this study shows that using different gain, it can affect the outcome greatly. Further research can be conducted by using different Prediction and Control Horizon in more details.

Overall, the best result is obtained when Prediction Horizon (Np) is 30 and Control Horizon (Nc) = 10 with Static Gain = 3 and Delay = 5. This setting can achieve a stable temperature of 30.2 °C which meeting the set point. It can be concluded that this setting has the best results because in this setting, the setpoint can be obtained quickly, compare with different settings. This setting has also minimum error steady state and minimum maximum overshoot. With a set point value of 30.0 °C in the Corn Green House temperature regulation system, it can be used to grow Corns. In the previous study, the effect of different Control and prediction horizon effects to analyze the performance if the controller is used in Green House system was not thoroughly analyzed.

5 Conclusion

The Objective of this research is to find the best parameter in using Model Predictive Control in terms of Prediction Horizon and Control Horizon related to Gain. The finding here is that different gain will greatly affect the outcome. Based on the results of testing data and discussion of temperature regulation in Green House systems using predictive control models, the following conclusions were obtained.

The temperature setting system on the Green House system using the Predictive Controller Model was successfully built using NI DAQ USB 6008 which connected to LabVIEW. Prediction Horizon and Control Horizon values give significant result to the output of Corn Green House system. The best parameter values obtained from many experiments on temperature settings in home systems using the Predictive Controller Model are found at Np = 30 and Nc = 10 and Static Gain = 3 and Delay = 5, with a stable temperature of 30.2 °C. Future works can be conducted by making a more detailed difference in parameters.

References

1. Hariadi TK (2007) Cahaya dalam rumah kaca. J Ilm Semesta Tek 10(1):82–93
2. Asnani B (2017) Foliages versus succulents: impact of houseplants indoor air foliages versus succulents . Int J Sci, Environ, Technol 6(1)
3. Moghaddam JJ, Zarei G, Momeni D, Faridi H (2022) Non-linear control model for use in greenhouse climate control systems. Res Agric Eng 68(1):9–17. https://doi.org/10.17221/37/2021-RAE

4. Chen WH, You F (2020) Efficient greenhouse temperature control with data-driven robust model predictive. In: Preceding American Control Conference, vol. 2020-July, pp 1986–1991, https://doi.org/10.23919/ACC45564.2020.9147701
5. Greaves JA (1996) Improving suboptimal temperature tolerance in maize—The search for variation. J Exp Bot 47(296):307–323. https://doi.org/10.1093/jxb/47.3.307
6. Coiera E (1993) Intelligent monitoring and control of dynamic physiological systems. Artif Intell Med 5(1):1–8. https://doi.org/10.1016/0933-3657(93)90002-K
7. Http D, Usm A, Theses EDU, Gaudet C (2003) Model Predictive Control for temperature dependent system. pp 1–2
8. Gough B, Kovac S, Devito L, Quick D (2004) Model predictive control of batch temperature. Forum Am Bar Assoc, pp 1–11
9. Van Straten G, Van Henten EJ (2010) Optimal greenhouse cultivation control: Survey and perspectives. IFAC Proc. 3(PART 1), doi: https://doi.org/10.3182/20101206-3-jp-3009.00004
10. Mady AED, Provan GM, Ryan C, Brown KN (2011) Stochastic model predictive controller for the integration of building use and temperature regulation. In: Proceedings of the National Conference on Artificial Intelligence 2:1371–1376
11. Jiaqiang Y, Yulong J, Jian G (2013) An Intelligent Greenhouse Control System. TELKOMNIKA Indones J Electr Eng 11(8):4627–4632. https://doi.org/10.11591/telkomnika.v11i8.3088
12. Mastalli C (2013) Model predictive control for robots. In: Proceedings Of The American Control Conference, 19(11), pp 0–1
13. Rehrl J, Schwingshackl D, Horn M (2014) Model predictive control of temperature and humidity in heating, ventilating and air conditioning systems. IFIP Adv Inf Commun Technol 443:285–295. https://doi.org/10.1007/978-3-662-45504-3_28
14. Lafont F, Balmat JF, Pessel N, Fliess M (2015) A model-free control strategy for an experimental greenhouse with an application to fault accommodation. Comput Electron Agric 110:139–149. https://doi.org/10.1016/j.compag.2014.11.008
15. Oravec J, Bakošová M, Meszáros A (2016) Robust model predictive control of heat exchangers in series. Chem Eng Trans, 52(Figure 1), pp 253–258. https://doi.org/10.3303/CET1652043
16. Martinčević A, Vasak M, Lesic V (2016) Model predictive control for energy-saving and comfortable temperature control in buildings. In: 24th Mediterranean Conference On Control And Automation MED 2016, pp. 298–303, https://doi.org/10.1109/MED.2016.7536001
17. Manonmani A, Thyagarajan T, Sutha S, Gayathri V (2016) Design of soft computing based optimal pi controller for greenhouse system. Circuits Syst 07(11):3431–3447. https://doi.org/10.4236/cs.2016.711292
18. Alamirew T, Balaji V, Gabbeye N (2017) Comparison of PID controller with model predictive controller for milk pasteurization process. Bull Electr Eng Informatics 6(1):24–35. https://doi.org/10.11591/eei.v6i1.575
19. Alyousif S, Zainuddin NF, Bin Hamzah B (2017) Intelligent temperature control system at greenhouse. Int J Appl Eng Res, 12(9), pp 1811–1814
20. Essahafi M, Lafkih MA (2018) Comparison between two adaptive controllers applied to greenhouse climate monitoring. Int J Adv Comput Sci Appl 9(1):341–346. https://doi.org/10.14569/IJACSA.2018.090147
21. Wahid A, Putra IGEP (2018) Multivariable model predictive control design of reactive distillation column for Dimethyl Ether production. In: IOP Conference Series: Materials Science and Engineering. 334(1), https://doi.org/10.1088/1757-899X/334/1/012018
22. Abderrahmane J, Sauter D, Alami K, Brahim C, Abdellah A (2018) Model predictive control (MPC) for building optimal temperature control. SSRN Electron J. https://doi.org/10.2139/ssrn.3186339
23. Mohamed S, Hameed IA (2018) A GA-Based adaptive neuro-fuzzy controller for greenhouse climate control system. Alexandria Eng. J. 57(2):773–779. https://doi.org/10.1016/j.aej.2014.04.009
24. Singh A, Singh AK (2019) Green house control system: A research. Int J Recent Technol Eng, 8(2) Special Issue 11, pp 2139–2142. https://doi.org/10.35940/ijrte.B1221.0982S1119

25. Jia Y, Li X (2021) Complex event processing methods for greenhouse control. Agric., 11(9). https://doi.org/10.3390/agriculture11090811
26. Hamad IH, Chouchaine A, Bouzaouache H (2021) Experimental validation of a dynamic analysis and fuzzy logic controller of greenhouse air temperature. IJCSNS 21, (5)
27. Hamidane H, El Faiz S, Guerbaoui M, Ed-Dahhak A, Lachhab A, Bouchikhi B (2021) Constrained discrete model predictive control of a greenhouse system temperature. Int. J. Electr. Comput. Eng, 11(2), pp 1223–1234, 2021, https://doi.org/10.11591/ijece.v11i2.pp1223-1234
28. Siskandar R, Santosa SH, Wiyoto W, Kusumah BR, Hidayat AP (2022) Control and automation: Insmoaf (Integrated Smart Modern Agriculture and Fisheries) on the greenhouse model. J. Ilmu Pertan. Indones., 27(1), pp 141–152, 2022, https://doi.org/10.18343/jipi.27.1.141
29. heat exchanger temperature control laboratory experiment (2022) Indones. J. Electr. Eng. Comput. Sci. 25(2):857–866. https://doi.org/10.11591/ijeecs.v25.i2.pp857-866
30. Lefebure N et al (2022) Distributed model predictive control of buildings and energy hubs. Energy Build. 259:111806. https://doi.org/10.1016/j.enbuild.2021.111806
31. He W, Xue F, Zheng F, Zhou Y, Liu K, Tian Y (2019) Research on AC & DC hybrid power supply system with high-proportion renewable energy of data centre. J Eng 2019(16):3230–3233. https://doi.org/10.1049/joe.2018.8925
32. Yudianto F (2018) Design monitoring of distribution transformer load by messenger based on microcontroller atmega 128. In: Proceeding 2017 4th International Conference on Computer Applications and Information Processing Technology. CAIPT 2017, 2018-January, pp 1–3, https://doi.org/10.1109/CAIPT.2017.8320696
33. Ilchmann A, Witschel J, Worthmann K (2022) Model predictive control for singular differential-algebraic equations. Int J Control 95(8):2141–2150. https://doi.org/10.1080/00207179.2021.1900604
34. Hadian M, Ramezani A, Zhang W (2021) Robust model predictive controller using recurrent neural networks for input–output linear parameter varying systems. Electron 10(13):1–20. https://doi.org/10.3390/electronics10131557
35. Sadi S (2015) Room temperature control system prototype industry based programmable logic controller zelio SR2 B121 BD. Innov. Syst. Des. Eng., 6(4), pp 52–68. www.iiste.org
36. Xu Z, Feng P, Zha H, Xu C, Ma Y, Feng F (1974) Research of multi-point temperature control method in the heating system of 3D glass hot bending machine. J Phys Conf Ser 1:2021. https://doi.org/10.1088/1742-6596/1974/1/012002
37. Sen N, Deb S, Sungoh D, Das S (2018) Automatic climate control of a greenhouse : a review. ADBU J Electr Electron Eng 2(1):14–16

DenseNet201 Model for Robust Detection on Incorrect Use of Mask

Faisal Dharma Adhinata, Nur Ghaniaviyanto Ramadhan, and Akhmad Jayadi

Abstract In 2022, the COVID-19 pandemic is still occurring. One of the optimal prevention efforts is to wear a mask properly. Several previous studies have classified the use of masks incorrectly. However, the accuracy resulting from the classification process is not optimal. This research aims to use the transfer learning method to achieve optimal accuracy. In this research, we used three classes, namely without a mask, incorrect mask, and with a mask. The use of these three classes is expected to be more detailed in detecting violations of the use of masks on the face. The classification method used in this research uses transfer learning as feature extraction and Global Average Pooling and Dense layers as classification layers. The transfer learning models used in this research are MobileNetV2, InceptionV3, and DenseNet201. We evaluate the three models' accuracy and processing time when using video data. The experimental results show that the DenseNet201 model achieves an accuracy of 93%, but the processing time per video frame is 0.291 s. In contrast to the MobileNetV2 model, which produces an accuracy of 89% and the processing speed of each video frame is 0.106 s. This result is inversely proportional to accuracy and speed. The DenseNet201 model produces high accuracy but slow processing time, while the MobileNetV2 model is less accurate but has faster processing. This research can be applied in the crowd center to monitor health protocols in the use of masks in the hope of inhibiting the transmission of the COVID-19 virus.

Keywords COVID-19 · Wearing mask · MobileNetV2 · InceptionV3 · DenseNet201

F. D. Adhinata (✉) · N. G. Ramadhan
Faculty of Informatics, Institut Teknologi Telkom Purwokerto, Purwokerto, Indonesia
e-mail: faisal@ittelkom-pwt.ac.id

A. Jayadi
Faculty of Engineering and Computer Science, Universitas Teknokrat Indonesia, Bandar Lampung, Indonesia

T. Triwiyanto et al. (eds.), *Proceeding of the 3rd International Conference on Electronics, Biomedical Engineering, and Health Informatics*, Lecture Notes in Electrical Engineering 1008, https://doi.org/10.1007/978-981-99-0248-4_18

1 Introduction

In November 2019, the first case of COVID-19 was found in China, where this virus has symptoms similar to pneumonia infection in human lungs [1, 2]. The spread of this virus is very fast. It can even spread through aerosols, namely particles of human respiratory droplets infected with COVID-19. These aerosols can stay in the air for hours and over long distances. Crowded, closed, and poorly ventilated public spaces are very vulnerable to the transmission of this virus [3]. For someone infected with this virus in the beginning, there are no symptoms that appear because this virus has an incubation period with an average of five days from the beginning of infection until the first symptoms appear [4]. Even humans are infected, but no symptoms are felt, so they are still free to travel in public spaces. This fact makes the COVID-19 virus spread to become a pandemic. The World Health Organization (WHO) concentrates on dealing with this outbreak. At the beginning of 2022, WHO recorded that 318,648,834 people were infected, and 5,518,343 people died due to the spite of this virus [5].

Countries continue to develop COVID-19 vaccines to increase immunity when infected and inhibit the mutation process of this virus [6, 7]. Indonesia is one of the countries that is actively vaccinating its citizens. Through the acceleration of the vaccination program, it is hoped that the community will return to normal life. However, a new variant immune to the COVID-19 vaccine has recently emerged, namely the Omicron variant [8]. Of course, this new variant made the world community panic. Several countries began to close the arrival of foreign tourists to their country. There is a face-to-face learning policy for students in Indonesia starting in early 2022 [9]. This face-to-face learning is carried out with strict health protocols, especially using masks. The correct use of masks is a solid effort to prevent transmission of this virus because even someone who has been vaccinated can still be infected with this new variant. In public places, especially in offices, schools, and shopping centers, masks use must be strictly controlled. Many people wear masks simply on their mouths or chins, leaving the nose uncovered. The security forces must continue to regulate and remind it. If there are a huge number of participants, security forces will have trouble controlling the use of these masks. As a result, we require a system that can detect inappropriate mask usage.

The detection system for incorrect use of mask can be made by utilizing the field of Artificial Intelligence (AI) [10]. AI techniques to process complex image data usually use deep learning as Convolutional Neural Network (CNN) [11]. As technology develops, transfer learning techniques are deep learning developments that use fewer data [12]. Several studies that use transfer learning models to detect the use of face mask include the MobileNetV2 [13], InceptionV3 [14], and DenseNet201 [15] models. Previous research classifying mask errors has not been optimally classified [16]. In this research, the accuracy results obtained were still below 85%. Previous research has not used a suitable feature extraction method, so the accuracy is not optimal. Good accuracy is needed to minimize error detection results. Therefore, the proposed research is expected to increase the accuracy of the results. We propose the use of a more accurate method. This research aimed to detect incorrect wearing mask, not wearing mask, and wearing mask correctly on face. In this case study, we will evaluate the three transfer learning models, namely MobileNetV2 [17], InceptionV3 [18], and DenseNet201 [19]. Hopefully, this research can provide new insights regarding the correct method of detecting the use of masks on face.

2 Materials and Methods

The detection system for incorrect wearing of mask consists of a training and testing stage. The training stage begins with input data without mask, incorrect mask, and mask on the face. The inputted dataset will be subjected to a training process for model formation. This research will use a dataset with RGB or grayscale color format. Before the training process is carried out, the data is resized to uniform the dataset size. Then, a data augmentation process is carried out to increase the diversity of data. Furthermore, the data is divided into training and validation data for feature extraction using the transfer learning model. In this research, the transfer learning models used are MobileNetV2, InceptionV3, and DenseNet201. Figure 1 shows the proposed system architecture. The result of the formation of the model is a model that will be used for matching using data testing or video data. We will evaluate the resulting model to get the best model out of the three transfer learning models. At the testing stage, data testing uses new image or video data. Testing data is used to measure accuracy, while video data is used to measure processing speed. Humans recorded on video will be detected by their facial area using the Haar Cascade Classifier. The detected face is resized. Next, the faces are matched with each model's best transfer learning models. The matching result is a bounding box with three classifications: without mask, incorrect mask, or with mask on the face.

2.1 Data Acquisition

This research used a dataset sourced from Kaggle [20]. The dataset consists of three classes: without mask, incorrect mask, and with mask. In this research, we compared the use of datasets with RGB and grayscale colors. The process of changing the color from RGB to grayscale using the Python library, namely OpenCV. Figure 2 shows an example of the dataset used in this research.

All the data we got had the extension.jpg with a total size of 1.89 GB. Table 1 shows the distribution of the dataset according to the three classes. The dataset in this research uses RGB or grayscale colors. The total data used in each color of this research was 11,171 images with class details without mask 4402, incorrect mask 2009, and with mask 4760. Then, training data distribution was 9308, and validation data were in 1863.

Fig. 1 Proposed system architecture

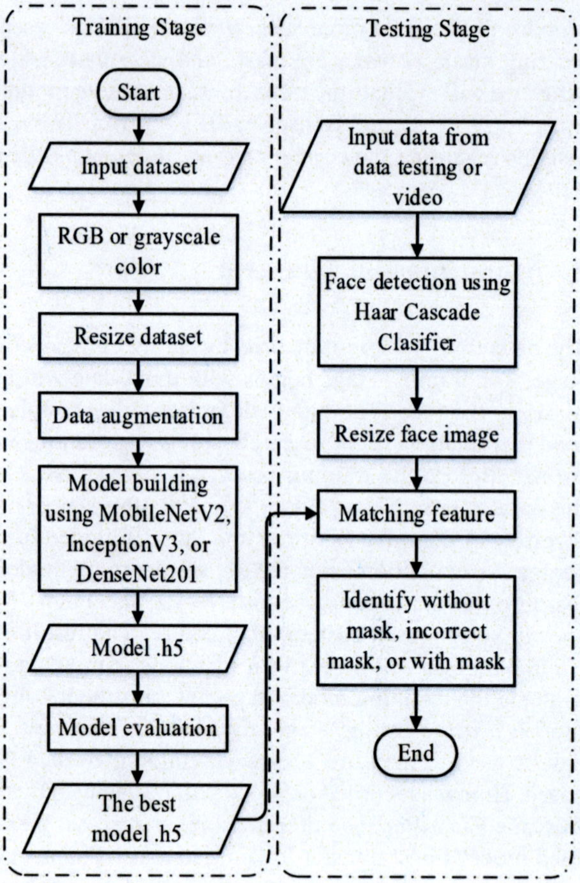

2.2 *Preprocessing Data*

The raw dataset is pre-processed using the transfer learning model before the training process. The pre-processing stage in this research is resizing and augmenting data. Resize is done to make it uniform with the transfer learning model used in this research. We resize 224 × 224 for the MobileNetV2 and DenseNet201 models, while 299 × 299 for the InceptionV3 models. Then for the data augmentation process, we use the ImageDataGenerator library in the Python programming language [21]. The configuration of augmentation data in this research is shown in Table 2. This study's generator or augmentation employs the rotation range option to randomly rotate images at 45 degrees, width shift range, and height shift range for a horizontal image shift of 0.3 and a vertical image shift of 0.3. Then, augmentation utilizes the horizontal flip parameter to flip the image along the vertical axis and the fill mode parameter with the "nearest" value to fill the vacant area with the nearest pixel values.

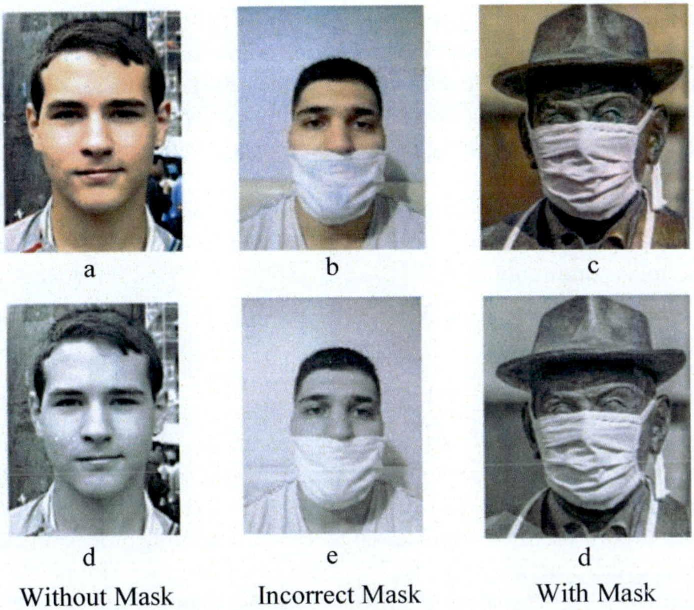

Fig. 2 Examples of data used in this research: **a**, **b**, **c** RGB dataset, **d**, **e**, **f** Grayscale dataset [20]

Table 1 Number of images in each class

Image class	Training	Validation	Testing	Total
Without mask	3668	734	489	4402
Incorrect mask	1674	335	223	2009
With mask	3966	794	528	4760

Table 2 Augmentation data configurations

Configuration	Value
Rescale	1./255
Rotation range	45
Width shift range	0.3
Height shift range	0.3
Horizontal flip	True
Fill mode	Nearest

2.3 Transfer Learning

In computer vision, object recognition aims to make decisions about real physical things using images from sensors such as cameras. Object recognition is frequently accomplished using machine learning technologies [22]. Machine learning is the process of an algorithm, or machine, comprehending and processing data from a given dataset. Such a machine can rapidly generate novel conclusions from data that humans could very well omit. The term "learning" refers to the machine's ability to improve its effectiveness through the training experience [23]. Machine learning transforms into deep learning as technology advances. Deep learning is a set of successive layer architectures. Each layer performs a nonlinear transformation on the input and give represents outputs. Deep learning is frequently used to process image data and is commonly referred to as Convolutional Neural Network [24]. The following Eq. (1) can be used to represent the convolution process.

$$S(i, j) = (I * K)(i, j) = \sum_m \sum_n I(m, n)K(i - m, j - n) \quad (1)$$

where I is the image input, K is the convolution kernel or filter, m is an array of images, and n is the image column. Subsamples or pooling are utilized to reduce feature maps. The input data convolution filter is conceptually equivalent to the pooling filter. In contrast to the convolution process, the pooling process in the shifting filter does not overlap between filters [25]. While deep learning is typically used for enormous amounts of data, there are times when the data is limited, like incorrect mask recognition. Transfer learning is one method for processing small amounts of data in which a model trained on one problem can be used in other situations due to the problem's interrelationships [26]. Transfer learning can reduce training time for neural network models and can result in lower generalization errors. Examples of transfer learning models are MobileNetV2, InceptionV3, and DenseNet201.

MobileNetV2. The model uses the ImageNet dataset, which results in better accuracy than MobileNetV1 with fewer parameters [27]. Figure 3 shows the architecture of MobileNetV2. Additional features in MobileNetV2 are linear bottlenecks and connections between bottlenecks. Between the models in the bottleneck, the component is an input and output section, while the inner layer contains the model's functions for converting the input from the lower layer (pixels) to the higher-level descriptors (image classification). Thus, like the residual connection in a classic CNN architecture, connecting the bottlenecks speeds up the training process and improves accuracy [28].

InceptionV3. The model is the first architecture with fewer parameters and is computationally efficient [29]. In InceptionV3, there is factorization to reduce parameters. Unlike the traditional convolutional layer, the InceptionV3 model architecture uses multiple filters on the convolutional layer. The results of several filters will be combined again using Channel Concat before entering the iteration in the next stage [30]. The inception model's objective is to execute a multi-level feature extractor using filter convolutions calculated within the same model. After stacking these filters into the channel dimensions, they are inserted into the next layer. Figure 4 shows the InceptionV3 architecture.

DenseNet201. The model takes advantage of the condensed network, making it simple to train and very parametrically efficient due to the potential of reusing

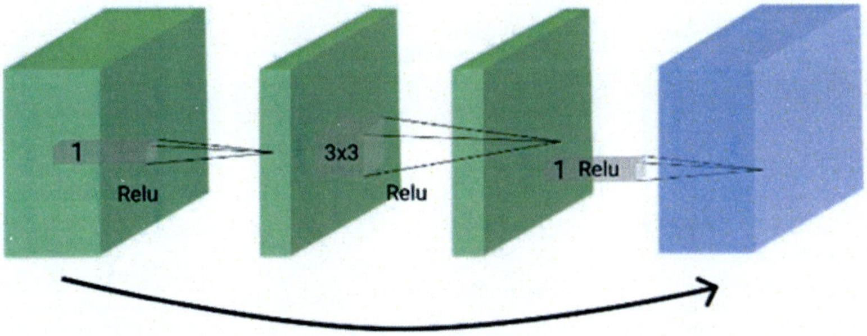

Fig. 3 MobileNetV2 architecture that skips connection

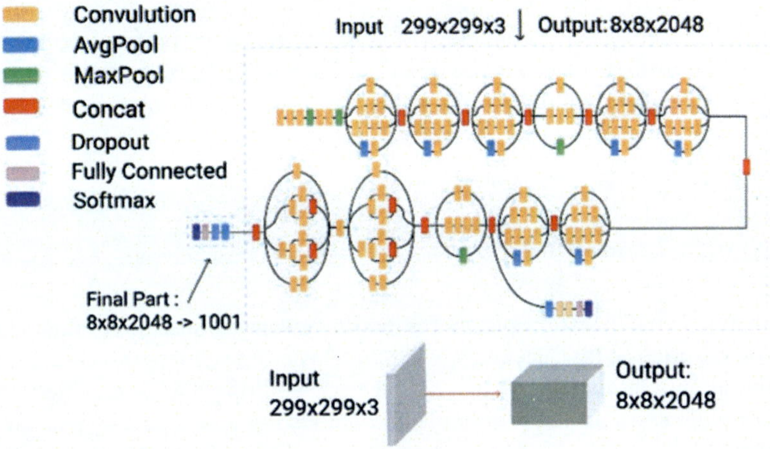

Fig. 4 InceptionV3 architecture

features across layers, which increases variety in subsequent layer input and enhances performance [31]. The DenseNet201 has demonstrated exceptional performance on various datasets, including ImageNet and CIFAR-100. For enhanced connectivity in the DenseNet201 model, the direct connections between all preceding and subsequent layers are improved. Figure 5 shows the layers in the DenseNet201 model.

$$x_l = H_l\left(\left[x_0, x_1, x_2, \ldots, x_{l-1}\right]\right) \tag{2}$$

where l is the layer index, and H is the nonlinear operation. Then, x_l is the characteristic of the l th layer. DenseNet made additional modifications to the model by concatenating all the output feature maps sequentially instead of summing them as it did in the prior version's Eq. (2).

The idea of downsampling dense blocks was proposed [32]. Figure 5 illustrates a Dense Block instance in which the number of layers is five, and the growth rate is

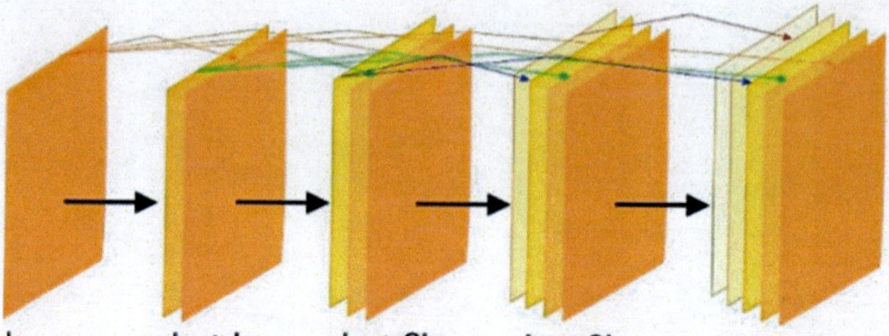

Fig. 5 DenseNet201 layer structure

k. Each layer receives the feature maps of all previous layers. Figure 4 demonstrates that H_l, k feature maps are generated for every operation. Figuring out $k_0 + 4k$ feature maps is possible given that Fig. 5 comprises five layers. The number k_0 relates to the previous layer's feature maps.

2.4 *System Evaluation*

The research on the detection system for incorrect wearing masks is evaluated using the following criteria: loss, accuracy, validation loss, and validation accuracy values. All training and validation results will be tracked throughout a specified period. Next, we will assess accuracy value from data testing and processing speed from video data.

3 Result and Discussion

This section will explain the method configuration used in this research. Furthermore, the training results will be provided along with the analysis. Finally, we will be testing using data testing and video data.

3.1 *Hardware and Method Configuration*

This research uses computer hardware with the specifications of the Intel® Core™ i3-9100F Processor, 8192 MB RAM, and 128 GB SSD. The programming language that we use is Python with CPU mode configuration. Then, this research uses transfer learning (MobileNetV2, InceptionV3, and DenseNet201) as feature extraction and

Global Average Pooling as classification. We start with transfer learning and freeze it to be the first layer to run the training process. We applied Global Average Pooling and the Dense layer four times, following the base layer.

3.2 Training Result

This research uses the Adam optimizer, and categorical crossentropy is used as the loss function for the training stage. We use categorical crossentropy because we have three classes of datasets. In this research, the experimental process is carried out by evaluating the number of epochs in each model. The number of epochs observed in this research is 12, 15, and 18. In this experiment, we used a batch size value of 64.

The graph of the training process is shown in Fig. 6. During the training process, none of the three models experienced overfitting. Even though the data used is imbalanced because the number of incorrect mask data is half the number of other classes. The loss value indicates no overfitting with validation loss, and the accuracy value with validation accuracy is not much different. Figure 6 shows a graph of the training results that do not occur overfitting as shown by the graph of training and validation accuracy. Using the Global Average Pooling layer also prevents the overfitting process, in line with the experimental results in previous studies with different cases [33].

The training results show that the DenseNet201 model achieves the best accuracy and validation accuracy than the MobileNetV2 and InceptionV3 models. Table 3 shows the experimental results of the effect of the number of epochs. The DenseNet201 model achieves optimal accuracy in the 15th epoch, as does the MobileNetV2 model. It differs from the InceptionV3 model, which has not achieved more than 98% accuracy in epoch 18. Then the results of using RGB and grayscale colors RGB color results are better in all models. The use of masks will be more visible when using RGB colors, especially those that distinguish between masks and skin colors. RGB colors also provide good contrast between mask colors and skin tones. Therefore, we use the RGB color training model to test using image data and video data. Each model with the best results will be used to test the image and video data.

3.3 Testing Result

In the testing stage, we use testing data, as shown in Table 2. Accuracy results are obtained by matching the image with the best model from each model of RGB color. Table 4 shows the average accuracy results (without mask, incorrect mask, and with mask) for each model and the processing time per frame. Then to get the value of processing time, we tested using video data with a resolution of 640×360.

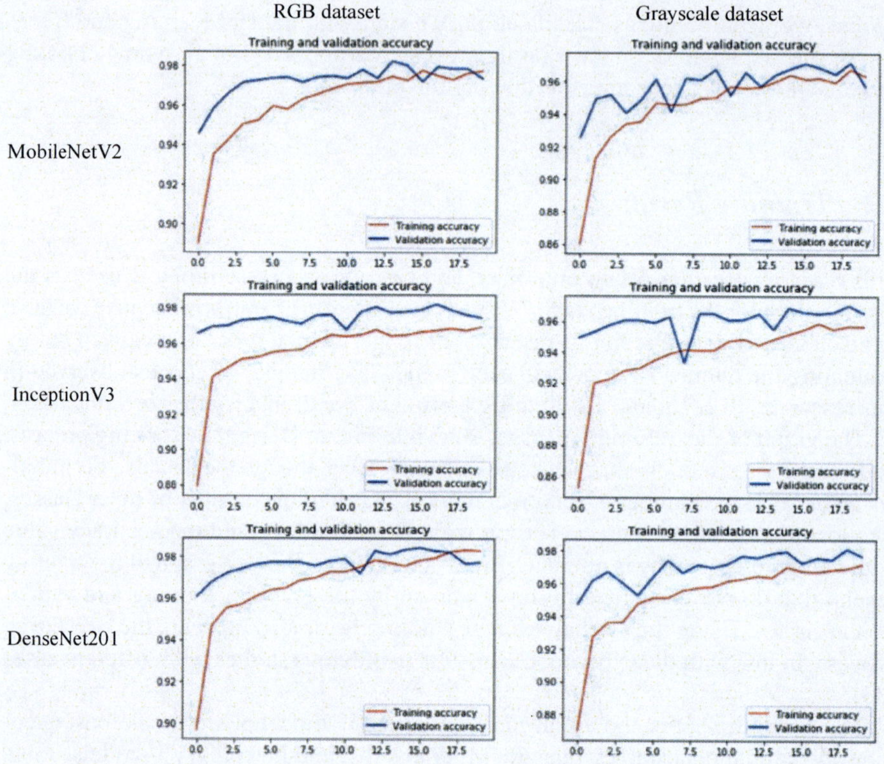

Fig. 6 Graphics of training process

Table 3 The experiment results influence the number of epochs

Epoch	Result	MobileNetV2		InceptionV3		DenseNet201	
		RGB	Grayscale	RGB	Grayscale	RGB	Grayscale
12	Loss	0.0790	0.1200	0.1019	0.1425	0.0777	0.1058
	Accuracy	0.9714	0.9563	0.9648	0.9486	0.9751	0.9628
	Val. loss	0.0740	0.1182	0.0707	0.1111	0.0766	0.0760
	Val. Accuracy	0.9779	0.9661	0.9779	0.9612	0.9720	0.9768
15	Loss	**0.0763**	**0.1019**	0.1010	0.1384	**0.0614**	**0.0870**
	Accuracy	**0.9726**	**0.9644**	0.9647	0.9517	**0.9783**	**0.9701**
	Val. loss	**0.0687**	**0.1081**	0.0696	0.1041	**0.0481**	**0.0811**
	Val. Accuracy	**0.9801**	**0.9682**	0.9779	0.9688	**0.9844**	**0.9795**
18	Loss	0.0746	0.1089	**0.0981**	**0.1241**	0.0551	0.0849
	Accuracy	0.9731	0.9598	**0.9685**	**0.9550**	0.9824	0.9685
	Val. loss	0.0864	0.1011	**0.0596**	**0.1008**	0.0609	0.0780
	Val. Accuracy	0.9784	0.9650	**0.9790**	**0.9661**	0.9822	0.9747

Table 4 Testing results using data testing and video data

Model	Accuracy	Processing time per frame (s)
MobileNetV2	0.89	0.106
InceptionV3	0.91	0.212
DenseNet201	0.93	0.291

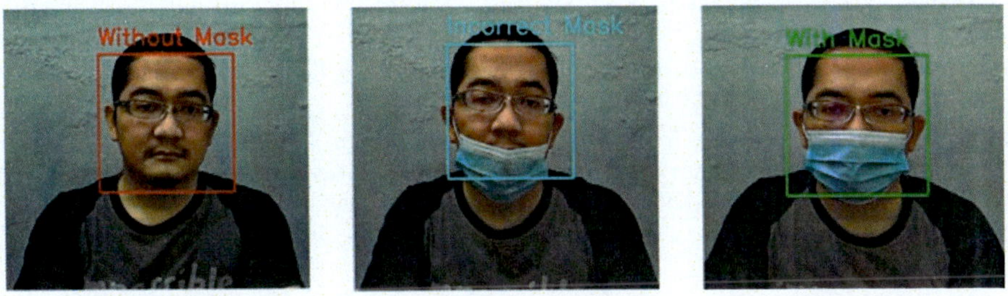

Without mask Incorrect mask With mask

Fig. 7 Example of matching model with video data

The use of the DenseNet201 model produces the best accuracy compared to the InceptionV3 and MobileNetV2 models. However, in running video data, the DenseNet201 model is the slowest. The MobileNetV2 model is the fastest because it has the fewest MobileNetV2 parameters, 3.5 million. Unlike the case with InceptionV3 and DenseNet201, the number of parameters reaches more than 20 million. The number of these parameters affects the result of accuracy and processing speed. These results show that the three models can be applied in real time. An example of matching results is shown in Fig. 7. There are three examples of the results of classifying the use of masks. Not wearing a mask on the face will be detected without mask, wearing a mask but not covering the nose area will be caught with an incorrect mask, and wearing a mask correctly will be detected with mask. In previous research [16], the accuracy of the results was less than 85%, so the results in the proposed research were better than in previous research. This research still has a weakness. The accuracy is inversely proportional to processing speed. Future research can use a combination of transfer learning and CNN layers to improve accuracy and processing speed.

4 Conclusion

The COVID-19 pandemic is not over yet. Even recently, a new variant that is immune to vaccines has emerged. The correct use of masks is an effective way to stop the transmission of this virus. Researchers have developed many applications to detect the wearing of masks, but most still detect wearing a mask or not wearing a mask. In this research, we added one class that used masks that did not fit or did not cover the nose area. The results showed that using transfer learning techniques resulted in the best accuracy of 93% using DenseNet201. Then the fastest processing time is 0.106 s using the MobileNetV2 model. In previous studies, the resulting accuracy value was only 85%. The proposed research can increase the resulting accuracy by 8%. This research still produces accuracy and speed that is inversely proportional. This opposite accuracy and computational speed make the real-time process not optimal. The proposed system has increased accuracy but cannot run in real-time for speed. Future research can modify the stages of feature extraction and classification using other combinations of transfer learning and CNN layers to achieve real-time processing.

Acknowledgements The author would like to thank the Lembaga Penelitian dan Pengabdian Masyarakat (LPPM) Institut Teknologi Telkom Purwokerto, which has provided funds to develop this research.

References

1. Roberts DL, Rossman JS, Jarić I (2021) Dating first cases of COVID-19. PLoS Pathog 17(6):1–10
2. Adhinata FD, Tanjung NAF, Widayat W, Pasfica GR, Satura FR (2022) Real-time masked face recognition using FaceNet and supervised machine learning. In: Proceedings of the 2nd international conference on electronics, biomedical engineering, and health informatics, pp 189–202
3. Morawska L et al (2020) How can airborne transmission of COVID-19 indoors be minimised? Environ Int 142:1–7
4. Pathak N (2021) Coronavirus incubation period: how long and when most contagious. WebMD
5. World Health Organization (2022) WHO coronavirus (COVID-19) dashboard with vaccination data. World Health Organization
6. Moore JP (2021) SARS-CoV-2 vaccines and the growing threat of viral variants
7. Tavilani A, Abbasi E, Kian Ara F, Darini A, Asefy Z (2021) COVID-19 vaccines: current evidence and considerations. Metabolism Open 12:1–5
8. Chen J, Wang R, Gilby NB, Wei G (2021) Omicron variant (B.1.1.529): infectivity, vaccine breakthrough, and antibody resistance. J Chem Inf Model 1–12
9. Jumeri J (2022) All schools must implement limited PTM in 2022. Direktorat Sekolah Dasar
10. Maity S, Das P, Jha KK, Dutta HS (2021) Face mask detection using deep learning. In: International conference on advances and applications of artificial intelligence and machine learning, pp 495–509
11. Patil A, Rane M (2021) Convolutional neural networks: an overview and its applications in pattern recognition. Smart Innov Syst Technol 195:21–30
12. Adhinata FD, Junaidi A (2022) Gender classification on video using FaceNet algorithm and supervised machine learning. Int J Comput Digit Syst 11(1):199–208
13. Joshi AS, Joshi SS, Kanahasabai G, Kapil R, Gupta S (2020) Deep learning framework to detect face masks from video footage. In: International conference on computational intelligence and communication networks (CICN), pp 435–440
14. Jignesh Chowdary G, Punn NS, Sonbhadra SK, Agarwal S (2020) Face mask detection using transfer learning of InceptionV3. Lecture notes in computer science (including subseries Lecture Notes in Artificial Intelligence and Lecture Notes in Bioinformatics), vol 12581, pp 81–90

15. Adhinata FD et al (2021) A deep learning using DenseNet201 to detect masked or non-masked face. JUITA: Jurnal Informatika 9(1):115–121
16. Tomás J, Rego A, Viciano-Tudela S, Lloret J (2021) Incorrect facemask-wearing detection using convolutional neural networks with transfer learning. Healthcare (Switzerland) 9(8):1–17
17. Hassan SM, Maji AK, Jasiński M, Leonowicz Z, Jasińska E (2021) Identification of plant-leaf diseases using CNN and transfer-learning approach. Electronics (Switzerland) 10(12):1–19
18. Ruvinga C, Malathi D, Dorathi Jayaseeli JD (2020) Human concentration level recognition based on vgg16 CNN architecture. Int J Adv Sci Technol 29(6):1364–1373
19. Khayyat MM, Elrefaei LA (2020) Towards author recognition of ancient Arabic manuscripts using deep learning: a transfer learning approach. Int J Comput Digit Syst 90(5):783–799
20. Rjouba R (2022) Face_mask_detector-with_without_incorrect_mask. Kaggle. Kaggle.com
21. Shorten C, Khoshgoftaar TM (2019) A survey on image data augmentation for deep learning. J Big Data 6(1):1–48
22. Wiley V, Lucas T (2018) Computer vision and image processing: a paper review. Int J Artif Intell Res 2(1):28–36
23. Koteluk O, Wartecki A, Mazurek S, Kołodziejczak I, Mackiewicz A (2021) How do machines learn? Artificial intelligence as a new era in medicine. J Pers Med 11(1):1–22
24. Syarief M, Setiawan W (2020) Convolutional neural network for maize leaf disease image classification. Telkomnika (Telecommun Comput Electron Control) 18(3):1376–1381
25. Anton A, Nissa NF, Janiati A, Cahya N, Astuti P (2021) Application of deep learning using convolutional neural network (CNN) method for women's skin classification. Sci J Inform 8(1):144–153
26. Gultom Y, Arymurthy AM, Masikome RJ (2018) Batik classification using deep convolutional network transfer learning. Jurnal Ilmu Komputer dan Informasi 11(2):59–66
27. Sandler M, Howard A, Zhu M, Zhmoginov A, Chen LC (2018) MobileNetV2: inverted residuals and linear bottlenecks. In: Proceedings of the IEEE computer society conference on computer vision and pattern recognition, pp 4510–4520
28. Huu PN, Thi Thu HN, Minh QT (2021) Proposing a recognition system of gestures using MobilenetV2 combining single shot detector network for smart-home applications. J Electr Comput Eng 1–18
29. Szegedy C, Vanhoucke V, Ioffe S, Shlens J, Wojna Z (2016) Rethinking the inception architecture for computer vision. In: 2016 IEEE conference on computer vision and pattern recognition (CVPR), pp 2818–2826
30. He K, Zhang X, Ren S, Sun J (2016) Deep residual learning for image recognition. In: 2016 IEEE conference on computer vision and pattern recognition (CVPR), pp 770–778
31. Huang G, Liu Z, Van Der Maaten L, Weinberger KQ (2017) Densely connected convolutional networks. In: Proceedings—30th IEEE conference on computer vision and pattern recognition, vol 2017, pp 2261–2269
32. Wang S-H, Zhang Y-D (2020) DenseNet-201-based deep neural network with composite learning factor and precomputation for multiple sclerosis classification. ACM Trans Multimedia Comput Commun Appl 16(2)
33. Adhinata FD, Fitriana GF, Wijayanto A, Pajar M, Putra K (2021) Corn disease classification using transfer learning and convolutional neural network. JUITA Jurnal Informatika 9(2):1–7

Comparison of Nutritional Status Prediction Models of Children Under 5 Years of Age Using Supervised Machine Learning

Mediana Aryuni, Eka Miranda, Meyske Kumbangsila, Richard, Alfi Yusrotis Zakiyyah, Albert Verasius Dian Sano, and Faqir M. Bhatti

Abstract The Indonesian government continues to deal with nutritional issues on Indonesian children, such as stunting and wasting. Stunting is a common symptom of children at risk of wasting, and they are more likely to develop long-term developmental issues. Malnutrition in children must be identified as soon as possible in order to prevent many instances and provide prompt, effective treatment to keep the condition from getting worse. The goal of this study is to create a model for predicting children's nutritional status using supervised machine learning algorithms. In order to create a nutritional status prediction model for kids under 5 based on physical examination, this study compares three supervised machine learning algorithms. C4.5 Decision Tree, K-Nearest Neighbors (KNN), and Naive Bayes are the machine learning models. Healthcare Sawah Besar Community Health Service provided its 360 patients with 4 attributes' worth of record information. A model's performance was evaluated using F1-Score and accuracy. The nutritional condition of children under the age of five can be predicted using the C4.5 Decision Tree, K-Nearest Neighbors, and Naive Bayes algorithms. The Sawah Besar Community Health Service can utilize the model to track the nutritional health of children under five years of age, and

M. Aryuni (✉) · E. Miranda · Richard
Information Systems Department, School of Information Systems, Bina Nusantara University, Jakarta, Indonesia
e-mail: mediana.aryuni@binus.ac.id

M. Kumbangsila
Head of Personal and Supporting Health Services Unit and Head of Maternal and Child Health, Sawah Besar Community Health Service, Jakarta, Indonesia

A. Y. Zakiyyah
Mathematics Department, School of Computer Science, Bina Nusantara University, Jakarta, Indonesia

A. V. D. Sano
Computer Science Department, School of Computer Science, Bina Nusantara University, Jakarta, Indonesia

F. M. Bhatti
Riphah Institute of Computing and Applied Sciences, Riphah International University, Raiwind, Lahore, Pakistan

T. Triwiyanto et al. (eds.), *Proceeding of the 3rd International Conference on Electronics, Biomedical Engineering, and Health Informatics*, Lecture Notes in Electrical Engineering 1008, https://doi.org/10.1007/978-981-99-0248-4_19

it can also assist mothers in understanding the nutritional condition of their children. The outcome reveals that the C4.5 Decision Tree performs best, with an accuracy rate of 89.87% and an F1-Score of 91.67%. The C4.5 Decision Tree approach is the best way for forecasting the nutritional status of children under the age of five, according to the experiment data.

Keywords Nutritional status · Children under 5 years of age · Machine learning

1 Introduction

Infants and children's cognitive development rely on getting enough nutrients. Lack of nutrition in children increases their chance of developing growth problems [1, 2] and death [3, 4]. For young children to grow as optimally as possible, adequate nutrition is crucial [5, 6]. Nutritional issues like stunting and wasting affect almost two million Indonesian children under the age of five [7]. In Indonesia, the prevalence of stunting in children has increased over the past ten years and is at 37% nationwide [8]. The number of children under the age of five who suffer from stunting is highest in Indonesia, where it ranks fifth globally [9]. Early life stunting has significant financial and human costs [10]. Moreover, the COVID-19 pandemic can provide various negative impacts on children in short, medium, or long term. UNICEF estimates show that the number of children who experiencing wasting or malnutrition increased by about 15% during the pandemic COVID-19. Children at risk of wasting will tend to experience stunting and vulnerable to long-term developmental disorders [11].

The key to effective prevention and treatment of child malnutrition is early detection [11–13]. Numerous cases of malnutrition can be averted and promptly and effectively treated if this exercise is carried out to its full potential [14]. Malnutrition in children under the age of five has been the subject of numerous earlier research [2, 4, 15–25]. The goals of this research are to identify the risk factors for stunting [18, 21, 26] and undernutrition [15–17] in children under the age of five.

A component of artificial intelligence called machine learning (ML) has the potential to improve the development of nonlinear relationships in nutritional data [27]. In a few research [19–22, 28–33], machine learning algorithms were applied to forecast malnutrition in young infants. Bitew et al. [19] describes a study that used five machine learning (ML) techniques to create undernutrition prediction models for Ethiopia. These methods included Extreme gradient boosting, k-nearest neighbors (k-NN), random forest, neural network, and generalized linear models. Talukder and Ahammed [20] used Five well-known ML techniques, including logistic regression (LR), support vector machines (SVM), random forest (RF), and k-nearest neighbors (k-NN), have been thought to successfully predict malnutrition status among Bangladeshi toddlers. Chilyabanyama et al. [21] used the Naive Bayes (NB), XG Boost (XgB), SV classification (SVC), Logistic regression (LR), Random Forest (RF), and SV classification (RF) algorithms to predict the likelihood of stunting among children under the age of five in Zambia.

Using the C4.5 decision tree, the study [30] constructed a nutritional status prediction model. While [24] used the J48 decision tree, Naive Bayes, and PART rule induction classifiers to predict nutritional status. The use of Random Forest, Support Vector Machine, K-Nearest Neighbors, and Logistic Regression to predict malnutrition was proposed in [34]. k-Nearest Neighbors (KNN) [19, 20, 29], C4.5 Decision Tree [30, 31], and Naive Bayes [21, 32, 33] are three commonly used algorithms.

KNN has independency regarding the underlying data with acceptable performance. The C4.5 Decision Tree algorithm is simply interpreted, able to deal with discrete and numeric attributes, and has good accuracy. In Naïve Bayes algorithm, each attribute is independent and has the same impact on the result and has good performance although the algorithm is simple. Therefore, the goal of this study is to create a prediction model for children's nutritional status using supervised machine learning techniques such as C4.5 Decision Tree, K-Nearest Neighbors (KNN), and Naive Bayes, and to evaluate how well these techniques perform.

2 Methodology

The study's methodology, which was adapted from Knowledge Discovery from Database (KDD) techniques [35], is shown in Fig. 1. Data from the Sawah Besar Community Health Service were initially collected, and the dataset was then preprocessed. Data cleansing, data transformation, and data selection made up data processing. Data splitting was used to partition the dataset into 30% for testing and 70% for training [19]. The C4.5 decision tree [30], K-nearest neighbors [19], and Naive Bayes [21] supervised machine learning techniques were utilized to create the nutritional status prediction modeling using training data. While testing, accuracy, precision, recall, and F1-score were utilized to assess and compare each model's performance.

2.1 Data Collection

The dataset of this study was collected from Healthcare Record data Sawah Besar Community Health Service using 360 Children patients' data. There were 7 attributes (as shown in Table 1) including age, gender, height, weight, address, religion, and doctor's name. The class labels of nutritional status prediction were good nutritional and nutritional problem.

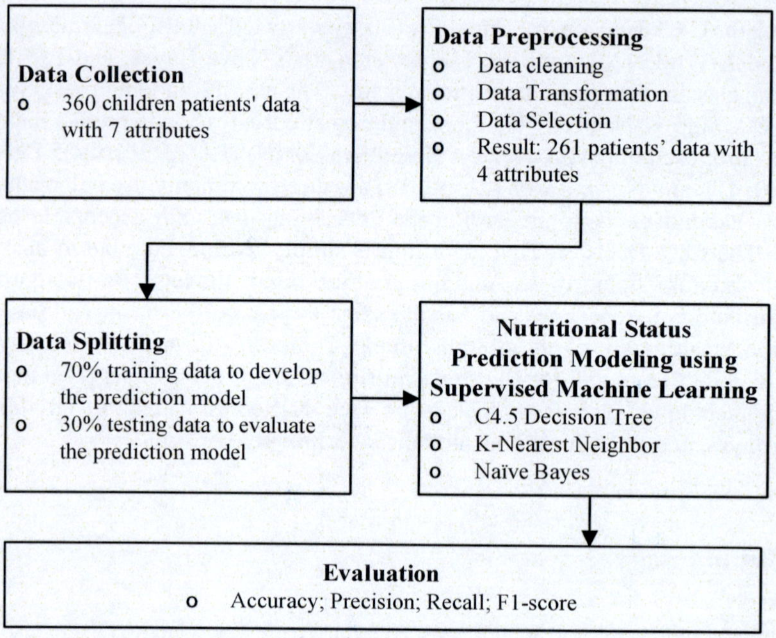

Fig. 1 Research methodology

Table 1 Attributes of nutritional status prediction

Attribute	Data type	Description
Age	Numeric	Children age in years and months
Gender	Text	Children gender (boy or girl)
Height	Numeric	Children height in centimeters
Weight	Numeric	Children weight in kilograms
Address	Text	Children address
Religion	Text	Children religion
Doctor's name	Text	The name of doctor who do examination

2.2 *Data Preprocessing*

Data transformation, data selection, and data cleaning were the processes in the preprocessing of data. Data cleansing was the first stage in the preprocessing of data. Table 2 displays the data cleaning procedure.

The age variable underwent data transformation by transforming the age's years and months into months. For instance, 15 months was substituted for 1 year, 3 months of age. Data transformation with the gender variable was also used to change the data

Table 2 Data cleansing process

Problem	Solution
There were outlier data (age > 5 years old)	Remove outlier data
There were missing values in some attributes	Remove data with missing values

Table 3 Attributes of nutritional status prediction model after data preprocessing

Attribute	Data type	Description
Age	Numeric	Children age in months
Gender	Numeric	Children gender (0 = boy and 1 = girl)
Height	Numeric	Children height in centimeters
Weight	Numeric	Children weight in kilograms

type from text (boy or girl) to numeric (value 0 represents boy and value 1 represents girl).

Attribute subset selection was the method used to choose the data. With the aim of doing research, attribute subset selection is a technique to exclude the qualities that are unnecessary or lack important information. In this study, the useless data elements, including the doctor's name, address, and religion, were eliminated. After data preprocessing, Table 3 displays the characteristics of the nutritional status prediction model. Based on Indonesian anthropometry standards [14, 36], 261 patients' data were utilized to estimate the nutritional health of children under the age of five. These qualities included age, gender, height, and weight.

2.3 *Nutritional Status Prediction Modeling*

C4.5 Decision Tree. Some research used the C4.5 Decision Tree for security intrusion detection systems [37] and the Management Information System of College Education & Teaching [38]. By calculating the values of Entropy, Information Gain, Split Information, and Gain Ratio, the C4.5 decision tree method organizes the data into categories [30]. Equation (1) contains the equation for entropy:

$$\text{Entropy (S)} = \sum_{i=1}^{n} -p_i * \log 2\ p_i \tag{1}$$

where S is the total datasets, n denotes the total partitions, and pi denotes the ratio of Si to S. Equation (2) contains the Information Gain equation:

$$\text{Gain (S, A)} = \text{Entropy(S)} - \sum_{i=1}^{n} \frac{|S_i|}{|S|} \tag{2}$$

where |Si| is the number of samples on the partition, |S| is the number of samples in S, S is the number of datasets, |A| is the attribute, and n is the number of partitions of the attribute set A. Equation (3) contains the Split Info equation:

$$\mathrm{SplitInfo}(S, A) = -\sum_{i=1}^{v} \frac{|S_i|}{|S|} \times \log 2\left(\frac{|S_i|}{|S|}\right) \tag{3}$$

where v is the subset obtained after employing attribute A, which has as many values as v, to solve the problem. Equation (4) contains the equation for the gain ratio:

$$\mathrm{GainRatio}(S, A) = \frac{\mathrm{Gain}(S, A)}{\mathrm{SplitInfo}(S, A)} \tag{4}$$

Finding the root node with the highest Gain Ratio value is the first step in tree creation. From there, leaf nodes are developed iteratively until a decision tree is produced [30].

K-Nearest Neighbors. In several instances, the K-Nearest Neighbors (KNN) method was used to construct security intrusion detection systems [37] and classify legal text data [39]. KNN is a non-parametric algorithm that doesn't rely on any underlying data assumptions [19]. The categorization is based on Euclidean distance between training and testing data. Equation (5) contains the Euclidean distance equation:

$$d_i = \sqrt{\sum_{i=1}^{p} (x_{2i} - x_{1i})^2} \tag{5}$$

where $\times 2$ is training data, $\times 1$ is testing data, and p is the number of attributes.

Naïve Bayes. For the classification of legal text data [39] and spam and ham [40], some studies created Naive Bayes. Based on the Bayes theorem, the Naive Bayes (NB) algorithm was created [21]. This method makes the following two key assumptions: Each attribute has the same effect on the outcome and is independent of the others. Equation (6) [21] contains the NB formula:

$$P(y|X) = \frac{P(X|y)\, P(y)}{P(X)} \tag{6}$$

where X is the independent predictors and P(X) is the predictors' prior probability. P(y|X) is the probability of label y given predictors X (posterior probability), and P(y) is prior probability of label y. P(X|y) is the likelihood.

Table 4 The confusion matrix

	Actual/True class		
	Confusion matrix	Positive	Negative
Predicted class	Positive	True positive (TP)	False positive (FP)
	Negative	False negative (FN)	True negative (TN)

2.4 Evaluation

Accuracy, precision, recall, and F1-score were the four metrics used to assess each model's performance. According to Table 4, the measurements were computed using the confusion matrix. The number of positive class data that are predicted to be in the positive class is known as True Positive (TP), while the number of positive class data that are predicted to be in the negative class is known as False Negative (FN), and the number of negative class data that are predicted to be in the positive class is known as True Negative (TN).

The equation of accuracy, precision, recall, and F1-score [41] are in Eqs. 7, 8, 9, and 10:

$$Accuracy = (TP + TN) / (TP + FP + FN + TN) \tag{7}$$

$$Precision = (TP) / (TP + FP) \tag{8}$$

$$Recall = TP / (TP + FN) \tag{9}$$

$$F1 - Score = (2 * Recall * Precision) / (Recall + Precision) \tag{10}$$

Both positive and negative class datasets were successfully predicted, as evidenced by accuracy [42]. A percentage of all truly positive expected observations is what is meant by the term "precision". Recall is the occurrence of an observation that is expected to belong to a positive class and does so. The F1-score is another name for the harmonic mean of evaluation metrics for precision and recall.

3 Results and Discussions

C4.5 Decision Tree Model. The C4.5 Decision Tree in this study was created by identifying the category that has the most influence on judgments regarding nutritional status. The decision tree model variable was necessary to specify a Decision Tree model in order to create a C4.5 Decision Tree model. Entropy is utilized as a node-division criterion in the Decision Tree model. There was also a random state parameter that produced the same outcomes. According to the test findings, the random_state parameter's value was the one that produced the best accuracy results. The max_depth parameter, another parameter in the Decision Tree model, was utilized to establish a maximum limit and ascertain the depth to which nodes might be divided. The decision_tree_predict variable, which was used to choose the Decision Tree model's prediction outcomes, was another factor in the development of the C4.5 Decision Tree model.

K-Nearest Neighbors Model. In this study, age, gender, height, and weight were the independent variables, and the dependent variable was an attribute of nutritional status. The K-Nearest Neighbors (KNN) model was developed using the knn_model variable, which was used to specify the KNN model. Additionally, the Euclidean Metric was used by the K-Nearest Neighbors (KNN) model in this study to determine the closest distance. The model's prediction outcomes were obtained using the knn_predict variable.

Naïve Bayes. The Gaussian Naive Bayes model was employed in this study to create the model. A straightforward Naive Bayes classification method, Gaussian Naive Bayes is predicated on the idea that each attribute is taken through a straightforward Gaussian distribution. A Naive Bayes model is declared by the variable naive_bayes_model. The outcome of the Naive Bayes model's prediction was stored in the variable naive_bayes_predict.

Table 5 displays the accuracy, precision, recall, and F1-score for each nutritional status prediction model.

Table 6 displays the confusion matrix for testing data for each C4.5 Decision Tree, K-Nearest Neighbors (KNN), and Naive Bayes nutritional status prediction model.

Based on Tables 5 and 6, the C4.5 Decision Tree approach accurately predicted 71 out of a total of 79 data, with a precision value of 89.80%, an F1-score of 91.67%, an accuracy value of 89.87%, a recall or sensitivity value of 93.62% on testing data, and a recall or sensitivity value of 89.80%. The experimental data mining classification methodology employing the C4.5 Decision Tree method gives good results and is thus included in the Good Classification category (accuracy with a range of value 80%–90%), according to the evaluation values obtained.

Entropy is used as a node-division criterion in the C4.5 Decision Tree Model. The weight attribute produced the best results, with age, gender, and height following. Using the data from Tables 5 and 6, the K-Nearest Neighbors approach was able to accurately predict 65 out of a total of 79 data, with an F1-score of 84.44%, an accuracy value of 82.28%, a precision value of 88.37%, a recall value or sensitivity of

Table 5 The performance comparation

Algorithm	Accuracy (%)	Precision (%)	Recall (%)	F1-score (%)
C4.5 decision tree	89.87	89.80	93.62	91.67
KNN	82.28	88.37	80.85	84.44
Naïve Bayes	73.42	96.43	57.45	72.00

Table 6 The confusion matrix for testing data

	Actual/True class		
	Confusion matrix C4.5 Decision Tree	Nutritional problem	Good nutritional
Predicted class	Nutritional problem	44	3
	Good nutritional	5	27

	Actual/True class		
	Confusion matrix KNN	Nutritional problem	Good nutritional
Predicted class	Nutritional problem	38	9
	Good nutritional	5	27

	Actual/True class		
	Confusion matrix Naïve Bayes	Nutritional problem	Good nutritional
Predicted class	Nutritional problem	27	20
	Good nutritional	1	31

80.85% on test data, and. The experimental data mining classification methodology employing the K-Nearest Neighbors (KNN) method generates good results and is included in the Good Classification category (Accuracy with a value range of 80–90%), according to the evaluation values obtained.

According to Tables 5 and 6, the prediction model utilizing the Naive Bayes approach was able to accurately predict 58 out of a total of 79 data, with a precision value of 96.43%, a recall value of 57.45% on test data, and an F1-score of 72.0%. The results of the accuracy value in the classification technique of the Naïve Bayes method tend to be low because the Naïve Bayes model is a simple method and has limited functions in the Python programming language. In this regard, the experimental test for predicting children's health using the Naïve Bayes model includes Fair Classification (Accuracy with a value range of 70–80%). We can conclude based on accuracy and F1-score, the result shows that C4.5 Decision Tree has the highest performance with 89.87% of accuracy and 91.67% of F1-Score. Since different dataset sets yield different results, we cannot declare that our study result was more accurate than previous studies. Moreover, our study's dataset had the key benefit for medical professionals' decisions as ground truth.

The data from the Sawah Besar Community Health Service's Healthcare Record were used in this study to expose the novelty covering theoretical and clinical significance. Additionally, a prediction model based on three supervised machine learning algorithms—the C4.5 Decision Tree, K-Nearest Neighbors (KNN), and Naive Bayes—was developed and tested. With 89.87% accuracy and 91.67% F1-Score, the C4.5 Decision Tree approach is the most accurate method for predicting the nutritional status of children under five years old. The accuracy of K-Nearest Neighbors (KNN) and Naive Bayes, in contrast, was 82.28% and 73.42%, respectively. K-Nearest Neighbors (KNN) and Naive Bayes have F1-scores of 84.44% and 72.0%, respectively.

C4.5 Decision Tree models in [30] have accuracy of 90.16%, 76.64%, and 83.83%. In our study, the C4.5 Decision Tree's accuracy was marginally higher than that of the two models in [30]. With 73% accuracy, the KNN algorithm in [19] showed the worst performance. While in our study, KNN's accuracy was marginally superior to [19]. The Naive Bayes model was eliminated based on [21] because it lacked precision even after calibration. Additionally, our analysis revealed that Naive Bayes has the lowest accuracy and F1-Score.

Additionally, the study demonstrated its relevance as a model for predicting children's nutritional status under the age of five and indicated that it could serve as the foundation for future prediction applications.

There were several weaknesses or limitations of this study, including the dataset was too small, no historical data in making predictions based on supervised machine learning, only used 4 attributes (age, gender, height, weight) based on anthropometry standard in Indonesia [36], and only had 2 nutritional status prediction classes (Good Nutritional and Nutritional Problem).

4 Conclusion

In order to examine the performance of three supervised machine learning algorithms, this research created a nutrition status prediction model for children under the age of five using C4.5 Decision Tree, K-Nearest Neighbors (KNN), and Naive Bayes.

The C4.5 Decision Tree approach, which has an accuracy rate of 89.87% and an F1-Score of 91.67%, is the best method for predicting the nutritional condition of children under the age of five, according to the results of the experiments. The accuracy of K-Nearest Neighbors (KNN) and Naive Bayes, in contrast, was 82.28% and 73.42%, respectively. K-Nearest Neighbors (KNN) and Naive Bayes have F1-scores of 84.44% and 72.0%, respectively.

The Sawah Besar Community Health Service can utilize the model to track the nutritional health of children under the age of five and to assist mothers in understanding the nutritional condition of their children.

Some future works are utilizing more datasets for better accuracy, using historical medical records for better predictive results, add more attributes such as demographic, and providing more specific information on the nutritional status prediction (stunting, wasting, or obesity).

Acknowledgements As a part of the BINUS Research Untuk Nusantara (BRUN) Research Grant titled "Rancang Bangun Aplikasi Berbasis Web Prediksi Kesehatan Ibu Hamil Dan Gizi Balita Dengan Pendekatan Data Mining" with contract number: No: 064/VR.RTT/IV/2022 and contract date: 8 April 2022, this work is supported by the Research and Technology Transfer Office, Bina Nusantara We also value the assistance provided by Puskesmas Kecamatan Sawah Besar, Jakarta Pusat, and our students during the research process (Shofi Rafiiola, Muhammad Dzaki Izza Romadhon, Muhammad Rafi Zhafransyah).

References

1. Roberts M, Tolar-Peterson T, Reynolds A, Wall C, Reeder N, Rico Mendez G (2022) The effects of nutritional interventions on the cognitive development of preschool-age children: a systematic review. Nutrients 14:532. https://doi.org/10.3390/nu14030532
2. Rahman SMJ, Ahmed NAMF, Abedin MdM, Ahammed B, Ali M, Rahman MdJ, Maniruzzaman Md (2021) Investigate the risk factors of stunting, wasting, and underweight among under-five Bangladeshi children and its prediction based on machine learning approach. PLoS One 16:e0253172. https://doi.org/10.1371/journal.pone.0253172
3. Khare S, Kavyashree S, Gupta D, Jyotishi A (2017) Investigation of nutritional status of children based on machine learning techniques using indian demographic and health survey data. Procedia Comput Sci 115:338–349. https://doi.org/10.1016/j.procs.2017.09.087
4. Methun MdIH, Kabir A, Islam S, Hossain MdI, Darda MA (2021) A machine learning logistic classifier approach for identifying the determinants of Under-5 child morbidity in Bangladesh. Clin Epidemiol Glob Health 12:100812. https://doi.org/10.1016/j.cegh.2021.100812
5. Ramli KEA, Inder KJ, Bowe SJ, Jacobs J, Dibley MJ (2009) Prevalence and risk factors for stunting and severe stunting among under-fives in North Maluku province of Indonesia. BMC Pediatr 9:64. https://doi.org/10.1186/1471-2431-9-64
6. Mukuku O, Mutombo AM, Kamona LK, Lubala TK, Mawaw PM, Aloni MN, Wembonyama SO, Luboya ON (2019) Predictive model for the risk of severe acute malnutrition in children. J Nutr Metab 2019:1–7. https://doi.org/10.1155/2019/4740825
7. UNICEF: Nutrition: tackling the "double burden" of malnutrition in Indonesia. https://www.unicef.org/indonesia/nutrition. Accessed 26 March 2022
8. Beal T, Tumilowicz A, Sutrisna A, Izwardy D, Neufeld LM (2018) A review of child stunting determinants in Indonesia. Matern Child Nutr 14:e12617. https://doi.org/10.1111/mcn.12617
9. Titaley CR, Ariawan I, Hapsari D, Muasyaroh A, Dibley MJ (2019) Determinants of the stunting of children under two years old in indonesia: a multilevel analysis of the 2013 Indonesia basic health survey. Nutrients 11:1106. https://doi.org/10.3390/nu11051106
10. Torlesse H, Cronin AA, Sebayang SK, Nandy R (2016) Determinants of stunting in Indonesian children: evidence from a cross-sectional survey indicate a prominent role for the water, sanitation and hygiene sector in stunting reduction. BMC Public Health 16:669. https://doi.org/10.1186/s12889-016-3339-8
11. UNICEF: Indonesia: Angka masalah gizi pada anak akibat COVID-19 dapat meningkat tajam kecuali jika tindakan cepat diambil. https://www.unicef.org/indonesia/id/press-releases/angka-masalah-gizi-pada-anak-di-indonesia-akibat-covid-19-dapat-meningkat-tajam
12. Shi H, Yang D, Tang K, Hu C, Li L, Zhang L, Gong T, Cui Y (2022) Explainable machine learning model for predicting the occurrence of postoperative malnutrition in children with congenital heart disease. Clin Nutr 41:202–210. https://doi.org/10.1016/j.clnu.2021.11.006
13. Raphaeli O, Singer P (2021) Towards personalized nutritional treatment for malnutrition using machine learning-based screening tools. Clin Nutr 40:5249–5251. https://doi.org/10.1016/j.clnu.2021.08.013
14. KEMKES: Standar operasional prosedur (SOP) deteksi dini dan rujukan balita gizi buruk atau yang berisiko gizi buruk. https://gizi.kemkes.go.id/katalog/sop-gibur-deteksi-dini.pdf
15. Kassie GW, Workie DL (2020) Determinants of under-nutrition among children under five years of age in Ethiopia. BMC Public Health 20:399. https://doi.org/10.1186/s12889-020-08539-2
16. Nhampossa T, Sigaúque B, Machevo S, Macete E, Alonso P, Bassat Q, Menéndez C, Fumadó V (2013) Severe malnutrition among children under the age of 5 years admitted to a rural district hospital in southern Mozambique. Public Health Nutr 16:1565–1574. https://doi.org/10.1017/S1368980013001080
17. Govender I, Rangiah S, Kaswa R, Nzaumvila D (2021) Malnutrition in children under the age of 5 years in a primary health care setting. South African Family Practice 63. https://doi.org/10.4102/safp.v63i1.5337

18. Habimana S, Biracyaza E (2019) Risk factors of stunting among children under 5 years of age in the eastern and western provinces Of Rwanda: analysis of rwanda demographic and health survey 2014/2015. Pediatric Health Med Ther 10:115–130. https://doi.org/10.2147/PHMT.S222198
19. Bitew FH, Sparks CS, Nyarko SH (2021) Machine learning algorithms for predicting undernutrition among under-five children in Ethiopia. Public Health Nutr 1–12. https://doi.org/10.1017/S1368980021004262
20. Talukder A, Ahammed B (2020) Machine learning algorithms for predicting malnutrition among under-five children in Bangladesh. Nutrition 78:110861. https://doi.org/10.1016/j.nut.2020.110861
21. Chilyabanyama ON, Chilengi R, Simuyandi M, Chisenga CC, Chirwa M, Hamusonde K, Saroj RK, Iqbal NT, Ngaruye I, Bosomprah S (2022) Performance of machine learning classifiers in classifying stunting among under-five children in Zambia. Children 9:1082. https://doi.org/10.3390/children9071082
22. Fenta HM, Zewotir T, Muluneh EK (2021) A machine learning classifier approach for identifying the determinants of under-five child undernutrition in Ethiopian administrative zones. BMC Med Inform Decis Mak 21:291. https://doi.org/10.1186/s12911-021-01652-1
23. Shahid M, Liu Y, Ameer W, Qureshi MG, Ahmed F, Tang K (2022) Comparison of different nutritional screening approaches and the determinants of malnutrition in under-five children in a marginalized district of Punjab province Pakistan. Children 9:1096. https://doi.org/10.3390/children9071096
24. Markos Z (2014) Predicting under nutrition status of under-five children using data mining techniques: the case of 2011 ethiopian demographic and health survey. J Health Med Inform 5. https://doi.org/10.4172/2157-7420.1000152
25. Hemo SA, Rayhan MdI (2021) Classification tree and random forest model to predict under-five malnutrition in Bangladesh. Int J Biostat. 10, 116–123
26. Khan JR, Tomal JH, Raheem E (2021) Model and variable selection using machine learning methods with applications to childhood stunting in Bangladesh. Inform Health Soc Care 46:425–442. https://doi.org/10.1080/17538157.2021.1904938
27. Russo S, Bonassi S (2022) Prospects and pitfalls of machine learning in nutritional epidemiology. Nutrients 14:1705. https://doi.org/10.3390/nu14091705
28. Kurniati I, Dewi CS, Juniantika R (2021) penerapan data mining dengan algoritma neural network pada sistem informasi prediksi kasus balita gizi buruk di provinsi nusa tenggara barat. Jurnal Rekayasa Informasi Swadharma. 1
29. Dwi Nugraha S, Putri RRM, Wihandika RC (2017) Penerapan fuzzy K-nearest neighbor (FK-NN) dalam menentukan status gizi balita. Jurnal Pengembangan Teknologi Informasi dan Ilmu Komputer 1:925–932
30. Pinaryanto K, Nugroho RA, Basilius Y (2021) Classification of toddler nutrition using C4.5 decision tree method. Int J Appl Sci Smart Technol 03:131–142. https://doi.org/10.24071/ijasst.v3i1.3366
31. Wajhillah R, Mutiara E (2016) Penerapan algoritma C4.5 untuk diagnosa status gizi pada anak balita berbasis website. Swabumi 4
32. Rahmawati N, Novianto Y, Jasmir J (2020) Klasifikasi kondisi gizi balita menggunakan metode naive bayes (studi kasus posyandu melati IV). Jurnal Ilmiah Mahasiswa Teknik Informatika 2:257–268
33. Sinaga ASR, Simanjuntak D (2020) Sistem pakar deteksi gizi buruk balita dengan metode naïve bayes classifier. Jurnal Inkofar 1. https://doi.org/10.46846/jurnalinkofar.v1i2.110
34. Kar S, Pratihar S, Nayak S, Bal S, Gururai HL, Ravikumar V (2021) Prediction of child malnutrition using machine learning. In: 2021 10th international conference on internet of everything, microwave engineering, communication and networks (IEMECON), pp 01–04. IEEE (2021). https://doi.org/10.1109/IEMECON53809.2021.9689083
35. Han J, Kamber M, Pei Y (2012) Data mining: concepts and technique. Morgan Kaufman
36. KEMKES: Standar Antropometri Anak

37. Elaeraj O, Leghris C, Renault É (2021) Performance evaluation of some machine learning algorithms for security intrusion detection. Presented at the (2021). https://doi.org/10.1007/978-3-030-70866-5_10
38. Chen F (2021) The management information system of college education and teaching based on C4.5 classification algorithm. Presented at the (2021). https://doi.org/10.1007/978-981-16-0115-6_253
39. Araújo DC, Lima A, Lima JP, Costa JA (2021) A comparison of classification methods applied to legal text data. Presented at the (2021).https://doi.org/10.1007/978-3-030-86230-5_6
40. Sastry JKR, Harika P, Dubey T, Vijay Ditya Y (2023) Spam and ham classification by multinomial naïve bayes classification in text data. Presented at the (2023). https://doi.org/10.1007/978-981-19-1484-3_26
41. Cho E, Chang T-W, Hwang G (2022) Data preprocessing combination to improve the performance of quality classification in the manufacturing process. Electronics (Basel) 11:477. https://doi.org/10.3390/electronics11030477
42. Van Siy VT, Antonio VA, Siguin CP, Gordoncillo NP, Sescon JT, Go CC, Miro EP (2022) Predicting undernutrition among elementary schoolchildren in the Philippines using machine learning algorithms. Nutrition 96:111571. https://doi.org/10.1016/j.nut.2021.111571

Stock Investment Modeling and Prediction Using Vector Autoregression (VAR) and Cross Industry Standard Process for Data Mining (CRISP-DM)

Agung Triayudi, Iskandar Fitri, Sumiati, and Iksal

Abstract Prediction investment share is one issue important right now, as many people now have to switch to digital investment. Many studies have been done to help Stock data prediction using machine learning. However, most machine learning models used complex and predictive only one variable row time. This research focuses on creating machine learning models using the VAR algorithm to predict several variables at a time with 1 model and provides recommendations, and uses the framework Cross Industry Standard Process for Data Mining (CRISP-DM) work in holding his research. The contribution of this research is to analyze whether the open, high, low, and close share price variables can be predicted based on each variable's past data. Then build a forecasting model using machine learning technology, the Vector Autoregression (VAR) algorithm, and the Cross Industry Standard Process for Data Mining (CRISP-DM) method. From the resulting study, the VAR model is able to produce a model capable of predicting three variables at a time, that is, price highs, lows, and closes with each R2 Score is 0.60, 0.51, 0.54 and uses an optimal lag of 273 but for the variable price opening make a separate model with the lag difference is two lags and the R2 Score is 0.63. Based on the results of testing and evaluation of the use of R2, MAE, and RMSE scores on the model that was successfully created, it can be concluded that VAR can be used to predict the highest, lowest, and closing stock prices at once and has a fairly good accuracy even though the opening price variable must make a separation.

Keywords Stock investment · Prediction · Variable · VAR algorithm · CRISP-DM

A. Triayudi (✉) · I. Fitri
Department of ICT, Universitas Nasional, Jakarta, Indonesia
e-mail: agungtriayudi@civitas.unas.ac.id

Sumiati
Informatics Department, Universitas Serang Raya, Serang, Indonesia

Iksal
Engineering Department, Universitas Faletehan, Kabupaten Serang, Indonesia

T. Triwiyanto et al. (eds.), *Proceeding of the 3rd International Conference on Electronics, Biomedical Engineering, and Health Informatics*, Lecture Notes in Electrical Engineering 1008, https://doi.org/10.1007/978-981-99-0248-4_20

1 Introduction

Investment is the commitment individual or group to give some of the money he has on something asset with the aim of getting future profits [1]. Return or profit investment share generated from sale share that. Sell and buy shares need literacy good finance _ because good literacy affects the return value or later profit day [2]. There are several how to get profit from investment stock, one of them that is forecasting with the help of machine learning [3–5].

Already many study forecasting uses machine learning, starting from ARIMA, XGBoost, LSTM, SVR, the combination of a number of algorithms, and still many again. The problem is that most models used complex and predictive only one variable course. Then Researcher wants to build a forecasting model that can predict more from one variable at a time with more simple models [6–8].

The CNN-BiLSTM-AM approach is suggested in this study as a way to forecast the closing price for the following day. Convolutional neural networks (CNN), bidirectional long short-term memory (BiLSTM), and an attention mechanism are used in this technique (AM). To extract features from input data, CNN is employed. To forecast the closing stock price for the following day, BiLSTM leverages extracted feature data. The gap from this study is that predictions are only accurate for the short term. For the long term, monthly or yearly, the prediction rate decreases or is less accurate [9].

In another study, there is a modeling of dynamic market conditions and trends using stock representations to produce dynamic correlations between stocks and the market, and then we combine these correlations with dynamic stock indicators to achieve more accurate stock predictions. The gap from this research, the resulting model is not detailed on stock prices in particular, but only up and down price movements [10].

Investing in stocks is means important for management finance in modern society, and how to forecast stock data has been one _ important issue [11]. Own stock is part ownership of something company where everyone on the sheet gives the right voice to the owner [12]. ICBP.JK is code share PT Indofood CBP Sukses Makmur Tbk, which is a company that produces light food, spice food, milk, miscellaneous drinks, biscuits, and food specials certain [13, 14].

The method used in this research is CRISP-DM [15]. Cross Industry Standard Process for Data Mining (CRISP-DM) large received as framework work for the data mining industry and data analytics for research or looking for knowledge data-based [14]. Multivariate Time Series (MTS) is the series score with an indicator of the same statistics arranged in order of the chronological incident. Function from past data could be used to predict future value variable if we change variable contained in the information from past data [16]. The algorithm used is Vector Autoregression (VAR). Vector Autoregression (VAR) is a calculation prediction used when two-row times or more impact one another [17].

In research previously in the article entitled Stock-Price Forecasting Based on XGBoost and LSTM, the researcher compares algorithm models such as Autoregressive Integrated Moving Average (ARIMA) or also called combination among algorithm autoregressive with moving averages and combinations XGBoost with LSTM to predict price stock. Datasets used were taken from the forex market from January 1, 2008 to March 19, 2018 with a total data of 709,314. Then the researcher uses price as the target. As a result, the ARIMA model scores a Mean Absolute Error (MAE) of 4.149×10^{-4}, whereas the combination XGBoost with an LSTM of 3.825×10^{-4} [18].

In another study in an article entitled Price Prediction of Seasonal Items Using Machine Learning and Statistical Methods, researchers compare a number of algorithms among them, namely Support Vector Machine (SVR), Linear Regression, Random Forest, Ridge Regression, and Autoregressive Integrated Moving Average (ARIMA). The method used in the research is to do data collection and preparation first. Then make, design, train, test, and deploy models. As a result, the Random Forest algorithm has the smallest Score, i.e., 2016, followed by ARIMA, which is 34, 44 [19].

Then, in an article titled "Stock Price Prediction Using Brown's Weighted Exponential Moving Average technique with Optimization," there is a study that is comparable to the prediction of stock data. Levenberg–Marquardt. This research uses the algorithm Brown's Weighted Exponential Moving Average (B-WEMA), then combines it with algorithm optimization Levenberg–Marquardt and compares them without Optimization. Method of the research is started from to do a literature study, then collecting data, designing the system, implementing the system, doing analysis results, and creating an interesting conclusion. Research results put forward that the B-WEMA algorithm with Optimization proved better compared to those without Optimization, that is, with error almost reached 0% [20, 21].

From several studies, two main problems can be drawn, and the first is how to make accurate stock price prediction modeling. Second, many methods have been used to predict stock prices but have not worked optimally.

The state of the art of this research is how the implementation of the Cross Industry Standard Process for Data Mining (CRISP-DM) method to the Vector Autoregression (VAR) algorithm and its application to a case study of predicting stock price movement modeling. Algorithm Autoregressive is often found to be an algorithm study, especially to do forecasting, however often combined with another algorithm. Besides that algorithm, it's just to predict one variable course. Election combination method or framework work CRISP-DM research is due to the flow easily understood and implemented, whereas election VAR algorithm because at the end study expected with the algorithm that could produce a model capable of predicting a number of variable row time at once.

The purpose of this study is to analyze whether the open, high, low, and close share price variables can be predicted at a time based on the past data of each variable. Then build a forecasting model using machine learning technology, the Vector Autoregression (VAR) algorithm, and the CRISP-DM research method so that it can provide price recommendations using the VAR algorithm.

The contribution of this research is (1) to find out whether the VAR algorithm can produce a model with good accuracy, especially using existing variables, so that it can be used to forecast stock data; (2) create a forecasting model that can predict more than one line time variable at a time using a machine learning model with the VAR algorithm; and (3) can provide recommendations to sell or buy ICBP.JK shares based on the predicted results.

The problem limitation of this research is only using open, high, low, and closed stock price data. The data used is daily data from the range of July 29, 2019–November 26, 2021. The next time limit is the results of the model made in this study only to predict future prices as far as 80 working days from November 26, 2021.

2 Research Methods

This study uses secondary data that gathers shares listed on the Indonesia Stock Exchange (IDX) of various issuers [22], but only ICBP.JK stock data is used. The data used to create this stock dataset was scraped from the official IDX website, IDX.co.id, and collected via the kaggle.com website. This study employs the CRISP-DM methodology. This approach comprises six phases: business comprehension, data comprehension, data preparation, modeling, evaluation, and implementation. [22]. The overview and description of the cycle phase can be shown in Fig. 1 as follows.

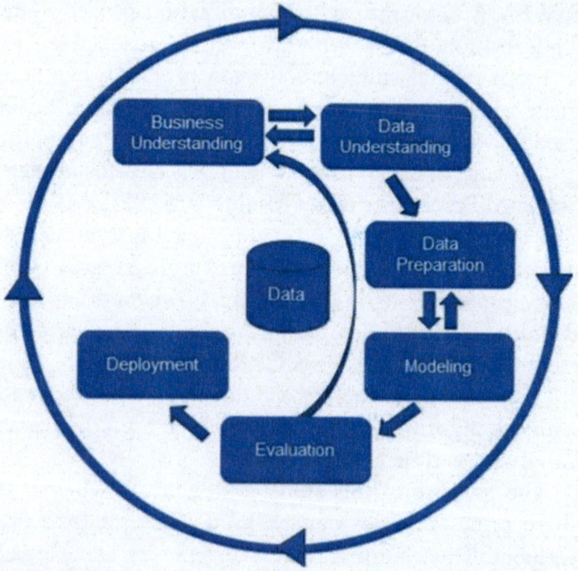

Fig. 1 CRISP-DM Siklus cycle [11]

Table 1 Column name description

Column name	Information
Date	Date the way trading
Open price	The day's initial purchase price
High	The day's highest price
Low	Best deal of the day
Close	Final value for the day

2.1 Business Understanding

In this study, the approach of Machine Learning aims to build a model for forecasting stock data to provide recommendation prices for dates certain based on past data. So that expected could assist in making decisions in transactions shared, specifically ICBP.JK shares [23, 24].

2.2 Data Understanding

Stock data set is obtained from the kaggle.com site, which method the collection is with scrapping data from the official IDX website IDX.co.id. The dataset consists of 565 lines meaning there are 565 lags. Here's the description of attributes that exist in the dataset used (Table 1).

2.3 Data Preparation

At this stage, the data will be prepared for processing as training data as well as test data. The following are the steps taken at this stage: (a) Creating Training and Test Data: The first step in stage data preparation is to create training data and test data from datasets with the amount of test data is five lags or time, whereas the rest used as training data. (b) Stationarity Test: Basically, VAR uses _ regression in its implementation. In regression, if the data is used non-stationary so will produce what is called spurious regression [25]. The stationarity test in this study was carried out using Augmented-Dickey Fuller (ADF). (c) Differentiated: If there are non-stationary time series data, then conduct differencing using the first difference in training data, then do a stationarity test return until all-time series stationary. (d) Granger Test-Casualty Granger test Among two which variable is the variable first said granger-causes variable second if Score variable second the could predictable with help information contained in past data variable first [14]. Granger-causality test was performed on training data [14, 25, 26].

2.4 Modeling

This research was conducted to make VAR estimation. VAR is an algorithm for calculating prediction used when at least two-row time impact on another. That is, the relationship between two directions among rows includes time. VAR algorithm basically has the same formula as Autoregressive AR(p) like the following:

$$Y_t = \alpha + \beta_1 Y_{t-1} + \beta_2 Y_{t-2} + \cdots + \beta_p Y_{t-p} + \varepsilon_t \tag{1}$$

where α is the intercept or constant and $\beta 1, \beta 2$ until $\beta \mathrm{p}$ is lag coefficient or hose time until order p while Y is the variable predictor and t is time [27].

Each variable at a given point in time is predicted by every variable (including the variable itself) at point $t - 1$ in a first-order vector autoregressive (VAR(1)) model. The VAR (1) model also includes cross-lag effects, which show how much the variable was predicted by all other variables at the prior time point, in addition to a set of intercept parameters. Autoregressive effects are shown as how much the variable was forecasted by itself at the prior time point.

Formally, the variable $X_t \in R^p$ at the time point, $t \in Z$ is modeled as a linear combination of the same variables at $t - 1$ [26].

$$X_t = \beta_0 + B X_{t-1} + \in = \begin{bmatrix} X_{t,1} \\ X_{t,p} \end{bmatrix} \tag{2}$$

where $\beta_{0,1}$ is the intercept of variable 1, $\beta_{1,1}$ is the autoregressive effect of $X_{t-1,1}$ is $X_{t,1}$, and $\beta_{p,1}$ is the cross-lag effect of $X_{t-1,1}$ is $X_{t,p}$, and we assume that $\in = \left\{ \in_1, \ldots, \in_\mathrm{p} \right\}$ independent samples (across time points) are taken from a multivariate Gaussian distribution with a variance–covariance matrix R [25].

2.5 Evaluation

At stage evaluation, the model has been evaluated using metrics. The mean absolute error (MAE) calculates the average error (difference score actual with results forecast) absolute, Root Mean Square Error (RMSE) calculates the total of difference results prediction with actual data squared, then calculates the average and rooted and finally, that is R2 to see performance of the built model [28–30].

$$\mathrm{MAE}(y - \hat{y}) = \frac{1}{N} \sum_{j=1}^{N} |y - \widehat{y}| \tag{3}$$

$$\mathrm{RMSE} = \sqrt{\frac{\sum_{j=1}^{N} (y - \hat{y})^2}{N}} \tag{4}$$

$$R2 = 1 - \frac{\sum_{j=1}^{N} (y_j - \widehat{y)}^2}{\sum_{j=1}^{N} (y_j - \overline{y})^2} \quad (5)$$

where average error has been assessed with $\gamma = 1$, which occurs only when |e1| = |e2| = ...|en| or e1 2 = e2 2 = ...en 2.

After doing all stages above, the next stage is to make a model so that it is more easily accessed. For that made the web page simple with date parameters, then it showed graphs and tables, resulting in predictions containing _ recommendations so that it could help make decisions in transactions.

3 Result and Discussion

Stationarity Test

The ratio of 495:80, or 495 lag for training data and 80 lag for test data, determines how shared data become training data and test data. The ADF test, more often known as the training data analysis, was then used to evaluate whether or not all variables were stationary or not at the level of 0.05 or 5% significance.

In Table 2 and Fig. 2, it can be seen that the whole data variable is not stationary. Stationarity test was carried out, that is, using ADF.

In Fig. 3 and Table 3, based on stationarity test results first found that there is number of variable that is not yet stationary. Because of that need conducted differencing with the first difference is to test the stationary back. The result is as follows:

Granger Test-Casualty

After all, the data is stationary. The next step is to perform the Granger-causality test to see the connection between the data and each variable. The focus of the Granger-causality test is to see what is past data and every variable the each other give influences to predict the Score of another variable.

Table 4 shows Granger-causality test results from all possible combinations from data series time every variable to other variables with $H_{0,}$ which means the variable predictor does not have information that can help predict response. The variable in the row is a variable response, while those in the column are the predictor, and the value

Table 2 The results of the training data test at the level

Variable name	P-value	Information
Open price	0.36	Non-stationary
High	0.8	Non-stationary
Low	0.61	Non-stationary
Close	0.73	Non-stationary

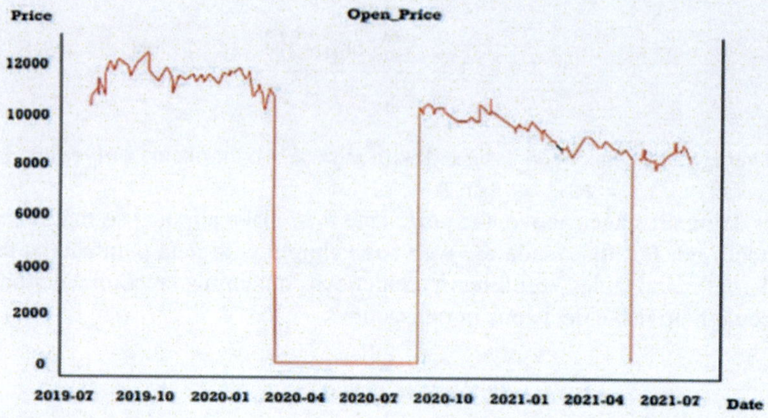

Fig. 2 Plot of training data

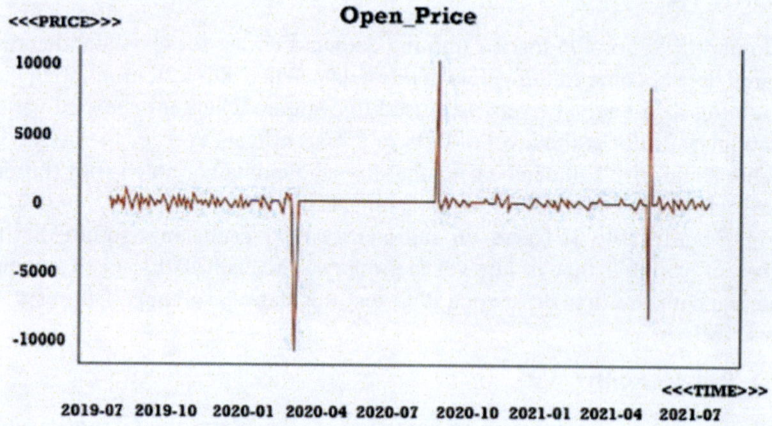

Fig. 3 Training data on the first difference

Table 3 Stationarity test results of training data on the first difference

Variable name	P-value	Information
Open price	0.0	Stationary
High	0.0	Stationary
Low	0.0	Stationary
Close	0.0	Stationary

in the table is P-Values. Almost all combination variables reject H_0, which mean that the data in the past each have influence between variable to predict Score another variable. Except for variable response, open price with predictor low and high, which

Table 4 Granger-Causality test results

	Open price	High	Low	Close
Open price	1.00	0.45	0.23	0.00
High	0.00	1.00	0.00	0.00
Low	0.00	0.00	1.00	0.00
Close	0.00	0.02	0.01	1.00

means not enough proof that second variable the give influence to predict variable open price.

Model Selection

In choosing a model, the first thing to do is look for optimal lag using a number of information criteria, among them Akaike Information Criteria (AIC), Bayesian Information Criteria (BIC), Final Prediction Error (FPE), and Hannan-Quinn information criterion (HQ). In Table 5, in the process is known that the optimal lag obtained is inconsistent if the changed maximum is given lag. Because of that, optimal search lag conducted with iterative with the maximum lag between 1 and 400 later gather all the existing optimal lag. Then estimate to make four models with Prioritize the lowest RMSE for each variable. Model results found with the lowest RMSE for each variable as follows:

In Table 6, based on optimal results, lag each of the above models needs conducting check their autocorrelation on the model using Durbin-Watson. To make it easier to understand the table, the following models that prioritize the variable Open Price will call the OP model, then the HL model for the variable High and Low, and the C model for the variable Close.

Table 5 Comparison of RMSE for all existing models

Variable name	RMSE	Optimal lag
Open price	217.16	2
High	228.29	273
Low	247.71	273
Close	236.78	291

Table 6 Autocorrelation check using Durbin-Watson

Variable	Open price	High	Low	Close
OP	2.0	2.04	2.07	1.99
HL	1.97	2.22	1.95	2.03
C	1.7	2.05	1.88	1.87

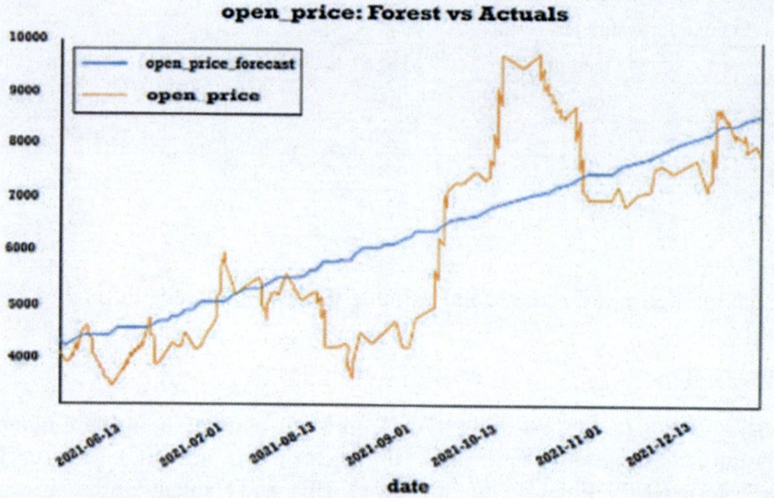

Fig. 4 The blue line is the prediction of the results, while the orange line is the actual data. Prediction results just follow a pattern trend but are not suitable with actual data except for variable Open Price

Figure 4 shows that all variables in these models are independent or don't have autocorrelation. To choose the right model researcher To do tests the above model to past test data and compares his R2 Score on each variable.

In Table 7, the R2 score for the variable Open Price big enough, which is 63% but not on other variables, especially variable Close, where is the R2 Score negative, showing that the model cannot yet predict variable Close.

In Table 8, it can be seen that good RMSE, MAE, and R2 scores are better than the OP's model except for the variable Open Price.

Table 7 Result score OP model testing

Variable	RMSE	MAE	R2
Open price	217.16	169.38	0.63
High	313.95	238.75	0.24
Low	339.47	265.94	0.07
Close	396.16	308.44	−0.22

Table 8 Result score HL model testing

Variable	RMSE	MAE	R2
Open price	4171.07	3940.63	−134.21
High	228.29	184.69	0.60
Low	247.71	212.5	0.51
Close	242.79	199.06	0.54

In Fig. 5, result pattern of all C model predictions almost approach or the same with actual data. The test results of model C in Table 9 show that the model is better than the OP's model but no better than the HL model except for the variable Close with not much significant difference. Based on the results test in Tables 7, 8, and 9, the Researcher decided to use the HL model to predict variables High, Low, and Close and the OP's model to predict variable Open Price.

Implementation

In this section, we will explain how implementation from the existing model was made. This implementation is part of the CRISP-DM deployment cycle that will use a simple page web to display results prediction. Here's a flowchart about the plot work page on the website:

In Fig. 6, there are charts showing the results prediction of all variables from the date tomorrow day (since the day page opens) until the target date is selected. Then underneath, there is a table showing only the number of all variables along with column addition recommendations that contain recommendation buy and sell ± MAE score of each variable.

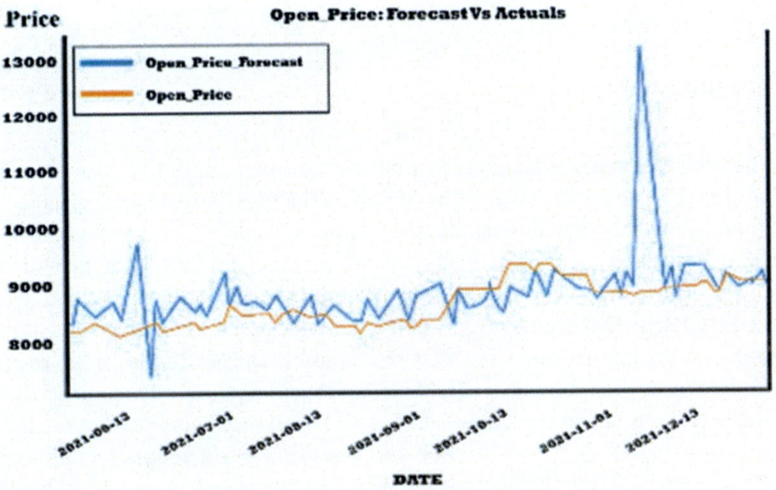

Fig. 5 Result pattern HL model prediction for variable Open Price does not follow actual data while the variable High, Low, and Close seen follow actual data pattern

Table 9 Result score C. model testing

Variable	RMSE	MAE	R2
Open price	615.30	338.125	−1.94
High	235.85	195.63	0.57
Low	261.93	225.63	0.45
Close	236.78	193.13	0.56

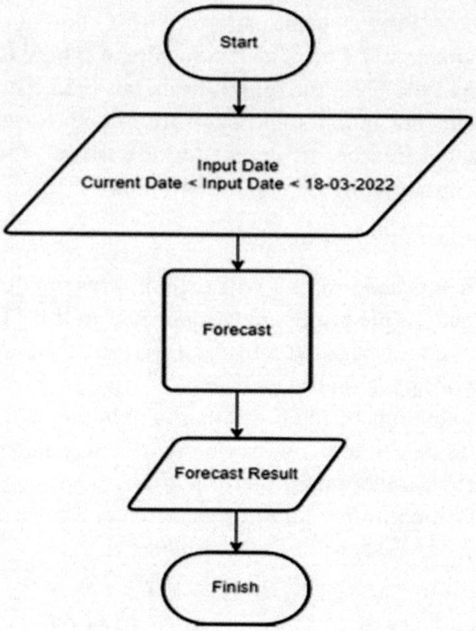

Fig. 6 Flowchart work web page. On the input data, the maximum limit prediction is March 18, 2022, and then only one can choose a date more from the day moment open page

4 Conclusion

The purpose of this study is to analyze whether the open, high, low, and close stock price variables can be predicted at a time based on the past data of each variable. Then build a forecasting model using machine learning technology, Vector Autoregression (VAR) algorithm, and the CRISP-DM research method. So that it can provide price recommendations using the VAR algorithm and the results of this study, and it can be seen that the CRISP-DM framework method has succeeded in conducting studies on data mining and is proven and easy to understand the cycle. Based on the results of testing and evaluation of the use of R2, MAE, and RMSE scores on the model that was successfully created, it can be concluded that VAR can be used to predict the highest, lowest, and closing stock prices at once and has fairly good accuracy, although the opening price variable must make a separation. But the permanent model has fairly good accuracy. The results of the created model can also be implemented in the form of a simple web page that displays graphs and tables of prediction results and recommendations (with $\pm$ MAE for each variable), with the desired input data being predictable. Suggestions for future research, there are many forecasting algorithms that can be tested in this case and, in other cases, can be developed for global stock exchanges.

References

1. Yasin H, Warsito B, Santoso R, Suparti (2018) Soft computation vector autoregressive neural network (VAR-NN) GUI-based. E3S Web Conf 73:13008. https://doi.org/10.1051/e3sconf/20187313008
2. Hushani P (2019) Using autoregressive modelling and machine learning for stock market prediction and trading. In: Third international congress on information and communication technology, pp 767–774. Springer, Singapore. https://doi.org/10.1007/978-981-13-1165-9_70
3. Gupta R, Huber F, Piribauer P (2020) Predicting international equity returns: evidence from time-varying parameter vector autoregressive models. Int Rev Financ Anal 68:101456. https://doi.org/10.1016/j.irfa.2020.101456
4. Farid S, Tashfeen R, Mohsan T, Burhan A (2021) Forecasting stock prices using a data mining method: evidence from emerging market. Int J Financ Econ. https://doi.org/10.1002/ijfe.2516
5. Mailinda I, Ruldeviyani Y, Tanjung F, Mikoriza T, Putra R, Fauziah AT (2021) Stock price prediction during the pandemic period with the SVM, BPNN, and LSTM algorithm. In: 2021 4th international seminar on research of information technology and intelligent systems (ISRITI), pp 189–194. IEEE. https://doi.org/10.1109/ISRITI54043.2021.9702865
6. Rohmawati AA, Gunawan PH (2019) The causality effect on vector autoregressive model: the case for rainfall forecasting. In: 2019 7th international conference on information and communication technology (ICoICT). IEEE, pp 1–5. https://doi.org/10.1109/ICoICT.2019.8835379
7. Chaiboonsri C, Wannapan S (2021) Applying quantum mechanics for extreme value prediction of VaR and ES in the ASEAN stock exchange. Economies 9:13. https://doi.org/10.3390/economies9010013
8. Suroso, Rusiadi, Purba br R, Siahaan APU, Sari AK, Novalina A, Lubis AIF (2018) Autoregression vector prediction on banking stock return using CAPM model approach and multi-factor apt. Int J Civ Eng Technol (IJCIET) 9:1093–1103
9. Lu W, Li J, Wang J, Qin L (2021) A CNN-BiLSTM-AM method for stock price prediction. Neural Comput Appl 33:4741–4753. https://doi.org/10.1007/s00521-020-05532-z
10. Chen C, Zhao L, Bian J, Xing C, Liu T-Y (2019) Investment behaviors can tell what inside. In: Proceedings of the 25th ACM SIGKDD international conference on knowledge discovery & data mining. ACM, New York, NY, USA, pp 2376–2384. https://doi.org/10.1145/3292500.3330663
11. Mauritsius T (201) Bank marketing data mining using CRISP-DM approach. Int J Adv Trends Comput Sci Eng 8:2322–2329. https://doi.org/10.30534/ijatcse/2019/71852019
12. Jaggia S, Kelly A, Lertwachara K, Chen L (2020) Applying the CRISP-DM framework for teaching business analytics. Decis Sci J Innov Educ 18:612–634. https://doi.org/10.1111/dsji.12222
13. Huber S, Wiemer H, Schneider D, Ihlenfeldt S (2019) DMME: data mining methodology for engineering applications—a holistic extension to the CRISP-DM model. Procedia CIRP 79:403–408. https://doi.org/10.1016/j.procir.2019.02.106
14. Majumder A, Rahman MdM, Biswas AA, Zulfiker MdS, Basak S (2022) Stock market prediction: a time series analysis. https://doi.org/10.1007/978-981-16-2877-1_35
15. Triayudi A, Sumiati S, Dwiyatno S, Karyaningsih D, Susilawati S (2021) Measure the effectiveness of information systems with the naïve Bayes classifier method. IAES Int J Artif Intell (IJ-AI) 10:414. https://doi.org/10.11591/ijai.v10.i2.pp414-420
16. Triayudi A, Widyarto WO, Rosalina V (2020) CLG clustering for mapping pattern analysis of student academic achievement. ICIC Express Lett 14:1225–1234
17. Exenberger E, Bucko J (2020) Analysis of online consumer behaviour—design of CRISP-DM process model. Agris On-Line Pap Econ Inform 12:13–22. https://doi.org/10.7160/aol.2020.120302
18. Nagashima H, Kato Y (2019) APREP-DM: a framework for automating the pre-processing of a sensor data analysis based on CRISP-DM. In: 2019 IEEE international conference on pervasive

computing and communications workshops (PerCom Workshops). IEEE, pp 555–560. https://doi.org/10.1109/PERCOMW.2019.8730785
19. Purbasari A, Rinawan FR, Zulianto A, Susanti AI, Komara H (2021) CRISP-DM for data quality improvement to support machine learning of stunting prediction in infants and toddlers. In: 2021 8th international conference on advanced informatics: concepts, theory and applications (ICAICTA). IEEE, pp 1–6. https://doi.org/10.1109/ICAICTA53211.2021.9640294
20. Ribeiro R, Pilastri A, Moura C, Rodrigues F, Rocha R, Cortez P (2020) Predicting the tear strength of woven fabrics via automated machine learning: an application of the CRISP-DM methodology. In: Proceedings of the 22nd international conference on enterprise information systems. SCITEPRESS—Science and Technology Publications, pp 548–555. https://doi.org/10.5220/0009411205480555
21. Rezki D, Mouss LH, Baaziz A (2018) Using a data mining CRISP-DM methodology for rate of penetration (ROP) prediction in oil well drilling. In: The second European international conference on industrial engineering and operations management. Proceedings of the international conference on industrial engineering and operations management, Paris, France
22. Schafer F, Zeiselmair C, Becker J, Otten H (2018) Synthesizing CRISP-DM and quality management: a data mining approach for production processes. In: 2018 IEEE international conference on technology management, operations and decisions (ICTMOD). IEEE, pp 190–195. https://doi.org/10.1109/ITMC.2018.8691266
23. Martinez-Plumed F, Contreras-Ochando L, Ferri C, Hernandez-Orallo J, Kull M, Lachiche N, Ramirez-Quintana MJ, Flach P (2021) CRISP-DM twenty years later: from data mining processes to data science trajectories. IEEE Trans Knowl Data Eng 33:3048–3061. https://doi.org/10.1109/TKDE.2019.2962680
24. Kristoffersen E, Aremu OO, Blomsma F, Mikalef P, Li J (2019) Exploring the relationship between data science and circular economy: an enhanced CRISP-DM process model. https://doi.org/10.1007/978-3-030-29374-1_15
25. Parot A, Michell K, Kristjanpoller WD (2019) Using artificial neural networks to forecast exchange rate, including VAR-VECM residual analysis and prediction linear combination. Intell Syst Account Financ Manag 26:3–15. https://doi.org/10.1002/isaf.1440
26. Azhar Z, Putra HS, Saputra D (2020) Effect of macroeconomic factors on the composite stock price index using the vector auto regression (VAR) method. In: Proceedings of the 4th Padang international conference on education, economics, business and accounting (PICEEBA-2 2019). Atlantis Press, Paris, France. https://doi.org/10.2991/aebmr.k.200305.081
27. Sathyanarayana S, Gargesa S (2019) Modeling cryptocurrency (Bitcoin) using vector autoregressive (Var) model. SDMIMD J Manag 10:47–64. https://doi.org/10.18311/sdmimd/2019/23181
28. Lu F, Qiao H, Wang S, Lai KK, Li Y (2017) Time-varying coefficient vector autoregressions model based on dynamic correlation with an application to crude oil and stock markets. Environ Res 152:351–359. https://doi.org/10.1016/j.envres.2016.07.015
29. Shahrestani P, Rafei M (2020) The impact of oil price shocks on Tehran Stock Exchange returns: application of the Markov switching vector autoregressive models. Resour Policy 65:101579. https://doi.org/10.1016/j.resourpol.2020.101579
30. Aydin AD, Cavdar SC (2015) Comparison of prediction performances of artificial neural network (ANN) and vector autoregressive (VAR) models by using the macroeconomic variables of gold prices, Borsa Istanbul (BIST) 100 index and US Dollar-Turkish Lira (USD/TRY) exchange rates. Procedia Econ Financ 30:3–14. https://doi.org/10.1016/S2212-5671(15)01249-6

Development Human Activity Recognition for the Elderly Using Inertial Sensor and Statistical Feature

Ismail, Istiqomah, and Husneni Mukhtar

Abstract The Elderly is a human being over 60 years old. Humans over the age of 60 years have the potential to fall due to balance and gait disturbances. The disturbance is caused by a decrease in the sensory system that focuses the view. This impact will result in the risk of developing fractures and even death if it cannot be treated quickly. Previous research has conducted tests on Human Activity Recognition. In this study, we will test the selection of feature extraction and machine learning methods regarding Human Activity Recognition. The extraction features tested in this study are the mean, median, maximum, minimum, skewness, kurtosis, and variance with Fast Fourier Transform from each value obtained by the IMU sensor. The machine learning methods studied were Stochastic Gradient Descent, Random Forest, K-Nearest Neighbor, Decision Tree, and Gaussian Naive Bayes. The test results demonstrate that Y-Axis Gyroscope means, X-Axis Acceleration skewness, X-Axis Gyroscope variance, and X-Axis Gyroscope max are the optimum extraction features for machine learning. The most accurate machine learning algorithm is Random Forest, which has a 99.59% accuracy rate. Therefore, the author made this Human Activity Recognition system to monitor the activities of the elderly. With this research, elderly monitors can keep track of the elderly's activities and concentrate more attention on all of the elderly's activities, especially fall activities. Thus, monitors can provide early assistance to the elderly.

Keywords The elderly · Fall · Machine learning · Extraction features · Human activity recognition

1 Introduction

Because more than 37 million falls each year necessitate medical attention, falls are a severe public health issue [1]. One of them is the elderly, who can put themselves in danger of serious harm which can be hip fractures or even death [2, 3]. In 2030, there

Ismail (✉) · Istiqomah · H. Mukhtar
Faculty of Electrical Engineering, Telkom University, Bandung, Indonesia
e-mail: ismailsir@student.telkomuniversity.ac.id

T. Triwiyanto et al. (eds.), *Proceeding of the 3rd International Conference on Electronics, Biomedical Engineering, and Health Informatics*, Lecture Notes in Electrical Engineering 1008, https://doi.org/10.1007/978-981-99-0248-4_21

will be 1.4 billion elderly, and by 2050, there will be 2.1 billion. Ages 65 and older have a higher risk of falling (by 28–35%) than seniors 65 and older. For those who are older than 70, this risk rises to 32–42% [4, 5]. This research was created to be able to do early prevention of the elderly in the case of a fall incident because it is a severe concern. There is a system that can detect human behaviors using a variety of algorithms has been developed through several experiments. The recognized target in this system has a human movement feature. Human Activity Recognition has been the subject of several investigations. There are a several research on HAR that using radar [6–9], a system of computer vision [10–14], and an inertial sensor [11, 15, 16]. Because it is inexpensive and suitable for use by the elderly during activities, the author employed an inertial sensor for HAR investigation.

Several academics have investigated the use of different algorithms to Utilize inertial sensors to detect human activity. In a study [17], deep neural network (DNN), bidirectional-long short-term memory (BLSTM), CNN, and CNN-LSTM algorithms were used to create a wearable device with an IMU sensor. In this study, the maximum accuracy obtained was 90%. According to research [18], the Hidden Markov model (HMM) method outperformed the k-nearest neighbor (KNN), Naïve Bayes (NB), and LSM methods (ANN) with an average accuracy classification rate was 93.2%. A dataset from 91 participants that were kept for 27.76 h was used in the research [19] used a dataset stored for 27.76 h from 91 people. The CNN approach was employed in this investigation. Extraction Features take part in these studies that impact the accuracy value. Because feature extraction may characterize data that provides information about the most prominent aspects, it has become absolutely important in terms of data-related issues [20].

The goal of this research is to develop a HAR that can detect the activities of the elderly using datasets. The dataset consists of each axis' acceleration and gyroscope data. This dataset was created from a sample of 10 individuals, split into 4 classes. Walking, Falling, Sitting to Standing, and Standing to Sitting are the four classes in question. From the collected dataset, it is continued with the preprocessing stage with an amount of data 28,958. Using the XGBoost method, the data from the preprocessing results will select the top 4 extraction features. The top 4 extraction features were chosen to improve system performance during classifying operations. The four most successful extraction characteristics will be used as the data for processing using stochastic gradient descent, random forest, K-nearest neighbor, decision tree, and Gaussian Naive Bayes. We will select one of the best machine learning methods from among the five by comparing the average accuracy values acquired. The best machine learning method produced will be followed by an evaluation of the training data results utilizing the confusion matrix.

2 Method and Material

This experiment uses a dataset that looks at the inertial sensor's acceleration and gyroscope values as an input. The position of inertial sensor is placed on the user's chest so that the measuring point of this inertia sensor is on the chest. This dataset will be preprocessed first using the fast Fourier transform method. After using the fast Fourier transform method is continued by looking at the mean, median, maximum, minimum, skewness, kurtosis, and variance values. From all the extraction features obtained, the selection of the best four feature extractions is carried out using the XGBoost algorithm. Training will be carried out on the four extraction features using the Stochastic Gradient Descent, Random Forest, K-Nearest Neighbor, Decision Tree, and Gaussian Naive Bayes methods to compare the average accuracy values of each machine learning method. The output of this system is the identification of human activity after selecting feature extraction and machine learning approaches. The drilling process is carried out as shown in Fig. 1.

2.1 Datasets

The dataset used is a dataset obtained from 10 samples of subjects for each movement. The dataset sample will be 4 classes. These 4 classes are walking, standing to sitting, sitting to standing, and falling as seen from the acceleration and gyroscope values for every 0.01 s. Each person performs the movement from standing to sitting ten times, sitting to standing ten times, walking for 1 min, and falling 15 times. From

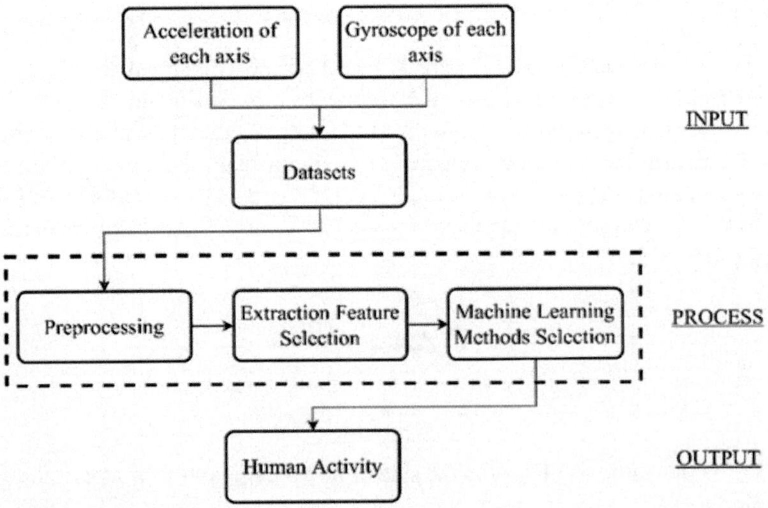

Fig. 1 Proposed method

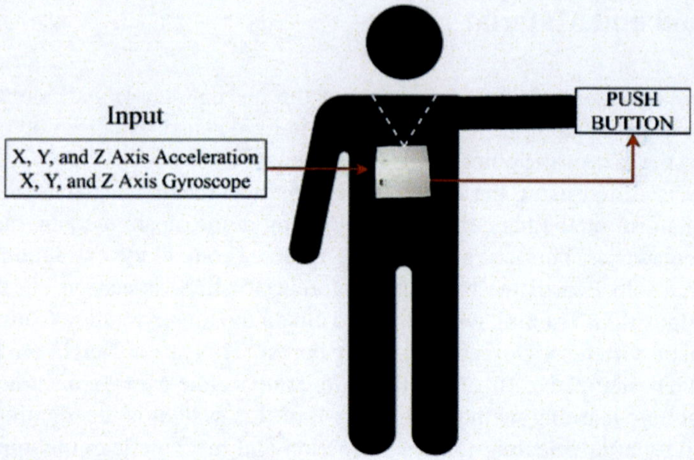

Fig. 2 Wearable device placement

the 15 falling activities, there are three variations of the falling movement, five times fall forward, five times fall on the right side, and five times fall on the left side. The method used for sampling is by connecting a push button to the wearable device. When the participant is doing an activity, the participant will press the push button until the activity is over. The wearable device placement system for participants is shown in Fig. 2.

2.2 Preprocessing

The preprocessing used in this system is Fast Fourier Transform (FFT). A signal is shifted from the time domain to the frequency domain using the fast Fourier transform. The first step in preprocessing is to analyze the data and utilize the Fast Fourier Transform technique to transform the signal from the time domain to the frequency domain [21]. The best technique for signal processing is called Fast Fourier Trans-form [22]. The general equations for the Fast Fourier Transform are in Eqs. (1) and (2) [23].

$$X_{(k)} = \sum_{n=0}^{N-1} x_n \left(W_n^{kn}\right) \tag{1}$$

$$W_n^{kn} = e^{-j\omega_0 kn} \tag{2}$$

where $X_{(k)}$ is the value of FFT, N is the size of its domain, and x_n is a periodic signal with period n.

2.3 Extraction Features

The preprocessing used in this system is a fast Fourier transform. The next process is grouping the data after collecting the acceleration and gyroscope data in the frequency domain. The data is grouped for every 1 s when frequency domain data is being processed. Using feature extraction, the mean, median, maximum, minimum, skewness, kurtosis, and variance values are obtained from the data every second.

Mean is the statistical formula to calculate the average value of the results of data collection with a formula shown in Eq. (3).

$$\overline{x} = \frac{\sum x}{N} \tag{3}$$

where $\sum x$ Sum of data and N Number of data.

Median is one of the statistical formulas that aim to get the median value of data collection that has been ordered. The formula for the median can be seen in Eq. (4).

$$Med(X) = \begin{cases} X\left[\frac{n}{2}\right], if\ n\ even \\ \frac{\left(X\left[\frac{n-1}{2}\right]+X\left[\frac{n+1}{2}\right]\right)}{2}, if\ n\ odd \end{cases} \tag{4}$$

Maximum is a statistical method that has a function in determining the highest value in the collected data.

Minimum is a statistical method with a function that is inversely proportional to the maximum, which is getting the lowest value from the data collected.

Skewness is a statistical method by looking at the level of asymmetry of the data obtained. The following is the formula for the Skewness method, which can be seen in Eq. (5).

$$\tilde{\mu_3} = \frac{\sum_i^N (x_i - \overline{x})^3}{(N-1) * \sigma^3} \tag{5}$$

where N is Number of data, x_i is Random variable, $\overline{x}$ is Mean of the data, and σ^3 is Standard Deviation.

Kurtosis is a method by looking at the sharpness of the collected data. To get the sharpness value, it can be shown in Eq. (6).

$$Kurt = \frac{\mu_4}{\sigma^4} \tag{6}$$

where μ_4 is Central moment and σ^4 is Standard Deviation.

Variance is a method to find out how far the data is spread. The value can be found in Eq. (7).

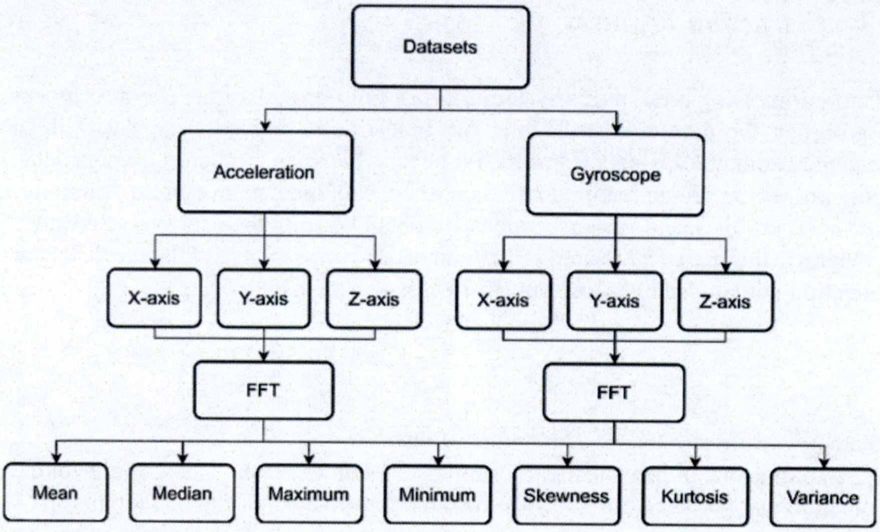

Fig. 3 Feature extraction diagram

$$S^2 = \frac{\sum (x_i - \overline{x})^2}{n - 1} \tag{7}$$

where S^2 is Variance, x_i is Data per index, $\overline{x}$ is Mean, and n is number of data.

With a dataset in the form of acceleration and gyroscope, Fig. 3 shows a representation of the feature extraction process used in this experiment. The acceleration and gyroscope dataset consists of 3 axes, namely the X, Y, and Z axes. Using the Fast Fourier Transform technique, each of these axes will be transformed into a frequency domain. The data that has been translated into the frequency domain will provide the mean, median, maximum, minimum, skewness, kurtosis, and variance. In order to achieve this, 42 extraction features were used in this experiment.

2.4 Feature Selection

From all the extracted features obtained, the extraction feature will be selected. This selection aims to reduce the number of feature extractions used for training data. In this selection, the XGBoost algorithm is used. XGBoost is a gradient boosted decision tree extension. It has been used to solve numerous classification issues in various fields [24]. One of these features is that it can determine the best extraction feature. This best feature extraction is obtained by calculating how many features are used to divide the data across all trees. So it will bring up the most dominating extraction features [25].

2.5 Classifier

From survey of classifier that was used for human activity recognition [11], there are several classifiers which have good accuracy modal. There are KNN, Decision tree, and Random Forest. Therefore in this study, it still used that classifier, but for com-parison, Gaussian NB is added. This research can be described whether the important feature will produce a good model with all classifiers.

Stochastic Gradient Descent. It is a simple statistical-based optimization technique that is efficiently used in finding coefficient values to minimize loss (error) functions on a large scale [26]. Generally, stochastic gradient methods are applied to solve optimization issues using Eq. (8).

$$\min_{x \in \mathbb{R}^d} f(x) := \mathbb{E} f_\gamma(x) \tag{8}$$

where $\{fr : r \in \Gamma\}$ is a family of functions from $\mathbb{R}^d$ to $\mathbb{R}$ and γ is a Γ-valued random variable, with respect to which the expectation is taken (these notions will be made precise in the following sections). In supervised learning applications, is typically a uniform random variable taking values in the range of $\{1, 2, \ldots, n\}$. f is the total empirical loss function in this case, while $\{fr : r \in \Gamma\}$ are the loss functions resulting from the rth training.

Decision Tree Classifier process consists of converting the data format (table) into a tree model, converting the tree model into rules and simplifying the rules. In building a decision tree using the CART algorithm, impurity or entropy and information gain are used to determine the root node [26]. Entropy and information gain in Decision Tree Classifier have a significant impact on the Decision Tree Classifier algorithm. According to Shannon, entropy is a measurement of the amount of data created and the level of uncertainty in that output. According to Shannon, a discrete system's entropy value is

$$H = -\Sigma_{P_i} \log_2 p_i \tag{9}$$

where p_i is the probability of the event occurring.

Knowing how much meaningful knowledge is gathered about the response variables from the explanatory variable is important to the building of a classification tree. This is known as information gain. Information gain can be used to determine how essential or influential an explanatory variable is in relation to the response variable. In terms of entropy, we can describe it as [27, 28]:

$$IG(Y|X) = H(Y) - H_X(Y) \tag{10}$$

Random Forest is an ensemble technique consisting of several decision trees as classifiers. Classes obtained from this classification process are taken from the most Classes generated by the decision tree in Random Forest [26]. Numerous branches of tree classification are possible as a result of the equation. The process known as "majority voting" is the most popular. This function will select the most frequent class that is classified using a tree [27].

K-Neighbors Classifier is a simple classification in classifying features based on the closest distance to adjacent features [26]. The main idea behind this approach is to determine the distance between two classes. The KNN function by default uses the Euclidean distance, which may be determined using the following equation.

$$D(a, b) = \sqrt{(a_i - b_1)^2 + (a_2 - b_2)^2 + \cdots + (a_n - b_n)^2} \tag{11}$$

where a is the position for the first class and b is the position for the second class [29].

Gaussian Naive Bayes is a Naive Bayes classification model that uses continuous data types, and each type is characterized by Gaussian multivariate or Normal Probability Density Function (PDF). Gaussian Naive Bayes has two parameters mean and variance [26]. Bayesian classifier can be seen in Eq. 12:

$$h_{nb} = argmax\, P(c)\Pi_{i=0}^{d} P(x_i|c)c \in Y \tag{12}$$

where c is a part of Y, which is the total number of activity categories, $Y = \{c_1, c_2, \ldots, c_N\}$. N is the number of activity categories overall. d is the total number of characteristics. The ith characteristic is represented by x_i [29].

3 Results and Analysis

3.1 Preprocessing

The goal of preprocessing is to change the incoming data's format so that it can be processed in the right way. The rapid Fourier transform method is used to first preprocess each axis' time domain acceleration and gyroscope data into frequency domain data. Following the acquisition of the frequency domain value, the feature extraction features of mean, median, maximum, minimum, skewness, kurtosis, and variance are recorded. XGBoost is used to choose the features from the extracted features. The extraction characteristics of Y-Axis Gyroscope mean, X-Axis Acceleration skewness, X-Axis Gyroscope variance, and X-Axis Gyroscope max are the best extraction features based on the results of selecting the most important extraction features. The feature extraction outcomes that most important affect HAR and the resulting Score are shown in Table 1.

Table 1 Score of each extraction feature

Extraction features	Score
Y-axis gyroscope mean	0.25406
X-axis acceleration skewness	0.14947
X-axis gyroscope variance	0.06053
X-axis gyroscope max	0.04188
Y-axis gyroscope variance	0.03490
Z-axis acceleration skewness	0.03284
X-axis gyroscope median	0.03148
X-axis acceleration kurtosis	0.02701
Z-axis acceleration kurtosis	0.00905
Y-axis acceleration max	0.00648

3.2 *Machine Learning*

Using the feature extraction from the outcomes of the preprocessing, compare the machine learning approach with the cross-validation result 3 and test size value 0.2. Table 2 displays a comparison of the average accuracy values for each machine learning method.

The average accuracy value while combining four feature extractions and just one feature extraction is displayed in Table 2. Based on the average accuracy results, the highest average accuracy value is Random Forest with combined feature and Random Forest has the lowest average accuracy value with only using the X-Axis Gyroscope maximum. The average accuracy value of the Random Forest with combined feature is 99.59%, and Random Forest with only using the X-Axis Gyroscope maximum average accuracy value is 61.15%. As a result of Random Forest's best accuracy with features combined, proceed by looking at the confusion matrix produced by

Table 2 Average accuracy results

Machine learning methods	Combined (%)	X-axis acceleration skewness (%)	X-axis gyroscope variance (%)	X-axis gyroscope max (%)	Y-axis gyroscope mean (%)
Stochastic gradient descent	89.66	81.43	67.04	62.09	78.42
Random forest	99.59	75.64	70.21	61.15	73.40
K-nearest neighbor	99.08	77.26	72.49	63.76	75.72
Decision tree	99.06	75.64	70.20	61.12	73.43
Gaussian Naive Bayes	86.75	81.22	71.81	69.30	78.38

this method. The confusion matrix of Random Forest with combined features can be shown in Fig. 4.

Figure 4 demonstrates several errors in the classification of activities in the confusion matrix data. This Figure shows that the test data utilized is a dataset from a 20% split with a total data of 5,791. The amount of each activity's inaccurate categories are 5 for falling, 0 for walking, 9 for standing to sitting, and 14 for sitting to standing. Table 3 displays the findings of the entire data evaluation.

For each class, Table 3 displays the list of precision, recall, F1-Score, and support values. The data shows that 0.97 and 0.99 correspondingly represent the lowest recall and precision values. The lowest F1 score from this value is 0.98, while the highest F1 score is 1.00. As a result, it can be said that the training results accurately detect HAR due to the value's high precision, recall, and f1 score. Additionally, it can classify data with a low rate of classification errors in every class.

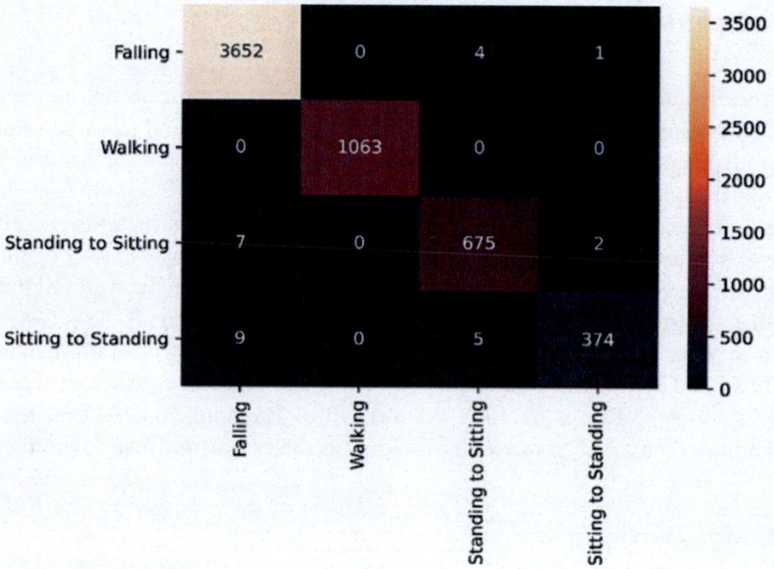

Fig. 4 Confusion matrix

Table 3 Data evaluation

Class	Precision	Recall	F1-score	Support
Falling	1.00	1.00	1.00	3657
Walking	1.00	1.00	1.00	1063
Standing to sitting	0.99	0.99	0.99	684
Sitting to standing	0.99	0.97	0.98	388

4 Discussion

These results show that an extraction feature has an impact on how elderly people will classify human activities. We can select the optimal extraction feature for classification using the XGBoost algorithm without using all the acceleration and gyro-scope information on every axis. Therefore, using this discovery, computations for activity classification can be done quickly. Research on HAR using the IMU Sensor has been conducted in the past, such as the [2, 15, 16] research with various inertial sensor placements. The preprocessing method used in this study separates it from that study's research by time domain to frequency domain conversion and applying statistical techniques. As a result, the dataset used in this study's training is not made up entirely of raw data for acceleration and gyroscope values from each axis. The mean Y-axis gyroscope, X-axis acceleration skewness, X-axis variance gyroscope, and X-max axis gyroscope are found to be the best combinations for feature extraction in this study using the Xgboost method.

The weakness of this research is that the training process takes a long time. The preprocessing required to obtain a value for machine learning is the explanation. Additionally, the performance of the system decreases with increasing statistical formula complexity. Therefore, a simpler statistical method and a limitation on the amount of extraction features employed during training are required to speed up system performance. Given that falls are frequently experienced by the elderly, the ability to recognize human movement in the elderly makes it possible to administer early treatment in the event of a fall. The consequences of falls in the elderly, which can lead to serious damage or death, necessitate early care.

5 Conclusion

According to the result of this research, this HAR can determine the activities of walking, falling, standing to sitting, and sitting to standing. Feature extraction and machine learning method that is very accurate at detecting HAR has been created. The mean Y-axis gyroscope, X-axis acceleration skewness, X-axis variance gyro-scope, and X-max axis gyroscope are the strongest extraction characteristics discovered in this research. The random forest technique is shown to have the highest average value using these 4 extraction features as training data. 99.59% is the average accuracy value. The training results exhibit high recall, precision, and F1-Score values in addition to high accuracy. The smallest recall value is 0.99, precisely 0.97, and the F1-score 0.98. As a result, using the strongest extraction characteristics and Random Forest method, it is possible to identify HAR, particularly when employed in the elderly with an inertial sensor. This HAR can provide early attention to the elderly by knowing the daily activities of the elderly that can keep track of elderly activities and concentrate more attention on elderly activities, particularly fall activities. Thus, monitors can provide early assistance to the elderly. This research can be expanded by selecting the optimal extraction feature to identify more activity categories, resulting in a better level of accuracy. As well as the installation of inertial sensors to enhance the elderly comfort.

References

1. Saleh M, Abbas M, Prud'Homm J, Somme D, Le Bouquin Jeannes R (2021) A reliable fall detection system based on analyzing the physical activities of older adults living in long-term care facilities. IEEE Trans Neural Syst Rehabil Eng 29:2587–2594. https://doi.org/10.1109/TNSRE.2021.3133616
2. Lee DW, Jun K, Naheem K, Kim MS (2021) Deep neural network-based double-check method for fall detection using IMU-L sensor and RGB camera data. IEEE Access 9:48064–48079. https://doi.org/10.1109/ACCESS.2021.3065105
3. Bekibele CO, Gureje O (2010) Fall incidence in a population of elderly persons in Nigeria. Gerontology 56:278–283. https://doi.org/10.1159/000236327
4. Ibrahim A, Chaccour K, Hassani AHE, Andres E (2021) Bed-fall detection and prediction: a generic classification and review of bed-fall related systems. IEEE Sens J 21:5678–5686. https://doi.org/10.1109/JSEN.2020.3037711
5. Howland J, Hackman H, Taylor A, O'Hara K, Liu J, Brusch J (2018) Older adult fall prevention practices among primary care providers at accountable care organizations: a pilot study. PLoS ONE 13:1–10. https://doi.org/10.1371/journal.pone.0205279
6. Cagliyan B, Karabacak C, Gurbuz SZ (2014) Indoor human activity recognition using BumbleBee radar. 1055–1058. https://doi.org/10.1109/siu.2014.6830414
7. Li X, He Y, Fioranelli F, Jing X (2022) Semisupervised human activity recognition with radar micro-doppler signatures. IEEE Trans Geosci Remote Sens 60:1–12. https://doi.org/10.1109/TGRS.2021.3090106
8. Cheng C, Ling F, Guo S, Cui G, Jian Q, Jia C, Ran Q (2020) A real-time human activity recognition method for through-the-wall radar. In: IEEE national radar conference—proceedings, 2020 Sept. https://doi.org/10.1109/RadarConf2043947.2020.9266393
9. Zhu JP, Chen HQ, Ye WB (2020) Classification of human activities based on radar signals using 1D-CNN and LSTM. Proceedings—IEEE international symposium on circuits and systems, 2020 Oct. https://doi.org/10.1109/iscas45731.2020.9181233
10. Babiker M, Khalifa OO, Htike KK, Hassan A, Zaharadeen M (2018) Automated daily human activity recognition for video surveillance using neural network. In: 2017 IEEE international conference on smart instrumentation, measurement and applications, ICSIMA 2017, 2017 Nov, pp 1–5. https://doi.org/10.1109/ICSIMA.2017.8312024
11. Gupta A, Gupta K, Gupta K, Gupta K (2020) A survey on human activity recognition and classification. In: Proceedings of the 2020 IEEE international conference on communication and signal processing, ICCSP 2020, pp 915–919. https://doi.org/10.1109/ICCSP48568.2020.9182416
12. Lamghari S, Bilodeau GA, Saunier N (2020) A grid-based representation for human action recognition. In: Proceedings—international conference on pattern recognition, pp 10500–10507. https://doi.org/10.1109/ICPR48806.2021.9413136
13. Abdul Manaf F, Singh S (2021) Computer vision-based survey on human activity recognition system, challenges and applications. In: 2021 3rd international conference on signal processing and communication, ICPSC 2021, pp 110–114. https://doi.org/10.1109/ICSPC51351.2021.9451736
14. Banjarey K, Prakash Sahu S, Kumar Dewangan D (2021) A survey on human activity recognition using sensors and deep learning methods. In: Proceedings—5th international conference on computing methodologies and communication, ICCMC 2021, pp 1610–1617. https://doi.org/10.1109/ICCMC51019.2021.9418255

15. Zebin T, Scully PJ, Ozanyan KB (2017) Evaluation of supervised classification algorithms for human activity recognition with inertial sensors. In: Proceedings of IEEE Sensors, 2017 Dec, pp 1–3. https://doi.org/10.1109/ICSENS.2017.8234222
16. Perez-Gamboa S, Sun Q, Zhang Y (2021) Improved sensor based human activity recognition via hybrid convolutional and recurrent neural networks. In: INERTIAL 2021—8th IEEE international symposium on inertial sensors and systems, proceedings, pp 0–3. https://doi.org/10.1109/INERTIAL51137.2021.9430460.
17. Bijalwan V, Semwal VB, Gupta V (2022) Wearable sensor-based pattern mining for human activity recognition: deep learning approach. Ind Robot 49:21–33. https://doi.org/10.1108/IR-09-2020-0187
18. Wang Z, Chen Y (2017) Recognizing human concurrent activities using wearable sensors: a statistical modeling approach based on parallel HMM. Sens Rev 37:330–337. https://doi.org/10.1108/SR-01-2017-0003
19. Shavit Y, Klein I (2021) Boosting inertial-based human activity recognition with transformers. IEEE Access 9:53540–53547. https://doi.org/10.1109/ACCESS.2021.3070646
20. Salau AO, Jain S (2019) Feature extraction: a survey of the types, techniques, applications. In: 2019 international conference on signal processing and communication, ICSC 2019, pp 158–164. https://doi.org/10.1109/ICSC45622.2019.8938371
21. Palupi IR, Raharjo W (2021) The utilization of signal analysis by using short time Fourier transform. In: RSF conference series: engineering and technology, vol 1, pp 30–36. https://doi.org/10.31098/cset.v1i1.445
22. Cooley JW, Lewis PAW, Welch PD (1969) The fast Fourier transform and its applications. IEEE Trans Educ 12:27–34. https://doi.org/10.1109/TE.1969.4320436
23. Islam MN, Sulaiman N, Rashid M, Bari BS, Hasan MJ, Mustafa M, Jadin MS (2020) Empirical mode decomposition coupled with fast Fourier transform based feature extraction method for motor imagery tasks classification. In: 2020 IEEE 10th international conference on system engineering and technology, ICSET 2020—proceedings, pp 256–261. https://doi.org/10.1109/ICSET51301.2020.9265370
24. Cherif IL, Kortebi A (2019) On using eXtreme gradient boosting (XGBoost) machine learning algorithm for home network traffic classification. In: IFIP wireless days, 2019 Apr, pp 1–6. https://doi.org/10.1109/WD.2019.8734193
25. Hsieh CP, Chen YT, Beh WK, Wu AYA (2019) Feature selection framework for XGBoost based on electrodermal activity in stress detection. In: IEEE workshop on signal processing systems, SiPS: design and implementation, 2019 Oct, pp 330–335. https://doi.org/10.1109/SiPS47522.2019.9020321
26. Géron A (2017) Hands-on machine learning
27. Baines O, Chung A, Raval R (2020) Random forest classification algorithm. Math Res J 500
28. Zhong Y (2016) The analysis of cases based on decision tree. 2016 7th IEEE international conference on software engineering and service science (ICSESS). https://doi.org/10.1109/icsess.2016.7883035
29. Shen J, Fang H (2020) Human activity recognition using Gaussian Naïve Bayes algorithm in smart home. J Phys Conf Ser 1631:0–5. https://doi.org/10.1088/1742-6596/1631/1/012059

Heart Abnormality Classification with Power Spectrum Feature and Machine Learning

Istiqomah, Achmad Rizal, and Herming Chiueh

Abstract Heart sounds are essential in diagnosing and analyzing heart disease and detecting abnormalities in the heart. Abnormalities in the heart can usually be detected when there is an additional sound during an incomplete valve opening. Additional sounds in cardiac abnormalities can be called murmurs. Normal and murmur heart sound happen in different frequency. Therefore, frequency-based feature extraction can be used to classify heart sound. One of frequency domains is power spectrum that can be calculated for power by two frequency of signal, and it can clearly show the pattern of murmur and normal heart sound. In this research, the proposed feature extraction based on the power spectrum feature is used to become another option feature extraction for heart sound classification, which is different from previous heart sound classification studies. There are five types of feature extraction that developed base power spectrum, which are Mean Frequency, Total Power, Maximum Peak Frequency, 1st Spectral Moment, and 2nd Spectral moment. Several classifiers also are used to get the best classier base that features. The best selection feature of this research is Mean Frequency, with best classifier are Stochastic Gradient Descent and logistic regression and accuracy 93%. When all features are used for classifier, almost all of the models have the highest accuracy especially when classifier with mean frequency, 1st Spectral, and 2nd Spectral moment has good accuracy too. Using all features, the best classifier for heart sound case is Gaussian Naïve Bayes with accuracy reaching 100%. These excellent outcomes can elevate feature extraction to the top contender and help machine learning generate effective classifiers.

Keywords Power Spectrum · Heart Abnormality · Machine Learning

---

Istiqomah (✉) · A. Rizal
School of Electrical Engineering, Telkom University, Bandung, Indonesia
e-mail: Istiqomah@telkomuniversity.ac.id

H. Chiueh
Departement Electronic and Electrical Engineering, NYCU, Hsinchu, Taiwan

T. Triwiyanto et al. (eds.), *Proceeding of the 3rd International Conference on Electronics, Biomedical Engineering, and Health Informatics*, Lecture Notes in Electrical Engineering 1008, https://doi.org/10.1007/978-981-99-0248-4_22

1 Introduction

Heart sounds are essential in diagnosing and analyzing heart disease and detecting abnormalities in the heart. The cardiovascular system process produces the heart sound. That process is opening and closing the heart valves for filling blood and flowing blood into and out of the heart. Two sounds can be heard through a stethoscope, namely lub-dub [1–4]. The lub sound is caused by the closure of the tricuspid and mitral valves so that blood can flow from the atria to the heart chambers and not back into the atria. That sound is known as the first heart sound (S1) with an interval of 20 to 30 ms (ms). The dub sound, also known as the second heart sound (S2), is caused by the closing of the semilunar from the aortic and pulmonary valves. The frequency that heart sound S2 happen in the range between 20 and 250 Hz with shortened interval period. S2 produce a higher-pitch sound than S1 [5]. The third heart sound (S3) co-occurs with the cessation of atrioventricular filling, while the fourth heart sound (S4) is correlated with atrial contraction and has a low amplitude and frequency component [6, 7].

Abnormalities in the heart can usually be detected when there is an additional sound during an incomplete valve opening. The heart forces blood through narrow openings or by regurgitation caused by incomplete closure of valves resulting in a backflow of blood. In each case, the sound produced results from high-velocity blood flow through the narrow opening. Additional sounds in cardiac abnormalities can be called murmurs [8]. Usually murmur sound can be observed in range frequency 20 and 600 Hz for intra-cardiac [5] Therefore, from the differences in the frequency characteristic of normal sound and murmur sound, a good model can be produced to classify both sounds if the feature extraction is used with the frequency domain.

The previous study used several feature extractions to classify heart sounds [9]. Discrete wavelet transform and Shannon entropy are applied to segment the heart sound and produce an accuracy of 97.7% with the DNN model [10]. Another research with a statistical frequency domain feature can create ANN Classified with an accuracy of 93% [8]. In another case, wavelet packet transform is used for phonocardiogram classification [11]. It produces the best SVM model, with an accuracy of 99.74. All previous studies highlight differences in range frequency between normal and murmur sound as reason feature extractions work well and be the feature that makes it easy to recognize the pattern for machine learning model.

In this research, it used power spectrum of frequency as basic feature extraction for heart sounds data. The power spectrum can be calculated as the square of the magnitude of the Fourier transform (or Fourier series) of the heart sound [12]. Several classifications use the power spectrum as an extraction feature. In this research [13, 14], that extraction feature is used for EEG classification and has an accuracy above 85%. In other applications, ECG classification [15–17] produces better accuracy for several methods, the highest is 92%. In heart sound classification [18], the power spectrum is used as a base extraction feature with a result of 88%. With that good result, it can be a possibility that the power spectrum can be a great choice to classify heart sounds, and it also supports differences in frequency of murmur and normal heart sound.

There are five types of feature extraction that be developed based on power spectrum, which are Mean Frequency, Total Power, Maximum Peak Frequency, 1st Spectral Moment, and 2nd Spectral moment. There are several methods of the classifier that can be compared, which are AdaBoost, Stochastic Gradient Descent (SGD), Gradient Boosting, Random Forest, Decision Tree (DT), Gaussian Naïve Bayes, KNN, SVM, and Logistic Regression [19]. This study will search best feature extraction with base power spectrum and look the best machine learning model. There are five sections in this paper, which consist of Introduction, method and material, result, discussion, and conclusion.

2 Method and Material

This section elaborates on all proposed methods and material data used in this study. There are sub-sections that explain the dataset's source, feature extraction, and classifier. The system classifies data into two classes: normal and murmur heart sounds.

2.1 Proposed Method

Figure 1 is the proposed method in this research, in which a dataset with the label is trained many times to get a good system to classify heart sounds become normal and murmur sounds. There are 132 heart sounds for all classes that are used. The first step is that data must convert from the time domain to the frequency domain in FFT Process. After that, the dataset is processed into some feature extractions developed from the power spectrum.

This study uses five feature extractions: Mean Frequency, Total Power, Maximum Peak Frequency, 1st Spectral Moment, and 2nd Spectral moment. After the data are processed in the feature extraction, data must be scaled before classifier training to make the model easier to learn [5]. There are several machine learning methods of the classifier, which are AdaBoost, Stochastic Gradient Descent (SGD), Gradient Boosting, Random Forest, Decision Tree (DT), Gaussian Naïve Bayes, KNN, SVM, and Logistic Regression [19].

2.2 Dataset

The heart murmur and normal heart sounds from this study's dataset [19] were chosen as the labels. This information was gathered from two different sources: clinical trials

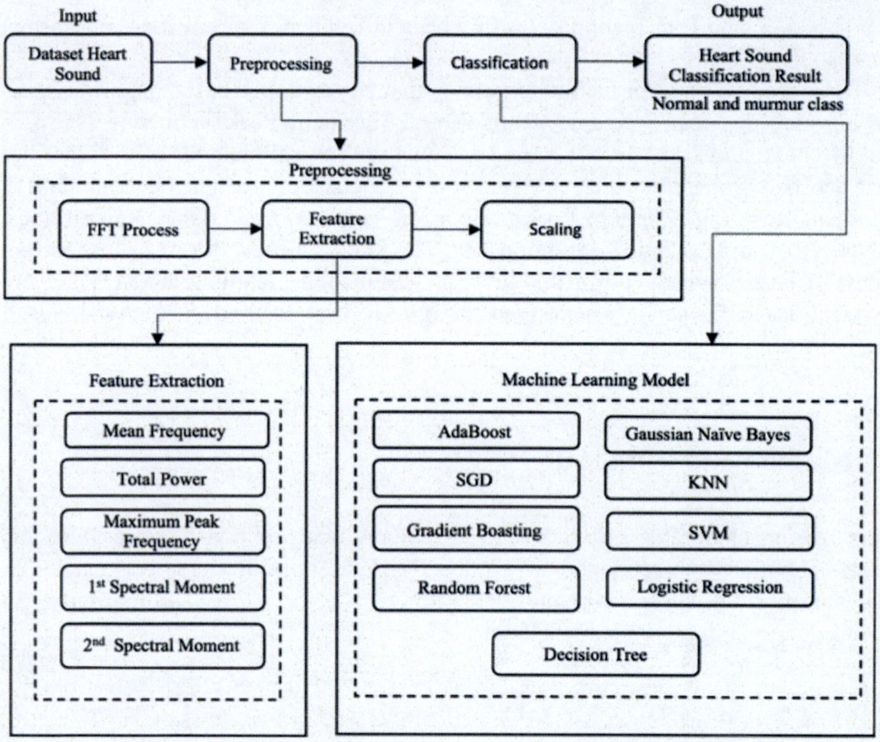

Fig. 1 Proposed method

Table 1 Dataset heart sounds

Heart sound class	Number of sample	Total duration
Normal	66	377,95
Murmur	66	505,57

conducted in hospitals using a DigiScope digital stethoscope and the general public using the iStethoscope Pro iPhone app. There are 132 heart sounds in total, divided into two categories. The sampling frequency for each data point is 4000 Hz. Table 1 contains more details on the data and duration. Figure 2 displays an example heart sound from the collection.

2.3 *Feature Extraction*

The results of a good classifier model require proper feature extraction. The data from the FFT, the data is continued to the feature extraction process. Power spectrum is the basis for feature extraction processing to be carried out. The power spectrum can

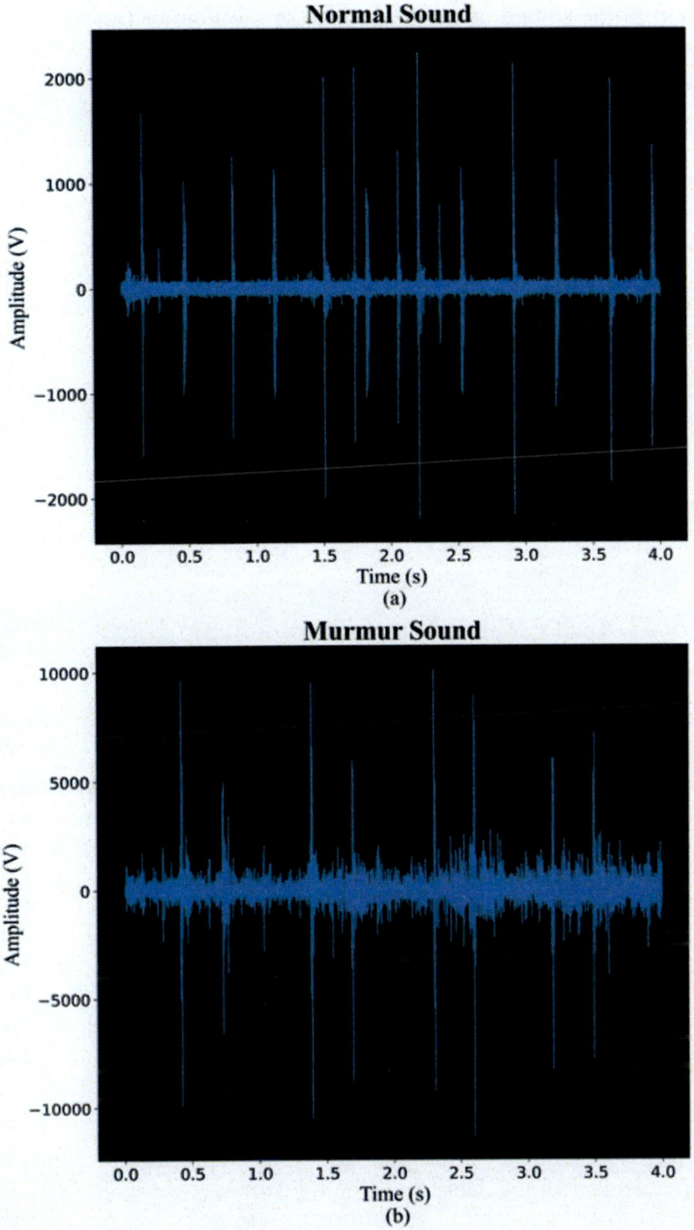

Fig. 2 Heart sound, **a** normal sound and **b** murmur sound

be calculated as the square of the magnitude of the Fourier transform (or Fourier series) of the heart sound. Equation (1) is a Power Spectrum calculation [12].

$$\text{Power spectrum }(f) = |X(f)|^2 \quad (v^2/Hz) \tag{1}$$

Mean Frequency, Total Power, Spectral Moments, and Maximum Peak Frequency are some characteristics used. The following is an explanation of each feature extraction used.

Mean Frequency is the average frequency resulting from the sum of the power spectrum times frequency divided by the total power spectrum, which is shown in Eq. (2).

$$\text{Mean Frequency} = \sum_{i=1}^{M} f_i P_i / \sum_{i=1}^{M} P_i(Hz), \quad i = 1, 2, 3, \ldots M \tag{2}$$

Total Power is the total power spectrum of the input data. Equation (3) is a total power calculation.

$$\text{Total Power} = \sum_{\mathrm{i}=1}^{\mathrm{M}} \mathrm{P_i}(\mathrm{v}^2/\mathrm{Hz}) i = 1, 2, 3, \ldots . M \tag{3}$$

Spectral Moment is a way to analyze statistics to extract the power spectrum of the input signal. 1st Spectral Moment and 2nd Spectral Moment will be used in this calculation. 1st Spectral Moment is the sum of the power spectrum timed by frequency. The formula for 2nd Spectral Moment is almost the same as 1st Spectral Moment, and the difference is frequency power by 2. Equations (4) and (5) are calculations for 1st Spectral Moment and 2nd Spectral Moment.

$$\text{1st Spectral Moment} = \sum_{i=1}^{M} P_i f_i (\mathrm{v}^2) i = 1, 2, 3, \ldots . M \tag{4}$$

$$\text{2nd Spectral Moment} = \sum_{i=1}^{M} P_i f_i^2 (\mathrm{v}^2\mathrm{Hz}) i = 1, 2, 3, \ldots . M \tag{5}$$

Maximum Peak Frequency is the maximum value of the peak frequency contained in a set of power spectrum values, shown in Eq. (6).

$$\text{Maximum Peak Frequency} = \max(P_i)(\mathrm{v}^2/\mathrm{Hz}), i = 1, 2, 3, \ldots . M \tag{6}$$

2.4 Classifier

In the previous study, some classifiers commonly used to create a good model of machine learning for heart sound is like SVM, KNN, ANN, and CNN [1, 5, 20–23]. Several classifiers have not been used for classifier heart sounds, such as AdaBoost, Stochastic Gradient Descent, Gradient Boosting, Random Forest, Decision Tree, Gaussian Naive Bayes, and Logistic Regression [19]. Therefore in this study, were tried several methods of machine learning such as which are AdaBoost, Stochastic Gradient Descent (SGD), Gradient Boosting, Random Forest, Decision Tree (DT), Gaussian Naïve Bayes, KNN, SVM, and Logistic Regression.

AdaBoost is the machine learning method used with the sequential predictor. The first fitting classifier is used in the original dataset, and the next classifier's misclassification data from the previous classifier is added. That procedure happens in the next classifier, so the sequential classifier is focused more on difficult cases and updated weight [24]. All predictor in AdaBoost make prediction and weigh them using the predictor weight α_j. Majority vote is used to decide predicted class from all predictors as shown in Eq. 8. Base predictor used in AdaBoost is decision tree.

$$\hat{y}(x) = \underset{k}{\text{argmax}} \sum_{\substack{j=1 \\ \hat{y}_{(x)=k}}}^{N} \alpha_j \text{where N is the number of predictors} \tag{7}$$

Stochastic Gradient Descent (SGD) is a type of gradient descent with an optimization algorithm to find an optional solution to minimize cost function with a random instance from all datasets [25]. In the learning process to get weight in the next iteration ($\theta_j^{(\text{Next})}$), the current weight (θ_j) is decreased by derivatives cost function from one random instance of dataset multiplied by learning rate (α), shown in Eq. 9 [19]. The learning process is stopped when the cost function reaches 0 or iteration has stopped.

$$\theta_j^{(\text{Next})} := \theta_j - 2\alpha\left(h_\theta\left(x^{(i)}\right) - y^{(i)}\right)x_j^{(i)}, \tag{8}$$

where$\left(h_\theta\left(x^{(i)}\right) - y^{(i)}\right)x_j^{(i)} is$derivativescostfunction.

Gradient Boosting is a sequential prediction technique similar to AdaBoost. Gradient Boosting differs in that it does not alter the weight but instead fits a new predictor using the residual error of the prior predictor [19, 26].

Decision Tree (DT) is a machine learning model that can be applied for classification and regression, defining a threshold to build a tree to predict the output. The decision tree used Gini impurity or Gini entropy to measure impurity in every tree node, which will be used in CART (Classification and Regression Tree) to define the threshold in the decision tree. Learning process that be used is look for the right threshold (t_k) in every single feature (k) with the minimum CART cost function is shown in Eq. 10 [19, 27].

$$J(k, t_k) = \frac{m_{\text{left}}}{m} G_{left} + \frac{m_{\text{right}}}{m} G_{\text{right}} \tag{9}$$

where $\begin{cases} \text{G}_{\text{left/right}}\, is\, measure\, impurity\, of\, the\, left\, and\, the\, right\, subset \\ \text{m}_{\text{left/right}}\, is\, number\, of\, instances\, in\, the\, left\, and\, the\, right\, subset. \end{cases}$

Random Forest is an ensemble learning of a decision tree, where the dataset for every predictor or decision tree classifier is defined using the bagging method. Random forest generates multiple decision trees, which is how the method makes a prediction using a majority vote for every predictor [28].

Gaussian Naive Bayes Gaussian Naive Bayes is the name of a machine learning technique that uses the Bayes theorem to assess the conditional independence between each pair of features under the assumption that the class variable's value is constant. Equation 11 illustrates the prediction result, which is the output class's greatest probability attained by multiplying each feature's likelihood by output [29].

$$\hat{y} = \underset{y}{\text{argmax}}\; P(y) \prod_{i=1}^{n} P(x_i|y) \tag{10}$$

K-Nearest Neighbors, or KNN, is a type of supervised learning that draws its knowledge from nearest-neighbor data. The number K refers to the number of data that must describe the criteria used to group data and vote on the class of that group. Equation 12 illustrates that Euclidean distance is used to calculate the distance between data neighbors [30].

$$\text{Euclideandistance}(a, b) = \sqrt{(a_i - b_1)^2 + (a_2 - b_2)^2 + \ldots + (a_n - b_n)^2} \tag{11}$$

SVM or Support Vector Machine is supervised learning with a boundary that separates data into two classes for classification or keeps data inside the boundary for regression. In this study, SVM is used for classification. Equation 13 is the way that SVM makes predictions [19].

$$\hat{y} \begin{cases} 0\, if\; w^T.x + b < 0 \\ 1 if w^T.x + b \geq 0 \end{cases} \tag{12}$$

Logistic Regression is a regression method that is used for binary classification. This method uses the probability of instances that measure with the sigmoid function to define the class output. Equation 14 is used to predict the output.

$$\hat{y} \begin{cases} 0\, if\; \hat{p} < 0.5 \\ 1 if \hat{p} \geq 0.5 \end{cases} \tag{13}$$

3 Result

Power spectrum is powered by two of magnitude frequency. Because range frequency murmur higher than normal heart sound, it makes the power spectrum murmur sound stronger than the normal heart sound. It can be shown in Fig. 3. Power spectral density murmur heart sound higher than normal heart sound. That characteristic can be basic pattern for classification model.

Figures 4 and 5 show boxplots of each feature of each heart sound class. Because the power spectral density of the murmur heart sounds higher than the normal one, so the feature of murmur data has a higher range than the normal one. In Fig. 4, it shows that mean frequency has the biggest differences in range data for each class compared to other features, as shown in Fig. 5. It can indicate that mean frequency can become the best feature that can produce a good classifier.

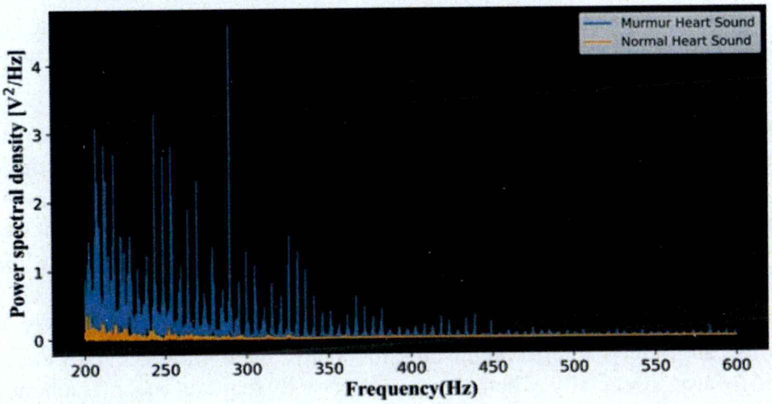

Fig. 3 Power spectrum

Fig. 4 Mean frequency

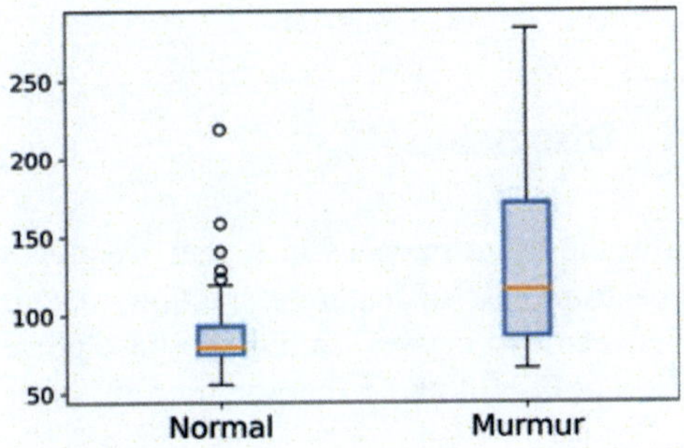

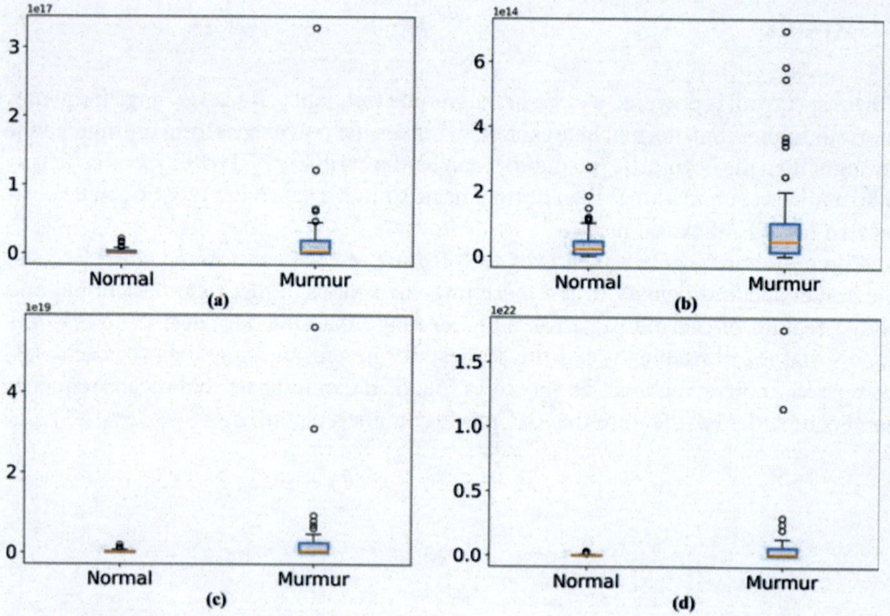

Fig. 5 The other feature extraction, **a** total power, **b** max. peak frequency, **c** 1st spectral power, **d** 2nd spectral power

Table 2 is the result of testing of classifier for each feature or all features with a different training size. Almost all classifiers have good accuracy with the mean frequency feature, with an average accuracy above 83%. The highest accuracy classifier with mean frequency feature is 93% with classifier Stochastic Gradient Descent and logistic regression. The other features that impact to classifier are 1st Spectral and 2nd Spectral moment. With that features good model still can be produced, it can be shown in some classifiers like KNN, AdaBoost, SVM, and Gaussian NB. When all features are trained, almost all the classifiers have the highest accuracy compared to each feature, especially when the classifier with features mean frequency, 1st Spectral, and 2nd Spectral moment has good accuracy too. Using all features, the best classifier for the heart sound case is Gaussian Naïve Bayes with an accuracy of 100%.

4 Discussion

Murmur class happens in higher frequency than normal class, so with the power spectrum base of feature extraction, machine learning can easily recognize pattern between two classes. In the five-base power spectrum used in this study, it can be seen in Figs. 4 and 5 that the murmur class has higher range data in every feature.

Table 2 Accuracy (%) for each classifier using different feature extraction or All feature with different train sizes

Classifier	Train size (%)	Mean frequency (%)	Total power (%)	Max. peak frequency (%)	1st spectral moment (%)	2nd spectral moment (%)	All feature (%)
KNN	90	85	50	50	71	78	92
	85	80	50	55	80	80	95
	80	81	59	51	77	62	92
AdaBoost	90	86	79	50	71	79	85
	85	75	45	55	70	80	75
	80	81	44	56	74	78	81
SVM	90	86	71	64	86	79	93
	85	90	70	65	85	75	95
	80	93	67	63	78	78	93
Random forest	90	86	57	57	71	79	71
	85	75	45	45	75	75	75
	80	85	41	52	67	56	89
Logistic regression	90	86	71	64	71	79	93
	85	90	65	55	70	75	95
	80	93	63	56	63	78	89
Decision tree	90	86	79	57	71	79	79
	85	80	50	55	75	75	70
	80	81	37	56	56	74	85
SGD	90	93	36	36	36	36	79
	85	90	70	45	75	75	100
	80	33	74	70	70	33	96
Gradient Boosting	90	86	57	50	79	79	93
	85	80	50	55	80	70	80
	80	81	44	63	70	67	70
Gaussian NB	90	86	79	79	86	86	100
	85	90	80	60	85	90	100
	80	89	74	63	78	81	89

The feature which has the highest differences in range data for the two classes is seen in Mean Frequency. That pattern data can produce better accuracy of the machine learning model than the other feature. It is supported with average accuracy for every machine learning model with Mean Frequency feature of 83%. Basically, the power spectrum feature shows pattern differences between the two classes. It can be shown that when all features are combined, and it produces higher accuracy than just using one feature. The best classifier for the heart sound case using all features is Gaussian Naive Bayes, with an accuracy of 100%.

In the previous study [18], the power spectrum also is used as feature extraction of the heart sound classification but has a different form. This research proposed method shows higher accuracy, better than the previous one, and even accuracy reaches 100%. The limitation of this model is that it could not be implemented in the real-time system because it has to buffer data first, so it will take time to collect. This study can be referenced heart sound classification, which wants excellent accuracy.

5 Conclusion

In this study, we tried to find feature extraction based on power spectrum to classify heart sound into normal and murmur heart sound. The proposed research is looking for best feature extraction with base power spectrum and look the best machine learning model. Feature extractions used in this research are Mean Frequency, Total Power, Maximum Peak Frequency, 1st Spectral Moment, and 2nd Spectral moment. From the result, Mean Frequency is the best feature that can be used for heart sound classification, with best classifier being Stochastic Gradient Descent and logistic regression and accuracy of 93%. When all features are used for classifier, almost all of the models as highest accuracy especially when classifier with mean frequency, 1st Spectral, and 2nd Spectral moment has good accuracy too. Using all features, the best classifier for heart sound case is Gaussian Naïve Bayes with accuracy reaching 100%. For the future work, this research can be an option for another feature extraction, mainly the classification of the signal with different frequencies for each class.

References

1. Li J, Ke L, Du Q (2019) Classification of heart sounds based on the wavelet fractal and twin support vector machine. Entropy 21(5)
2. Shi K et al (2020) Automatic signal quality index determination of radar-recorded heart sound signals using ensemble classification. IEEE Trans Biomed Eng 67(3):773–785
3. Nivitha Varghees V, Ramachandran KI (2017) Effective heart sound segmentation and murmur classification using empirical wavelet transform and instantaneous phase for electronic stethoscope. IEEE Sens J 17(12):3861–3872
4. Majety P, Umamaheshwari V (2016) An electronic system to recognize heart diseases based on heart sounds. In: 2016 IEEE international conference on recent trends in electronics, information & communication technology (RTEICT), pp 1617–1621
5. Dwivedi AK, Imtiaz SA, Rodriguez-Villegas E (2019) Algorithms for automatic analysis and classification of heart sounds: a systematic review. IEEE Access 7:8316–8345
6. Topal T, Polat H, Güler I (2008) Software development for the analysis of heartbeat sounds with LabVIEW in diagnosis of cardiovascular disease. J Med Syst 32(5):409–421
7. Rizal A, Handzah VAP, Kusuma PD (2022) Heart sounds classification using short-time fourier transform and gray level difference method. Ingénierie des systèmes d information 27(3):369–376

8. Milani MGM, Abas PE, de Silva LC, Nanayakkara ND (2021) Abnormal heart sound classification using phonocardiography signals. Smart Health 21
9. Ren Z et al (2022) Deep attention-based neural networks for explainable heart sound classification. Mach Learn Appl 9:100322
10. Chowdhury TH, Poudel KN, Hu Y (2020) Time-frequency analysis, denoising, compression, segmentation, and classification of PCG signals. IEEE Access 8:160882–160890
11. Safara F, Ramaiah ARA (2021) RenyiBS: Renyi entropy basis selection from wavelet packet decomposition tree for phonocardiogram classification. J Supercomput 77(4):3710–3726
12. Brunton SL, Nathan Kutz J (2019) Fourier and wavelet transforms. In: Data driven science & engineering machine learning, dynamical systems, and control. Cambridge University Press, Washington, pp 54–70
13. Fernando J, Saa D, Sotaquira M, Delgado Saa JF, Sotaquirá Gutierrez M (2010) EEG signal classification using power spectral features and linear discriminant analysis: a brain computer interface application
14. Hasan MJ, Shon D, Im K, Choi HK, Yoo DS, Kim JM (2020) Sleep state classification using power spectral density and residual neural network with multichannel EEG signals. Appl Sci (Switzerland) 10(21):1–13
15. Muthuvel K, Padma Suresh L, Jerry Alexander T, Krishna Veni SH (2015) Spectrum approach based Hybrid Classifier for classification of ECG signal. In: 2015 international conference on circuit, power and computing technologies, pp 1–6
16. Khazaee A, Ebrahimzadeh A (2010) Classification of electrocardiogram signals with support vector machines and genetic algorithms using power spectral features. Biomed Signal Process Control 5(4):252–263
17. Mahajan R, Bansal D (2015) Identification of heart beat abnormality using heart rate and power spectral analysis of ECG. In: 2015 international conference on soft computing techniques and implementations (ICSCTI), pp 131–135
18. Kristomo D, Hidayat R, Soesanti I, Kusjani A (2016) Heart sound feature extraction and classification using autoregressive power spectral density (AR-PSD) and statistics features. In: AIP conference proceedings, vol 1755
19. Géron A (2017) Hands-on machine learning. 53(9)
20. Tiwari S, Jain A, Sharma AK, Mohamad Almustafa K (2021) Phonocardiogram signal based multi-class cardiac diagnostic decision support system. IEEE Access 9:110710–110722. https://doi.org/10.1109/ACCESS.2021.3103316
21. Fernando T, Ghaemmaghami H, Denman S, Sridharan S, Hussain N, Fookes C (2020) Heart sound segmentation using bidirectional LSTMs with attention. IEEE J Biomed Health Inform 24(6):1601–1609
22. Dominguez-Morales JP, Jimenez-Fernandez AF, Dominguez-Morales MJ, Jimenez-Moreno G (2018) Deep neural networks for the recognition and classification of heart murmurs using neuromorphic auditory sensors. IEEE Trans Biomed Circ Syst 12(1):24–34
23. Mishra M, Menon H, Mukherjee A (2019) Characterization of S1 and S2 heart sounds using stacked autoencoder and convolutional neural network. IEEE Trans Instrum Meas 68(9):3211–3220
24. Freund Y, Schapire RE (1997) A decision-theoretic generalization of on-line learning and an application to boosting
25. Bottou L (2022) Stochastic gradient descent. https://leon.bottou.org/projects/sgd. Last accessed 11 Dec 2022
26. Friedman JH (2001) Greedy function approximation: a gradient boosting machine. Ann Stat 29(5):1189–1232
27. Breiman L, Friedman J, Olshen R, Stone C (2017) Classification and regression trees
28. Breiman L (2001) Random forests
29. Zhang H (2004) The optimality of naive bayes
30. Zhang Z (2016) Introduction to machine learning: K-nearest neighbors. Ann Transl Med 4(11)

Classification of Epileptic EEG Signal Using MSLD Entropy

Achmad Rizal, Inung Wijayanto, Sugondo Hadiyoso, Yunendah Nur Fuadah, Ki Moo Lim, and Triwiyanto Triwiyanto

Abstract Epilepsy is the most common neurological disorder characterized by recurrent seizures due to the abnormality of brain neuronal discharge. One of the tools to help neurologists diagnose epilepsy relies on EEG signals extensively because it can represent the brain's neuron activity. Due to the EEG signal being considered a complex biological signal, the signal complexity-based feature extraction method is suitable for characterizing epileptic EEG signals. One method for extracting EEG signals is entropy which is able to quantify signal complexity. Several previously proposed methods were wavelet entropy and IMF entropy. This study proposed multi-distance signal level difference (MSLD) entropy as a feature extraction method to extract the EEG signal complexity. The decomposed signal from MSLD was then extracted using entropy measurement. In the classification process, a Support Vector Machine (SVM) was applied to classify the normal, pre-ictal, and ictal signals of EEG signals. The highest accuracy of 96% was obtained using cubic SVM as the classifier. The proposed method provides an alternative method for analyzing EEG or other biomedical signals based on signal complexity.

Keywords Multi-distance signal level difference · Entropy · EEG · Seizure · Epileptic

---

A. Rizal (✉) · I. Wijayanto
School of Electrical Engineering, Telkom University, Bandung, Indonesia
e-mail: achmadrizal@telkomuniversity.ac.id

S. Hadiyoso
School of Applied Science, Telkom University, Bandung, Indonesia

Y. N. Fuadah
Computational Medicine Lab, Department of IT Convergence Engineering, Kumoh National Institut of Technology, Gumi, South Korea

K. M. Lim
Computational Medicine Lab, Department of Medical IT Convergence Engineering, Kumoh National Institute of Technology, Gumi, South Korea

T. Triwiyanto
Departement of Medical Electronics Technology, Poltekkes Kemenkes, Surabaya, Indonesia

T. Triwiyanto et al. (eds.), *Proceeding of the 3rd International Conference on Electronics, Biomedical Engineering, and Health Informatics*, Lecture Notes in Electrical Engineering 1008, https://doi.org/10.1007/978-981-99-0248-4_23

1 Introduction

Epilepsy is one of the most common nervous system disorders characterized by seizures due to the over-discharge activity of brain neurons [1–3]. Electroencephalogram (EEG) is one of the medical modalities as one of the gold standards in the diagnosis and analysis of epilepsy [4]. The EEG signal represents how neurons activity when a person has a seizure, even before the seizure. Until now, EEG processing in epilepsy cases is still an interesting issue to be developed in detecting epileptic EEG conditions. Numerous methods for automatic detection of seizures have been developed [5, 6].

Feature extraction methods with single or multi-domain features play an essential role in detecting epileptic EEG [7, 8]. The feature vector becomes a predictor in the classification stage using machine learning methods. Since the nature of EEG signal is the result of complex neuronal activity, the signal complexity-based feature extraction method is the best approach to characterize epileptic EEG signals [9].

Signal complexity methods have been widely used in detecting abnormalities of the EEG signal. They include statistics [10, 11], chaos [12, 13], and entropy [14, 15]. However, in processing EEG signals, they are often faced with a large amount of noise which can reduce the detection accuracy because the main characteristics of the signal can be disrupted. Signal decomposition or multiscale analysis is one way to get the intrinsic characteristics of a noise-mixed signal [16]. Several methods are proposed, such as coarse-grain procedure, wavelet transformation (WT), empirical mode decomposition (EMD), and multi-distance signal level difference (MSLD). The feature is then calculated for each signal level [17–20].

In previous studies, the signal resulting from the MSLD process was calculated several metrics which would later be used as features. The characteristics used include the Hjorth descriptor [21, 22], sample entropy [14], and fractal dimensions [23]. This feature cannot display interactions between signals at various levels of decomposition.

In previous studies, entropy was calculated on the MSLD signal separately. Thus, we cannot see the interaction between MSLD signals at any distance. In this study, we propose a calculation of entropy based on the relative energy of each signal decomposition of MSLD results. This method will measure the entropy by utilizing the signal energy distribution due to the MSLD process. This method was tested to distinguish normal pre-ictal and ictal signals on EEG signals. Classification is done using SVM with multiple kernels [24]. The proposed method is expected to be an alternative for processing EEG signals in particular and biomedical signals in general.

The rest of this paper is organized as follows. Section 2 describes the EEG signal dataset, the MSLD entropy concept, and the classification method. Section 3 presents the result and analysis of the study, while the conclusion is presented in Sect. 4.

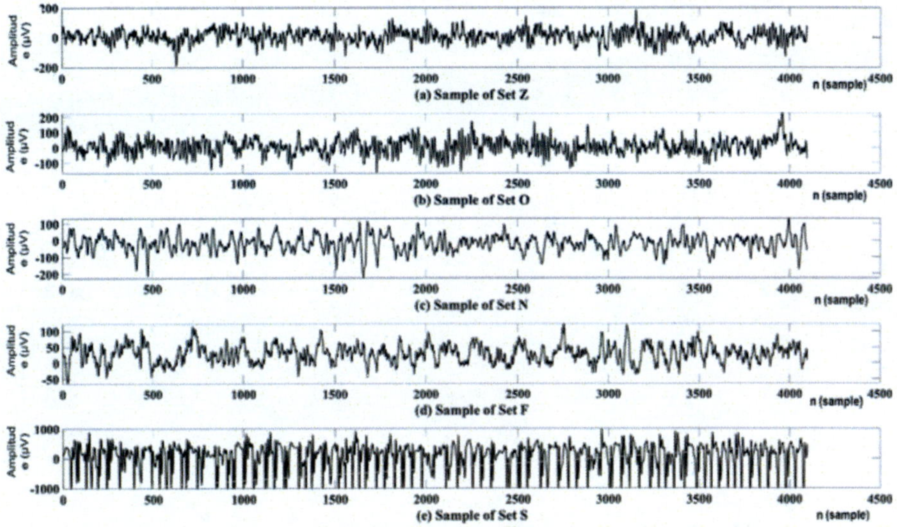

Fig. 1 Sample of EEG signals from Bonn University Dataset

2 Material and Method

2.1 EEG Signal Dataset

Public dataset was used in this study. The dataset was proved by Andrzejak et al. from Bonn University, Germany [25]. The dataset was created using scalp EEG in accordance with the international electrode placement standard of 10–20. In the recording process, an average standard reference and a 128-channel amplifier system are used. This dataset is classified into five categories: normal (open and closed eyes), interictal (open and closed eyes), ictal (open and closed eyes), and ictal conditions. In this dataset, volunteers' normal conditions are recorded with their eyes open (set Z) and closed (set O). Intracranial electrodes from the hippocampal formation (set F) and the epileptogenic zone are used to record the interictal state (set N). The ictal condition, as recorded in seizure activity, is the final category (S). Figure 1 provides an example of the Bonn University dataset for each class.

2.2 MSLD Entropy

Multidistance signal level difference (MSLD) is intended to calculate the joint occurrence of two signals at a certain distance [21]. This joint event is measured by calculating the difference between two signal samples over a certain distance. For signal $x(i)$ with N samples and distance $d = 1, \ldots, K$, the MSLD signal is calculated using

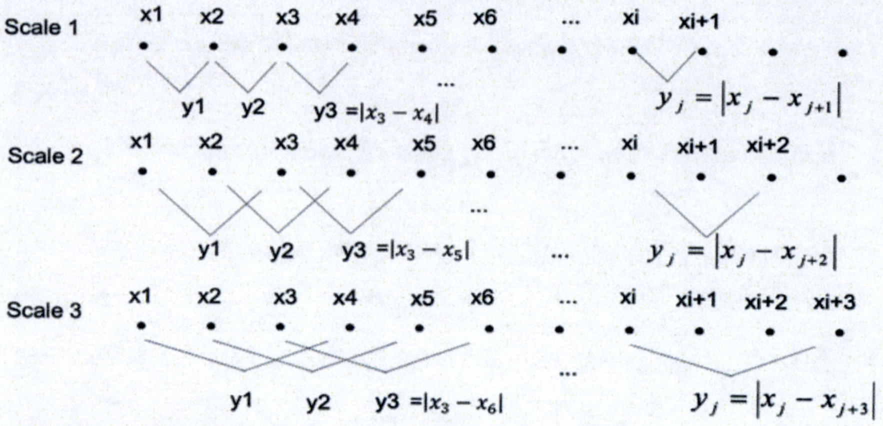

Fig. 2 MSLD process in scale of 3

Eq. 1. Figure 2 presents the visualization of The MSLD process.

$$y_d(i) = |x(i) - x(i+d)|,\ i = 1, 2, \ldots, N - d \text{ and } d = 1, 2, \ldots, K \quad (1)$$

This study proposes the MSLD entropy method as a feature for classifying seizures on EEG signals. For example, for d = 2, two MSLD signals will be obtained, namely y_1 and y_2 as in Eq. 2. The energy of y_1 and y_2 are expressed in Eq. 3. While ET is the total energy for y_1 and y_2 as in Eq. 4. Using relative energy of P_1 and P_2 (Eq. 5), we can calculate MSLD entropy as in Eq. 5.

$$y_1(i) = |x(i) - x(i+1)| \text{ and } y_2(i) = |x(i) - x(i+2)| \quad (2)$$

$$E_1 = \sum (y_1)^2 \text{meanwhile } E_2 = \sum (y_2)^2 \quad (3)$$

$$E_T = E_1 + E_2 \quad (4)$$

$$P_1 = \frac{E_1}{E_T} \text{and } P_2 = \frac{E_2}{E_T} \quad (5)$$

where E_T is total energy, E_1 and E_2 are energy of y_1 and y_2 respectively. P_1 and P_2 are relative energy of y_1 and y_2.

Then MSL entropy is expressed as Eq. 6.

$$MSLD\_ent_2 = -\sum_{j=1}^{2} p_j \ln p_j \quad (6)$$

In general, it can be written as Eq. 7 [26]:

$$MSLD\_ent_d = -\sum_{j=1}^{d} p_j \ln p_j \tag{7}$$

With $P_j = \frac{E_j}{E_T}$ and $E_j = \sum (Y_j)^2$, $j = 1, 2, \ldots, d$, here d is the distance of sample signal.

2.3 *Classification*

The last part of the proposed method is the classification of feature vectors generated from MSLD entropy. To evaluate the performance of MSLD entropy, we employ a support vector machine (SVM). This study observes the use of several kernels of SVM to see which is suitable for the classification process. SVM is chosen for this study because it has been shown to perform well in classifying cases, particularly biomedical signals [8]. SVM, introduced by Vapnik [27], has been used to find the best separation plane between two classes. SVM has an imaginary separation line called a hyperplane with supporting vectors [28]. SVM is mostly used to implement in linear cases, but due to a large number of non-linear classification cases, a non-linear kernel was developed to address the issue. The Support Vector Machine has several classifiers, including Linear, Quadratic, Cubic, Fine Gaussian, Medium Gaussian, and Coarse Gaussian [29]. Because SVM is a supervised learning method, it requires cross-validation to distinguish between training and test data. It is also been used to keep classification result from overfitting. The performance was tested using fivefold cross-validation in this study.

3 Results

Figure 3 shows the results of the MSLD processing the epileptic EEG signal at d = 1–5. The figure shows that all signal samples' values are positive because the absolute value is taken from the calculation result of the signal difference as in Eq. 1. MSLD is a modification of the gray level difference matrix (GLDM) that was initially used to measure texture in the image [21].

Since the pixel value in the image cannot have a negative value, the MSLD calculates the absolute value of the difference between two signal samples at a certain distance. The result of MSLD displayed signal fluctuations, where signals that have low fluctuations produce a relatively flat MSLD signal. MSLD can be combined using signal complexity measurement. Previous studies obtained features by calculating the fractal dimension [23] or sample entropy [14, 15]. Figure 4 shows the mean value of the MSLD entropy calculation in the five data classes. From the graph, it can be seen that the greater the distance *d*, the greater the MSLD entropy value. It means the signal complexity increases when using a higher distance. This increasing

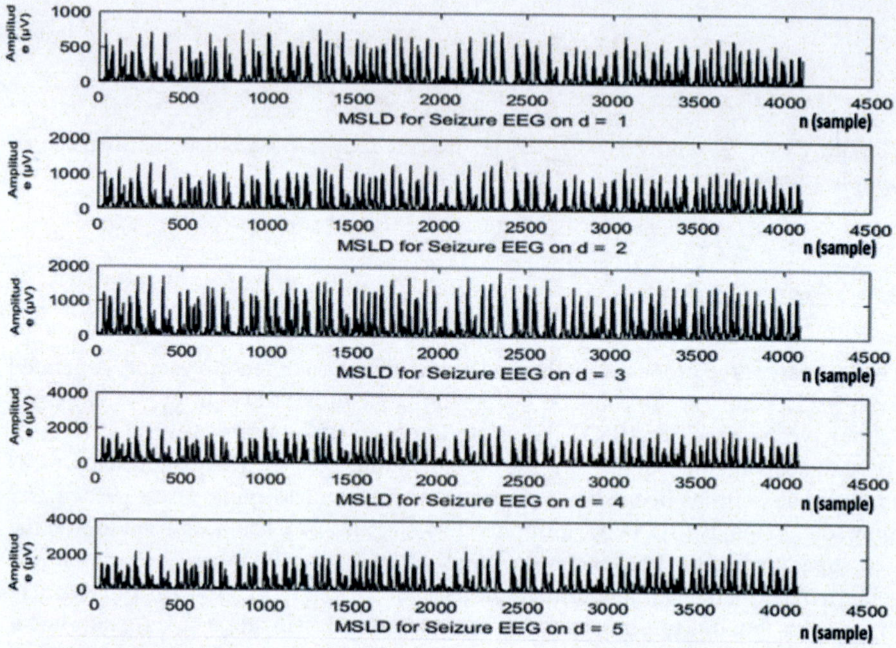

Fig. 3 Result of MSLD Process for Epileptic EEG (set S) using $d = 1 - 5$

pattern is similar to multilevel wavelet packet entropy (MWPE), which uses the same calculation principle [30]. This MWPE method has also been tested on epileptic EEG cases with the highest accuracy reaching 94.3% for classifying three data classes.

Even though the characteristics produced by the MSLD entropy used are similar and close together, using the *f* classifier, it is hoped that a reasonably high accuracy

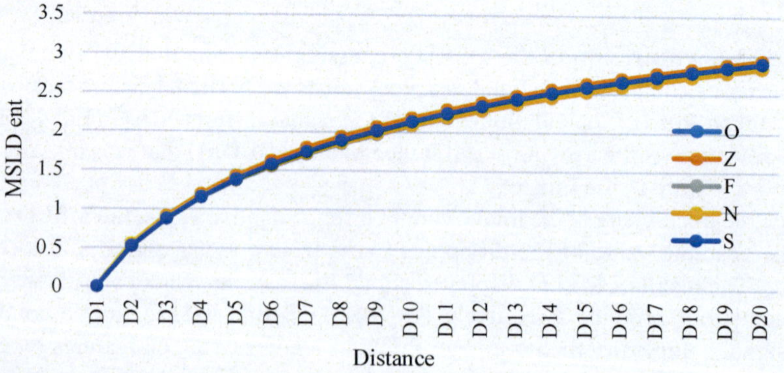

Fig. 4 MSLD entropy for $d = 1–20$

will be obtained. In this study, testing is carried out using several MSLDs at different distances to get the best accuracy.

The accuracy test is carried out using three scenarios. The first is a five-class classification, where each data set is considered as a separate data class. The second scenario is a classification using two normal conditions and two pre-ictal conditions combined into one class, while the seizure data set stands alone. The third scenario consists of three data classes: normal, pre-ictal, and seizure.

The result of the first scenario is shown in Table 1. In Table 1, the highest accuracy of 79.4% is achieved using cubic SVM with 20 features generated by MSLD entropy with d = 1–20. The results show that 20 features may result in higher accuracy than fewer features for SVM with multiple kernels.

Table 2 shows accuracy using the second scenario. There are three data classes: normal (Z + O), interictal (N + F), and seizure (S). In this scenario, the highest accuracy is 94.4% using 20 features and cubic SVM as a classifier. This result is similar to the first scenario. The difference between the new data classes seems to increase when more features are used. Table 3, 4, 5 and 6 results from accuracy testing using the third scenario. The classification is performed on three data classes: one normal dataset, one interictal dataset, and seizures. The highest accuracy achieved is 96% when tested using the O-N-S dataset, as shown in Table 3. This result is higher than the previous two scenarios because the normal and interictal datasets have the same characteristics. The highest accuracy is achieved using 20 features and cubic SVM. This is consistent with the feature plot in Fig. 4, where the characteristic value of each data set differs for the larger *d* value.

Table 1 Classification accuracy (%) of five classes' data (O-Z-F-N-S)

Classifier	D = 1–20	D = 1–15	D = 1–10	D = 1–5
Linear SVM	75	74.4	71.4	61.8
Quadratic SVM	77.2	75.2	71.8	67.8
Cubic SVM	79.4	78.2	76.4	68.6
Fine Gaussian SVM	72.8	72.2	71.8	65.8
Medium Gaussian SVM	67.4	66	64	5.8
Coarse Gaussian SVM	57.8	52.6	51.6	49.8

Table 2 Classification accuracy (%) of three classes' data (%) ((O + Z)-(F + N)-S)

Classifier	D = 1–20	D = 1–15	D = 1–10	D = 1–5
Linear SVM	90	89	86.2	80.6
Quadratic SVM	92.8	91	89	88.8
Cubic SVM	94.4	92.6	91.4	90.2
Fine Gaussian SVM	89.6	89	88.6	84.2
Medium Gaussian SVM	86.2	86.2	86	81.6
Coarse Gaussian SVM	83.4	80.8	79.2	76.8

Table 3 Classification accuracy (%) of three classes' data (%) (O-N-S)

Classifier	D = 1–20	D = 1–15	D = 1–10	D = 1–5
Linear SVM	93.3	92.7	90.3	76
Quadratic SVM	94.3	93.3	90	88.7
Cubic SVM	96	94	92.7	87.7
Fine Gaussian SVM	93.3	93	90.7	81
Medium Gaussian SVM	89.3	87.7	86.7	75.3
Coarse Gaussian SVM	79.7	77.3	70.3	66.7

Table 4 Classification accuracy (%) of three classes' data (%) (O-F-S)

Classifier	D = 1–20	D = 1–15	D = 1–10	D = 1–5
Linear SVM	92	89.7	87.7	73
Quadratic SVM	93.3	90.7	86	84.7
Cubic SVM	95	92.3	92	86
Fine Gaussian SVM	91	87.3	85.7	75
Medium Gaussian SVM	88.7	83.3	83	71.7
Coarse Gaussian SVM	77.7	73	68.3	64.7

Table 5 Classification accuracy (%) of three classes' data (%) (Z-N-S)

Classifier	D = 1–20	D = 1–15	D = 1–10	D = 1–5
Linear SVM	93.7	93	92.7	94
Quadratic SVM	92.7	92.7	92.7	93.7
Cubic SVM	94.3	94.3	93.3	93.3
Fine Gaussian SVM	94.3	94.3	93.3	94.7
Medium Gaussian SVM	91.7	91.7	91.3	91.7
Coarse Gaussian SVM	81.7	83	85.7	84.3

Table 6 Classification accuracy (%) of three classes' data (%) (Z-F-S)

Classifier	D = 1–20	D = 1–15	D = 1–10	D = 1–5
Linear SVM	92	92.3	89.3	89.7
Quadratic SVM	92	91	92	89.7
Cubic SVM	92.7	93.3	89	92
Fine Gaussian SVM	88.7	90.7	88.7	90.3
Medium Gaussian SVM	90.3	88.7	83.3	88.3
Coarse Gaussian SVM	80	82	90.7	79.3

4 Discussion

The proposed method using MSLD entropy generally produces characteristics similar for each class compared to the MWPE method in previous study [30]. However, MWPE achieved the highest accuracy of 94.3% for the three data classes, while MSLD entropy achieved the highest accuracy of 96% for the same condition. MSLD entropy results in lower accuracy than the EEG epileptic classification using a combination of MSLD and fractal dimensions as reported by Silalahi et al., reaching 99% for the three data classes [23]. Another study similar to this paper is MSLD using sample entropy, where sample entropy is calculated on the new signal resulting from the MSLD process. The highest accuracy reached 97.7% for the three data classes [14].

Table 7 presents a comparison of our proposed method to other previous studies. The result shows that MSLD entropy has a competitive result compared to other researches. The MSLD entropy method uses the same approach as the calculation of wavelet entropy [31] and IMF entropy [32]. Entropy is calculated from the relative energy of the subband or IMF. In MSLD entropy, the energy signal is unpredictable because it is influenced by signal shift, noise, and magnitude. In contrast to wavelet entropy, the energy signal can be predicted by looking at the spectrum of each subband signal [33]. This condition is similar to IMF entropy, where the IMF signal is also strongly influenced by signal shifts [34]. Determining the distance on the MSLD entropy also significantly affects the resulting entropy. This study uses d = 1 -20 according to previous studies using multiscale entropy and its derivative methods [35, 36]. For signals with a high sampling frequency (e.g., 200 samples/second), the distance d = 1 sample will equal 1/200 s. This change in a rapidly fluctuating signal will not be significant, so the MSLD signal tends to be flat. For this reason, an experiment to find the value of the distance d in the signal will be an exciting research topic in the next project. The results indicate that the proposed method can enrich the selection of EEG processing methods for detecting epilepsy. There are opportunities to use this method for other biomedical signal processing.

5 Conclusion

This study proposes a feature extraction method called MSLD entropy. MSLD is calculated based on the relative energy of the signal resulting from the MSLD process. The proposed method is tested in the case of classification of EEG epileptic signals. The accuracy test resulted in the highest accuracy of 96% for the three data classes and cubic SVM as the classifier. These results were obtained using 20 features from entropy calculations on the MSLD signal with a distance of d = 1–20. This accuracy is competitive with other similar methods in previous studies. The distance selection determines MSLD entropy. This study used a distance of 1–20 according to previous studies, which can be compared directly. The selection of the proper distance with

Table 7 Comparison with previous research using other entropy or MSLD + entropy

Reference	Method	Number of classes	classifier	Number of features	Accuracy
[30]	Multilevel Wavelet packet entropy	3	SVM	5	94.3%
[32]	IMF Entropy	3	SVM	5	86.3%
[14]	MSLD + sample entropy	3	SVM	20	97.7%
[23]	MSLD + fractal dimension	3	SVM	10	99%
Proposed method	MSLD entropy	3	SVM	20	96%

a broader range and the use of a more sophisticated classifier became the focus of the following study. In the next research, the performance of MSLD entropy will be tested using other biomedical signals.

References

1. Beghi E (2020) The Epidemiology of Epilepsy. Neuroepidemiology 54:185–191. https://doi.org/10.1159/000503831
2. Weinstein, S.: Seizures and epilepsy: An overview. Epilepsy: The Intersection of Neurosciences, Biology, Mathematics, Engineering, and Physics, Boca Raton (2011). https://doi.org/10.1201/b10866.
3. Rizvi S, Ladino LD, Hernandez-Ronquillo L, Téllez-Zenteno JF (2017) Epidemiology of early stages of epilepsy: Risk of seizure recurrence after a first seizure. Seizure. 49:46–53. https://doi.org/10.1016/j.seizure.2017.02.006
4. Nakano, R.H.S.J.E.-H.: Basic Electroencephalogram and Its Common Clinical Applications in Children. Presented at the (2020). https://doi.org/10.5772/intechopen.94247.
5. Sharmila A (2018) Epilepsy detection from EEG signals: a review. J Med Eng Technol 42:368–380. https://doi.org/10.1080/03091902.2018.1513576
6. Siddiqui MK, Morales-Menendez R, Huang X, Hussain N (2020) A review of epileptic seizure detection using machine learning classifiers. Brain Informatics. 7:1–18. https://doi.org/10.1186/s40708-020-00105-1
7. Miao, Y., Cao, J.: Comparison of EMD, MEMD and 2T-EMD by analyzing standard artificial signals and EEG. In: 2017 International Joint Conference on Neural Networks (IJCNN). pp. 1367–1371. IEEE (2017). https://doi.org/10.1109/IJCNN.2017.7966012.
8. Wijayanto I, Hartanto R, Nugroho HA (2020) Comparison of empirical mode decomposition and coarse-grained procedure for detecting pre-ictal and ictal condition in electroencephalography signal. Informatics Med. Unlocked. 19:100325. https://doi.org/10.1016/j.imu.2020.100325
9. Wijayanto, I., Hartanto, R., Nugroho, H.A., Setiawan, N.A.: A Study on Signal Complexity Measurement for Epileptic Seizure Detection. In: 2019 IEEE 9th International Conference on System Engineering and Technology (ICSET). pp. 320–325. IEEE (2019). https://doi.org/10.1109/ICSEngT.2019.8906319.

10. Frolov NS, Grubov VV, Maksimenko VA, Lüttjohann A, Makarov VV, Pavlov AN, Sitnikova E, Pisarchik AN, Kurths J, Hramov AE (2019) Statistical Properties and Predictability of Extreme Epileptic Events. Sci Rep 9:7243. https://doi.org/10.1038/s41598-019-43619-3
11. Sayeid MIE, Gemeay E, Khames S (2016) Statistical Analysis of EEG Signals in Wavelet Domain for Efficient Seizure Prediction. Am. J. Biomed. Eng. 6:32–41. https://doi.org/10.5923/j.ajbe.20160601.05
12. Khoa, T.Q.D., Thi Minh Huong, N., Toi, V. Van: Detecting Epileptic Seizure from Scalp EEG Using Lyapunov Spectrum. Comput. Math. Methods Med. 2012, 1–11 (2012). https://doi.org/10.1155/2012/847686.
13. Kannathal, N., Chee, J., Er, K., Lim, K., Tat, O.H.: Chaotic Analysis of Epileptic EEG Signals BT - The 15th International Conference on Biomedical Engineering. Presented at the (2014).
14. Rizal A, Hadiyoso S (2018) Sample Entropy on Multidistance Signal Level Difference for Epileptic EEG Classification. Sci World J 2018:1–6. https://doi.org/10.1155/2018/8463256
15. Li P, Karmakar C, Yearwood J, Venkatesh S, Palaniswami M, Liu C (2018) Detection of epileptic seizure based on entropy analysis of short-term EEG. PLoS ONE 13:e0193691. https://doi.org/10.1371/journal.pone.0193691
16. Muñoz-Gutiérrez PA, Giraldo E, Bueno-López M, Molinas M (2018) Localization of active brain sources from EEG signals using empirical mode decomposition: a comparative study. Front Integr Neurosci 12:1–14. https://doi.org/10.3389/fnint.2018.00055
17. Chen G, Xie W, Bui TD, Krzyżak A (2017) Automatic Epileptic Seizure Detection in EEG Using Nonsubsampled Wavelet-Fourier Features. J. Med. Biol. Eng. 37:123–131. https://doi.org/10.1007/s40846-016-0214-0
18. Shaikh, M.H.N., Farooq, O., Chandel, G.: EMD Analysis of EEG Signals for Seizure Detection BT - Advances in System Optimization and Control. Presented at the (2019).
19. Ji, N., Ma, L., Dong, H., Zhang, X.: EEG Signals Feature Extraction Based on DWT and EMD Combined with Approximate Entropy. Brain Sci. 9, (2019). https://doi.org/10.3390/brainsci9080201.
20. Akbari, H., Esmaili, S.S., Zadeh, S.F.: Classification of seizure and seizure-free eeg signals based on empirical wavelet transform and phase space reconstruction. arXiv. (2019).
21. Rizal A, Hidayat R, Nugroho HA (2017) Hjorth descriptor measurement on multidistance signal level difference for lung sound classification. J. Telecommun. Electron. Comput. Eng. 9:23–27
22. Rizal, A., Hidayat, R., Nugroho, H.A.: Comparison of multi-distance signal level difference Hjorth descriptor and its variations for lung sound classifications. Indones. J. Electr. Eng. Informatics. 7, 345–356 (2019). https://doi.org/10.11591/ijeei.v7i2.771.
23. Silalahi DK, Rizal A, Rahmawati D, Sri Aprillia B (2021) Epileptic seizure detection using multidistance signal level difference fractal dimension and support vector machine. J Theor Appl Inf Technol 99:909–920
24. Kumar, N., Alam, K., Siddiqi, A.H.: Wavelet transform for classification of EEG signal using SVM and ANN. Biomed. Pharmacol. J. 10, 2061–2069 (2017). https://doi.org/10.13005/bpj/1328.
25. Andrzejak RG, Lehnertz K, Mormann F, Rieke C, David P, Elger CE (2001) Indications of nonlinear deterministic and finite-dimensional structures in time series of brain electrical activity: Dependence on recording region and brain state. Phys Rev E 64:061907. https://doi.org/10.1103/PhysRevE.64.061907
26. Lei L, Kun S (2017) Speaker Recognition Using Wavelet Packet Entropy, I-Vector, and Cosine Distance Scoring. J Electr Comput Eng 2017:1735698. https://doi.org/10.1155/2017/1735698
27. Boser, B.E., Guyon, I.M., Vapnik, V.N.: A training algorithm for optimal margin classifiers. In: Proceedings of the fifth annual workshop on Computational learning theory - COLT '92. pp. 144–152. ACM Press, New York, New York, USA (1992). https://doi.org/10.1145/130385.130401.
28. Cevikalp H (2017) Best Fitting Hyperplanes for Classification. IEEE Trans Pattern Anal Mach Intell 39:1076–1088. https://doi.org/10.1109/TPAMI.2016.2587647

29. Jain, U., Nathani, K., Ruban, N., Joseph Raj, A.N., Zhuang, Z., G.V. Mahesh, V.: Cubic SVM Classifier Based Feature Extraction and Emotion Detection from Speech Signals. In: 2018 International Conference on Sensor Networks and Signal Processing (SNSP). pp. 386–391. IEEE (2018). https://doi.org/10.1109/SNSP.2018.00081.
30. Wijayanto, I., Rizal, A., Hadiyoso, S.: Multilevel Wavelet Packet Entropy and Support Vector Machine for Epileptic EEG Classification. In: 2018 4th International Conference on Science and Technology (ICST). pp. 1–6. IEEE (2018). https://doi.org/10.1109/ICSTC.2018.8528634.
31. Rosso OA, Blanco S, Yordanova J, Kolev V, Figliola A, Schürmann M, Başar E (2001) Wavelet entropy: a new tool for analysis of short duration brain electrical signals. J Neurosci Methods 105:65–75. https://doi.org/10.1016/S0165-0270(00)00356-3
32. Yu, Y., YuDejie, Junsheng, C.: A roller bearing fault diagnosis method based on EMD energy entropy and ANN. J. Sound Vib. 294, 269–277 (2006). https://doi.org/10.1016/j.jsv.2005.11.002.
33. Zunino, L., Pérez, D.G., Garavaglia, M., Rosso, O.A.: Wavelet entropy of stochastic processes. Phys. A Stat. Mech. its Appl. 379, 503–512 (2007). https://doi.org/10.1016/j.physa.2006.12.057.
34. Das, A.B., Bhuiyan, M.I.H.: Discrimination and classification of focal and non-focal EEG signals using entropy-based features in the EMD-DWT domain. Biomed. Signal Process. Control. 29, 11–21 (2016). https://doi.org/10.1016/j.bspc.2016.05.004.
35. Gu, R.: Multiscale Shannon entropy and its application in the stock market. Phys. A Stat. Mech. its Appl. 484, 215–224 (2017). https://doi.org/10.1016/j.physa.2017.04.164.
36. Hu M, Liang H (2017) Multiscale Entropy: Recent Advances BT - Complexity and Nonlinearity in Cardiovascular Signals. Presented at the. https://doi.org/10.1007/978-3-319-58709-7_4

Comparison Performance of Deep Learning Models for Brain Tumor Segmentation Based on 2D Convolutional Neural Network

Dian Nova Kusuma Hardani, Hanung Adi Nugroho, and Igi Ardiyanto

Abstract A brain tumor is a lump of aberrant brain cells whose formation can interfere with the brain's normal functioning and adversely affect the patient's health. Brain tumor segmentation is a fundamental step for quantitatively analyzing tumor masses and extracting infected areas of brain tissue. Accurate and reliable segmentation is helpful in clinical diagnosis and treatment planning so that the probability of survival can be improved. The deep learning technique showed a significant performance improvement in brain tumor segmentation. The objectives of this study are to comprehensively investigate and compare the effectiveness of multiple deep learning based on 2-dimensional Convolutional Neural Networks for clustering brain tumors on MRI images. This study implements a simple U-Net model and modifies it with different backbones as encoders, including VGG19, ResNet50, InceptionV3, and InceptionResnetV2. This model was trained and tested on the BraTS 2020 dataset. The tumor area was segmented into three main areas: necrotic, edematous, and enhancing tumors. The predicted image is weighed against the ground truth for validation. The predictive performance of each model was analyzed using quantification metrics. The results showed that the five models tested, including Simple U-Net, VGG19-UNet, Res-UNet, InceptionV3-UNet, and InceptionResnetV2-UNet, achieved 98.8% to 99.3% pixel accuracy. However, when the evaluation was carried out on the three sub-areas, each model showed comparable performance, except for the VGG19-UNet model, which performed significantly lower. It shows that performance can be influenced by many factors, such as the amount of training data, loss function, parameter tuning, and the hyperparameters of each model. The proposed model can be implemented well. Thus, this research needs to be developed further.

D. N. K. Hardani · H. A. Nugroho (✉) · I. Ardiyanto
Department of Electrical and Information Engineering, Faculty of Engineering, Universitas Gadjah Mada, Yogyakarta, Indonesia
e-mail: adinugroho@ugm.ac.id

D. N. K. Hardani
Department of Electrical Engineering, Faculty of Engineering and Science, Universitas Muhammadiyah Purwokerto, Purwokerto, Indonesia

T. Triwiyanto et al. (eds.), *Proceeding of the 3rd International Conference on Electronics, Biomedical Engineering, and Health Informatics*, Lecture Notes in Electrical Engineering 1008, https://doi.org/10.1007/978-981-99-0248-4_24

Keywords Brain tumor segmentation · Deep learning model · Convolutional neural network · Performance · Quantification metrics

1 Introduction

A brain tumor, also known as glioma, is an unrestrained brain disorder that causes clusters of aberrant brain cells in or near the brain. The formation of these irregular cells can interfere with the brain's normal functioning and hurt the patient's health [1]. Early diagnosis of brain tumors is essential in increasing the possibility of optimal treatment [2–4]. Suppose the tumor can be detected correctly and accurately at an early stage. In that case, the chances of survival can be increased [5–8], and patients also get information about the judgment, action planning, and prediction of patient outcomes [9, 10].

Magnetic Resonance Imaging (MRI) scanning is among the most well-liked prevalent approaches for resectioning and examining irregularities in the brain form, size, or placement of tissue that helps detect tumors [11]. MRI imaging is considered more valuable and precise for tumors [12] and safe because it uses radio frequency signals, so it is not exposed to any radiation [7] and has higher contrast features [13]. In addition, MRI has still been considered the standard gold imaging for diagnosing brain tumors [12, 14].

MR image segmentation is a fundamental step with many applications in neurology, such as analyzing quantitative tumor masses to recognize their dynamic expansion over time [15], operational planning, and functional imaging [16]. Extracting infected brain tissue areas from MRI images [1] and localization of abnormalities [17] used segmentation. Although MRI images can accurately describe brain structures, segmenting medical images is difficult. It is due to low spatial resolution, low contrast, ambiguous borders, inhomogeneity, partial volume effects, noise, variable object shape, and the lack of anatomical models that fully capture the possible deformation in each structure [10, 16, 18]. The clinical need for tumor segmentation is paramount, including planning radiotherapy doses, assessing tumor volume changes while keeping track of low to high-grade glial tumor transformation, and monitoring therapy response [4].

Deep learning techniques have significant performance improvements in the medical healthcare sectors [19] and computer vision [20]. Deep learning can provide a more precise explanation of extremely complicated phenomena than classical statistical methods if the available dataset is of high dimension, its performance directly corresponds to the input size, and a high degree of flexibility [21]. Deep learning methods have succeeded in various aspects of computer vision, including object recognition, localization, and segmentation in usual images. Many studies have carried out the segmentation of brain tumors using deep learning. Segmentation technique using deep learning In 2013, Convolutional Neural Network (CNN) won the Brain Tumor Segmentation (BraTS) Challenge, and in 2015, it placed second [22]. Havaei et al. [23] present the CNN architecture simultaneously by exploiting local and global contextual features. This work examines a cascade design where the output of the base CNN serves as an additional information source for succeeding CNNs. Razzak et al. [24] also embed the cascade architecture into a dual-path CNN group where the output from the base CNN is considered a secondary source and combined in the final layer. Wang et al. [25] suggested a CNN cascade to group brain tumors by tier-based subregions of multimodal MRI images. FCNN and dense micro-block difference feature (DMDF) were fully integrated to create the brain tumor segmentation method, which produced consistent and spatial presence segmentation results [26]. The average Dice coefficient can reach 90.98% and has a very high real-time performance. Ribalta Lorenzo et al. [27] also utilize FCNN and are equipped with augmentation techniques. The system is resistant to poor data quality and short training set variability. Nawaz et al. [28] proposed VGG19-UNET for brain tumor segmentation and a collaborative learning model for survival analysis. Segmentation using BraTS 2020, which consists of 371 image files. The algorithm yielded dice coefficient scores of 0.81, 0.86, and 0.88 for enhancing tumors, core tumors, and whole tumors.

Saha et al. [29] proposed a new multi-pathway U-Net coupled with residual tissue and skip connection to divide multimodal MR images into three glioma subregions. They employ a shared encoder followed by a different decoder for each class. The residual connection used in the model facilitates increased performance. AboElenein et al. [30] proposed the Inception Residual Dense Nested U-Net (IRDNU-Net) encoder-decoder architecture. Modules Residual and Inception are utilized instead of the typical U-Net convolution layer in this model to boost model width without increasing computational complexity. Encoder and decoder are coupled via Inception Residual densely nested path sequences in the proposed architecture to excerpt more data and increase network depth while decreasing the total quantity of network parameters. The suggested segmentation structure was assessed utilizing two large benchmark data sets for brain tumor subdivision, BraTS'2019 and BraTS'2020. IRDNU-Net outperformed U-Net by 1.8%, 11.4%, and 11.7% in all cancers, core tumors, and boosting tumors, respectively, according to the experimental findings.

Nitesh et al. [31] demonstrate an algorithm for segmenting brain tumors using a modified U-Net using Inception as a backbone. The U-Net modification increased the F1-Score and IoU scores in brain tumor segmentation. The study did not specify which Inception model was used for segmentation. Recently, Sandhya et al. [32] developed a highly automated method for segmenting multimodality MRI brain tumors using the neural network architecture of stratified anisotropic neural networks, 3D U-Net, and H-DenseNet. This study applies the rule of majority voting to the architecture of the ensemble neural network to evaluate brain tumor segmentation.

Based on the benefits shown in previous studies in improving brain tumor segmentation performance, the primary goal of this investigation is to determine the performance of deep learning models in brain tumor segmentation using a 2D ConvNet. This paper investigates several models specifically, including the ResNet model used in ResNet50 and the inception model used in InceptionV3 and InceptionResNetV2. We focus on the U-Net model's architecture as a decoder. This study compares the simple U-Net model with the modified U-Net model with several pre-trained classifier models as encoders, including VGG19, ResNet50, Inception-V3, and InceptionResNetV2. These strengths and weaknesses of each model can be evaluated and developed for different research purposes. Models were trained and evaluated using the BRATS 2020 dataset.

This paper is structured as follows. Section 1 contains the background of this study. Data, methods used for segmentation, and performance measurements are explained in Sect. 2. Section 3 explains the result of all segmentation processes. Section 4 presents a discussion of the result. Finally, the conclusions of this investigation are presented in the last section.

2 Materials and Method

This section describes the methodology conducted in this paper, including the public dataset used, deep learning models, and research methods, including preprocessing, segmentation process, and performance evaluation.

2.1 Data

The dataset on brain tumors utilized in this investigation is generally available, namely Brain Tumor Segmentation (BraTS) 2020.[1] The Multimodal BRATS Challenge standard benchmarks dataset derived from the International Conference on Medical Image Computing, and Computer-Assisted Interventions (MICCAI) is the most popular and frequently used dataset by researchers [33]. This data contains the scan results before and after therapy. The BraTS 2020 dataset consists of 369 samples of training data and 125 samples of validation data. Four MR images, comprising T1-weighted (T1), post-contrast T1-weighted (T1ce), T2-weighted (T2), and fluid-attenuated inversion recovery (FLAIR) sequences, are acquired for each sample. The sizes of 3 dimensions image files are 240 × 240 × 155 voxels. Figure 1 shows an example of a sequence, namely a FLAIR image with a different plotting function.

2.2 Deep Learning Models

U-Net. U-Net is a convolutional network technique for efficient and precise image segmentation [34]. Within the scope of the International Symposium on Biomedical Imaging (ISBI) segmentation challenge for neural structures in electron microscopic stacks, it outperformed the previous best answer (a sliding-window convolutional

[1] https://www.med.upenn.edu/cbica/brats2020/data.html.

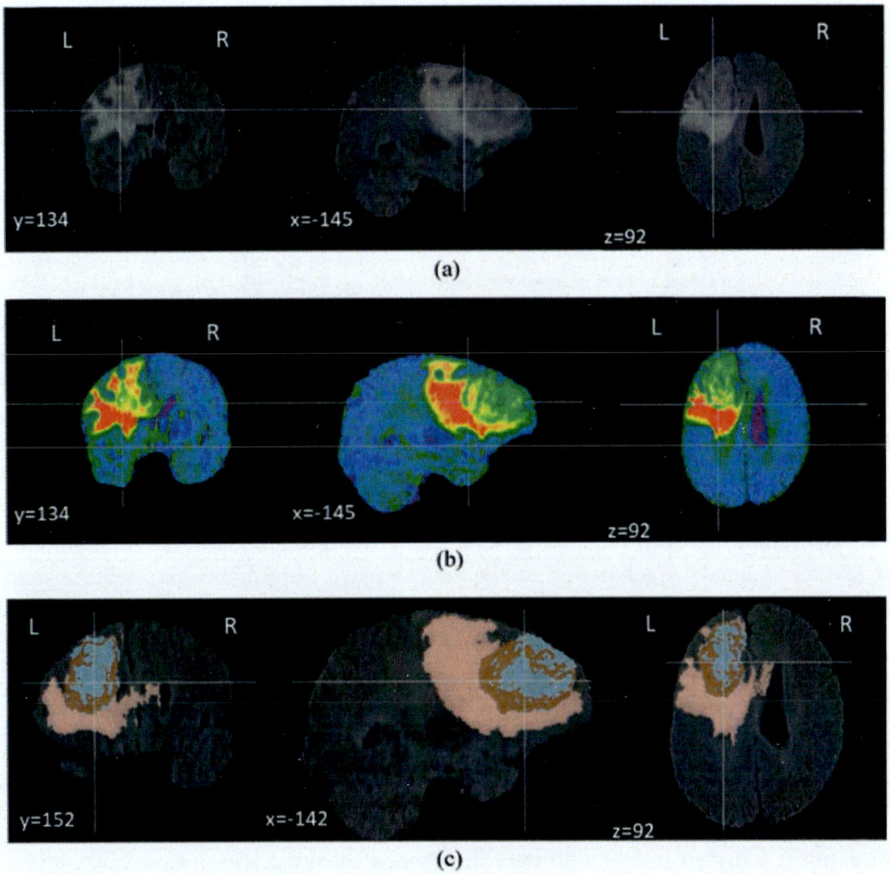

Fig. 1 Example of FLAIR image data with different plotting functions. **a** Plotting an anatomical image, **b** plot cuts of an EPI image (by default cuts: frontal, lateral, and axial), and **c** Plotting ROIs or a mask with an optional background. *x*, *y*, and *z* are the axes. *L* is the left side, and *R* is the right side

network) to date. The two most difficult types of conveyed light microscopy (Phase contrast and DIC microscopy) triumphed by a wide boundary in ISBI 2015 hosted the Grand Challenge for Computer-Automated Detection of Caries in Bitewing Radiography and the Cell Tracking Challenge.

U-Net comprises a constricting path (the left side) and an increasing path (the right side). The path of constricting conforms to the standard construction of a convolutional network. It is composed of repeated applications as described in [34]. Figure 2 shows the basic U-Net network architecture. The arrows symbolize many operations. The blue squares indicate the feature maps in each layer, whereas the white squares represent the feature maps removed from the constricting path. It is composed of the recurrent use of two 3 × 3 convolutions (bearingless convolutions), each after a rectified linear unit (ReLU) and a 2 × 2 maximum pooling operation with two steps

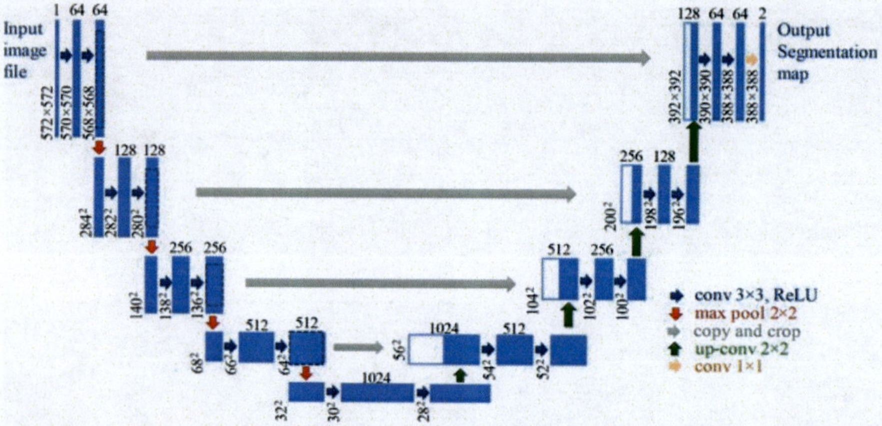

Fig. 2 Basic U-Net architecture [34]

for downsampling. Each successive step of downsampling doubles the total amount of feature channels. Each action along the extensive route includes a feature map upsample. This 2 × 2 ("up-convolution") convolution separations the total amount of specialized channels, a merge with an appropriately trimmed map of features from the contract pathway, and two 3 × 3 convolutions, each accompanied by a ReLU. Trimming is necessary because of the loss of boundary pixels during each convolution. In the topmost layer, the 1 × 1 convolution is utilized to convert each feature vector with 64 components into the necessary categories. The network consists of twenty-three convolutional layers in total.

This study uses a convolution network topology with a 2-dimensional type because the input is a digital image with two dimensions from the slices. Convolution is a mathematical process that requires two function inputs. The convolution operation in the time domain function (t) is usually denoted by an asterisk shown in Eq. 1 [35].

$$s(t) = (x * w)(t) \tag{1}$$

The initial argument to convolution (in this example, function x) is typically mentioned as input and the kernel's second parameter (w). Sometimes, the output is represented as a map of features.

The time index is restricted to integer values. We may now describe discrete convolutions if we adopt that x and w are specified solely on integers t. Equation 1 can then be rewritten as Eq. 2, known as a discrete convolution.

$$s(t) = (x * w)(t) = \sum_{a=-\infty}^{\infty} x(a)w(t-a) \tag{2}$$

Typically, a data array with multiple dimensions is the input. The kernel is a multi-dimensional range of learning algorithm-adapted parameters in machine learning applications. Since each member of the input and kernel must be independently and specifically saved, these functions are always believed to be null other than in the stored points. In reality, infinite addition can be implemented as the sum of a finite number of array members employing a kernel with two dimensions, K, when a two-dimensional image is utilized, I as input. Convolution is commutative, so Eq. 3 can be rewritten as Eq. 4.

$$S(i, j) = (I * K)(i, j) = \sum_m \sum_n I(m, n)K(i - m, j - n) \tag{3}$$

$$S(i, j) = (K * I)(i, j) = \sum_m \sum_n I(i - m, j - n)K(m, n) \tag{4}$$

The following formulation is simpler to incorporate in artificial intelligence libraries because the range of valid m and n values is less variable.

Backbones. Backbone is the name of the classification model (without the final dense layer) used to extract segmentation model features [36]—Keras models for image segmentation with pre-trained backbones. The backbones used in this study are:

VGG-19. Visual Geometry Group Network (VGG-Net) is a CNN co-created by the Visual Geometry Group at the University of Oxford and Google DeepMind [37]. VGG-Net thoroughly evaluated the depth enhancement network using an architecture with 3 × 3 convolutional kernels and 2 × 2 pooling layers. The VGG-19 is a refinement of the VGG-16 model. It is a CNN model with 19 layers. It is built by stacking convolutions, but the model's depth is limited due to a diminishing gradient problem. Figure 3 shows networks of deep convolutional neurons based on VGG-19 architecture.

ResNet50. A residual Neural Network (ResNet) is a type of Artificial Neural Network (ANN) that contains residual blocks stacked in a network [38]. A ResNet transforms a standard network into its residual counterpart by inserting shortcut connections. The ResNet-50 model is one of CNN's popular deep residual networks with a depth of 50 layers. Along with 1 Max Pool layer and 1 Average Pool layer, ResNet50 features 48 Convolution layers. Table 1 shows the ResNet-50 architecture in detail.

Inception-V3. In the 2014 ImageNet Large-Scale Visual Recognition Challenge (ILSVRC14), Szegedy et al. [39] developed a deep convolutional neural network architecture dubbed Inception, which set a new benchmark for classification and detection. This design is distinguished by its greater exploitation of network computing resources. Inception-V3 is a CNN design that adds label smoothing and factored 7 × 7 convolutions, among other enhancements [40]. The Inception-V3 model, which has 42 layers and a lower error rate than its precursors, was released in 2015. Table 2 depicts the Inception-V3 network's construction with Inception modules in Fig. 4.

Inception-ResNetV2. Inception-ResNet-V2 is a convolutional neural architecture based on the Inception architecture family. That replaces the filter concatenation step

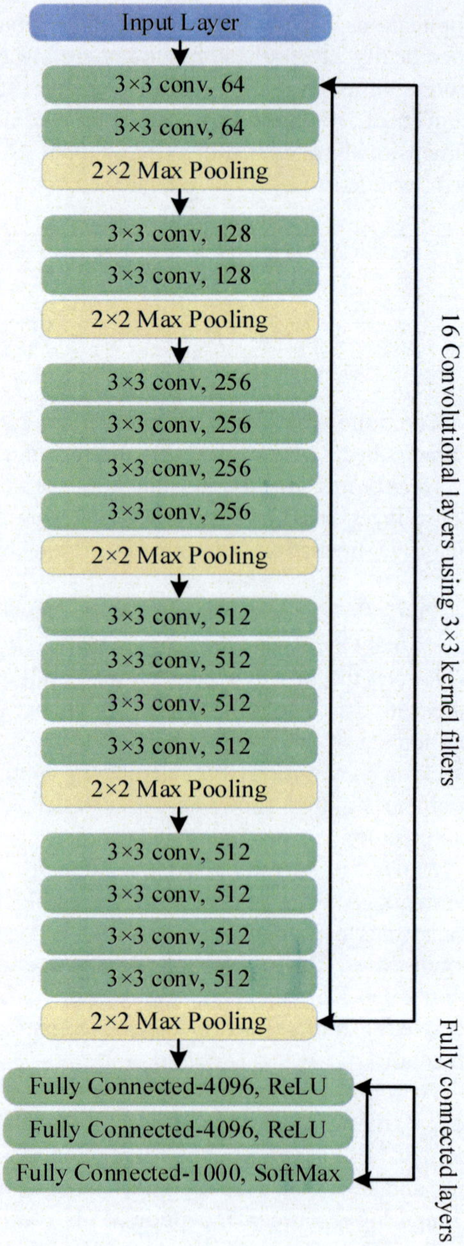

Fig. 3 VGG-19 architecture [42] based on conv-net configuration in [37]

Table 1 Construction for ResNet-50 [38]

Layer name	Output size	50-layer
conv1	112 × 112	7 × 7, 64, stride 2
conv2_x	56 × 56	3 × 3 max pool, stride 2
		$\begin{bmatrix} 1 \times 1, 64 \\ 3 \times 3, 64 \\ 1 \times 1, 256 \end{bmatrix} \times 3$
conv3_x	28 × 28	$\begin{bmatrix} 1 \times 1, 128 \\ 3 \times 3, 128 \\ 1 \times 1, 512 \end{bmatrix} \times 4$
conv4_x	14 × 14	$\begin{bmatrix} 1 \times 1, 256 \\ 3 \times 3, 256 \\ 1 \times 1, 1024 \end{bmatrix} \times 6$
conv5_x	7 × 7	$\begin{bmatrix} 1 \times 1, 512 \\ 3 \times 3, 512 \\ 1 \times 1, 2048 \end{bmatrix} \times 4$
	1 × 1	Average pool, 1000d-FC, SoftMax

Table 2 The construction of the Inception-V3 network [40]. The size of each output module equals the input size of the following module

Type	Patch size/stride	Input size
Conv	3 × 3/2	299 × 299 × 3
Conv	3 × 3/1	149 × 149 × 32
Conv padded	3 × 3/1	147 × 147 × 32
Pool	3 × 3/2	147 × 147 × 64
Conv	3 × 3/1	73 × 73 × 64
Conv	3 × 3/2	71 × 71 × 80
Conv	3 × 3/1	35 × 35 × 192
3 × Inception	Figure 4a	35 × 35 × 288
5 × Inception	Figure 4b	17 × 17 × 768
2 × Inception	Figure 4c	8 × 8 × 1280
Pool	8 × 8	8 × 8 × 2048
Linear	Logits	1 × 1 × 2048
Softmax		1 × 1 × 1000

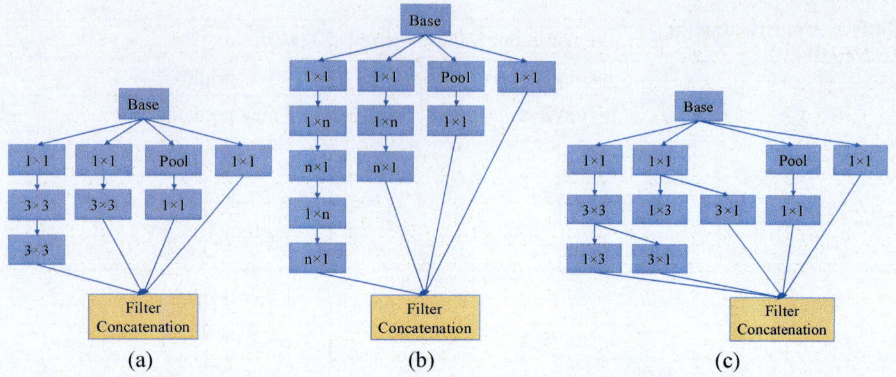

Fig. 4 Inception modules [40]. **a** Replacing each 5 × 5 convolution with two 3 × 3 convolutions. **b** Following factoring of the n × n convolutions. **c** With more significant outputs from the filter bank

of the Inception architecture with residual networks [41]. In the Inception-Resnet chunk, residual connections integrate different sizes of convolutional filters. Not only does the introduction of residual networks eliminate the issue of deterioration induced by deep structures, but it also saves training time. The large-scale structure of Inception-Resnet-V2 has seen in Fig. 5. The stem block refers to the initial operations executed before introducing the Inception blocks. A filter-expansion layer follows each Inception block (1 × 1 convolution devoid of stimulation) that is used to enhance the previous dimension of the filter bank to correspond with the input's depth. In Inception-ResNet, batch-normalization is only applied in addition to the normal layers, not summations. The main Inception module's pooling operation in the reduction block is replaced to identify the remaining connections.

2.3 Research Methods

The research method describes the performance of deep learning in the segmentation of brain tumors. Brain tumor images are segmented using U-Net-based architectures after preprocessing enhances the input images.

Preprocessing. 2D Convolutions are essential for developing CNN and for standard image processing filters, such as blurring, sharpening, and edge identification. They utilize a kernel and iterate through an input image to generate an output image. 2D convolution blocks offer layers that can identify spatial information in an image and work directly with image data or output from previous convolution blocks. This study creates a 2D convolution and then uses it to segment an image using the kernel.

The amount of BraTS2020 dataset is organized into T1, T2, T1ce, and FLAIR sequences. 2D slices from the axial, coronal, and sagittal perspectives comprise 3D MRI images. Only 2D slices of axial anatomic visualization were used as input in

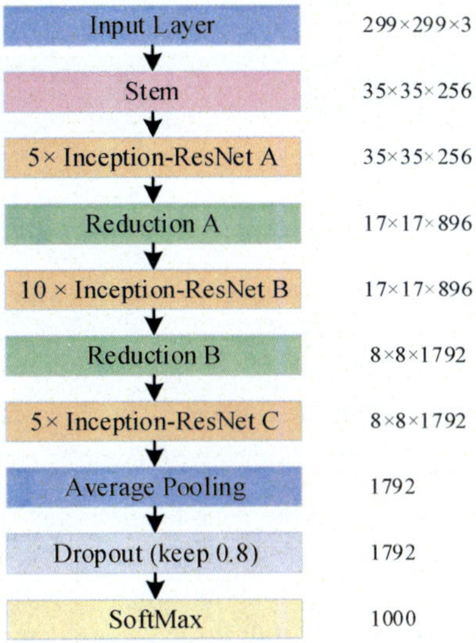

Fig. 5 Schema for InceptionResNet-v2 networks [41]

this study because only these slices had the information needed to differentiate tumor tissue. There are 155 slices per volume. Each 2D image slice is segmented using a variety of image modalities. Therefore, patches of 128 × 128 pixels were created. The patches were all focused on a single pixel that was categorized. The initial and end slices of a completely black MR image and no brain image do not apply. Therefore, black slices are removed during the initial phase of preprocessing. So, to start at five and use 145 slices means we skip the first five and last five slices. Each input was composed of patches with four modalities. Then, image normalization is conducted due to the relatively high-intensity levels across MRI slices. The slices are shown in four sequences, and the ground truth is displayed in Fig. 6.

The types of brain tumors are as follows: (1) necrotic, (2) edema, (3) not enhancing tumor, and (4) enhancing tumor. The tumor is divided into three groups for segmentation analysis: (1) the Whole tumor containing all four tumor areas, (2) The tumor's core section arranged of necrotic, enhancing tumor, and decreasing tumors, and (3) Enhancing tumor composed only of the enhancing area. Background or not tumor (label 0), Non-enhancing Tumor (label 1), Edema (label 2), and Enhancing tumor

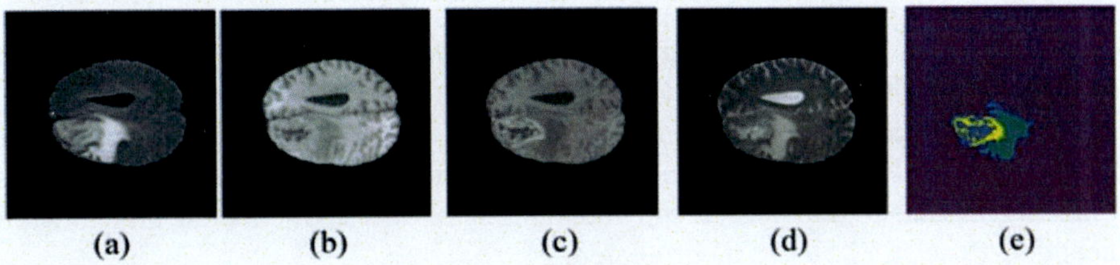

Fig. 6 Samples of brain tumors using four MRI sequences **a** FLAIR, **b** T1, **c** T1ce, **d** T2, and **e** the ground truth of tumor boundaries drawn by the doctors

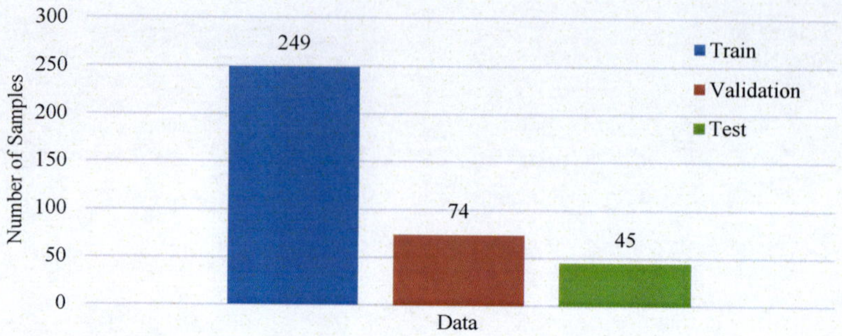

Fig. 7 Distribution of data

(label 4) are the four labeled classes that Jiang et al. [43] apply to the segmented images. In the implementation, the enhancing tumor label 4 was changed to label 3 to sort the labels during computation. In addition, the training data was divided automatically into three parts in the training process, with details of 20% of the data chosen for validation, 15% for model testing, and the rest for training. Figure 7 shows the distribution of data for the training stage.

Training and Implementation. U-Net is trained in the GPU. First, the training was carried out on a simple U-Net model. Then, the next stage combines the popular deep CNN model U-Net with classifier models pre-trained as a backbone, such as VGG19, ResNet50, Inception-V3, and InceptionResnetV2. VGG19-UNet is a pre-trained combination of VGG19 with U-Net. The VGG19 is pre-trained on a larger dataset. ImageNet, making learning new and complicated designs straightforward and efficient. The encoder component of UNET is the pre-trained VGG19, subsequently, the decoder component.

ResNet50-UNet is a model for semantic segmentation inspired by deep residual learning and U-Net [44], an architecture that utilizes both the Residual and U-Net models. The residual unit will facilitate network training. There are three components to the ResNet50-UNet network: encoding, bridging, and decoding. First, the input image is encoded into a compact form. The middle region serves as a link between the encoding and decoding paths. The last component restores the representation to a pixel-based categorization. A residual unit composed of two 3 × 3 convolution blocks and identity mapping is utilized to generate the three components. Each convolution block contains a layer of batch normalization, a layer of ReLU activation, and a layer of convolution. Identification mapping links the units' inputs and outputs.

The following model is a novel end-to-end U-Net-based brain tumor segmentation architecture that incorporates the Inception module InceptionV3-UNet is the theoretical method for reaching a solution employing InceptionV3 as the backbone with ImageNet-trained weights and U-Net as the segmentation technique. The following U-Net architecture is the foundation for the segmentation model with Inception-ResNet-v2 blocks incorporated.

We have utilized the loss function with categorical cross-entropy, Adam optimizer with 0.001 learning rate, and batch normalization to boost the network's normalization and stability in every layer of our model. The model was trained using an NVIDIA DGX-1 equipped with Tesla V100 GPUs. Our project was built with Keras with a Tensorflow backend. Keras Applications are available deep learning models that include pre-trained weights. Even the widely used programming language Python is compatible with these libraries and uses the Jupyter notebook.

During the testing phase, testing data are added to the model in order to identify tumors in brain images. The proposed model is compared to different methods using assessment measures. Pixel accuracy, mean IoU, dice similarity coefficient, precision, sensitivity, and specificity were occupied to assess the effectiveness of the proposed approach for predicting tumor areas. Conceptually, pixel accuracy is likely the simplest to grasp. It is the percentage of correctly categorized pixels in an image. The Jaccard index, another name for intersection-over-union (IoU), is a widely used metric for assessing the accuracy of a proposed image segmentation relative to a known/ground-truth segmentation. IoU is preferred over accuracy in segmentation tasks because the underlying class imbalance negatively impacts foreground/background segmentation tasks. The dice represent the region of overlap between the input and target images. Precision represents the proportion of anticipated entire tumors with a matching ground truth segment.

3 Result

We simulate the BraTS 2020 dataset for segmenting brain tumors from MRI images. Simple U-Net, VGG19-UNet, ResNet50-UNet, InceptionV3-UNet, and InceptionResnetV2-UNet were among the deep learning models whose performance was compared. The test results were analyzed from various perspectives to confirm the proposed network's performance for segmenting images of brain tumors.

During the training process, 65% of the sample is chosen randomly for training, and the remainder is used to test and validate. It was repeated ten times for each architecture, and the average scores for the evaluation criteria were published. Figure 8 represents a graph of the training accuracy and validation of the suggested model. This graph shows that The suggested model succeeds with excellent accuracy during training, although the convergence is different. The loss function is computed for the datasets for training and validation.

Figure 9 shows training and validation loss in a different model. The number of computational mistakes in the validation data also increases as the number of epochs in the proposed network training buildups. Therefore, the optimal number of training the proposed model's epochs is twenty. It suggests that convergence is more rapid than the U-Net structure.

After the training process is complete, the next step is to perform tests to predict the segmented area. Tests are carried out randomly on the selected test data. The preparation of data for prediction is done before testing. The data used for testing

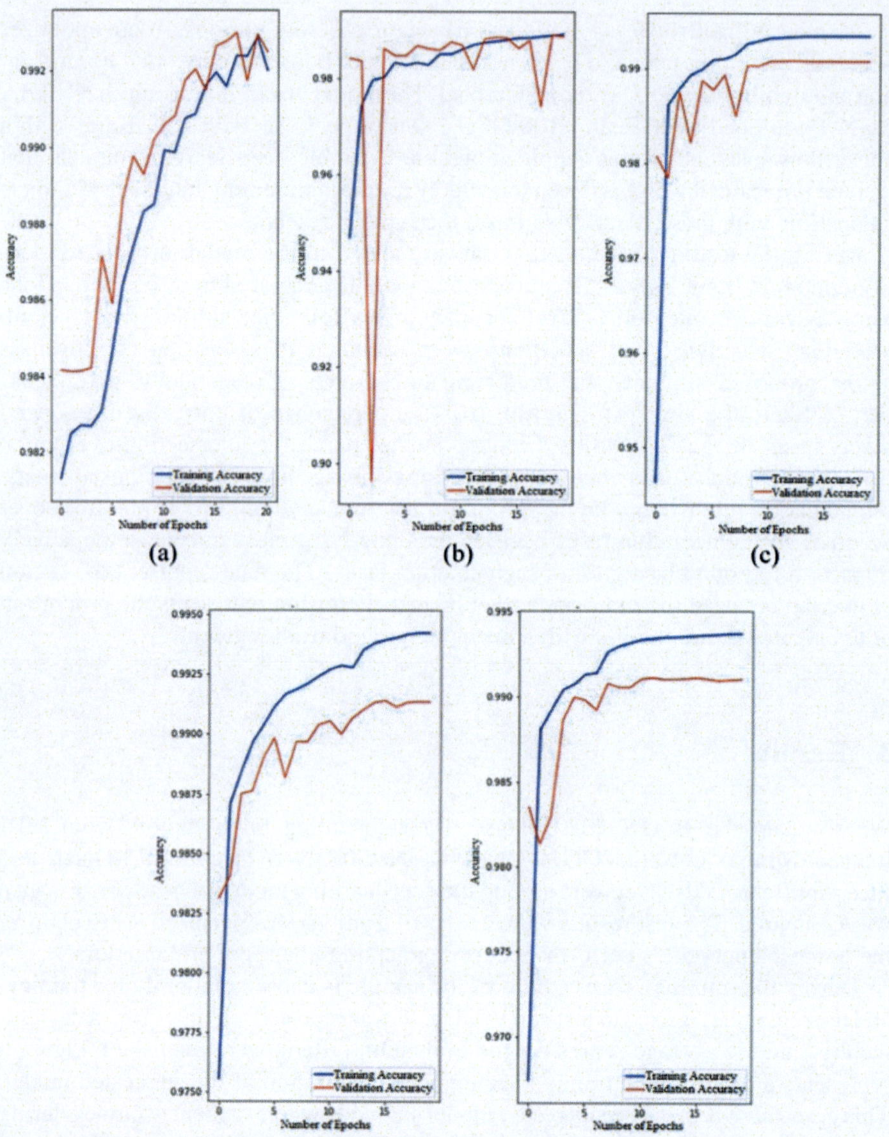

Fig. 8 Accuracy in training and validation in different models. **a** Simple U-Net, **b** VGG19-UNet, **c** ResNet50-UNet, **d** InceptionV3-UNet, and **e** InceptionResnetV2-UNet

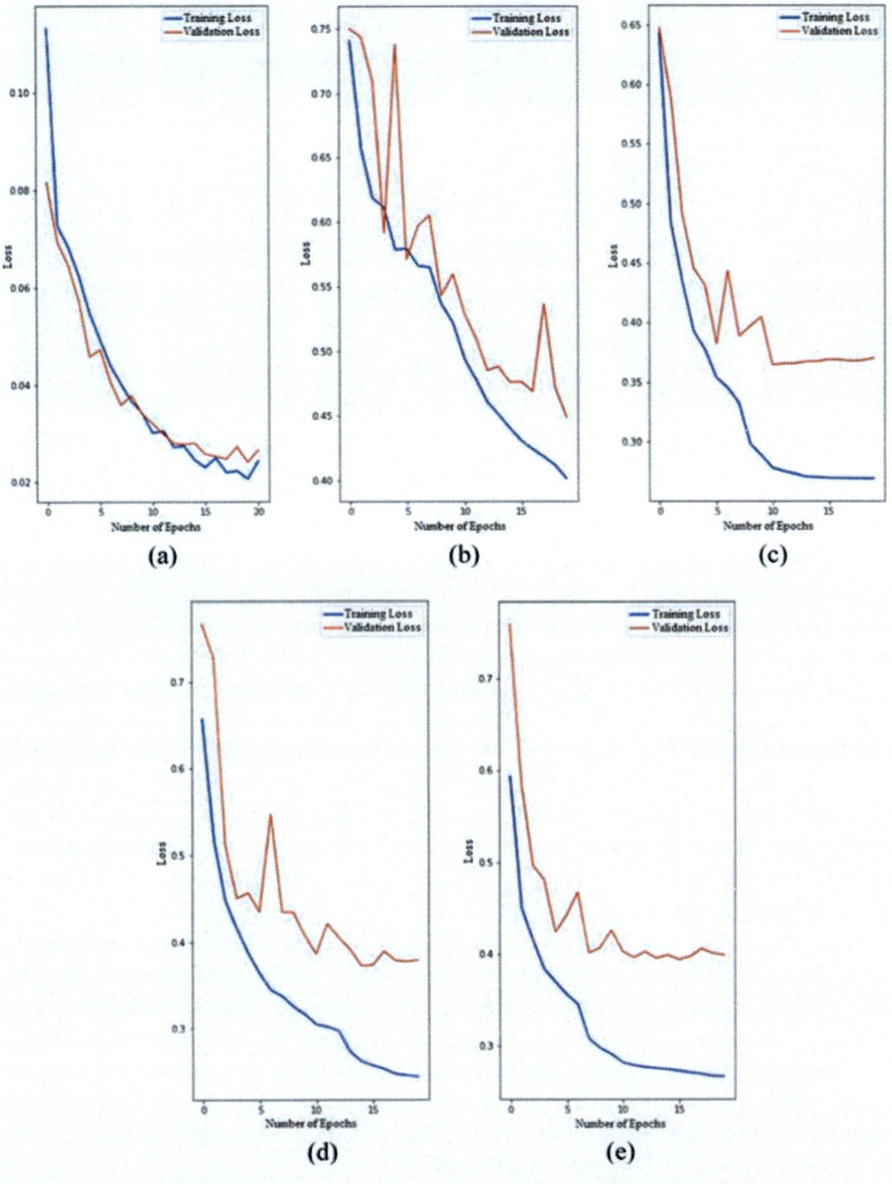

Fig. 9 Training and validation loss in different models. **a** Simple U-Net, **b** VGG19-UNet, **c** ResNet50-UNet, **d** InceptionV3-UNet, and **e** InceptionResnetV2-UNet

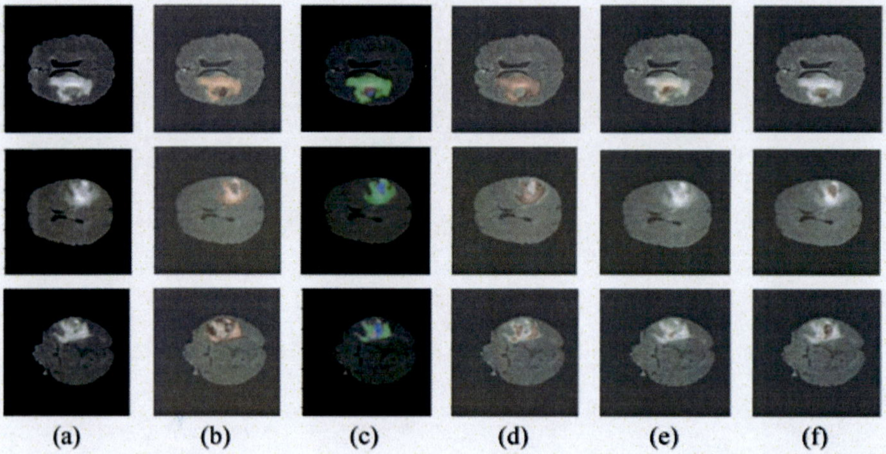

Fig. 10 Result of segmentation. **a** Original FLAIR, **b** the ground truth, **c** all predicted classes, **d** necrotic/core predicted, **e** edema predicted, and **f** enhancing tumor predicted

include sequences from FLAIR, T1ce, and ground truth. FLAIR and T1ce were the most significant sequences to see the presence of tumors. Almost all brain imaging protocols include the FLAIR sequence, which is particularly beneficial for detecting tiny alterations in the hemispheres' perimeter and the periventricular region adjacent to the Cerebrospinal Fluid (CSF). While the T1ce sequence is a T1 signal given by gadolinium-based contrast agents to provide a contrast-enhancing effect on tumors, the area of inflammation/infection appears brighter than the surrounding tissue. Then, show the predicted data using the FLAIR sequence because the whole tumor area is visible in the FLAIR sequence. Figure 10 shows three samples of random test results. The tumor is segmented as a whole and divided into three sub-areas: necrotic/core tumor, edema, and enhancing.

Experiments were carried out on the proposed model with the previously indicated optimizations on training and validation images, and the model was validated using the test dataset. The model's performance is assessed using six metrics: metric accuracy, mean IoU, dice coefficient, precision, sensitivity, and specificity. Table 3 contains the evaluation metrics determined from all the assessment measures for whole tumor segmentation in the model used in this paper. Table 4 compares the deep learning model performance of the two similarity metrics used in the comparison set, including the mean IoU and dice coefficient.

From Table 3, it can be seen that all models have satisfactory performance above 98.8% during the segmentation process. However, in different conditions, when looking at the mean IoU performance in Table 4, simple U-Net and InceptionResnetV2-UNet show comparable performance, which is 0.838 and 0.859, respectively. Meanwhile, when viewed from the dice coefficient, VGG19-UNet showed the worst performance with a dice of 0.557. When segmenting three tumor sub-areas (necrotic, edema, and tumor enhancing), VGG19-UNet also showed the

Table 3 Evaluation metrics of deep learning models on the test dataset

Model	Accuracy (%)	Precision (%)	Sensitivity (%)	Specificity (%)
Simple U-Net	99.3	99.4	99.2	99.8
VGG19-UNet	98.8	98.8	98.8	99.6
ResNet50-UNet	99.2	99.2	99.1	99.7
InceptionV3-UNet	99.2	99.2	99.2	99.7
InceptionResnetV2-UNet	99.1	99.2	98.9	99.7

Table 4 The mean IoU and dice coefficient of segmentation results

Model	Mean IoU	Dice
Simple U-Net	0.838	0.621
VGG19-UNet	0.518	0.557
ResNet50-UNet	0.429	**0.698**
InceptionV3-UNet	0.623	0.660
InceptionResnetV2-UNet	**0.859**	0.600

worst performance, as shown in Fig. 11. It can be influenced by a considerable number of variables owned by VGG19, thus affecting the prediction results.

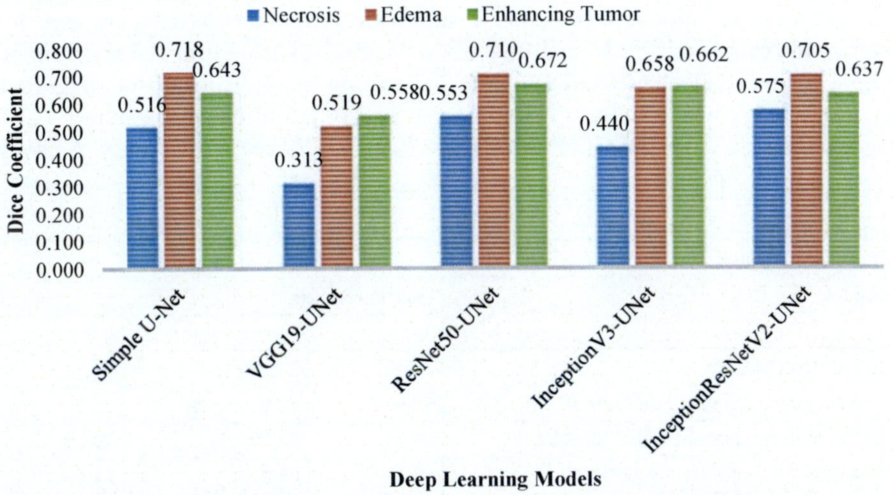

Fig. 11 Dice coefficient for three areas of brain tumor are shown: necrosis, edema, and enhancing tumor on different backbones

4 Discussion

Based on the quantification metrics shown in Table 3, the whole tumor segmentation showed an outstanding performance. However, based on Table 4 regarding similarity metrics, the performance is not excellent. Many factors can influence it.

Table 5 compares model performance with the most recent techniques for dice coefficient scores on the BraTS 2020 dataset. In an article [45], Ullah et al. introduced a wholly automated segmentation approach for identifying areas of brain tumors utilizing multi-scale residual attention-UNet (MRA-UNet). MRA-UNet uses three successive slices as inputs to arrange information in sequential order. In addition, the adaptive region of interest was utilized in conjunction with cascade multi-scale learning to segment improved and specific core tumor regions. This method yielded cutting-edge results on the BraTS2020 dataset, with mean dice scores of 90.18%, 87.22%, and 86.7%, respectively, for the overall tumor, tumor core, and enhanced tumor region. Jun et al. [46] suggested an additional automatic method for segmenting brain tumors with a diversity of 3D U-Net. This model uses a redesigned attention block to fine-tune the rendering of the feature map along a passing bond consisting of a spatial attention block and a channel with parallel connections. Enhancing tumor, entire tumor, and tumor core dice coefficients reached 0.752, 0.879, and 0.779, respectively. Utilizing densely coupled blocks encoding and decoding paths, Ahmad et al. [47] modified the UNet architecture for brain tumor segmentation. This section pulls multi-contextual data from the notion of feature reuse. Furthermore, to excerpt local and global information, residual-inception blocks (RIB) are used by integrating characteristics from different-sized kernels. The multimodal brain tumor segmentation challenge (BRATS) for the 2020 assay dataset validated the suggested architecture. A whole tumor (WT), tumor core (TC), and enhancing tumor (ET) each had a dice score (DSC) of 89.12%, 84.74%, and 79.0%, respectively. A novel

Table 5 Comparison of proposed models to previous deep learning segmentation models on the BraTS 2020 dataset

Model	Dice coefficient (%)		
	WT	TC	ET
MRA-UNet [45]	90.18	87.22	86.74
U-Net with dual path attention [46]	87.9	77.9	75.2
U-Net with residual-inception blocks [47]	89.12	84.74	79.12
Modality-Pairing Network [48]	89.1	84.2	81.6
Proposed	Edema	Necrotic/TC	ET
Simple U-Net	71.8	51.6	64.3
VGG19-UNet	51.9	31.3	55.8
ResNet50-UNet	71.0	55.3	67.2
InceptionV3-UNet	65.8	44.0	66.2
InceptionResnetV2-UNet	70.5	57.5	63.7

end-to-end learning approach based on modalities for brain tumor segmentation was projected by Wang et al. [48]. Paralleled branches are designed to exploit the unique characteristics of each modality, and numerous layer dealings are used to imprison the intricate interactions and copious amounts of data between sense modalities. They employ a loss of constancy to reduce the difference in calculation between the two branches.

The model proposed in this study uses a 2D CNN-based U-Net architecture for brain tumor segmentation. The performance generated by the proposed model shows a difference. In deep learning, many factors can affect a model's performance, including optimization, loss functions, parameter initialization, hyperparameter tuning, and regularization.

In most deep learning tasks, training and validation accuracy and training and validation losses are usually visualized together in a graph. The goal is to diagnose the model's performance and identify which aspects need to be tuned. Training accuracy and validation were measured to evaluate model fitting. The model is overfitting when there is a significant difference between the two. The validation accuracy must be equal to or slightly less than the training accuracy to be a better model. Figure 8 shows the training and validation accuracy where two simple U-Net models and VGG19-UNet are overfitting.

Meanwhile, the ResNet50-UNet, InceptionV3-UNet, and InceptionResnetV2-UNet models do not converge. Figure 9 shows that the validation loss is greater than the training loss in almost all models except the simple U-Net model. It may indicate that the model does not fit properly. Underfitting occurs when the model cannot accurately model the training data, resulting in a significant error. The amount of data used during training has a significant effect. In this study, 249 samples of 3D MR images were used for training data sliced into 2D images. An insufficient amount of data affects accuracy and loss during training. These results indicate that further training is needed to reduce losses incurred during training or increase training data by obtaining more samples or adding data. The success of the training largely determines the performance of the testing.

In addition to data, the loss function is an essential component of deep learning model training. They measure the extent to which the trained model completes the designated task. In part, the loss function determines the characteristics studied by the model and can be used to train models capable of delivering impressive clinical outcomes when matched to the task. This study looked at the type of loss function used as categorical cross-entropy. Considering that not all loss functions are substantial for all segmentation tasks, the solution to this problem, the loss function used, must be examined.

The model parameters are studied as part of the training process. Tuning parameters can affect the training process. It can be beneficial by increasing model accuracy and reducing model run time.

On the other hand, hyperparameter settings are essential for the model. Hyperparameter values are set before the training and do not change during training. Hyperparameters play an essential function in the research of models because they straight influence the deep learning model's training behavior and positively impact training performance. For example, if the model's learning rate is remarkably rapid, it will likely collide. The required data pattern will likely be lost if it is low. Therefore, selecting appropriate hyperparameters is essential for successful deep learning architecture training because poor choice of hyperparameters can result in inaccurate learning. Before doing the training, many things need to be adjusted.

This study has limitations in training data because the augmentation process is not carried out. Whereas the availability of data significantly affects the training process. Before choosing a model, it also significantly influences factors that affect the training process, as explained earlier in this discussion section. It has implications for the segmentation model's performance. For example, VGG-19 has the largest hyperparameter as opposed to other models. The outcomes suggest that the model's performance is the lowest among others.

5 Conclusion

In this paper, we compare the performance of deep learning models for brain tumor segmentation. The deep learning architecture model is based on U-Net with two dimensions of a CNN. The simple U-Net model is compared with the modified model of the pre-trained classifier as the encoder and U-Net as the decoder. The outcomes demonstrated that the efficiency of the five models tested to segment the whole tumor area achieved a high level of pixel accuracy of 98.8–99.3%, a precision of 98.8–99.4%, the sensitivity of 98.8–99.2%, and a specificity of 99.6–99.8%. For similarity metrics, simple U-Net, VGG19-UNet, ResNet50-UNet, InceptionV3-UNet, and InceptionResNetV2-UNet attained mean IoU values of 0.838, 0.518, 0.429, 0.623, and 0.859, respectively. Meanwhile, the dice coefficient metrics for each model respectively reached 0.621, 0.557, 0.698, 0.660, and 0.600. In conclusion, all models can be implemented effectively for brain tumor segmentation in the BraTS2020 dataset. When the model segmented area by class, the VGG19-UNet, when compared to other models, this model performed the worst. It could be due to the many hyperparameters owned by VGG19. The amount of training data, loss function, parameter tuning, and hyperparameters greatly affect the performance of the segmentation model.

This research still has many inadequacies, so it needs to be developed again to get better performance. The following research is to perform dataset augmentation to increase the training data and modify the network architecture.

Acknowledgements This research work is funded by The Directorate of Research, Universitas Gadjah Mada, through the Research Grant of "Program Rekognisi Tugas Akhir". The authors would like to thank the Intelligent Systems Research Group in the Department of Electrical and Information Engineering for inspiring discussion and motivation.

References

1. Mittal M, Goyal LM, Kaur S, Kaur I, Verma A, Jude Hemanth D (2019) Deep learning based enhanced tumor segmentation approach for MR brain images. Appl Soft Comput 78:346–354. https://doi.org/10.1016/j.asoc.2019.02.036
2. Işın A, Direkoğlu C, Şah M (2016) Review of MRI-based brain tumor image segmentation using deep learning methods. Procedia Comput Sci 102:317–324
3. Wadhwa A, Bhardwaj A, Singh Verma V (2019) A review on brain tumor segmentation of MRI images. Magn Reson Imaging 61:247–259. https://doi.org/10.1016/j.mri.2019.05.043
4. Soltaninejad M, Yang G, Lambrou T, Allinson N, Jones TL, Barrick TR, Howe FA, Ye X (2018) Supervised learning based multimodal MRI brain tumour segmentation using texture features from supervoxels. Comput Methods Programs Biomed 157:69–84. https://doi.org/10.1016/j.cmpb.2018.01.003
5. Li YM, Suki D, Hess K, Sawaya R (2016) The influence of maximum safe resection of glioblastoma on survival in 1229 patients: can we do better than gross-total resection? J Neurosurg 124:977–988. https://doi.org/10.3171/2015.5.JNS142087
6. Abd-Ellah MK, Awad AI, Khalaf AAM, Hamed HFA (2019) A review on brain tumor diagnosis from MRI images: Practical implications, key achievements, and lessons learned. Magn Reson Imaging 61:300–318. https://doi.org/10.1016/j.mri.2019.05.028
7. Abdel-Maksoud E, Elmogy M, Al-Awadi R (2015) Brain tumor segmentation based on a hybrid clustering technique. Egypt Informatics J 16:71–81. https://doi.org/10.1016/j.eij.2015.01.003
8. Varuna Shree N, Kumar TNR (2018) Identification and classification of brain tumor MRI images with feature extraction using DWT and probabilistic neural network. Brain Informatics 5:23–30. https://doi.org/10.1007/s40708-017-0075-5
9. Sun L, Zhang S, Chen H, Luo L (2019) Brain tumor segmentation and survival prediction using multimodal MRI scans with deep learning. Front Neurosci 13:1–9. https://doi.org/10.3389/fnins.2019.00810
10. Kamnitsas K, Ledig C, Newcombe VFJ, Simpson JP, Kane AD, Menon DK, Rueckert D, Glocker B (2017) Efficient multi-scale 3D CNN with fully connected CRF for accurate brain lesion segmentation. Med Image Anal 36:61–78. https://doi.org/10.1016/j.media.2016.10.004
11. Tiwari A, Srivastava S, Pant M (2020) Brain tumor segmentation and classification from magnetic resonance images: Review of selected methods from 2014 to 2019. Pattern Recognit Lett 131:244–260. https://doi.org/10.1016/j.patrec.2019.11.020
12. Meola A, Rao J, Chaudhary N, Sharma M, Chang SD (2018) Gold nanoparticles for brain tumor imaging: a systematic review. Front Neurol 9:328
13. Amin J, Sharif M, Yasmin M, Fernandes SL (2020) A distinctive approach in brain tumor detection and classification using MRI. Pattern Recognit Lett 139:118–127. https://doi.org/10.1016/j.patrec.2017.10.036
14. Brindle KM, Izquierdo-García JL, Lewis DY, Mair RJ, Wright AJ (2017) Brain tumor imaging. J Clin Oncol 35:2432–2438. https://doi.org/10.1200/JCO.2017.72.7636
15. Ilunga–Mbuyamba E, Avina–Cervantes JG, Cepeda–Negrete J, Ibarra–Manzano MA, Chalopin C (2017) Automatic selection of localized region-based active contour models using image content analysis applied to brain tumor segmentation. Comput Biol Med 91:69–79. https://doi.org/10.1016/j.compbiomed.2017.10.003
16. Rabeh AB, Benzarti F, Amiri H (2017) Segmentation of brain MRI using active contour model. Int J Imaging Syst Technol 27:3–11. https://doi.org/10.1002/IMA.22205
17. Prashantha SJ, Poornima KM (2019) Automatic pattern discovery of neonatal brain tumor segmentation and abnormalities in MRI sequence. Lect Notes Electr Eng 545:107–116. https://doi.org/10.1007/978-981-13-5802-9_10/COVER
18. Vaishnavee KB, Amshakala K (2015) An automated MRI brain image segmentation and tumor detection using SOM-clustering and proximal support vector machine classifier. ICETECH 2015—2015 IEEE international conference engineering and technology. https://doi.org/10.1109/ICETECH.2015.7275030

19. Spinner T, Schlegel U, Schäfer H, El-Assady M (2020) explAIner: a visual analytics framework for interactive and explainable machine learning. IEEE Trans Vis Comput Graph 26:1064–1074. https://doi.org/10.1109/TVCG.2019.2934629
20. Sun J, Li J, Wang Q, Yang J, Yang T, Huang K, Li J (2020) A deep learning method for MRI brain tumor segmentation. Lect Notes Electr Eng 551:161–169. https://doi.org/10.1007/978-981-15-3250-4_19/COVER
21. Piccialli F, Somma VD, Giampaolo F, Cuomo S, Fortino G (2021) A survey on deep learning in medicine: why, how and when? Inf Fusion 66:111–137. https://doi.org/10.1016/J.INFFUS.2020.09.006
22. Cao C, Liu F, Tan H, Song D, Shu W, Li W, Zhou Y, Bo X, Xie Z (2018) Deep learning and its applications in biomedicine. Genom Proteomics Bioinform 16:17–32. https://doi.org/10.1016/J.GPB.2017.07.003
23. Havaei M, Davy A, Warde-Farley D, Biard A, Courville A, Bengio Y, Pal C, Jodoin P-M, Larochelle H (2017) Brain tumor segmentation with deep neural networks. Med Image Anal 35:18–31. https://doi.org/10.1016/j.media.2016.05.004
24. Razzak MI, Imran M, Xu G (2019) Efficient brain tumor segmentation with multiscale two-pathway-group conventional neural networks. IEEE J Biomed Heal Informatics 23:1911–1919. https://doi.org/10.1109/JBHI.2018.2874033
25. Wang G, Li W, Ourselin S, Vercauteren T (2019) Automatic brain tumor segmentation based on cascaded convolutional neural networks with uncertainty estimation. Front Comput Neurosci 13:56. https://doi.org/10.3389/fncom.2019.00056
26. Deng W, Shi Q, Luo K, Yang Y, Ning N (2019) Brain tumor segmentation based on improved convolutional neural network in combination with non-quantifiable local texture feature. J Med Syst 43. https://doi.org/10.1007/s10916-019-1289-2
27. Ribalta Lorenzo P, Nalepa J, Bobek-Billewicz B, Wawrzyniak P, Mrukwa G, Kawulok M, Ulrych P, Hayball MP (2019) Segmenting brain tumors from FLAIR MRI using fully convolutional neural networks. Comput Methods Programs Biomed 176:135–148. https://doi.org/10.1016/j.cmpb.2019.05.006.
28. Nawaz A, Akram U, Salam AA, Ali AR, Ur Rehman A, Zeb J (2021) VGG-UNET for brain tumor segmentation and ensemble model for survival prediction. In: 2021 international conference on robotics and automation in industry. ICRAI 2021. https://doi.org/10.1109/ICRAI54018.2021.9651367
29. Saha A (2021) Brain tumour segmentation with a muti-pathway ResNet based UNet. J Grid Comput 19. https://doi.org/10.1007/s10723-021-09590-y
30. AboElenein NM, Songhao P, Afifi A (2022) IRDNU-Net: inception residual dense nested u-net for brain tumor segmentation. Multimed Tools Appl 81:24041–24057. https://doi.org/10.1007/S11042-022-12586-9/TABLES/10
31. Nitesh B, Madhuri A, Manogna BS, Babu KNJ, Ishwarya N, Trivendra GM (2022) Brain tumor segmentation using U-net based on inception. In: Proceedings of the 2nd international conference on artificial intelligence and smart energy. ICAIS 2022, pp 908–914. https://doi.org/10.1109/ICAIS53314.2022.9743122
32. Sandhya S, Senthil Kumar M, Chidhambararajan B (2022) Ensemble DNN for the brain tumor segmentation—a hybrid framework centric on layer level and decision level fusion of multi-modal medical images. Lect Notes Electr Eng 905:63–73. https://doi.org/10.1007/978-981-19-2177-3_7
33. Menze BH, Jakab A, Bauer S, Kalpathy-Cramer J, Farahani K, Kirby J, Burren Y, Porz N, Slotboom J, Wiest R, Lanczi L, Gerstner E, Weber MA, Arbel T, Avants BB, Ayache N, Buendia P, Collins DL, Cordier N, Corso JJ, Criminisi A, Das T, Delingette H, Demiralp Ç, Durst CR, Dojat M, Doyle S, Festa J, Forbes F, Geremia E, Glocker B, Golland P, Guo X, Hamamci A, Iftekharuddin KM, Jena R, John NM, Konukoglu E, Lashkari D, Mariz JA, Meier R, Pereira S, Precup D, Price SJ, Raviv TR, Reza SMS, Ryan M, Sarikaya D, Schwartz L, Shin HC, Shotton J, Silva CA, Sousa N, Subbanna NK, Szekely G, Taylor TJ, Thomas OM, Tustison NJ, Unal G, Vasseur F, Wintermark M, Ye DH, Zhao L, Zhao B, Zikic D, Prastawa M, Reyes M, Van Leemput K (2015) The multimodal brain tumor image segmentation benchmark (BRATS). IEEE Trans Med Imaging 34:1993–2024. https://doi.org/10.1109/TMI.2014.2377694

34. Ronneberger O, Fischer P, Brox T (2015) U-Net: Convolutional networks for biomedical image segmentation. Lect Notes Comput Sci (including Subser Lect Notes Artif Intell Lect Notes Bioinformatics) 9351:234–241. https://doi.org/10.1007/978-3-319-24574-4_28
35. Goodfellow I, Bengio Y, Courville A (2016) Deep learning. MIT Press
36. Iakubovskii P (2019) Segmentation models
37. Simonyan K, Zisserman A (2014) Very deep convolutional networks for large-scale image recognition. In: 3rd international conference on learning representation (ICLR) 2015—conference track proc. https://doi.org/10.48550/arxiv.1409.1556
38. He K, Zhang X, Ren S, Sun J (2015) Deep residual learning for image recognition. In: Proceedings of the IEEE computer society conference on computer vision and pattern recognition, pp 770–778. https://doi.org/10.48550/arxiv.1512.03385
39. Szegedy C, Liu W, Jia Y, Sermanet P, Reed S, Anguelov D, Erhan D, Vanhoucke V, Rabinovich A (2015) Going deeper with convolutions. In: Proceedings of the IEEE computer society conference on computer vision and pattern recognition, pp 1–9. https://doi.org/10.1109/CVPR.2015.7298594
40. Szegedy C, Vanhoucke V, Ioffe S, Shlens J, Wojna Z (2015) Rethinking the inception architecture for computer vision. In: Proceedings of the IEEE computer society and conference on computer vision and pattern recognition, pp 2818–2826. https://doi.org/10.1109/CVPR.2016.308
41. Szegedy C, Ioffe S, Vanhoucke V, Alemi AA (2016) Inception-v4, inception-ResNet and the impact of residual connections on learning. In: 31st AAAI conference on artificial intelligence, AAAI 2017, pp 4278–4284. https://doi.org/10.48550/arxiv.1602.07261
42. Leonardo MM, Carvalho TJ, Rezende E, Zucchi R, Faria FA (2019) Deep feature-based classifiers for fruit fly identification (Diptera: Tephritidae). In: Proceedings of the 31st conference on graphics, patterns and images (SIBGRAPI 2018), pp 41–47. https://doi.org/10.1109/SIBGRAPI.2018.00012
43. Jiang M, Zhai F, Kong J (2021) A novel deep learning model DDU-net using edge features to enhance brain tumor segmentation on MR images. Artif Intell Med 121:102180. https://doi.org/10.1016/J.ARTMED.2021.102180
44. Zhang Z, Liu Q, Wang Y (2017) Road extraction by deep residual U-Net. IEEE Geosci Remote Sens Lett 15:749–753. https://doi.org/10.1109/lgrs.2018.2802944
45. Ullah Z, Usman M, Jeon M, Gwak J (2022) Cascade multi-scale residual attention CNNs with adaptive ROI for automatic brain tumor segmentation. Inf Sci (Ny) 608:1541–1556. https://doi.org/10.1016/J.INS.2022.07.044
46. Jun W, Haoxiang X, Wang Z (2021) Brain tumor segmentation using dual-path attention U-net in 3D MRI images. Lect Notes Comput. Sci. (including Subser. Lect. Notes Artificial Intelligence on Lecture Notes Bioinformatics), vol 12658. LNCS, pp 183–193. https://doi.org/10.1007/978-3-030-72084-1_17/COVER
47. Ahmad P, Qamar S, Shen L, Saeed A (2021) Context aware 3D UNet for brain tumor segmentation. Lect. Notes Comput. Sci. (including Subser. Lecture Notes on Artificial Intelligence on Lecture Notes Bioinformatics). 12658 LNCS, pp 207–218. https://doi.org/10.1007/978-3-030-72084-1_19/COVER
48. Wang Y, Zhang Y, Hou F, Liu Y, Tian J, Zhong C, Zhang Y, He Z (2021) Modality-pairing learning for brain tumor segmentation. Lecture Notes on Computer Science (including Subser. Lecture Notes on Artificial Intelligence on Lecture Notes Bioinformatics). 12658 LNCS, pp 230–240. https://doi.org/10.1007/978-3-030-72084-1_21/COVER

Hand Gesture Recognition Using FMCW Radar and Deep Learning for Understanding Deaf Sign Language

Bagas Wibisono, Fiky Y. Suratman, and Istiqomah

Abstract People have difficulty in understanding sign language of deaf people therefore a technology is needed to translate sign language to help deaf people. In Indonesia, society lacks fluency in national sign languages like Indonesian Sign Language (SIBI), which can affect their self-confidence and social interaction skills with others. Previous studies generally used a camera in dataset retrieval in sign language recognition. There is a weakness in using the camera because it has to pay attention to environmental conditions, such as being influenced by light intensity. Radar can correct this deficiency because it uses electromagnetic waves. In this study proposed, the use of uRAD radar by Antheral based on radar Frequency Modulated Continuous Wave (FMCW) to detect and then collect words of SIBI for raw data that is IQ signals. The proposed technique applies the preprocessing methods for the frequency-domain IQ signals of radar echoes as input to a convolutional neural network (CNN). The system designed is able to classify five words of Indonesian Sign Language into five classes. Thereafter compare three self-constructed architectures to find the best model with differences in the number of convolution and pooling layers in each architecture. The results of the proposed architectural classification show the movement classification accuracy exceeds more than 98%. This study has high accuracy because of the proposed preprocessing method and compares several CNN architectures whose accuracy is higher than previous studies which also used radar. Based on the results, the proposed system can be helpful in understanding deaf sign language with SIBI.

Keywords Indonesian sign language recognition · uRAD radar · Convolution neural network

B. Wibisono (✉) · F. Y. Suratman · Istiqomah
School of Electrical Engineering, Telkom University, Bandung, Indonesia
e-mail: bagaswibisono@student.telkomuniversity.ac.id

T. Triwiyanto et al. (eds.), *Proceeding of the 3rd International Conference on Electronics, Biomedical Engineering, and Health Informatics*, Lecture Notes in Electrical Engineering 1008, https://doi.org/10.1007/978-981-99-0248-4_25

1 Introduction

Hand gesture, a natural and instinctive form of interpersonal communication, is considered an ideal method of human–computer interaction (HCI) [1–3]. In the field of HCI, human hand gesture recognition (HGR) has tremendous significance in facilitating applications in different areas, from biomedical engineering [4] to smart houses [5], and sign language recognition. The lack of knowledge of Sign Language in society made the deaf have communication difficulties. So, to ruin this barrier of communication, there needs to be a system that can allow the conversion of sign language. Indonesia has 2 types of sign language, one of which is Indonesian Sign Language (SIBI), the commonly and officially used sign language in Indonesia [6]. SIBI is basically Indonesian language which is expressed by gestures, and SIBI is based on Indonesian grammar [7].

Research on building a model to recognize SIBI gestures has been proposed several times. Several techniques have been developed to create a high-accuracy system, such as computer vision [8, 9] and leap motion [10–12]. Those techniques have achieved high accuracy with a combined machine or deep learning. But there are weaknesses such as with different backgrounds and light conditions, may be less accurate, causing high reliance on environmental conditions and being susceptible to conditions of low visibility [13, 14]. Compared with the techniques mentioned above, radar has been proposed as an alternate technique for recognizing sign language because it can detect targets without light conditions.

Some studies have been carried out in sign language recognition using radar. In [15], gesture recognition used IQ signals preprocessed by the doppler radar signal amplitude threshold detection and spectral analysis. The final result showed five gestures with an average accuracy of 95%. There are two convolutional layers and two fully connected layers for designing only one architecture CNN network to classify the proposed hand gestures. In [16], gesture recognition used radar based on X-band Doppler radar transceiver to capture and extracted with DAQ system. Comparison between deep convolution neural network (DCNN) and VGG-16 algorithm. The accuracy was 87.5 and 95% in each algorithm. In [17] used the CW radar system for hand gesture recognition. To classify using the CNN method with one architecture. The result achieved high accuracy of 96.6%. However, in this study, the preprocessing is not thoroughly explained, and there is no comparison with various architectures of CNN.

To provide solutions to the above problems, this study proposes to be able to develop recognizing an Indonesian Sign Language system using uRAD radar by Anteral based on FMCW radar using in-phase (I)-quadrature (Q) signals for raw data. The IQ signal will go through preprocessing before it can use as a dataset in CNN. The preprocessing stage is signal attenuation from dc components, windowed by Fast Fourier Transform (FFT) to change from a time domain to a frequency domain and then statics clutter must be removed. The spectrograms will be cropped for the only target, i.e., hand gesture information. Then the results will be cropped into multiple spectrograms as input for training using CNN. Deep learning algorithms, Convolution Neural Network for classification, looking for the best model by comparing 3 architectures with the differences in the number of convolutional and pooling layers. The results of the proposed architectural classification show the movement classification accuracy exceeds more than 98%.

The rest of this paper is structured as follows. Section 1 describes the introduction to this paper and relevant studies. Section 2 introduces the radar system, methodology and preprocessing proposed. Section 3 presents experimental results and analysis of CNN architectural design. And discusses study's results are presented in Sect. 4. Finally, we conclude this study in Sect. 5.

2 Materials and Method

2.1 Material

Radar System. The FMCW radar adopted for sign language HGR in this study is the uRAD Raspberry Pi v1.2 radar device by Anteral. uRAD radar is a shield for the Raspberry Pi. uRAD radar is small and can be used as a portable radar. Therefore, it only works in conjunction with a compatible Raspberry Pi [18]. Raspberry Pi 4 is used in radar operations for this study. Figure 1 presents the uRAD Raspberry Pi v1.2 radar board that includes onboard etched antennas with receivers and transmitters, which enables distance information tracking. A frequency ramp is transmitted [19]. Used a FMCW radar transmitter and receiver signals are sawtooth waves [20, 21]. Frequency Modulated Continuous Wave (FMCW) is a radar system that transmits a continuous electromagnetic signal that increases or decreases from a particular frequency value [22]. In uRAD, the radar has an MTI mode, all static objects are ignored, and only moving target information associated with the uRAD is provided. The total reflected signal of the uRAD radar is decomposed in two arrays. There are the In-phase (I) and Quadrature (Q) signals for advanced data signal processing are classified.

SIBI Dataset. There are two main parts of gestures in SIBI, namely the word and finger gestures [23, 24]. In this study, we used word gestures and have prepared our own datasets.

The dataset used in this proposed is five classes on Indonesian Sign Language (SIBI) and a total of 6550 with 1310 for each class which was 400 × 70 matrix for the CNN model. The five classes are: (a) "push", (b) "safe", (c) "worry", (d) "good", (e) "bad". The specific gestures are shown in Fig. 2. The data is split into 75% for training and 25% for testing.

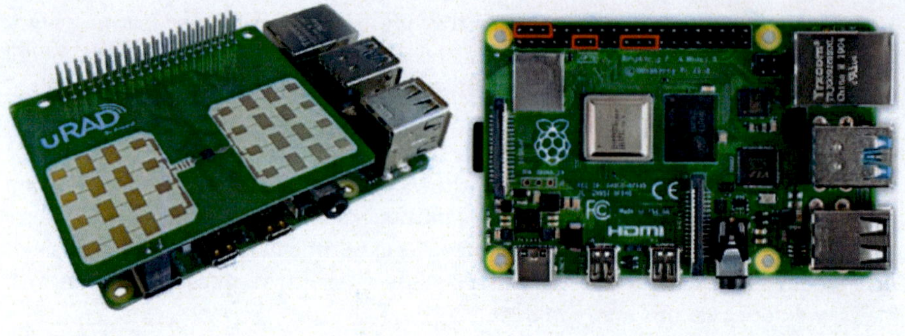

Fig. 1 The uRAD Raspberry Pi v1.2 is based on an FMCW radar board. Topside has the transmitter and receiver antennas. The bottom side consists of power supply and signal processing elements, which are managed by a microcontroller

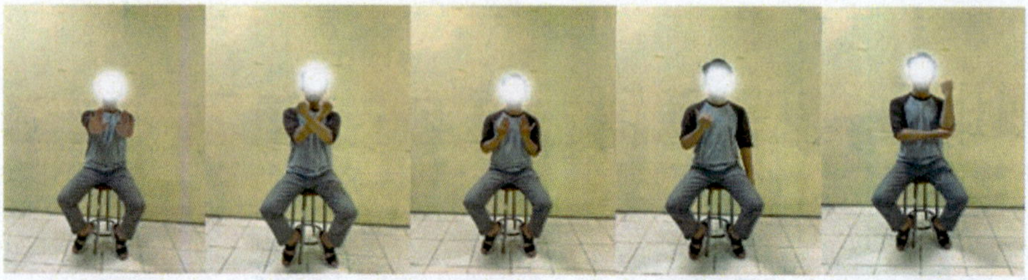

(a) Push (b) Safe (c) Worry (d) Good (e) Bad

Fig. 2 Illustrations of five kinds of word gestures in SIBI

2.2 Experimental Procedures

In this study, we use The FMCW uRAD Raspberry Pi v1.2 radar as a sensor for detecting targets. The radar will send a transmit signal through the transmitter antenna and receive a reflected signal to the receiver antenna from the target hand gesture in the form of an IQ signal. Signal processing will go through preprocessing stages as input for the classification method. We used the CNN method to classify 5 Indonesian sign language (SIBI) words, which will compare 3 CNN architectures to get the best model. Radar system and methods are proposed, which is shown in Fig. 3.

Hand Gesture Data Acquisition. In this study, we set up the radar with a configuration of the uRAD radar that connected with the raspberry pi 4. The bandwidth of the uRAD radar used is 240 MHz, and the operating frequency of 24.005 GHz with a number of samples (Ns) in one capture/period is 50. The radar was placed on a tripod to achieve optimal measurements as high as 100 cm, with the movement carried out at a distance of 120 cm from the antenna at a zero-aspect angle as shown in Fig. 4. Each gesture is measured 15 times and lasts about 10 s or 200 periods because in one period takes 50 mS. MTI mode in uRAD radar is active to eliminate static clutter experimental environment. We used mode 2 (sawtooth signal) in uRAD

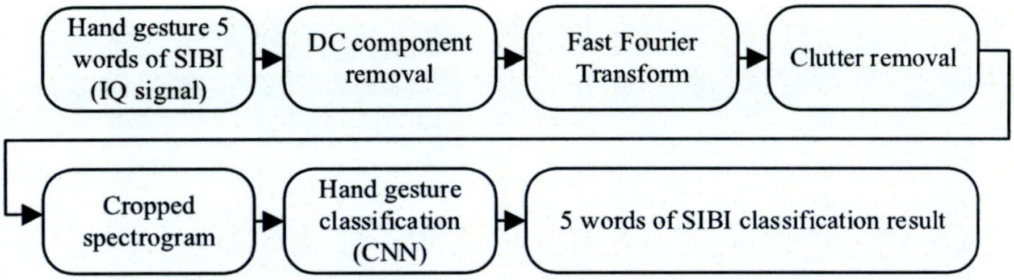

Fig. 3 The diagram of the proposed radar system and methods

radar because we only need information about distance. The output of uRAD radar is in-phase (I)-quadrature (Q) signals. The IQ signal from the radar will go through preprocessing as input for CNN model.

Pre-Processing. After the data collection, the output from the radar is a complex I/Q signal. The real and imaginary portions of the filtered signal are separated into two channels. The real part is the In-phase (I) channel, while the imaginary is the Quadrature (Q) channel. Then both will be converted into voltage because this raw data has arbitrary units from 0 to 4095 [18]. This conversion uses the maximum voltage issued by GPIO on the Raspberry Pi, which makes the maximum voltage it has to 3.3 V.

The output of uRAD radar is in-phase (I)-quadrature (Q) signals with a complex number I + Qj, which can use to extract the backscatter signal magnitude. Figure 5

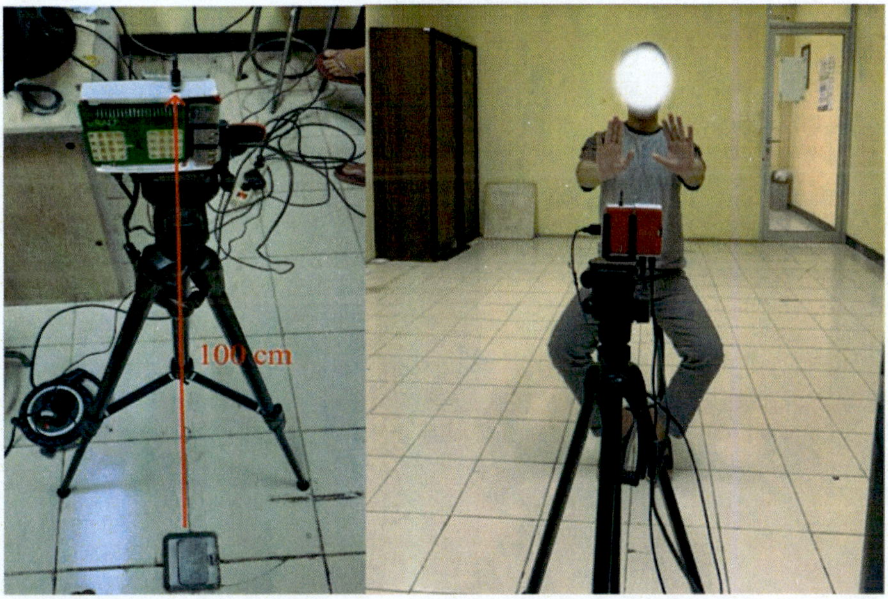

Fig. 4 Photograph of the measurement setup and a seated participant

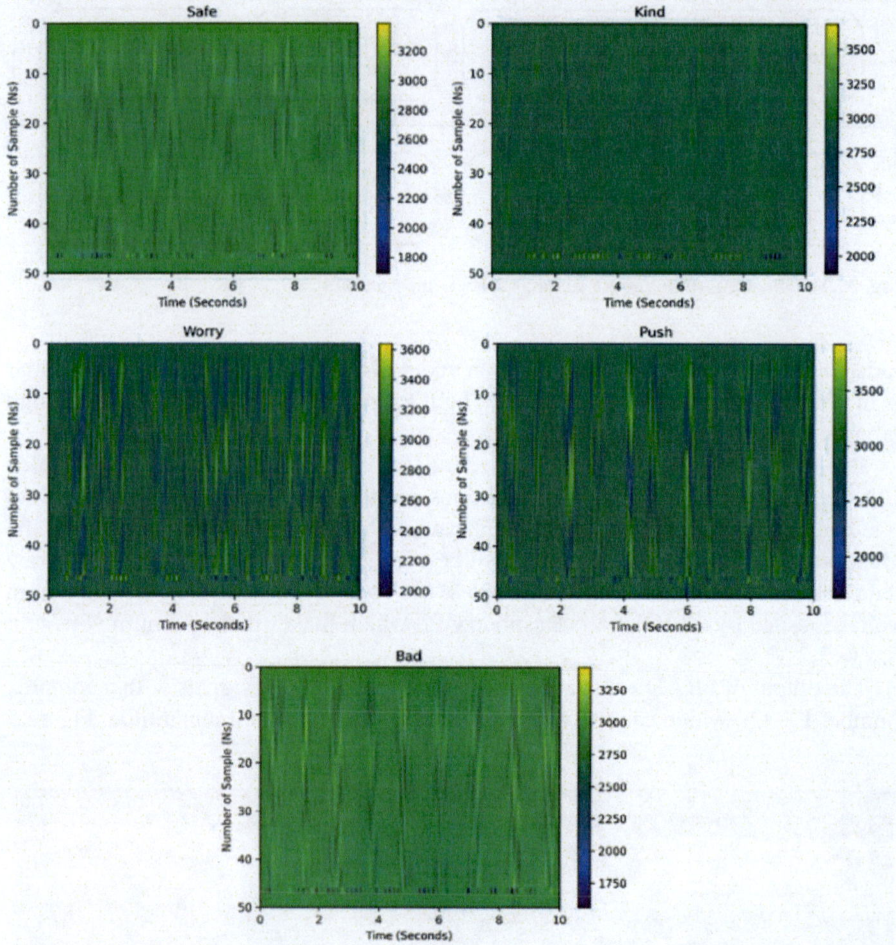

Fig. 5 Magnitude of IQ signals from reflected signal in form 2D, five hand gestures measured using FMCW radar

is a form of raw data that can be combined into a matrix form where rows denote Ns and columns denotes frames per capture. In one frame or period, it takes 50 ms to convert into seconds.

DC Component Removal. I and Q signals have noise from DC Component, which has a DC Component that can interfere with the classification results therefore the DC Component removal is needed [25]. DC Component removal is also required to eliminate interference at 0 Hz frequency. The DC component expresses in Eq. (1).

$$\mathbb{Y}^{(N_p)} = \mathbb{X}^{(N_p)} - J_{K,1}x\frac{1}{K}\left|\sum_{k=0}^{K-1} X^{(1)}|k], \sum_{k=0}^{K-1} X^{(2)}|k], \ldots, \sum_{k=0}^{K-1} X^{(N_p)}|k],\right] \quad (1)$$

Fast Fourier Transform. The raw complex time-domain signal is processed to a time frequency by Fast Fourier transform (FFT) [26, 27]. It can be seen that the time–frequency spectrum of the five-handed movements differs from each other. The IQ results from DC Component removal are converted into voltage before through the FFT method, with the number of frequency indexes used being 4096. The next step is to take only the necessary data. In data processing, only positive values are taken from the radar, so the frequency index is between 2048 and 4096 because this range has information about the distance between the radar and the target. The FFT method can be calculated using the following Eq. (2).

$$X[k] = \sum_{n=0}^{N-1} x[n] \mathrm{e}^{-j2\pi \frac{n}{N} k} \tag{2}$$

Figure 6 shows the FFT result, where the spectrogram's column part is the frequency index that has been converted to maximum distance. The maximum distance is 15.625 m.

Clutter removal. This clutter can come from walls or other static objects. In this study, clutter is removed using two steps. First, activate the MTI mode [28], a feature of the uRAD radar. The second eliminates clutter through Eq. (3).

$$\mathbb{Z}^{(N_p)} = \mathbb{Y}^{(N_p)} - \frac{1}{N_p}\left|\sum_{i=1}^{N_p} X^{(i)}|0], \sum_{i=1}^{N_p} X^{(i)}|1], \ldots, \sum_{i=1}^{N_p} X^{(i)}|K-1]\right]^T x J_1, N_p \tag{3}$$

Cropped Spectrograms. After that, it takes data at a radar distance, so the computation is not high. It is known that the frequency index used is between 2048 and 4096. Next, we will crop the spectrogram that contains only target information, namely the frequency index ranges from 2048 to 2448 (in the range of 400 index frequency) or if it is converted to a distance of 0–3.05 m. Further, cropped according to the target distance only as depicted in Fig. 7. Rows denote the distance information target and columns denote the time each data retrieval is 10 s.

Furthermore, the resulting spectrogram will be cropped every 70 frames or 3.5 s to increase the number of datasets so it will form a rectangular matrix with a value of 400 × 70. The result of this cropping will be input into CNN.

2.3 *Proposed CNN Design*

Convolutional neural networks are used to develop sign classifiers and allow for processing of two-dimensional data. Typically, a CNN consists of an input and output layer in a combination of several layers: convolution layer, pooling layer, and fully connected [29]. Convolution layers and input values will be filtered and produce

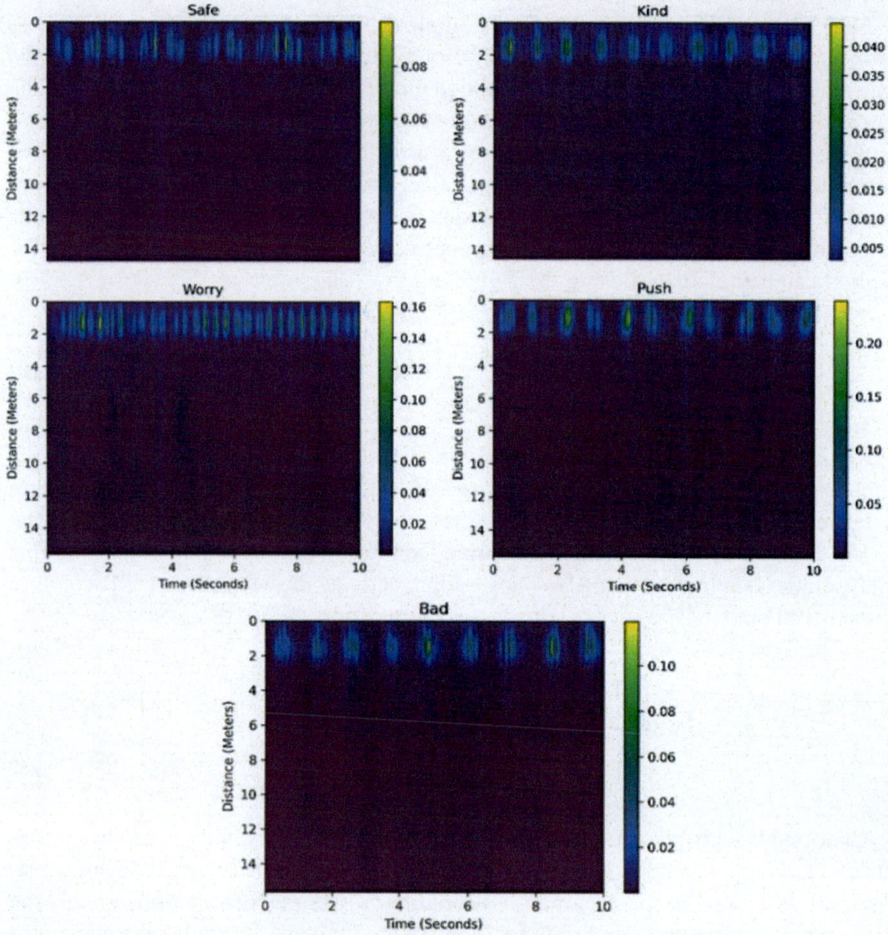

Fig. 6 The time–frequency spectrograms of five hand gestures

feature maps. The pooling layer will reduce the dimensions of the feature maps [9]. The fully connected layer will convert multidimensional arrays of feature maps into a one-dimensional array to classify data. In this study, we used three different architectures. All three architectures are self-constructed and consist convolution layer, pooling layer and are fully connected. We changed number of layers for the differences of each architecture, particularly convolution layer and pooling layer with the activation function of ReLU. In the classification of this study in the output of a fully connected layer we use softmax activation function. We want to compare all architectures for getting highest accuracy.

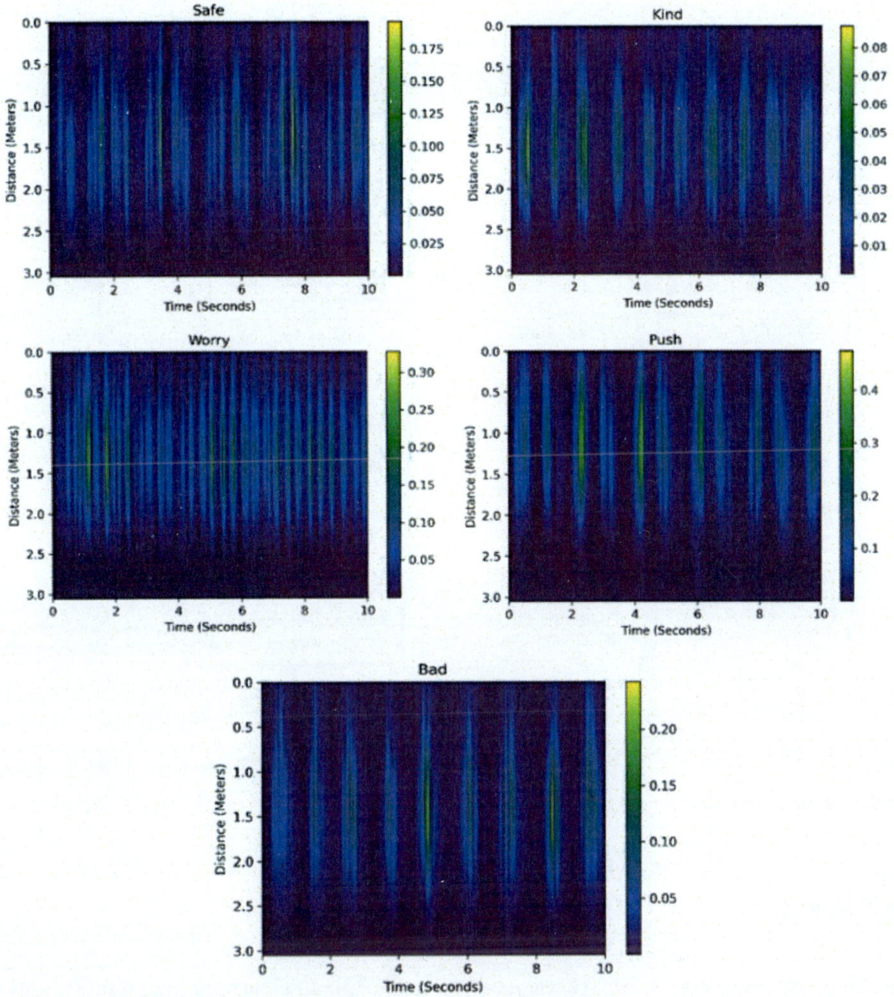

Fig. 7 Cropped spectrograms

2.4 *Proposed CNN Design*

In this study, the workings of this uRAD radar in data collection are shown in Fig. 8. The system will start by giving a set time lag in data retrieval. Then do the configuration on the radar. Then the raspberry pi 4 is connected to the radar for data retrieval. If an error occurs, the raspberry pi reconnects to the radar. If successful, the radar will emit an FMCW radar signal and get the raw data, namely I/Q signal. Data collection will continue until the specified time limit. If the time limit is not reached, the radar will continue to emit an FMCW signal. The resulting raw data is collected in a 2D array.

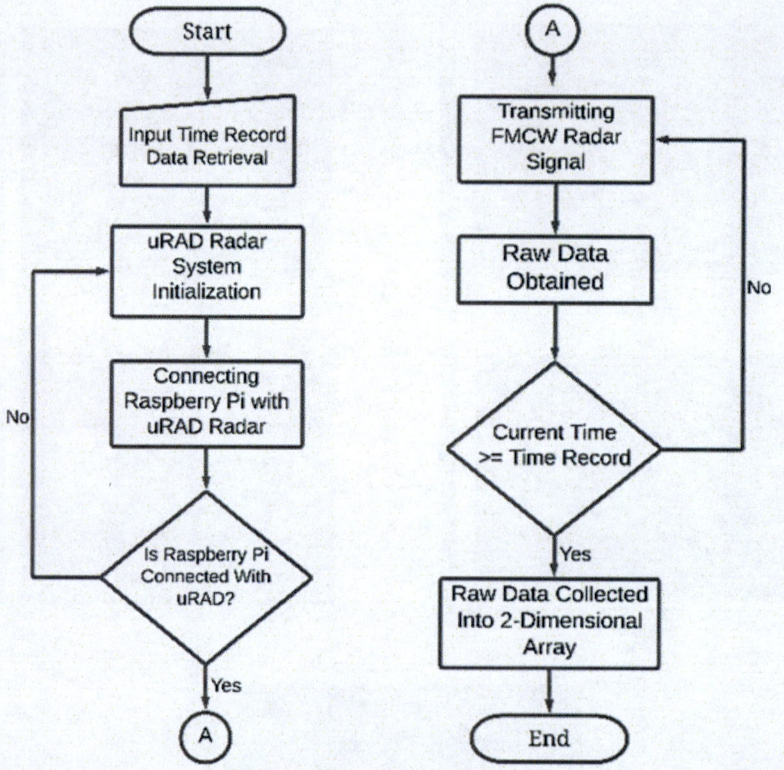

Fig. 8 Flowchart radar system integrated with raspberry pi 4 for retrieves raw data IQ signal data in 2-dimensional arrays

3 Results

The input value is 400 × 70. We use a batch size of 256 and learning rate of 0.001 and the optimizer is Adam [30]. We execute the same combination of hyperparameters in three architectures and then obtain the results from training different epoch values 20, 30 and 40. In this study, we used three different architectures. All three architectures are self-constructed. For the loss function we used Categorical Cross-Entropy because of our multiclass classification system. This loss function will train a CNN to have an output of a probability over the classes for each gesture [31]. The table below summarizes the result of accuracy and loss level (Table 1).

As the given results above, we can see that epoch values affect the testing results in this case. In all architecture, epoch values of 40 make increase accuracy. And the more layers, the higher the accuracy that we got. Based on the result, we also state that five layers with epoch values of 40 work best for the classification SIBI dataset cause got the highest accuracy, 99.88%. Likewise, with the loss value, the failure rate decreases as the number of epochs increases and the number of layers increases.

Table 1 Classification result from the CNN-based classifier

Architecture	Epoch	Accuracy (%)	Loss (%)
I 1 Layers	20	99.39	9.51
	30	99.21	3.97
	40	99.57	3.3
II 2 Layers	20	98.9	8.01
	30	99.57	1.75
	50	99.82	1.32
III 3 Layers	20	98.66	6.32
	30	99.57	1.79
	40	99.88	1.16

Loss value is 1.16%. However, if the number of epochs continues to increase, there is a possibility that there will be overfitting which reduces the accuracy of the training process which is too much. A summary of the third architecture can be seen in Fig. 9.

A confusion matrix evaluation is carried out to analyze classification quality in recognizing existing classes. The modelling of this system uses the CNN method. The testing process uses 4912 test data and randomly selects different types of hand gestures. In Fig. 10, there is an error in the classification of 5 test data. In Fig. 11, it is known that the training and test processes are not overfitting and good stability pattern. Furthermore, in Table 2 are the results of the calculation of the overall accuracy, precision value, recall value, and f1—score from the CNN method used with the best scenario model, namely in the third architecture, which consists of three convolution layers and three pooling layers.

4 Discussion

We get high results in this study, which is 99.88% accurate. We also have three scenarios for determining the outcome. In our case, it is known that the effect of the epoch value and the number of layers can increase the accuracy. In its implementation, according to the results obtained, our system can help the deaf communicate with the society. This result is also obtained because the preprocessing stage reduces the DC component, changing the time domain to the frequency domain using the FFT method, reducing clutter, and cropping the spectrogram, which aims to retrieve data according to the target distance only and multiply the dataset.

There are related studies on the classification of sign language from computer vision, leap motion, and radar. Radar has the advantage of not being sensitive to the environment, such as light. And also, easy to implement. In classification using radar, previous research uses an existing architecture. In our study, we use a self-constructed architecture. It should be made with simple architecture first.

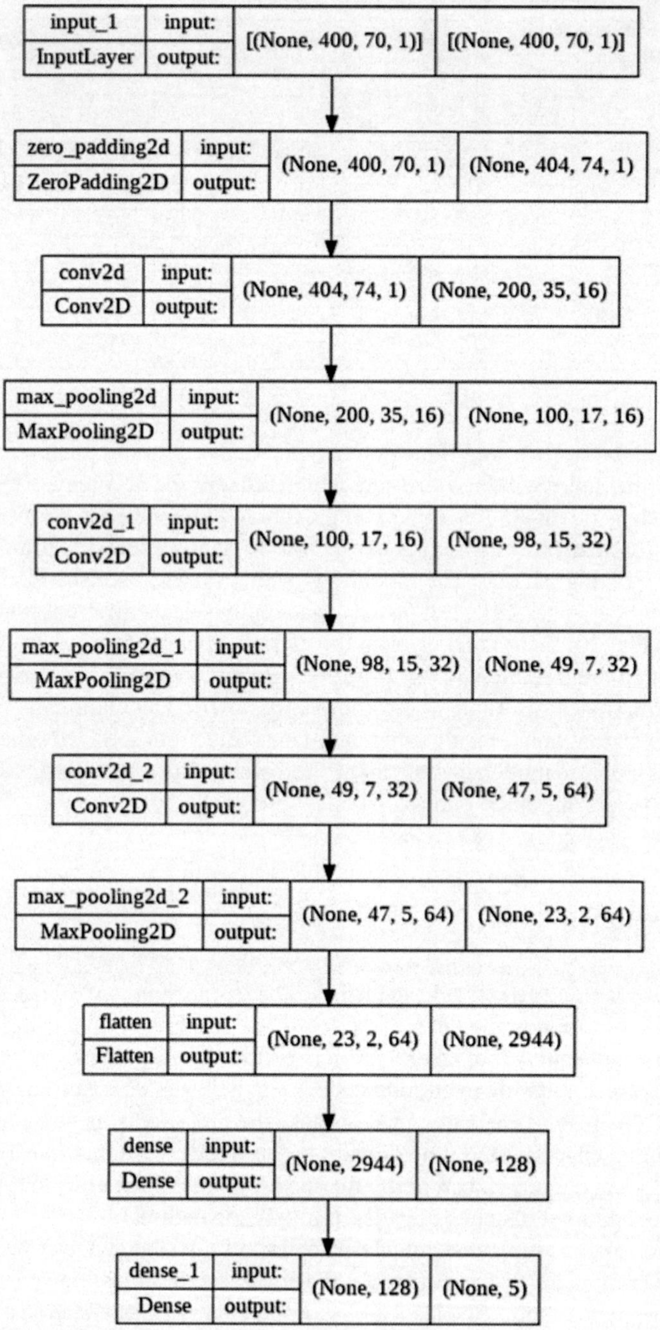

Fig. 9 Block diagram of the architecture III

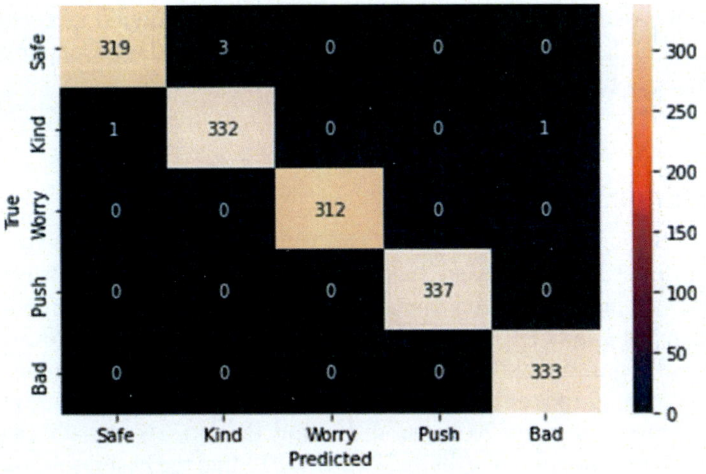

Fig. 10 Confusion matrix from best model

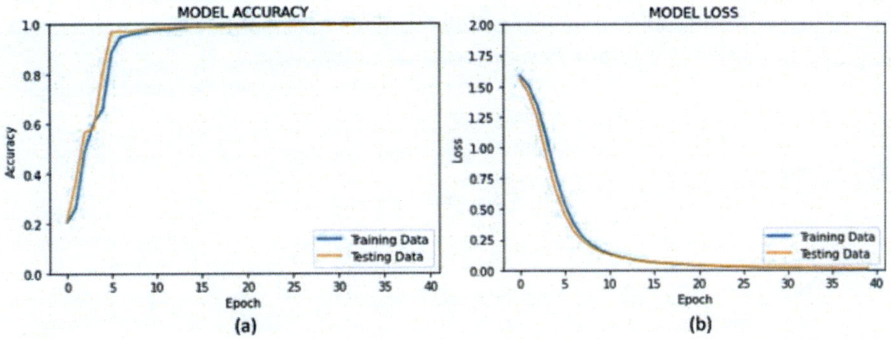

Fig. 11 Graph of **a** accuracy and **b** loss from best architectures

Table 2 Classification reports

Gesture	Precision	Recall	F1-score
Safe	1.00	0.99	1.00
Kind	1.00	1.00	1.00
Worry	1.00	1.00	1.00
Push	1.00	1.00	1.00
Bad	1.00	1.00	1.00

In this study, there are several shortcomings. Detection of differences in angles and distances is not explored. This study implies that during data collection, clutter often appears even though it has been removed by the removes DC Component and Clutter method. The drawback of the radar system used is the presence of interference if there are too many objects. This is because the reflected signal received will be divided between the target and the object that is not needed. However, the accuracy is high compared to previous studies classifying hand gestures.

5 Conclusion

This study proposed Indonesia sign language (SIBI) classification system using CNN. This study uses a radar output that operates with a raspberry pi 4. The output is an IQ signal, which consists of DC Component removal, Fast Fourier Transform (FFT) in converting the output signal I and Q into the frequency domain, noise reduction from clutter, and cropping spectrogram by only target information (400 frames) then will cropping spectrograms every 70 frames to multiply the datasets so that it can be used as input in CNN in the form of a 400 $\times$ 70 matrix. To find the best result, we applied CNN with three different architectures. There are self-construct architecture, which consists of three convolution layers and three pooling layers, resulting in an accuracy of 99.88% with epoch values is 40. Since sign language classification is one of the critical parts of communications, the following study can continue to recognize sign language in translator's system based on mobile in Indonesia.

References

1. Zhang ZT, Zhou M (2018) Latern: dynamic continuous hand gesture recognition using FMCW radar sensor. IEEE Sens J 18(8):3278–3289. https://doi.org/10.1109/JSEN.2018.2808688
2. Jiang W, Ren Y, Liu Y, Wang Z, Wang X (2021) Recognition of dynamic hand gesture based on mm-wave FMCW radar micro-Doppler signatures. In: ICASSP, IEEE international conference on acoustics, speech and signal processing—proceedings, vol 2021, pp 4905–4909. https://doi.org/10.1109/ICASSP39728.2021.9414837
3. Xuhao Z, Qisong W, Dixian Z (2018) Dynamic hand gesture recognition using FMCW radar sensor for driving assistance. https://doi.org/10.1109/WCSP.2018.8555642
4. Benatti S, Giovanni R, Fabio M, Elisabetta F (2017) A sub-10mW real-time implementation for EMG hand gesture recognition based on a multi-core biomedical SoC. In: Proceedings—2017 7th international workshop on advances in sensors and interfaces, IWASI 2017, pp 139–144. https://doi.org/10.1109/IWASI.2017.7974234
5. Trong KN, Bui H, Pham C (2019) Recognizing hand gestures for controlling home appliances with mobile sensors. https://doi.org/10.1109/KSE.2019.8919419
6. Zikky M, Rizky YH, Ahmad FAR, Abdulloh H, Achmad B (2018) Development of educational game for recognizing Indonesian sign language (SIBI) and breaking down the communication barrier with deaf people. https://doi.org/10.1109/ICSEC.2017.8443936
7. Franceschini S, Ambrosanio M, Vitale S, Baselice F, Gifuni A, Grassini G, Pascazio V (2020) Hand gesture recognition via radar sensors and convolutional neural networks. In: IEEE national radar conference—proceedings, vol 2020. https://doi.org/10.1109/RadarConf2043947.2020.9266565
8. Tanuj B, Shaunak S, Krish P, Purva R (2020) Real-time two way communication system for speech and hearing impaired using computer vision and deep learning. https://doi.org/10.1109/ICSSIT46314.2019.8987908

9. Dissanayake ISM, Wickramanayake PJ, Mudunkotuwa MAS, Fernando PWN (2020) Utalk: Sri Lankan sign language converter mobile app using image processing and machine learning. In: ICAC 2020—2nd international conference on advancements in computing, proceedings, pp 31–36. https://doi.org/10.1109/ICAC51239.2020.9357300
10. Hein Z, Htoo TP, Aye B, Htet SM, Ye KZ (2021) Leap motion based Myanmar sign language recognition using machine learning. In: Proceedings of the 2021 IEEE conference of Russian young researchers in electrical and electronic engineering, ElConRus 2021, pp 2304–2310. https://doi.org/10.1109/ElConRus51938.2021.9396496
11. Keumala A, Erdefi R, Lim YS (2020) Recognizing the components of inflectional word gestures in Indonesian sign system known as SIBI (Sistem Isyarat Bahasa Indonesia) by using lip motion. https://doi.org/10.1109/ICEEI47359.2019.8988806
12. Chairi NI, Ingrid N, Amil AI (2020) The effect of light on leap motion controller in the classification of sign language translator system. https://doi.org/10.1109/ISRITI48646.2019.9034602
13. Lin M, Octavian P, Haiqing Y, Yongsheng Y (2020) Short-range detection scheme based on FMCW doppler radar and wavelet denoising with adapted threshold function. In: 2019 international conference on sensing and instrumentation in IoT Era (ISSI). https://doi.org/10.1109/issi47111.2019.9043666
14. Shao Y, Guo S, Sun L, Chen W (2017) Human motion classification based on range information with deep convolutional neural network. In: Proceedings—2017 4th international conference on information science and control engineering, ICISCE 2017, pp 1519–1523. https://doi.org/10.1109/ICISCE.2017.317
15. Takuya S, Xiaomeng G, Ehsan Y, Ashikur R, Olga B, Victor ML (2018) Radar-based hand gesture recognition using I-Q echo plot and convolutional neural network. https://doi.org/10.1109/CAMA.2017.8273461
16. Hovannes K, Prakshi S, Michel K, Claude D (2020) Sign language gesture recognition using doppler radar and deep learning. https://doi.org/10.1109/GCWkshps45667.2019.9024607
17. Gao X, Jia X, Ashikur R, Ehsan Y, Alexander L, Victor L, Olga B (2016) Barcode based hand gesture classification using AC coupled quadrature doppler radar. In: IEEE MTT-S international microwave symposium digest, vol 2016. https://doi.org/10.1109/MWSYM.2016.7540013
18. uRAD by Anteral, User Manual Raspberry Pi version Software SDK v1.1
19. Liu D, Meng H (2020) Application of FMCW radar for the recognition of hand gesture using time series convolutional neural networks. https://doi.org/10.1109/ICMMT49418.2020.9386392
20. Winarko OD, Hidayat R, Nugroho HA, Anggara R, Lestari AA (2018) Mitigation methods of sawtooth modulations effect on FMCW radar INDERA MX-4. https://doi.org/10.1109/ICRAMET.2017.8253142
21. Jung DH, Kim DH, Azim MT, Park J, Park SO (2021) A novel signal processing technique for Ku-band automobile FMCW fully polarimetric SAR system using triangular LFM. IEEE Trans Instrum Meas 70. https://doi.org/10.1109/TIM.2020.3011601
22. Pal S (2019) FMCW—radar design. 65(4). https://doi.org/10.1080/03772063.2019.1615392
23. Nurilman BM, Med I, Fariani IH (2020) Morphological analysis of speech translation into Indonesian sign language system (SIBI) on android platform. https://doi.org/10.1109/ICACSIS47736.2019.8980000
24. Kustiawanto H, Erdefi R (2019) Sign language system for Bahasa Indonesia (known as SIBI) recognizer using TensorFlow and long short-term memory. https://doi.org/10.1109/ICACSIS.2018.8618134
25. Kang SW, Jang MH, Lee S (2012) Identification of human motion using radar sensor in an indoor environment. 21(7). https://doi.org/10.3390/s21072305
26. Wang Y, Shu Y, Jia X, Zhou M, Xie L, Guo L (2022) Multifeature fusion-based hand gesture sensing and recognition system. IEEE Geosci Remote Sens Lett 19. https://doi.org/10.1109/LGRS.2021.3086136
27. Wang Y, Ren A, Zhou M, Wang W, Yang X (2020) A novel detection and recognition method for continuous hand gesture using FMCW radar. IEEE Access 8:167264–167275. https://doi.org/10.1109/ACCESS.2020.3023187

28. Sungwon Y, Sungmoon C, Dong-Min S, Sung CH (2018) Adaptive clutter suppression algorithm for detection and positioning using IR-UWB Radar. https://doi.org/10.1109/UWBUSIS.2018.8520164
29. Mittal A, Kumar P, Roy PP, Balasubramanian R, Chaudhuri BB (2019) A modified LSTM model for continuous sign language recognition using leap motion. IEEE Sens J 19(16):7056–7063. https://doi.org/10.1109/JSEN.2019.2909837
30. Kodali RK, Dhanekula R (2021) Face mask detection using deep learning. https://doi.org/10.1109/ICCCI50826.2021.9402670
31. Harikrishnan A, Sourabh S, Rashi P (2020) Handwritten digit recognition with feed-forward multi-layer perceptron and convolutional neural network architectures. https://doi.org/10.1109/ICIMIA48430.2020.9074916

The Performance of Various Concise Convolutional Neural Network Configurations in Classifying Tomato Diseases Based on Leaf Images

Arnes Sembiring, Yuwaldi Away, Fitri Arnia, and Rusdha Muharar

Abstract Early detection of plant diseases requires a monitoring system that can classify plants accurately and run automatically in the agricultural field. Convolutional Neural Network offers better classification accuracy than various other classification methods but its implementation in agricultural monitoring system faces various challenges. The main challenge is the large amount of resources required to run various existing Convolutional Neural Network architectures. This study proposed a concise Convolutional Neural Network architecture and investigated the performance of its configuration in classifying tomato diseases based on leaf images. The proposed architectural model has a much smaller number of parameters compared to the 5 comparative architectural models in this study. The proposed architecture has 109.8k parameters while Squeezenet and Shufflenet as the most concise comparison CNN architectures in this study have 1.24M and 1.4M parameters, respectively. All comparison models and proposed architecture were trained and tested on the same dataset, namely the image of tomato leaves from PlantVillage Dataset. The results revealed that SqueezeNet was the fastest comparison CNN with 98.70% accuracy while Shufflenet achieved 98.89% accuracy. This accuracy is slightly higher than the proposed architecture, which is 98.64% but the proposed architecture is 7.9 times faster than SqueezeNet and 8.7 times than Shufflenet in classifying each image. Classification speed, small number of parameters and competitive classification accuracy indicate that the proposed architecture is feasible to be applied in agricultural monitoring system.

Keywords Classification of plant diseases · Convolutional neural network · Filter size · Number of parameter · PlantVillage tomato dataset

A. Sembiring (✉) · Y. Away · F. Arnia · R. Muharar
Doctoral Program, School of Engineering, Universitas Syiah Kuala, Banda Aceh, Indonesia
e-mail: arnessembiring@gmail.com

R. Muharar
Department of Electrical and Computer Engineering, Universitas Syiah Kuala, Banda Aceh, Indonesia

T. Triwiyanto et al. (eds.), *Proceeding of the 3rd International Conference on Electronics, Biomedical Engineering, and Health Informatics*, Lecture Notes in Electrical Engineering 1008, https://doi.org/10.1007/978-981-99-0248-4_26

1 Introduction

The agricultural sector is responsible for providing food for the community. It also plays a great role in the economic growth of a country. The contribution of this sector has been reported to reach 6.4% of the total world economic production in 2018 [1].

Many factors determine an increase in agricultural productivity. Environmental factors such as weather, temperature, humidity, and availability of production resources, such as labor, are the main factors. However, the factors that can reduce the production of yields are also very important to note. Among the factors found to reduce 20–30% of the world's agricultural productivity are plant diseases. They are among the major threats in ensuring food supply [2, 3].

Monitoring plant conditions is therefore an important task that will allow early detection of plant diseases, more effective control of spread, and handling [4]. However, crop supervision costs are not cheap. Monitoring a large agricultural area or the areas located in separate locations will require more labors and time [5]. However, reducing the cost of supervision can make the monitoring process slower and the management of plant diseases more difficult.

Automation of the monitoring process is one way to meet the growing demand for plants (both as food and as a source of energy). Automation will make it easier to increase the production at a lower cost and to preserve the environment at the same time because rapid disease identification will help to reduce the use of chemicals in the treatment of plant diseases. Identification and the ability to classify plants using a computer system based on imagery is an important part of this automation [6].

Image processing and artificial intelligence have performed the task of identifying and classifying plants using various algorithms and the classification accuracy becomes very high, even close to 100% when deep learning, especially Convolutional Neural Network (CNN), begins to be implemented [7]. This very high accuracy makes CNN widely applied in many fields, such as business, agriculture, automotive industry and other fields, especially for object detection and image classification [8]. CNN's main strength in obtaining high accuracy comes from its ability to automatically extract important and interesting features from an image, a video, and sound datasets without the need for feature selection from an expert [9, 10].

The main limitation in implementing and developing CNN in various fields is the availability of resources for the development of CNN itself. A considerable number of parameters involved in computation using CNN raises the need for abundant computing resources and long training time [11]. On the other hand, most of the tasks of identification and classification of objects in the field, such as classification in the agricultural fields and mobile applications, work on resource-constrained environments, limited data sources, low memory, and certain time limit [12, 13]. Therefore, one of the major challenges in deploying the CNN model in a real agriculture field for real time identification and classification tasks is to achieve a trade-off between the computational burden and accuracy [14]. There should be a CNN model with a smaller number of parameters, high accuracy, reasonable cost, and feasibility to be applied for automatic monitoring at a large scale. A small number of parameters in a

CNN model will provide many benefits; one of which is the ease of model updating [15, 16].

To solve the issue, a concise CNN architecture is proposed in this study. The performance of the proposed CNN will then be compared with some well-known CNN architectures, namely ShuffleNet, MobileNet-V2, GoogleNet, NASNet and SqueezeNet. The contribution of this paper is threefold:

1. It proposes a concise CNN model, namely Conf_Ch_7 with a smaller number of parameters and faster classification performance than those of the comparison architectures, even though the accuracy of the proposed model is slightly lower.
2. Due to its small number of parameters, the proposed model only needs fewer computing resources. In other words, it can achieve a trade-off between the need for computational resources and accuracy.
3. It provides a detailed investigation of several configurations of the proposed model. The investigation in this study shows that the filter size 7×7 is better than other filter sizes in extracting features from the leaf dataset used. The other information provided, such as activation functions used and optimization functions, can be useful for further similar research.

2 Material and Methods

2.1 Related Works

The Convolutional Neural Network (CNN) is a network type in the deep learning algorithm which is widely used for image-based classification, including plant disease classification. The main structure of a CNN is the convolutional layer, the pooling layer and the fully connected layer. The convolution layer extracts features with two operations, namely linear operations through convolution operations and non-linear operations through activation functions [9, 17]. The most important difference between a fully connected layer and a convolution layer is that a fully connected layer learns all feature patterns from its input layer while the convolution layer learns local patterns according to the filter size [18].

CNN is one of the best techniques currently in object detection, pattern recognition and classification in images. CNN offers better accuracy than other methods [17]. Many studies have been conducted to detect plant diseases based on the images of plant leaves using the well-known CNN architecture. AlexNet and VGGNet (VGG16) were used for disease classification in tomato plants in [19]. The dataset used consisted of 13,262 images of tomato leaves grouped into 7 classes: 1 for healthy leaf class while the others were for late blight, leaf mold, two-spotted spider mite, target spot, tomato yellow leaf curl virus, and tomato mosaic virus. AlexNet's fine-tuning results achieved 97.49% accuracy while VGG16 reached 97.29% accuracy.

Tomato plant disease detection based on leaf images was also carried out in [11]. AlexNet, VGGNet, and GoogleNet were fine-tuned as CNN models to classify 10 classes of tomato leaves from the PlantVillage dataset consisting of 1 healthy leaf class and 9 exposed classes with 9 types of disease. VGGNet achieved the best accuracy rate (95.24%), followed by AlexNet (91.52%), and GoogleNet (89.68%).

An assessment of the performance of many well-known CNN architectures for image classification of tomato leaves was also carried out in [20]. The dataset used has 10 classes from the PlantVillage with 18,160 images in total. The best validation accuracy was achieved by GoogleNet (99.39%). AlexNet, Inception V3, ResNet 18, and ResNet 50 achieved validation accuracy of 98.93%, 98.65%, 99.06%, and 99.16%, respectively.

Another architecture used for plant classification is MobileNet [21]. MobileNet has fewer parameters than AlexNet, VGGNet, and GoogleNet. The PlantVillage dataset used in the study comprised 10 classes of tomato leaf images with a total of 7176 images and achieved a validation accuracy of 90.3% at a learning rate of 0.001.

Other studies have chosen to use the CNN architecture that is more concise for plant classification that could run on computers with limited resources. Some studies developed their own proposed CNN architecture while others modified the existing CNN architectures.

A compact CNN architecture based on the GoogleNet architecture was developed in [22]. This architecture, called AgNet, involved 250,000 parameters. Agnet was used to classify grasses and new plants that grew on the weed/crop dataset [23] with an accuracy rate of 88.9 $\pm$ 0.4% and was implemented in agricultural robots which had limited computing resources named AgBot II.

D-CCN was used to detect cave leaf diseases in [24]. The proposed D-CNN model consisted of 4 layers of convolution. The first layer consisted of 32 kernels with 3 $\times$ 3 dimensions, stride 4, and a ReLu activation function. This first layer was followed by a max-pooling layer with dimensions of 2 $\times$ 2 and stride 1. The second, third, and fourth convolutional layers were constructed by kernels with the same dimensions as those of the first layer, but differ in the number of kernels which were 64, 128, and 256, respectively. Stride 1 was applied to the second and third convolutional as well as to the max-pooling layers, while the fourth layer was used in stride 2. The fully connected layer on D-CNN consisted of 3 layers with 64, 128 and 256 in size. D-CNN used 2,705 guava leaf images which were divided into 4 classes, namely healthy, whitefly, algal leaf spot, and rust. D-CNN achieved 98.74% testing accuracy while LeNet-5 and AlexNet as the comparison architectures obtained 96.97 and 97.92%, respectively.

2.2 Dataset

The dataset used in this study was taken from the PlantVillage dataset which is the open access dataset from the PlantVillage project [25]. This dataset is one of the most popular datasets in the study of image-based classification of plant diseases [26].

Originally the PlantVillage dataset consisted of 38 classes containing images of 14 crop species. This study used only tomato leaf datasets grouped into 10 classes. The first class contained images of healthy tomato leaves, whereas the other nine classes had images of tomato leaves affected by nine types of diseases, namely septoria leaf spot, early blight, late blight, bacterial spot, tomato mosaic virus, leaf mold, spider mites, target spot, and yellow leaf curl virus. All images in the dataset were RGB images at a resolution of 256×256. This original resolution was maintained for the proposed architecture in this study. Meanwhile, the resolutions of the input images for the comparison architectures were resized to their default resolutions. Figure 1 shows the exact number and sample images of each class used in this study.

Originally, there were 18,160 images in total, as in [20]. However, this study did not use all of the images. A careful selection was carried out, with some poor images being discarded, such as the overexposed ones. This left the total number of images at 17,641. This number was used for training and testing of the proposed CNN and all comparison architectures in this study. The dataset was divided into 80% for training and 20% for testing.

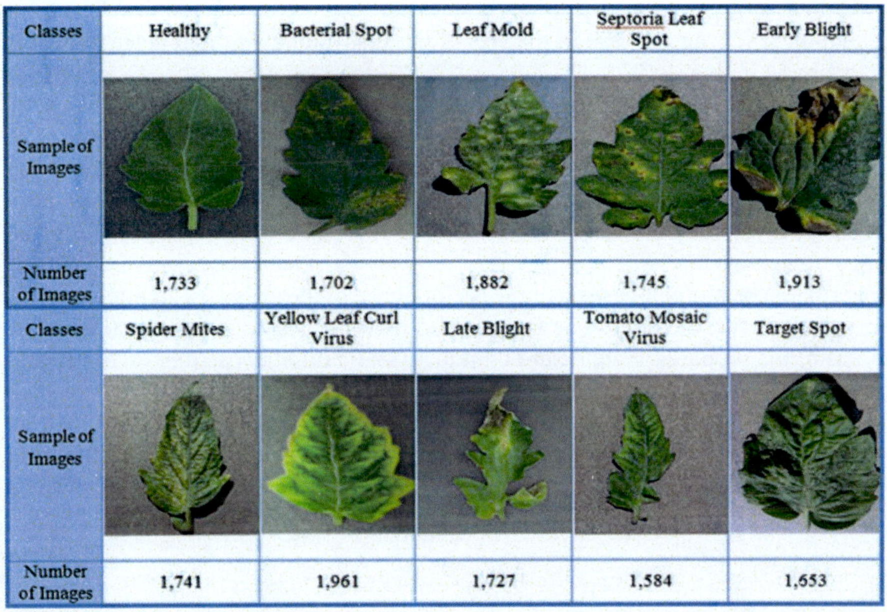

Fig. 1 The exact number and sample images from the PlantVillage dataset used in this work

2.3 The Proposed Architecture and Its Configurations

Figure 2 shows the architectural structure of the proposed CNN named Conf_Ch_7. The architecture consisted of 6 convolution layers. The first convolution layer comprised eight filters, whereas the second layer contained 16 filters. The third layer consisted of 32 filters, whereas the fourth to the sixth convolution layers had 64 filters.

The use of 6 layers of convolution was intended to keep the number of parameters involved low. The motivation for using this architecture comes from the baseline architecture proposed in [27] which consisted of 4 convolution layers and achieved a testing accuracy of 97.15% on the same dataset as the dataset used in this study. The achievement of this accuracy with only 4 layers of convolution shows that the architecture has great potential for development and performance improvement. Furthermore, in this study, three developments were proposed. The first was the addition of two convolution layers with each consisting of 64 filters aimed at increasing feature extraction capabilities with a deeper convolution layer so that accuracy is better. The second was the change in filter size in the first and second convolution layers from 3×3 to 7×7, also intended to increase feature extraction capabilities. The third development was an increase in the size of the first fully connected layer from 1×32 to 1×64 in this study.

Figure 2 also shows that the first to fifth convolution layers were followed by the normalization batch layer, the activation function and the maxPooling layer. The sixth convolution layer was followed by the batch normalization layer, the activation function, and the averagePooling layer. The classification layer consisted of two fully connected layers with the size of 1×64 and 1×10, respectively. It was also followed by a softmax layer.

Furthermore, the comparison of the performance of the proposed architecture was carried out in two methods. The first method used investigation of several configurations of the proposed architecture on tomato leaf dataset consisting of 10 classes. The first class contained images of healthy tomato leaves, whereas the other nine classes had images of tomato leaves affected by the diseases. The second method was to compare the performance of the proposed architecture with the performance of several well-known CNN architectures.

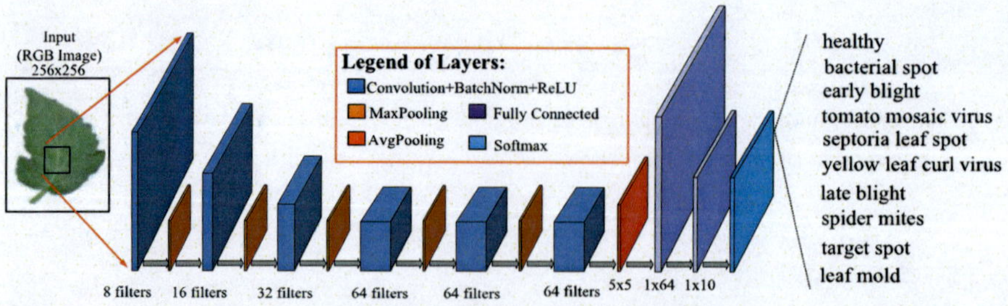

Fig. 2 Basic structure of the proposed architecture

Table 1 Configurations of the proposed architecture

Architecture	Filter size	Batch normalization	Activation function	Optimization function
Conf_Ch_9	9×9	Yes	ReLU	sgdm
Conf_Ch_7	7×7	Yes	ReLU	sgdm
Conf_Ch_5	5×5	Yes	ReLU	sgdm
Conf_Ch_3	3×3	Yes	ReLU	sgdm
Conf_LeakyRelu	7×7	Yes	LeakyReLU	sgdm
Conf_elu	7×7	Yes	ELU	sgdm
Conf_No_batch_norm	7×7	No	ReLU	sgdm
Conf_adam	7×7	Yes	ReLU	adam
Conf_rmsprop	7×7	Yes	ReLU	rmsprop

The first aspect investigated in this study was different filter sizes applied to the first and second convolution layers of each configuration. Meanwhile, the third to sixth convolution layers had the same size, namely 3×3. The application of different filter sizes to the configurations resulted in different sharpness of features to be extracted in the next convolution layer.

The first and second convolution layers of the first configuration used a filter size of 9×9. The architecture in this configuration was named Conf_Ch_9, as presented in Table 1. A different filter size was applied to the first and second convolution layers of the second configuration, namely 5×5. The architecture in this configuration was named Conf_Ch_5. The last configuration used a filter size of 3×3 and was called Conf_Ch_3.

The second aspect investigated was the effects of a batch normalization layer on the performance of the concise CNN. There were two different configurations used here; one was with a batch normalization layer (Conf_Ch_7 as shown in Fig. 2), while the other one was without a batch normalization layer called Conf_No_batch_norm.

The use of the batch normalization layer introduced in [28] is intended to accelerate the training of a network to reach convergence. This acceleration is obtained because the batch normalization layer reduces the internal covariate shift (ICS) in deep learning networks [29]. The use of the batch normalization layer also results in smoother network optimization and results in more stable gradient updates. This more stable condition then allows the deep learning network to use a higher learning rate, thereby accelerating the training process towards convergence [30].

The third investigated aspect was the difference in the activation functions used in each convolution layer. There were three activation functions used in this study, namely Rectified Linear Unit (ReLU), Leaky ReLU and exponential linear unit (ELU). The ReLU activation function was introduced using Eq. (1) [31]. Since 2015, ReLU has become the most widely used activation function in CNNs because it outperforms sigmoid and tanh, the most popular activation functions earlier [10].

$$f(x) = \max(0, x) \tag{1}$$

where x is the input signal of the ReLU layer. The LeakyReLU activation function is a variant of ReLU introduced using Eq. (2) [32]. The use of LeakyReLU activation function in several studies has shown an increase in classification accuracy [33, 34].

$$f(x) = \begin{cases} x & \text{if } x \geq 0 \\ \propto \times x & \text{otherwise} \end{cases} \quad (2)$$

where, x is the input signal of the LeakyReLU layer and $\propto$ is a constant set when the CNN network is used. LeakyReLU allows negative $f(x)$ values, as shown in Eq. (2), unlike ReLU which holds a minimum value of $f(x)$ at 0.

The ELU introduced in [35] is another variant of ReLU which often shows better performance than that of LeakyReLU and ReLU. ELU is derived from the following Eq. (3):

$$f(x) = \begin{cases} x & \text{if } x > 0 \\ \propto (\exp(x) - 1) & \text{if } x \leq 0 \end{cases} \quad (3)$$

where x is the input signal of the ELU layer.

In the third aspect investigation, three concise CNNs were run. The only difference among the three was the activation functions they used. The first and second layer of each CNN used a filter size of 7 × 7, while the third to sixth layer had a filter size of 3 × 3. Conf_Ch_7 was the configuration that used the ReLu activation function while Conf_elu was the one that used the ELU activation function. The configuration that used the Leaky ReLu activation function was named Conf_LeakyRelu.

The last aspect investigated was the effects of optimization functions to select the best weight and bias values to increase the performance of the proposed CNN. The optimization functions investigated in this study were stochastic gradient descent with momentum (sgdm) [36] derived from adaptive moment estimation (adam) [37], and root mean square propagation (rmsprop). The CNN configuration that applied the sgdm optimization function was Conf_Ch_7. The configuration that used the adam optimization function was called Conf_adam while the one using the rmsprop optimization function was named Conf_rmsprop.

2.4 Comparison Architectures

The architectures used for comparison in this study were ShuffleNet, MobileNet-V2, GoogleNet, NASNet and Squeezenet. They were chosen to represent reliable CNN architectures with the number of parameters being smaller than 10M.

In [20], the performances of GoogleNet, AlexNet, Inception V3, ResNet 18, and ResNet 50 on the PlantVillage tomato leaf dataset were evaluated. However, this research used GoogleNet only for two reasons. First, GoogleNet has the best performance with the highest accuracy and the second shortest training time after AlexNet at 30 training epochs. Second, the number of GoogleNet's parameters is smaller than 10M, whereas the parameters of the other architectures are greater than 10M.

2.5 Training and Evaluation

Performance evaluation was carried out by comparing the training accuracy, testing accuracy, training loss, testing loss, number of parameters involved, and classification time of each configuration. Classification accuracy is the most used metric in assessing the performance of a CNN [20]. Meanwhile, the selection of the number of parameters and classification time was done based on the purpose of this study, namely to find a concise CNN architecture that can classify leaf images quickly and automatically in an agricultural field.

The training and testing of all the architectures were carried out on a computer with an Intel Core i5-6400 CPU @ 2.70 GHz, 16 GB RAM and Matlab R2020a. No graphics memory device was involved in this process. The dataset was divided into 80% for training and 20% for testing. The input images for all configurations of the proposed CNN architecture were maintained in their original size, namely 256 × 256. However, for the comparison architectures, the images were resized to their default sizes.

All configurations of the proposed CNN and comparison CNN architectures were trained and tested sequentially using the dataset and the same computer. The performances of the proposed configurations (Table 1) were compared by looking at their performance trends. These trends were obtained after training the configurations gradually, starting from the configuration consisting of only 1 convolution layer, 2 layers, to 12 layers. A configuration consisting of 6 convolution layers is shown in Fig. 2 while the settings are presented in Table 1. A configuration consisting of 1–5 convolution layers was created by cutting the last convolution layer in the architecture, as shown in Fig. 2. Meanwhile, a configuration consisting of 7–12 convolution layers was made by duplicating the last convolution layer of each configuration.

This investigation aimed to test the stability of the configuration performance and find out the ideal number of convolution layers for the configuration's architecture. Testing of all the architectures was carried out at each completion of the training epoch. The best training and testing accuracy of each architecture was presented in Table 2 along with the lowest loss values, numbers of parameters, and classification time per image.

Table 2 The performance of Conf_Ch_7, its configurations and five comparison architectures

Architecture	Highest Accuracy Achieved (%)		Lowest Loss Achieved		Number of Parameters	Classification Time/ image (s)
	Training	Testing	Training	Testing		
Conf_Ch_9	100	97.76	0.0004	0.0774	114.6k	0.00307
Conf_Ch_7	100	98.64	0.0004	0.0452	109.8k	0.00283
Conf_Ch_5	100	98.58	0.0004	0.0447	106.1k	0.00260
Conf_Ch_3	100	97.68	0.0002	0.0751	103.7k	0.00233
Conf_LeakyRelu	100	98.44	0.0003	0.0448	109.8k	0.00310
Conf_elu	100	98.64	0.0004	0.0442	109.8k	0.00347
Conf_No_batch_norm	82.81	75.14	0.6711	0.796	109.3k	0.00250
Conf_adam	98.44	93.65	0.0784	0.1825	109.8k	0.00460
Conf_rmsprop	96.09	91.72	0.107	0.2352	109.8k	0.00283
Shufflenet	100	98.89	0.0008	0.0579	1.4M	0.0226
Mobilenet-v2	100	99.14	0.0003	0.0623	3.5M	0.0446
Googlenet	100	99.20	0.0002	0.0282	7.0M	0.0356
NASNet	100	99.12	0.0004	0.0632	5.3M	0.0775
Squeezenet	100	98.70	0.0002	0.0477	1.24M	0.0224

3 Results and Discussion

3.1 *Investigation of the Proposed Architectural Configuration*

Table 2 shows the performance comparison of Conf_Ch_7, the eight configurations and five comparison architectures. Of all the proposed configurations, Conf_Ch_7 and Conf_elu achieved the highest testing accuracy (98.64%). This accuracy was slightly higher than the accuracy of Conf_Ch_5 (98.58%) and Conf_LeakyRelu. The other configurations were found to not achieve above 98% accuracy.

Figure 3 shows the performance of the four configurations with different filter sizes applied to the convolution layers. Conf_Ch_7 and Conf_Ch_5 were found to outperform Conf_Ch_3 and Conf_Ch_9 in classifying images in the PlantVillage dataset. The best classification accuracy was achieved by Conf_Ch_7 with 6 convolution layers. Conf_Ch_5 achieved nearly the same accuracy as that of Conf_Ch_7, with 6 convolution layers as well. It was also found that adding the number of convolution layers did not increase the classification accuracy of the four configurations.

From Table 2, it can be seen that a CNN architecture without a batch normalization layer cannot achieve satisfactory performance. Figure 4 shows the poor performance of the Conf_No_batch_norm when its convolution layers were below 7. The performance improved when the convolution layers were increased to 8. However, this performance was still far below the performance of the other configurations.

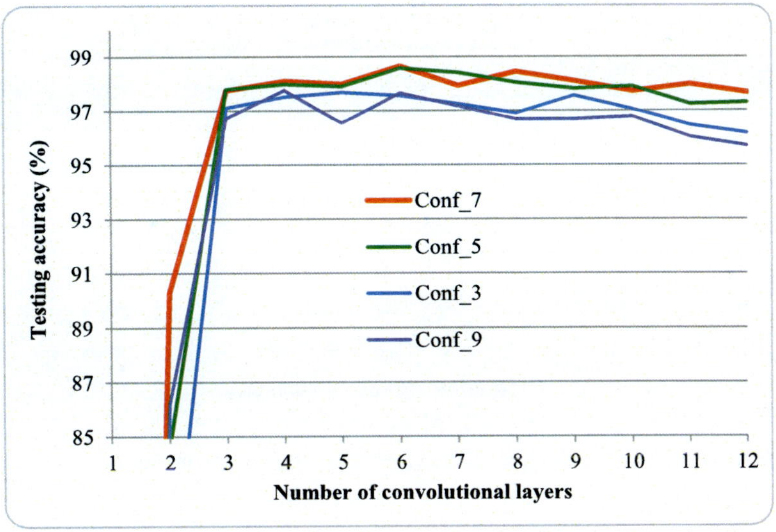

Fig. 3 Configuration performance based on filter size at 12 convolution layers

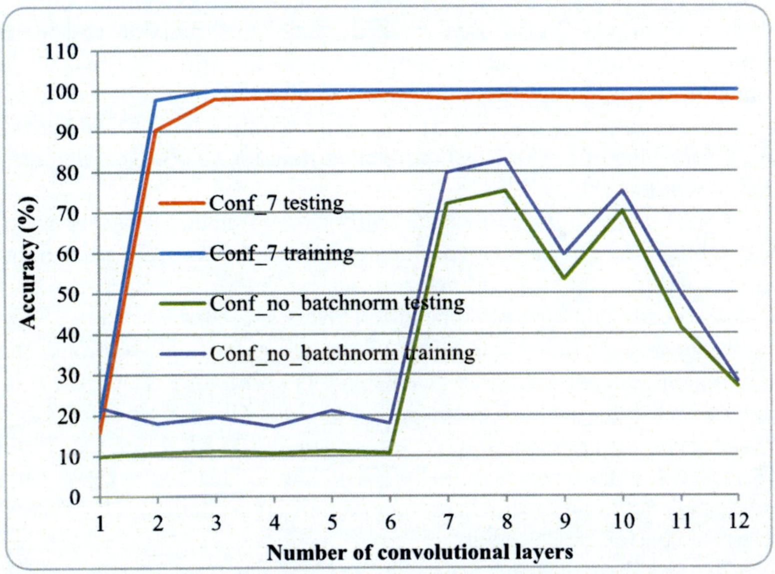

Fig. 4 Configuration performance based on the presence of a batch normalization layer

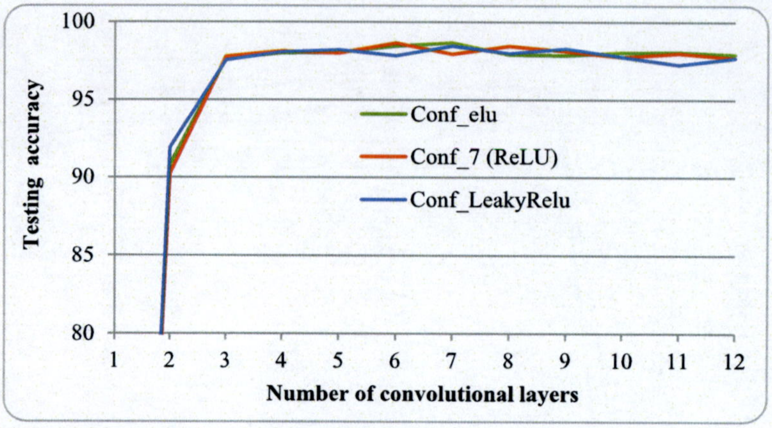

Fig. 5 Performance of each configuration based on the activation function used

Figure 5 shows each configuration performance based on the activation function used. Conf_Ch_7 used the ReLU activation function and achieved nearly the same and stable performance as that of Conf_elu and Conf_LekyRelu. Table 2 also confirms this. Conf_Ch_7 also used the sgdm activation function and reached a slightly higher accuracy and faster classification time than the other two configurations, which makes it the most recommended architecture of all. Based on the test data in Table 2, Conf_Ch_7 can classify one image within 0.00283 s, which is faster than the performance of Leaky ReLU activation function (0.00310 s) and the ELU activation function (0.00347 s).

Figure 6 shows the comparison of the optimization function performance on the proposed architecture. The performance of architecture that used the adam optimization function and rmsprop was still not satisfactory. The performance also declined significantly when the number of convolution layers exceeded 7.

Thus, it can be concluded that some of the proposed configurations, such as Conf_Ch_7, Conf_elu and Conf_Ch_5, have good performance. Conf_Ch_7 is 1.22 times faster than Conf_elu and is almost as fast as Conf_Ch_5. Both Conf_Ch_7 and Conf_elu have the same number of parameters, namely 109.8 k. Conf_Ch_7's testing accuracy is also slightly better than that of Conf_Ch_5. This makes Conf_Ch_7 the most promising and recommended configuration of all, as indicated by Table 2 and the investigated performance trends.

Figure 7 shows the confusion matrix of the Conf_Ch_7 architecture which was the best configuration of the proposed architecture. The highest misclassification value occurred during the classification of the Target Spot class. The classification accuracy of this class was 97% with 4 images classified as Spider Mites, 2 images classified as Tomato Mosaic Virus and 4 other images each in different classes. The Late Blight class was also quite difficult to classify with an accuracy of only 97.4%. Classes that can be classified without error were Healthy and Tomato Mosaic Virus classes.

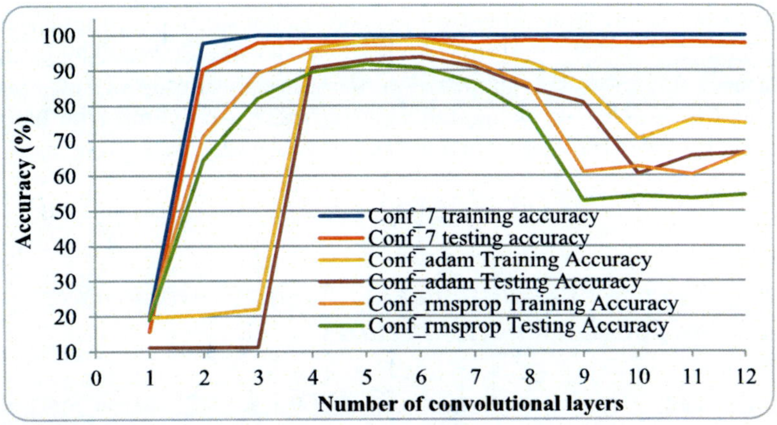

Fig. 6 Performance of the proposed configurations based on different optimization functions

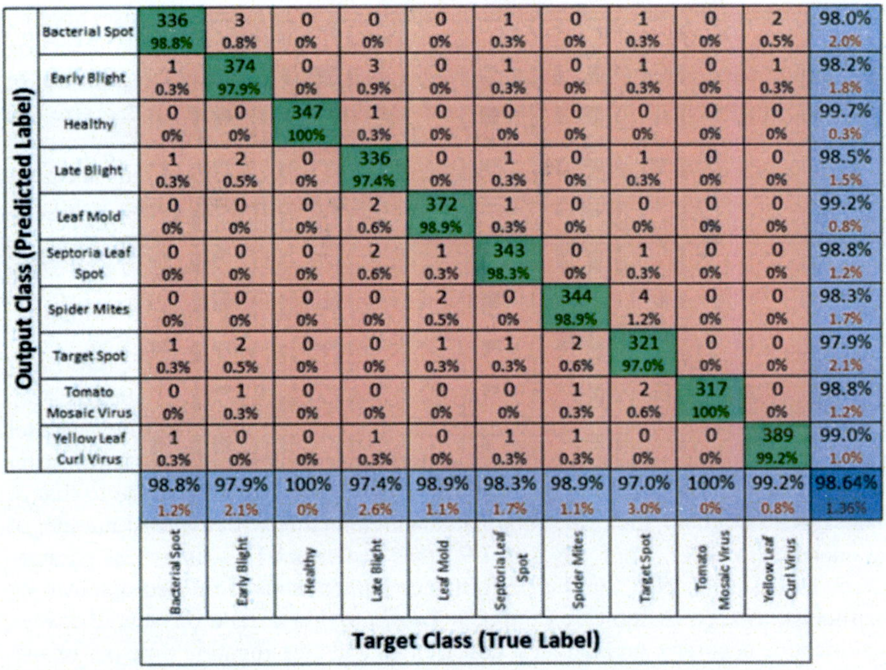

Fig. 7 Confusion matrix of Conf_Ch_7

The tests in this study also provided some additional information. First, using filter sizes of 9×9 and 3×3 did not result in a good performance for image classification in the dataset. The testing accuracy of configurations that used these two filter sizes also did not reach 98%. Second, the configurations that did not use a batch normalization layer provided the poorest classification performance with 82.81% training classification accuracy and 75.14% testing accuracy. Configuration performance using the Adam optimization function and rmsprop was also poor in classifying the dataset. The configurations using these two optimization functions did not achieve 100% training accuracy. The testing accuracy rates were also below 95%.

3.2 *Performance Comparison of the Proposed Architecture and the Comparison Architectures*

As shown in Table 2, GoogleNet achieved the best testing accuracy (99.20%), which is nearly the same as that of GoogleNet in [20] namely 99.39%. As mentioned earlier, the accuracy of GoogleNet in [11] was 89.68% even though the study also used a dataset of 10 tomato leaf images of PlantVillage class. This difference in accuracy is caused by the difference in the number of images in the dataset used by the two studies. The study in [20] used an input image of 224 × 224, the same size used in this study as well. The study in [11] reduced the image size to 64 × 64, of course the sharpness and completeness of the features are reduced at that size and the classification accuracy decreased.

Table 2 also shows that Mobilenet-v2 achieves 99.14% accuracy. This accuracy is quite different when compared to the accuracy shown in [21] which is 90.3%. This difference in accuracy stems from the difference in the number of images in the dataset even though the number of classes is both 10. This study used 17,641 while [21] used 7176 images. Differences in accuracy due to significant differences in the number of images in the dataset are also shown by [17].

The most recommended configuration of the proposed architecture is Conf_Ch_7 with 98.64% accuracy. Although Conf_Ch_7 has a slightly lower classification accuracy than that of GoogleNet, its number of parameters is 63.75 times smaller than that of GoogleNet. Its classification performance is also 12.58 times faster than GoogleNet. The accuracy of Conf_Ch_7 is 98.64%, which is close to that of SqueezeNet (98.70%), the fastest comparison architecture with the least number of parameters. However, Conf_Ch_7 is 7.9 times faster and 11.3 times less parameterized than SqueezeNet. Similar performance comparisons were also obtained by ShuffleNet, as seen in Table 2. Conf_Ch_7 can provide a trade-off value between classification accuracy, architectural conciseness and classification time per image, which makes it feasible for implementation in an agricultural field with limited resources.

4 Conclusion and Future Work

Having investigated and compared several proposed configurations, it can be concluded that Conf_Ch_7 has the best performance of all configurations. Conf_Ch_7 can achieve an accuracy rate of 98.64%, a classification speed of 0.00283 s per image on the test computer in the study, and 109.8k parameters.

The classification accuracy value of Conf_Ch_7 is acceptable after comparing it with the comparison architectures and trends in classification accuracy shown by other studies in this field. Conf_Ch_7 has two advantages. First, its classification time per image is the fastest of all. Second, it has the smallest number of parameters. These indicate that the Conf_Ch_7 architecture has competitive performance and provides a trade-off between accuracy, architectural conciseness, and classification time per image.

Our next research goal is to implement Conf_Ch_7 for classification in agriculture. A small number of parameters and short classification time will facilitate its implementation in a reliable and inexpensive real-time monitoring system of agricultural land at a large scale. The performance of the other proposed configurations in the current study can also be improved by future researchers.

Acknowledgements This work was supported by the Ministry of Research and Technology/National Research and Innovation Agency of Republic Indonesia (Kementerian Riset Dan Teknologi/Badan Riset Dan Inovasi Nasional Republik Indonesia) under the scheme of Penelitian Disertasi Doktor (PDD) 2021 with contract number of 56/SP2H/LT/DPRM/2021.

The authors would like to thank all colleagues at Multimedia Signal Processing Research Group at the Data Laboratory, Universitas Syiah Kuala, and the Research Group at The Robotic Laboratory, Universitas Harapan Medan for assistance and facilities during this research.

References

1. CIA (2018) The world factbook (GDP)
2. Khamparia A, Saini G, Gupta D, Khanna A, Tiwari S, Albuquerque VHC. Seasonal crops disease prediction and classification using deep convolutional encoder network. https://doi.org/10.1007/s00034-019-01041-0
3. Park H, JeeSook E, Kim S-H (2018) Crops disease diagnosing using image-based deep learning mechanism. https://doi.org/10.1109/CoCoNet.2018.8476914
4. Lu J, Hu J, Zhao G, Mei F, Zhang C (2017) An in-field automatic wheat disease diagnosis system. https://doi.org/10.1016/j.compag.2017.09.012
5. Ma J, Du K, Zheng F, Zhang L, Gong Z, Sun Z (2018) A recognition method for cucumber diseases using leaf symptom images based on deep convolutional neural network. Comput Electron Agric 154:18–24. https://doi.org/10.1016/j.compag.2018.08.048
6. Knoll FJ, Czymmek V, Poczihoski S, Holtorf T, Hussmann S (2018) Improving efficiency of organic farming by using a deep learning classification approach. Comput Electron Agric 153:347–356. https://doi.org/10.1016/j.compag.2018.08.032
7. Mohanty SP, Hughes DP, Salathé M (2016) Using deep learning for image-based plant disease detection. Front Plant Sci 7:1–10. https://doi.org/10.3389/fpls.2016.01419

8. Too EC, Yujian L, Njuki S, Yingchun L (2019) A comparative study of fine-tuning deep learning models for plant disease identification. Comput Electron Agric 161:272–279. https://doi.org/10.1016/j.compag.2018.03.032
9. Yamashita R, Nishio M, Do RKG, Togashi K (2018) Convolutional neural networks: an overview and its applications in pattern recognition. Smart Innov Syst Technol. https://doi.org/10.1007/978-981-15-7078-0_3
10. Lecun Y, Bengio Y, Hinton G (2015) Deep learning. Nature 521:436–444. https://doi.org/10.1038/nature14539
11. Suryawati E, Sustika R, Yuwana RS, Subekti A, Pardede HF (2018) Deep structured convolutional neural network for tomato diseases detection. In: 2018 International conference on advanced computer science and information systems (ICACSIS), pp 385–390. https://doi.org/10.1109/ICACSIS.2018.8618169
12. Khan A, Sohail A, Zahoora U, Qureshi AS (2020) A survey of the recent architectures of deep convolutional neural networks. Springer Netherlands. https://doi.org/10.1007/s10462-020-09825-6
13. Shakeel MF, Bajwa NA, Anwaar AM, Sohail A, Khan A, Haroon-ur-Rashid (2019) Detecting driver drowsiness in real time through deep learning based object detection. Lecture notes in computer science (including Subseries Lecture notes in artificial intelligence, Lecture notes in bioinformatics). LNCS, vol 11506, pp 283–296 (2019). https://doi.org/10.1007/978-3-030-20521-8_24
14. Karthik R, Hariharan M, Anand S, Mathikshara P, Johnson A, Menaka R (2020) Attention embedded residual CNN for disease detection in tomato leaves. Appl Soft Comput J 86:105933. https://doi.org/10.1016/j.asoc.2019.105933
15. Wu Y, Wang Z, Shi Y, Hu J (2020) Enabling on-device CNN training by self-supervised instance filtering and error map pruning. IEEE Trans Comput Des Integr Circuits Syst 39:3445–3457. https://doi.org/10.1109/TCAD.2020.3012216
16. Durmus H, Gunes EO, Kirci M (2017) Disease detection on the leaves of the tomato plants by using deep learning. In: 2017 6th International conference on agro-geoinformatics 2017. https://doi.org/10.1109/Agro-Geoinformatics.2017.8047016
17. Lu J, Tan L, Jiang H (2021) Review on convolutional neural network (CNN) applied to plant leaf disease classification. Agric 11:1–18. https://doi.org/10.3390/agriculture11080707
18. Chollet F (2018) Deep learning with python. Manning Publications Co., New York
19. Rangarajan AK, Purushothaman R, Ramesh A (2018) Tomato crop disease classification using pre-trained deep learning algorithm. Procedia Comput Sci 133:1040–1047. https://doi.org/10.1016/j.procs.2018.07.070
20. Maeda-Gutiérrez V, Galván-Tejada CE, Zanella-Calzada LA, Celaya-Padilla JM, Galván-Tejada JI, Gamboa-Rosales H, Luna-García H, Magallanes-Quintanar R, Guerrero Méndez CA, Olvera-Olvera CA (2020) Comparison of convolutional neural network architectures for classification of tomato plant diseases. https://doi.org/10.3390/app10041245
21. Elhassouny A, Smarandache F (2019) Smart mobile application to recognize tomato leaf diseases using convolutional neural networks. In: 2019 International conference of computer science and renewable energies (ICCSRE), pp 1–4. https://doi.org/10.1109/ICCSRE.2019.8807737
22. McCool C, Perez T, Upcroft B (2017) Mixtures of lightweight deep convolutional neural networks: applied to agricultural robotics. IEEE Robot Autom Lett 2:1344–1351. https://doi.org/10.1109/LRA.2017.2667039
23. Haug S, Ostermann J (2015) A crop/weed field image dataset for the evaluation of computer vision based precision agriculture tasks BT. Presented at the Computer vision—ECCV 2014 workshops
24. Howlader MR, Habiba U, Faisal RH, Rahman MM (2019) Automatic recognition of guava leaf diseases using deep convolution neural network. In: 2nd International conference on electrical, communication and computer engineering, ECCE 2019, pp 1–5. https://doi.org/10.1109/ECACE.2019.8679421

25. Hughes DP, Salathe M (2015) An open access repository of images on plant health to enable the development of mobile disease diagnostics
26. Abade A, Ferreira PA, de Barros Vidal F (2021) Plant diseases recognition on images using convolutional neural networks: a systematic review. Comput Electron Agric 185. https://doi.org/10.1016/j.compag.2021.106125
27. Sembiring A, Away Y, Arnia F, Muharar R (2020) Development of concise convolutional neural network for tomato plant disease classification based on leaf images. J Phys Conf Ser 1845. https://doi.org/10.1088/1742-6596/1845/1/012009
28. Ioffe S, Szegedy C (2015) Batch normalization: accelerating deep network training by reducing internal covariate shift
29. Awais M, Iqbal MT, Bin, Bae SH (2021) Revisiting internal covariate shift for batch normalization. IEEE Trans Neural Netw Learn Syst 32:5082–5092. https://doi.org/10.1109/TNNLS.2020.3026784
30. Bjorck J, Gomes C, Selman B, Weinberger KQ (2018) Understanding batch normalization. Adv Neural Inf Process Syst 7694–7705
31. Hahnloser RHR, Sarpeshkar R, Mahowald MA, Douglas RJ, Seung HS (2000) Digital selection and analogue amplification coexist in a cortex-inspired silicon circuit. Nature 405:947–951. https://doi.org/10.1038/35016072
32. Maas AL, Hannun AY, Ng AY (2013) Rectifier nonlinearities improve neural network acoustic models. In: ICML Workshop on deep learning for audio, speech and language processing, vol 28
33. Jiang D, Li F, Yang Y, Yu S (2020) A tomato leaf diseases classification method based on deep learning. In: Proceedings of the 32nd Chinese control and decision conference, CCDC 2020, pp 1446–1450. https://doi.org/10.1109/CCDC49329.2020.9164457
34. Prajapati R, Khatri U, Kwon GR (2021) An efficient deep neural network binary classifier for Alzheimer's disease classification. In: International conference on artificial intelligence in information and communication, ICAIIC 2021, pp 231–234. https://doi.org/10.1109/ICAIIC51459.2021.9415212
35. Clevert DA, Unterthiner T, Hochreiter S (2016) Fast and accurate deep network learning by exponential linear units (ELUs). In: 4th International conference on learning representations, ICLR 2016—conference track proceedings, pp 1–14
36. Murphy KP (2012) machine learning: a probabilistic perspective. The MIT Press, Cambridge, Massachusetts
37. Kingma DP, Ba JL (2015) Adam: a method for stochastic optimization. In: 3rd International conference on learning representations, ICLR 2015—conference track proceedings, pp 1–15

An Advanced Data Augmentation Scheme on Limited EEG Signals for Human Emotion Recognition

Dwi Wahyu Prabowo, Hanung Adi Nugroho, Noor Akhmad Setiawan, and Johan Debayle

Abstract EEG signals are the modality that is widely used to recognize human emotions. However, the limited data on EEG signals remains challenging because of the small recording participants, the need for an expert to interpret EEG signals, and the expensive cost of tools to record EEG signals. This research proposed the data augmentation schemes on the EEG datasets to overcome the limited available data problem. Augmenting the data will help the generalizability of the emotion recognition model. The EEG signals on the DEAP and SEED datasets are transformed into image samples using a recurrence plot and spectrogram. Then, the artificial recurrence plot and the artificial spectrogram samples are generated using Pix2pix. This research used these artificial samples to conduct the data augmentation process. LeNet5, ResNet50, MobileNet, and DenseNet121 are used to conduct the classification. The best four data augmentation schemes are as follows: Appending 20,000 artificial recurrence plot samples to DEAP and SEED training datasets, appending 20,000 artificial spectrogram samples to the DEAP training dataset, and appending 15,000 artificial spectrogram samples to the SEED training dataset. The kappa coefficient for each classification model based on the best data augmentation schemes is computed. It is found that among the compared classifiers, LeNet5 achieved the best accuracy in both SEED (98.58%) and DEAP (86.12%) datasets when spectrogram was used. Therefore, LeNet5 trained on the spectrogram samples is a reliable and robust classification model. This finding implies that the use of spectrogram is more promising than the recurrence plot in human emotion recognition.

Keywords EEG · Human emotion · Data augmentation · Pix2pix · Classification

D. W. Prabowo · H. A. Nugroho (✉) · N. A. Setiawan · J. Debayle
Department of Electrical and Information Engineering, Faculty of Engineering, Universitas Gadjah Mada, Yogyakarta, Indonesia
e-mail: adinugroho@ugm.ac.id

D. W. Prabowo
Department of Information System, Faculty of Computer Science, Universitas Darwan Ali, Sampit, Indonesia

J. Debayle
UMR 5307 LGF, Centre SPIN, MINES Saint-Etienne, CNRS, Saint-Etienne, France

T. Triwiyanto et al. (eds.), *Proceeding of the 3rd International Conference on Electronics, Biomedical Engineering, and Health Informatics*, Lecture Notes in Electrical Engineering 1008, https://doi.org/10.1007/978-981-99-0248-4_27

1 Introduction

Human–computer interaction (HCI) is a field that studies the interaction between computers and humans. The ability of computer devices to interact with humans supports various activities in various fields. This ability has led to the emergence of many studies that examine more deeply the interactions between humans and computers. If computers can interpret human emotional conditions, the HCI application will be more intuitive, fluent, and effective [1].

Humans express their emotions in several ways, such as intonation speech [2, 3], facial expressions [4], hand movements, and eye contact. Based on these several ways, information about the emotions felt by humans when interacting with computers will be utilized in several ways in the field of HCI [5]. In HCI, many modalities can be used to identify human emotions. These modalities are in the form of a database for recording psychological signals like electrocardiogram (ECG), galvanic skin response (GSR), respiration, and electroencephalogram (EEG) [6].

As an application of HCI, BCI uses EEG signals to recognize human emotions. EEG signal is a representation of activity patterns in the human brain in the form of a recording of an electric field. The choice of EEG signal as a modality for recognizing emotions is due to its noninvasive superiority, making it safe for use in humans. EEG is also cheaper and easier to implement when compared to other modalities used for BCI, such as fMRI and MEG [5]. However, the availability of data on EEG signals is still one of the challenges in emotional recognition. The amount of data recorded on an EEG signal is limited. This problem is due to several reasons, such as the small recording participants and the need for an expert to interpret EEG signals. The duration of the recording of an EEG signal also cannot last long because the preparation process is time-consuming. Furthermore, participants can experience fatigue during an extended recording series [7–9]. The expensive cost of a tool to record EEG signals also caused this problem [10–12].

The limited data availability tends to be the main generalization problem in developing machine learning models. The easiest technique to improve the generalization of a machine learning model is to train it on augmented data [13]. Many studies have conducted data augmentation on the recognition of human emotions. Wang et al. [14] used a non-generative-based technique. They generate more EEG signal samples by adding Gaussian noise to the original EEG signals. Luo & Lu [15] used a conditional Wasserstein Generative Adversarial Network (cWGAN) scheme to generate new artificial samples through the differential entropy feature of EEG signals. Luo et al. [10] adopted conditional Boundary Equilibrium GAN (cBEGAN), and Zhang et al. [16] proposed Multi-generator conditional Wasserstein GAN (MG-cWGAN) to address the instability and non-convergence problems of the original GAN. Then, they utilized the DE features to generate new artificial EEG signals. Luo et al. [17] used selective variational autoencoder (sVAE) and selective Wasserstein GAN (sWGAN) to generate new artificial EEG signals based on DE features. Then, they trained a classifier to select the appropriate artificial EEG signals.

This research aims to augment EEG signals to tackle the limited available data problem. The augmentation process is conducted by appending new artificial samples to the training set. Goodfellow et al. [13] explain that it is challenging to generate new artificial samples if the density estimation problem is not solved yet. Since EEG signals have a non-stationary property [18], the EEG signal's statistical values are different each time, and the location where signal values cluster tightly also changes. It makes it challenging to conduct the density estimation.

On the other hand, based on these recent studies, all the work utilized EEG signal values directly to generate artificial samples. They have not utilized another input formulation, such as transforming 1D-EEG signals into a 2D image representation of EEG signals to exploit the hidden texture features in the image classification task. Therefore, in this research, the image samples are preferred instead of using EEG signals value to avoid the density estimation problem.

This research proposed the recurrence plot (RP) and the spectrogram (SP) to provide the image samples generated from EEG signals. A recurrence plot is a signal analysis tool based on nonlinear and non-stationary data. A recurrence plot is appropriate for nalysing the hidden patterns and structural changes in time series data over time [19]. Therefore, it is suitable for nalysing the characteristic patterns of EEG signals. The spectrogram is used to characterize the continuous EEG brain oscillation activity fluctuations. This indicates that the spectrogram can reveal patterns of brain activity while the person performs a task [20].

The recent studies did not provide a scheme to reveal which data augmentation process provided the best accuracy improvement. It is difficult to assess the best data augmentation process since they conduct a different data augmentation scheme based on the number of samples appended into the data training set. Therefore, this research proposed a systematic accuracy comparison of data augmentation schemes to highlight which data augmentation scheme has the best accuracy improvement.

This research conducts emotion recognition by classifying the image samples generated from EEG signals using Convolutional Neural Network (CNN) based classifiers, such as LeNet5, ResNet50, MobileNet, and DenseNet121. CNN-based classifiers are used in this research because they perform well in image classification [21]. Then, the data augmentation schemes are proposed by appending the artificial recurrence plot samples and the artificial spectrogram sample to the training set to tackle the limited available data problem. Pix2pix is used to generate the artificial recurrence plot samples and the artificial spectrogram samples. The accuracy metric and the kappa coefficient are used as a classification performance evaluation.

2 Materials and Method

This section describes the methodology conducted in this research, including the public datasets used, the transformation of EEG signals into images sample using recurrence plots (RP) and spectrogram (SP); Pix2pix; research design, including data augmentation, classification strategy, and performance evaluation.

2.1 Dataset

DEAP. The DEAP[1] [22] dataset contains 40 EEG signal recording experiments from 32 subjects. Music video clips are used to stimulate the emotions of each subject during the recording of the EEG signal. The video clips used in the DEAP dataset are 60 s long. The emotion labels used in the DEAP dataset are within the range of valence and arousal value pairs. The emotion recognition conducted in this research is a multiclass classification task. Therefore, this binary class label must be transformed into a multiclass label. Suppose θ is the mid value on the range [1, 9] of DEAP class label. If the value on the range [1, 9] is greater than θ, it will be set as a high value. If the value on the range [1, 9] is lower than θ, it will be set as a low value. Based on this basis, four classes of DEAP, including LALV (low arousal-low valence), LAHV (low arousal-high valence), HALV (high arousal-low valence), and HAHV (high arousal-high valence), can be generated.

SEED. Zheng and Lu [23] proposed the SEED[2] dataset to classify human emotion based on three emotional states Positive, Neutral, and Negative. They use a 62-channel EEG system to record EEG signals from 15 subjects. Each subject is required to conduct a total of 15 trials. At first, the subjects are asked to watch four minutes of movie clips to elicit their emotional states. During the watching activity, the signals are recorded.

Self-assessment is necessary to provide the ground truth of the labeled emotional state. In this research, the preprocessed DEAP and SEED datasets were used. Each subject conducted a self-assessment after completing the recording session to verify the emotion value in both datasets.

The datasets used in this research have different characteristics. The DEAP dataset used music video clips to elicit the subject emotional states; meanwhile, the SEED dataset used movie clips. The DEAP dataset used four different emotional state labels (HAHV, HALV, LAHV, LALV), and the SEED dataset used three different emotional state labels (Negative, Neutral, Positive). They also used different EEG channel systems to record the signals. The DEAP dataset used a 32-channel EEG system, and the SEED dataset used a 62-channel EEG system. Table 1 shows the DEAP and SEED content summary.

2.2 Signal to Image Transformation

Recurrence plot. A recurrence plot is a nonlinear and non-stationary signal analysis technique. Suppose $x(t)$ is a one-dimensional signal in the time domain t where $t = 1, 2, ..., n$. The m dimensional trajectories can be generated by using the time delay embedding τ. The m-dimensional trajectories are formulated in Eq. 1 [24].

[1] https://www.eecs.qmul.ac.uk/mmv/datasets/deap/index.html.

[2] https://bcmi.sjtu.edu.cn/home/seed/seed.html.

Table 1 DEAP and SEED dataset summary

	DEAP	SEED
Subject	32 subjects	15 subjects
Trial	40 trials	15 trials
Data	Raw and preprocessed data	Raw and preprocessed data
Channel	32-channel EEG system	62-channel EEG system
Sampling rate	Sampling rate 128 Hz	Sampling rate 200 Hz
Label	Valence, arousal, and liking rated using a continuous scale between 1 to 9	Positive, neutral, Negative

$$\vec{s_i} = \left(x_i, x_{i+r}, \ldots, x_{i+(m-1)\tau}\right), \forall_i \in \{1, \ldots, n-(m-1)\tau\} \tag{1}$$

The recurrence plot $R_{i,j}$ plots an image representing the pairwise distance between the trajectories in Eq. 1. The recurrence plot $R_{i,j}$ is formulated in Eq. 2 [24].

$$R_{i,j} = \Theta\left(\varepsilon - \left\| \vec{s_i} - \vec{s_j} \right\|\right), \forall_{i,j} \in \{1, \ldots, n-(m-1)\tau\} \tag{2}$$

where s_i is a state in m-dimensional, Θ is a Heaviside function, a step function with zero negative value arguments and one for positive argument, and ε is the threshold.

Spectrogram. A spectrogram represents the spectrum of signal frequencies that vary in time. Suppose $x(t)$ is a one-dimensional signal in the time domain (t), ω is the angular frequency, $w(t-\tau)$ is the window function, and τ is the window translation parameter. A spectrogram $S_x(\tau, \omega)$ is formulated in Eq. 3 [25].

$$\begin{aligned} X(\tau, \omega) &= \sum_{t=-\infty}^{\infty} x(t) w(t-\tau) e^{-i\omega t} \\ S_x(\tau, \omega) &= |X(\tau, \omega)|^2 \end{aligned} \tag{3}$$

$|X(n, \omega)|^2$ is also called the short-time Fourier transform (STFT) [25].

2.3 *Pix2pix*

This research used the pix2pix [26] technique to generate new artificial data. Pix2pix is used to ensure that every pair of original-artificial samples are evaluated. Pix2pix consists of three components: U-Net [27] as the generator, PatchGAN [26] as the discriminator, and an optimization model. Figure 1 shows the pix2pix architecture with the recurrence plot/spectrogram generated from EEG signals as input.

Suppose that EEG image samples as an original input. Figure 1a shows that the U-Net generator takes the original input to generate artificial output. The PatchGAN discriminator creates a classification matrix using the original input and the fake

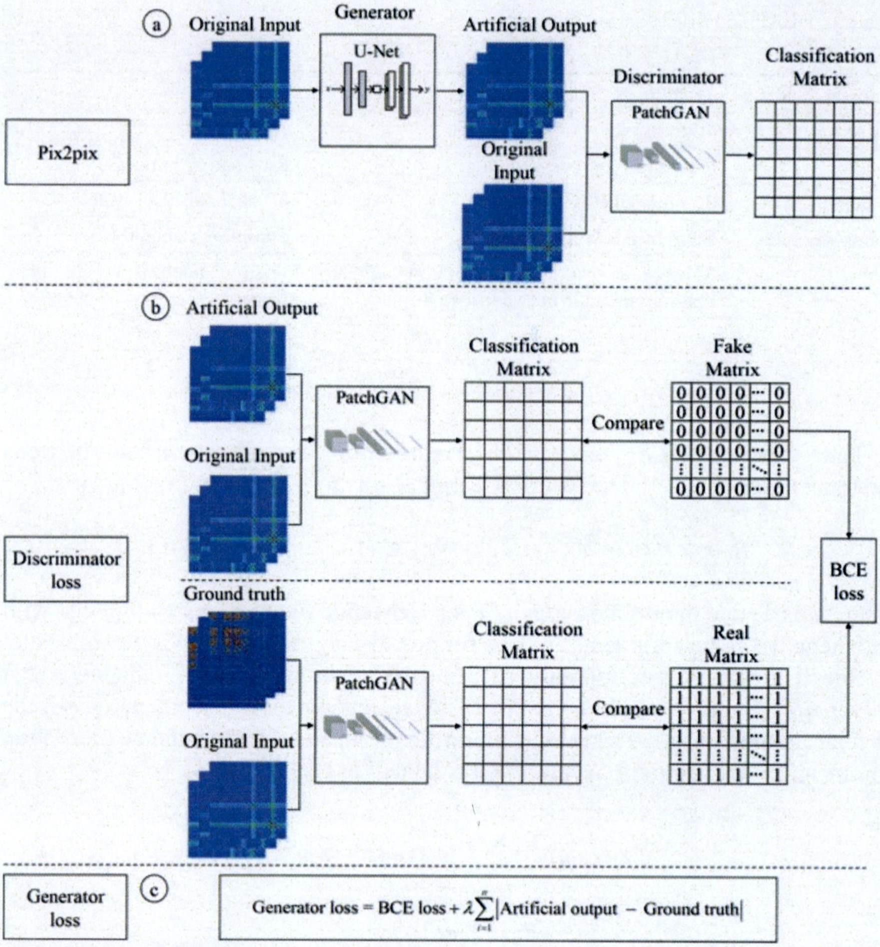

Fig. 1 (**a**) Pix2pix architecture; (**b**) Discriminator loss calculation; (**c**) Generator loss calculation (Compiled from [26, 28])

output. This classification matrix consists of element values in the range [0, 1]. Figure 1b shows the procedure to compute the discriminator loss. For the artificial output, the output of concatenating the artificial output with the original input is compared to the fake matrix label, the all-zeros matrix. The true matrix label is compared to the concatenating output between the ground truth and the original input for the original input. Then BCE loss is computed based on these comparisons. Figure 1c shows the equation to compute the generator loss. The generator loss is computed using BCE loss plus the distance between the artificial output and the ground truth multiplied by the parameter.

2.4 Cohen's Kappa Coefficient

Cohen's kappa coefficient is a tool to measure the agreements between two raters. Suppose P_0 is the observed agreement proportion and P_e is the expected agreement proportion; the kappa coefficient (κ) can be calculated using the formula in Eq. 4 [29].

$$\kappa = \frac{P_0 - P_e}{1 - P_e} \tag{4}$$

Landis and Koch [30] state that the kappa coefficient in the range of 0.81–1.00 has an almost perfect agreement. Therefore, this research used this range of kappa coefficients to evaluate the classification models.

2.5 Research Design

Data augmentation. The data augmentation process aims to increase the number of EEG signal data so that the size of the training data used by the classifier will be more significant. This research implemented the data augmentation based on Luo et al. [17] work. Luo et al. conducted data augmentation using EEG signals as input. In this research, the data augmentation was performed by appending the recurrence plot/spectrogram samples generated from EEG signals. Figure 2 shows the data augmentation framework. Based on Fig. 2, Pix2pix utilized the original training samples to generate artificial samples. The artificial samples were then appended into original training samples to produce augmented training samples.

Since the pix2pix method is a paired image-to-image translation method, the samples fed into the architecture must be pairwise of the original image and its ground truth. Figure 3 shows the pairwise input and ground truth of the recurrence plot and spectrogram sample. The original inputs were image samples generated using a distance threshold for the recurrence plots, so the recurrence plot is binarized. The ground truth samples were image samples generated using the distance threshold not applied. Both the recurrence plot and spectrogram samples apply colormap: Binary for the original input and colormap: Jet for the ground truth.

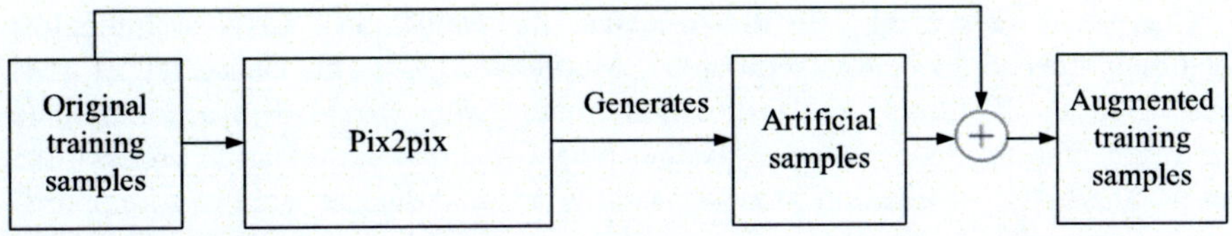

Fig. 2 Data augmentation framework

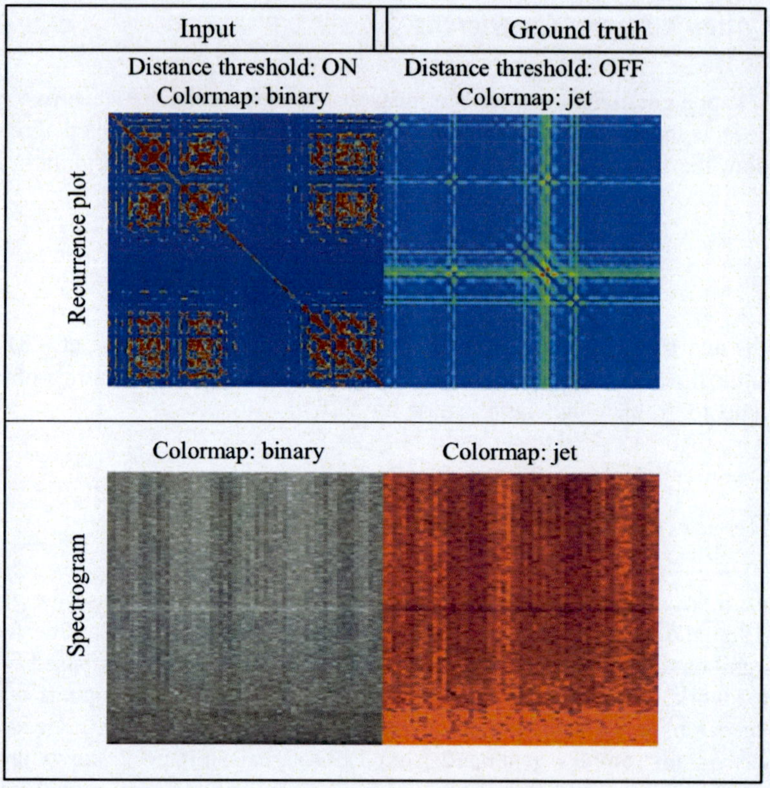

Fig. 3 Pairwise of input and ground truth of recurrence plot sample

The generation of the artificial sample is conducted based on the label provided on the DEAP and SEED datasets. This treatment procedure ensures that generated artificial samples are correct regarding the dataset labels. The assessment was then conducted to evaluate the artificial samples before appending them to the training data. First, a classifier was trained to compute the confident classification score for each artificial sample in the different labels. Then, the artificial samples which have high classification confidence were selected. In this research, LeNet5 was used as a classifier to compute the confident classification score since LeNet5 has a simpler architecture network than other classifiers.

Classification strategy. In this research, the well-known CNN architectures including LeNet5 [31], ResNet50 [32], MobileNet [33], and DenseNet121 [34] were used as classifiers. A classification strategy was provided to accommodate the augmentation process. Each classifier performed the classification process five times. The first classification process used the original dataset without adding artificial samples. The second classification process used the original dataset plus 5000 artificial samples. The third to the fifth classification process was carried out by adding artificial samples in multiples of 5000. The artificial samples were added evenly according to the labels for each dataset.

The hyperparameter settings used in this research were as follows: (1) The input size was 150×150. . (2) Learning rate is 0.0001. (3) The optimizer for all classifiers was Adam. (4) The loss function for the multiclass classification task was sparse categorical cross-entropy. (5) The number of epochs was 350 for LeNet5 and 50 for ResNet50, MobileNet, and DenseNet121.

Performance evaluation. The final step was performance evaluation. The dataset was split into training, validation, and testing parts to validate the classification model. 60% of the dataset was used as the training set, 20% of the dataset was used as a validation set, and 20% of the dataset was used as a testing set. The kappa coefficient metric was used in this research to evaluate the classification models. The McNemar [35] statistical test with $\alpha = 0.05$ was also conducted to show which data augmentation scheme significantly improved accuracy.

3 Result

3.1 Performance on Different Number of Appended Training Data

This section provides the classification performance analysis based on the used signal's transformation method and the used dataset. Each performance analysis provides the classification accuracy result on different artificial samples appended to the training set. The paired statistical test was conducted between the classifier trained on the original training set and the classifier trained on the augmented training set. Then the sign ($^+$) was put next to the accuracy value to indicate that the augmentation process improved the accuracy significantly and statistically.

Classification performance on the use of recurrence plot on DEAP. Based on Table 2, the accuracy of LeNet5, MobileNet, and DenseNet121 improved significantly by adding 10,000 to 20,000 artificial recurrence plot samples to the DEAP training set. However, the augmentation process took no effect on ResNet50. LeNet5 reaches the highest accuracy by appending 10,000 artificial recurrence plots (87.06%).

Classification performance on the use of recurrence plot on SEED. The classifier accuracy in Table 3 was enhanced by the varying number of added artificial samples on the SEED dataset. Adding 15,000 and 20,000 artificial recurrence plot samples considerably improved the accuracy of ResNet50. Adding artificial recurrence plot samples of 10,000, 15,000, and 20,000 significantly increased MobileNet's accuracy. In every augmentation method, DenseNet121's accuracy increased significantly. Meanwhile, applying data augmentation using artificial recurrence plot samples to the LeNet5 had no significant effect on accuracy. The highest accuracy is reached by ResNet50 by appending 20,000 artificial recurrence plots (91.02%).

Table 2 Classification accuracy (%) on the use of recurrence plots on the DEAP dataset

	DEAP + 0 (%)	DEAP + 5000 (%)	DEAP + 10,000 (%)	DEAP + 15,000 (%)	DEAP + 20,000 (%)
LeNet5	86.12	86.75	87.06⁺	86.67	86.89⁺
ResNet50	84.45	83.69	84.15	83.96	84.02
MobileNet	78.69	79.19	79.96⁺	80.52⁺	81.02⁺
DenseNet121	81.36	82.09	83.12⁺	82.25⁺	83.30⁺

⁺Sign shows the accuracy improvement is statistically significantly different

Table 3 Classification accuracy (%) on the use of recurrence plots on the SEED dataset

	SEED + 0 (%)	SEED + 5000 (%)	SEED + 10,000 (%)	SEED + 15,000 (%)	SEED + 20,000 (%)
LeNet5	90.41	89.19	90.47	90.18	90.39
ResNet50	89.41	89.74	90.01	90.61⁺	91.02⁺
MobileNet	82.58	82.71	83.86⁺	84.60⁺	84.87⁺
DenseNet121	87.54	88.28⁺	88.94⁺	89.93⁺	90.47⁺

⁺Sign shows the accuracy improvement is statistically significantly different

Classification performance on the use of spectrogram on DEAP. In Table 4, the data augmentation process significantly affects the accuracy of the classifier. All data augmentation schemes significantly improved each classifier's accuracy when the classification was conducted on the DEAP using spectrogram samples. The highest accuracy is reached by ResNet50 by appending 20,000 artificial spectrograms (91.53%).

Classification performance on the use of spectrogram on SEED. Table 5 showed the data augmentation method considerably impacts the classifier's accuracy. Each classifier's accuracy was significantly enhanced by all data augmentation schemes when conducted on the SEED dataset using spectrogram. Except for the ResNet50, adding 10,000 artificial samples did not result in a substantial gain in accuracy. LeNet5 reaches the highest accuracy by appending fifteen thousand artificial spectrograms (98.58%).

Table 4 Classification accuracy (%) on the use of spectrogram on the DEAP dataset

	DEAP + 0 (%)	DEAP + 5000 (%)	DEAP + 10,000 (%)	DEAP + 15,000 (%)	DEAP + 20,000 (%)
LeNet5	74.39	80.69⁺	82.92⁺	85.25⁺	86.12⁺
ResNet50	82.19	86.78⁺	89.12⁺	90.81⁺	91.53⁺
MobileNet	76.25	80.46⁺	83.25⁺	83.82⁺	87.20⁺
DenseNet121	81.57	84.68⁺	87.37⁺	89.12⁺	90.76⁺

⁺Sign shows the accuracy improvement is statistically significantly different

Table 5 Classification accuracy (%) on the use of spectrogram on the SEED dataset

	SEED + 0 (%)	SEED + 5000 (%)	SEED + 10,000 (%)	SEED + 15,000 (%)	SEED + 20,000 (%)
LeNet5	93.49	97.61+	98.10+	98.58+	98.23+
ResNet50	97.35	97.81+	97.77	97.98+	97.84+
MobileNet	81.89	83.11+	84.35+	85.09+	84.74+
DenseNet121	95.79	96.44+	96.79+	97+	97.16+

+Sign shows the accuracy improvement is statistically significantly different

Based on the classification results, when appending 5000 artificial samples using artificial spectrogram samples, the accuracies were improved significantly in both DEAP and SEED datasets. Meanwhile, the classifier accuracies were not significantly enhanced using DEAP and SEED datasets when appending 5000 artificial samples using artificial recurrence plot samples except for DenseNet121. This finding shows that using spectrogram samples as input is more promising than using a recurrence plot when classifying human emotion. This is because the recurrence plots have a redundant region in their image. The recurrence plot diagonal line shows that the divided areas have the same pattern. This redundant part will affect the classification performance.

3.2 The Best Data Augmentation Scheme

Based on the classification mentioned above for performance analysis, comparing many accuracy values was tedious work. Therefore, a systematic accuracy comparison using win-loss terminology was designed to ease the assessment of which data augmentation scheme was the best. The win means that in the same classifier, the accuracy in the specific data augmentation scheme performs better than in other data augmentation schemes. The loss has the opposite meaning.

The proposed systematic accuracy comparison was as follows: (1) Select the data augmentation scheme for each classifier and select only the classifier with significant accuracy improvement. (2) Compare the classifier accuracies on the other augmentation schemes and count the number of wins and losses. (3) Compute the merit values by subtracting the number of wins over the number of losses and then rank the data augmentation schemes based on the merit values. (4) Select the data augmentation scheme with the highest merit value as the best data augmentation. This proposed systematic accuracy comparison was encouraged by the work of Hall and Holmes [36].

Data Augmentation Schemes on the use of Recurrence Plot on DEAP. Table 6 shows the best data augmentation scheme by appending the DEAP training set with 20,000 artificial recurrence plot samples..

Table 6 Data augmentation rank on the use of recurrence plots on the DEAP dataset

Data augmentation scheme	Win	Loss	Merit (win-loss)
DEAP + 20,000	11	1	10
DEAP + 10,000	9	3	6
DEAP + 15,000	5	3	2
DEAP + 5000	0	0	0

Table 7 Data augmentation rank on the use of recurrence plots on the SEED dataset

Data augmentation scheme	Win	Loss	Merit (win-loss)
SEED + 20,000	12	0	12
SEED + 15,000	9	3	6
SEED + 10,000	4	4	0
SEED + 5000	1	7	− 6

Data augmentation schemes on the use of recurrence plot on SEED. Table 7 shows the best data augmentation scheme by appending the SEED training set with 20,000 artificial recurrence plot samples.

Data augmentation schemes on the use of spectrogram on DEAP. Table 8 shows the best data augmentation scheme by appending the DEAP training set with 20,000 artificial spectrogram samples.

Data augmentation schemes on the use of spectrogram on SEED. Table 9 shows the best data augmentation scheme by appending the SEED training set with 15,000 artificial spectrogram samples.

Table 8 Data augmentation rank on the use of spectrogram on the DEAP dataset

Data augmentation scheme	Win	Loss	Merit (win-loss)
DEAP + 20,000	16	0	16
DEAP + 15,000	12	4	8
DEAP + 10,000	8	8	0
DEAP + 5000	4	12	− 8

Table 9 Data augmentation rank on the use of spectrogram on the SEED dataset

Data augmentation scheme	Win	Loss	Merit (win-loss)
SEED + 15,000	15	1	14
SEED + 20,000	13	3	10
SEED + 10,000	6	6	0
SEED + 5000	5	11	− 6

4 Discussion

Based on the research result, appending 20,000 artificial samples to the training set was the best data augmentation scheme applied to the DEAP recurrence plots, DEAP spectrogram, and SEED Recurrence plots. Appending 15,000 artificial samples to the training set was the best data augmentation scheme for the SEED spectrogram. This research also explored the other performance matrices, including the accuracy improvement value and the kappa coefficient, to give a comprehensive performance analysis based on the best data augmentation scheme. Then these performance matrices were presented for each classifier.

4.1 Accuracy Improvement

Figure 4 presents the accuracy improvement for each classier based on the best data augmentation scheme. For the data augmentation scheme by appending 20,000 artificial recurrence plot (RP) samples on the DEAP training set, the best classifier with the highest accuracy improvement was MobileNet (2.33%), followed by DenseNet121 (1.94%) and LeNet5 (0.77%). However, the ResNet50 has a negative accuracy improvement value (–0.43%). It can be concluded that the artificial recurrence plot samples appended to the DEAP training set could not improve the model generalizability trained by ResNet50.

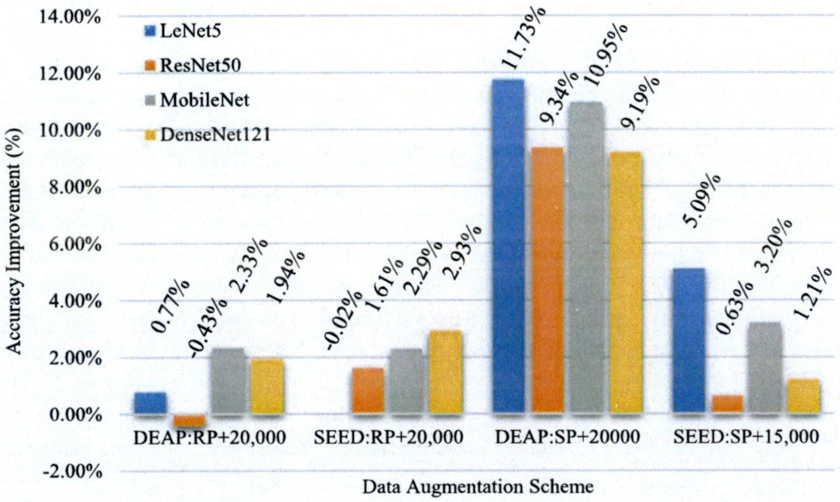

Fig. 4 Accuracy improvement

In the data augmentation scheme by appending 20,000 artificial recurrence plot (RP) samples to the SEED training set, the best classifier with the highest accuracy improvement was DenseNet121 (2.93%), followed by MobileNet (2.29%) and ResNet50 (1.61%). Meanwhile, the LeNet5 classifier has a negative accuracy improvement value (–0.02%). It can also conclude that the artificial recurrence plot samples appended to the SEED training set could not improve the model generalizability trained by LeNet5.

For the data augmentation scheme by appending 20,000 artificial spectrograms (SP) samples to the DEAP training set, the best classifier with the highest accuracy improvement was LeNet5 (11.73%), followed by MobileNet (10.95%), ResNet50 (9.34%), and DenseNet121 (9.19%).

For the data augmentation scheme by appending 15,000 artificial spectrograms (SP) samples to the SEED training set, the best classifier with the highest accuracy improvement was LeNet5 (5.09%), followed by MobileNet (3.20%), DenseNet121 (1.21%), and ResNet50 (0.63%).

4.2 *Kappa Coefficient*

The accuracy improvement analysis mentioned in the previous section obtained the four best classifiers for each data augmentation scheme. Then, the kappa coefficient for each classifier was computed. The kappa coefficient is used to measure the agreement degree between two raters. The kappa coefficient can be used to evaluate the classification model by assuming the ratings conducted by raters were the values of the label predicted by the classifier and the values of the actual label in the testing set.

A high level of agreement between raters will increase the confidence that the classification model was reliable and robust. Table 10 shows the kappa coefficient for each classifier based on the data augmentation scheme. Using the SEED dataset, classification models trained by LeNet5 and DenseNet121 have a kappa coefficient higher than 0.81. LeNet5 was trained on the appended spectrogram samples set, and Densenet121 was trained on the appended recurrence plot samples set. Then, it can be concluded that both classifiers were reliable and robust classification models.

Regarding the DEAP dataset, classification models trained by LeNet5 have a kappa coefficient higher than 0.81. Meanwhile, classification models trained by MobileNet have a kappa coefficient lower than 0.81. Therefore, LeNet5 trained on

Table 10 Kappa coefficient for each classifier based on data augmentation scheme

Data augmentation scheme	Classifier	Kappa coefficient
SEED: SP + 15,000	LeNet5	0.98
SEED: RP + 20,000	DenseNet121	0.86
DEAP: SP + 20,000	LeNet5	0.81
DEAP: RP + 20,000	MobileNet	0.74

the appended spectrogram samples set was a more reliable and robust classifier than MobileNet trained on the appended recurrence plot samples set.

4.3 Accuracy Benchmarking with Other Results

This section provides an accuracy benchmarking with other data augmentation results. The studies mentioned earlier that are compared are Wang et al. [14], Luo & Lu [15], Luo et al. [10], Zhang et al. [16], and Luo et al. [17]. Table 11 compares the accuracy of these studies as mentioned earlier with this study.

For fair accuracy benchmarking, the number of appended artificial samples used to compare in the SEED dataset is 5000 and in the DEAP dataset is 15,000 because these numbers are the closest number of appended artificial samples to other studies' results. Based on Table 11, this study has the best accuracy (97.81%) compared to other studies using the SEED dataset. On the use of the DEAP dataset, this study also has the best accuracy (90.81%) compared to another study.

Table 11 Accuracy benchmarking with other results

Studies	Dataset	Input	No. of appended	Methods	Accuracy (%)
Wang et al. [14]	SEED	Signal values	30-time of the training set	Gaussian noise + ResNet18	75
Luo & Lu [15]	SEED	Signal values	1-time of the training set	cWGAN + SVM	86.96
Luo et al. [10]	SEED	Signal values	2000 artificial samples	cBEGAN + SVM	87.56
Zhang et al. [16]	SEED	Signal values	900 artificial samples	MG-cWGAN + SVM	84
Luo et al. [17]	SEED	Signal values	1000 artificial samples	sWGAN + DNN	93.5
This study	SEED	Spectrogram	5000 artificial samples	Pix2pix + ResNet50	97.81
Luo et al. [17]	DEAP	Signal values	15,000 artificial samples	sWGAN + SVM	50.8
This study	DEAP	Spectrogram	15,000 artificial samples	Pix2pix + ResNet50	90.81

4.4 *Limitation and Implication*

In this study, the method used to assess the artificial recurrence plot and spectrogram samples is only through the confident classification score. The confident classification score is computed using a trained classifier (LeNet5). Therefore, the use of this trained classifier will affect the classification accuracy. This is confirmed by the experiment result in Table 10. The use of LeNet5 as a classifier has a superior performance based on the kappa coefficient compared with the other classifiers. This implies that the artificial recurrence plot and spectrogram samples evaluated by the trained LeNet5 produce a homogeneous training set. This homogeneous training set will only be beneficial for the LeNet5 classifier, not for other classifiers.

Based on this limitation, elaborating the evaluation of the artificial sample technique using a non-trained classifier is needed. Several mathematical quantitative-based methods can be used to evaluate the artificial samples, such as Inception Score (IS) [37], FID [38], structural similarity (SSIM) index [39], etc. The pross of mathematical quantitative-based methods is their objective assessment [40]. Therefore, the assessment process provides a relevant quality result regarding the artificial samples.

5 Conclusion

This research aims to overcome the limited available data problem in human emotional recognition by augmenting the EEG datasets. Since EEG signals have the density estimation problem because of their non-stationary property, they were transformed using a recurrence plot and spectrogram in this research. Pix2pix was used to generate the artificial recurrence plot and the spectrogram samples. Then, these artificial samples were utilized to conduct the data augmentation process.

This research found the best four data augmentation schemes in emotion recognition. The best four data augmentation schemes were as follows: Appending 20,000 artificial recurrence plot samples to DEAP and SEED training datasets, appending 20,000 artificial spectrogram samples to the DEAP training dataset, and appending 15,000 artificial spectrogram samples to the SEED training dataset.

This research also found the best classifier with the highest accuracy improvement based on the best data augmentation schemes. For the data augmentation scheme by appending 20,000 artificial recurrence plot samples on the DEAP training set, the best classifier with the highest accuracy improvement was MobileNet (2.33%). For the data augmentation scheme by appending 20,000 artificial recurrence plot samples to the SEED training set, the best classifier with the highest accuracy improvement was DenseNet121 (2.93%). For the data augmentation scheme by appending 20,000 artificial spectrogram samples to the DEAP training set, the best classifier with the highest accuracy improvement was LeNet5 (11.73%). For the data augmentation scheme by appending 15,000 artificial spectrogram samples to the SEED training set, the best classifier with the highest accuracy improvement was LeNet5 (5.09%).

Moreover, this research found that just using the accuracy metric was not enough to evaluate classification models. Therefore, the kappa coefficient for each classification model was computed. Based on this kappa coefficient, when using the SEED dataset, LeNet5 (accuracy 98.58%) trained on the appended spectrogram samples set and DenseNet121 (accuracy 90.47%) trained on the appended recurrence plot samples set were reliable and robust classification models. Regarding the DEAP dataset, LeNet5 (accuracy 86.12%) trained on the appended spectrogram samples set was a more reliable and robust classifier than MobileNet (81.02%) trained on the appended recurrence samples set.

This research also found that using spectrogram samples as input is more promising than using a recurrence plot when classifying human emotion. This is because the recurrence plots have a redundant region in their image. The recurrence plot diagonal line shows that the divided areas have the same pattern. This redundant part will affect the classification performance.

For future works, elaborating the evaluation of the artificial sample technique using a mathematical quantitative-based method is encouraged. This research only used a trained classifier to evaluate the quality of artificial samples generated by pix2pix.

Acknowledgements This work is supported by an Indonesian Doctoral Dissertation Research Grant from DIKTI. The authors would like to thank the Intelligent Systems Research Group at the Department of Electrical and Information Engineering for contributing to stimulating discussion and inspiration.

References

1. Ren F, Dong Y, Wang W (2019) Emotion recognition based on physiological signals using brain asymmetry index and echo state network. Neural Comput Appl 31:4491–4501. https://doi.org/10.1007/s00521-018-3664-1
2. Ziye L, Yan W, Derui S, Yiwen Q, Xiaofei S (2021) Speech emotion recognition based on transfer learning of spectrogram. In: Lecture Notes in Electrical Engineering. pp 1963–1967. Springer Singapore, Singapore. https://doi.org/10.1007/978-981-15-8411-4_259
3. Wang Y, Wang X, He C (2021) Speech emotion recognition algorithm for school bullying detection based on MFCC-PCA-SVM classification. In: Lecture Notes in Electrical Engineering. pp 1088–1093. Springer Singapore, Singapore. https://doi.org/10.1007/978-981-15-8411-4_143
4. Gu H, Chen Q, Xing X, Zhao J, Li X (2019) Facial emotion recognition in deaf children: Evidence from event-related potentials and event-related spectral perturbation analysis. Neurosci Lett 703:198–204. https://doi.org/10.1016/j.neulet.2019.01.032
5. Abhang PA, Gawali BW, Mehrotra SC (2016) Introduction to EEG and Speech-based emotion recognition. Elsevier. https://doi.org/10.1016/C2015-0-01959-1
6. Song T, Zheng W, Lu C, Zong Y, Zhang X, Cui Z (2019) MPED: A Multi-Modal physiological emotion database for discrete emotion recognition. IEEE Access. 7:12177–12191. https://doi.org/10.1109/ACCESS.2019.2891579
7. Lotte F, Bougrain L, Cichocki A, Clerc M, Congedo M, Rakotomamonjy A, Yger F (2018) A review of classification algorithms for EEG-based brain–computer interfaces: a 10 year update. J Neural Eng 15:031005. https://doi.org/10.1088/1741-2552/aab2f2

8. Harada S, Hayashi H, Uchida S (2018) Biosignal Data augmentation based on generative adversarial networks. In: 2018 40th Annual International Conference of the IEEE Engineering in Medicine and Biology Society (EMBC). IEEE. pp 368–371. https://doi.org/10.1109/EMBC.2018.8512396.
9. Chai X, Wang Q, Zhao Y, Liu X, Liu D, Bai O (2018) Multi-subject subspace alignment for non-stationary EEG-based emotion recognition. Technol Heal Care 26:327–335. https://doi.org/10.3233/THC-174739
10. Luo Y, Zhu L-Z, Lu B-L (2019) A GAN-Based data augmentation method for multimodal emotion recognition. In: Advances in Neural Networks—ISNN 2019. ISNN 2019. Lecture Notes in Computer Science. pp 141–150. Springer, Cham, Shanghai. https://doi.org/10.1007/978-3-030-22796-8_16
11. Zhao W, Zhao Z, Li C (2018) Discriminative-CCA promoted By EEG signals for physiological-based emotion recognition. In: 2018 First Asian Conference on Affective Computing and Intelligent Interaction (ACII Asia). IEEE, College of Computer and Information Engineering, Tianjin Normal University, Tianjin, China, pp 1–6. https://doi.org/10.1109/ACIIAsia.2018.8470373.
12. Ma, X, Liu Z, Jiang T, Zhang X (2019) Study of the algorithm for the classification of brain waves. In: Lecture Notes in Electrical Engineering. Springer Verlag, China, pp 2325–2331. https://doi.org/10.1007/978-981-10-6571-2_283
13. Goodfellow I, Bengio Y, Courville A (2016) Deep learning. MIT Press
14. Wang F, Zhong S, Peng J, Jiang J, Liu Y (2018) Data augmentation for EEG-Based emotion recognition with deep convolutional neural networks. In: Lecture Notes in Computer Science. Springer, Cham, Shenzhen, pp 82–93. https://doi.org/10.1007/978-3-319-73600-6_8
15. Luo Y, Lu B-L (2018) EEG data augmentation for emotion recognition using a conditional wasserstein GAN. In: 2018 40th Annual International Conference of the IEEE Engineering in Medicine and Biology Society (EMBC). IEEE, Shanghai, pp 2535–2538. https://doi.org/10.1109/EMBC.2018.8512865
16. Zhang A, Su L, Zhang Y, Fu Y, Wu L, Liang S (2022) EEG data augmentation for emotion recognition with a multiple generator conditional Wasserstein GAN. Complex Intell Syst 8:3059–3071. https://doi.org/10.1007/s40747-021-00336-7
17. Luo Y, Zhu L-Z, Wan Z-Y, Lu B-L (2020) Data augmentation for enhancing EEG-based emotion recognition with deep generative models. J Neural Eng 17:056021. https://doi.org/10.1088/1741-2552/abb580
18. Klonowski W (2009) Everything you wanted to ask about EEG but were afraid to get the right answer. Nonlinear Biomed Phys 3:2. https://doi.org/10.1186/1753-4631-3-2
19. Shankar A, Khaing HK, Dandapat S, Barma S (2021) Analysis of epileptic seizures based on EEG using recurrence plot images and deep learning. Biomed Signal Process Control 69:102854. https://doi.org/10.1016/j.bspc.2021.102854
20. Vrbancic G, Podgorelec V (2018) Automatic Classification of motor impairment neural disorders from EEG signals using deep convolutional neural networks. Elektron ir Elektrotechnika 24:1–7. https://doi.org/10.5755/j01.eie.24.4.21469
21. Craik A, He Y, Contreras-Vidal JL (2019) Deep learning for electroencephalogram (EEG) classification tasks: a review. J Neural Eng 16:031001. https://doi.org/10.1088/1741-2552/ab0ab5
22. Koelstra S, Muhl C, Soleymani M, Jong-Seok Lee, Yazdani A, Ebrahimi T, Pun T, Nijholt A, Patras I (2012) DEAP: A database for emotion analysis ;using physiological signals. IEEE Trans Affect Comput 3, 18–31. https://doi.org/10.1109/T-AFFC.2011.15
23. Zheng W, Lu B-L (2015) Investigating critical frequency bands and channels for EEG-Based emotion recognition with deep neural networks. IEEE Trans Auton Ment Dev 7:162–175. https://doi.org/10.1109/TAMD.2015.2431497
24. Eckmann J-P, Kamphorst SO, Ruelle D (1987) Recurrence plots of dynamical systems. Europhys Lett 4:973–977. https://doi.org/10.1209/0295-5075/4/9/004
25. Sanei S, Chambers JA (2007) EEG signal processing. John Wiley & Sons Ltd, West Sussex, England. https://doi.org/10.1002/9780470511923

26. Isola P, Zhu J-Y, Zhou T, Efros AA (2017) Image-to-Image translation with conditional adversarial networks. In: 2017 IEEE Conference on Computer Vision and Pattern Recognition (CVPR). pp 5967–5976. IEEE. https://doi.org/10.1109/CVPR.2017.632
27. Ronneberger O, Fischer P, Brox T (2015) U-Net: Convolutional networks for biomedical image segmentation. In: Medical Image Computing and Computer-Assisted Intervention—MICCAI 2015. MICCAI 2015. Springer, Cham. pp 234–241. https://doi.org/10.1007/978-3-319-24574-4_28
28. Generative Adversarial Networks (GANs) | Coursera, https://www.coursera.org/specializations/generative-adversarial-networks-gans, last accessed 2022/07/19.
29. Cohen J (1960) A coefficient of agreement for nominal scales. Educ Psychol Meas 20:37–46. https://doi.org/10.1177/001316446002000104
30. Landis JR, Koch GG (1977) The measurement of observer agreement for categorical data. Biometrics 33:159. https://doi.org/10.2307/2529310
31. Lecun Y, Bottou L, Bengio Y, Haffner P (1998) Gradient-based learning applied to document recognition. Proc IEEE 86:2278–2324. https://doi.org/10.1109/5.726791
32. He K, Zhang X, Ren S, Sun J (2016) Deep residual learning for image recognition. In: 2016 IEEE Conference on Computer Vision and Pattern Recognition (CVPR). IEEE. pp 770–778. https://doi.org/10.1109/CVPR.2016.90
33. Howard AG, Zhu M, Chen B, Kalenichenko D, Wang W, Weyand T, Andreetto M, Adam H (2017) MobileNets: Efficient convolutional neural networks for mobile vision applications. arXiv Prepr. arXiv1704.04861
34. Huang G, Liu Z, Van Der Maaten L, Weinberger KQ (2017) Densely connected convolutional networks. In: 2017 IEEE Conference on Computer Vision and Pattern Recognition (CVPR). IEEE. pp 2261–2269. https://doi.org/10.1109/CVPR.2017.243
35. McNemar Q (1947) Note on the sampling error of the difference between correlated proportions or percentages. Psychometrika 12:153–157. https://doi.org/10.1007/BF02295996
36. Hall MA, Holmes G (2003) Benchmarking attribute selection techniques for discrete class data mining. IEEE Trans Knowl Data Eng 15:1437–1447. https://doi.org/10.1109/TKDE.2003.1245283
37. Salimans T, Goodfellow I, Zaremba W, Cheung V, Radford A, Chen X (2016) Improved techniques for training GANs. In: Proceedings of the 30th International Conference on Neural Information Processing Systems. Curran Associates Inc., Barcelona, Spain. pp 2234–2242
38. Heusel M, Ramsauer H, Unterthiner T, Nessler B, Hochreiter S (2017) GANs trained by a two time-scale update rule converge to a local nash equilibrium. In: Proceedings of the 31st International Conference on Neural Information Processing Systems. Curran Associates Inc., California. pp 6629–6640
39. Wang Z, Bovik AC, Sheikh HR, Simoncelli EP (2004) Image quality assessment: from error visibility to structural similarity. IEEE Trans Image Process 13:600–612. https://doi.org/10.1109/TIP.2003.819861
40. Borji A (2019) Pros and cons of GAN evaluation measures. Comput Vis Image Underst 179:41–65. https://doi.org/10.1016/j.cviu.2018.10.009

Comparison of KNN and SVM Methods for the Accuracy of Individual Race Classification Prediction Based on SNP Genetic Data

Prihanto Ngesti Basuki, J. P. Sri Yulianto, and Adi Setiawan

Abstract A single nucleotide polymorphism (SNP) is a DNA sequence variation in a population. SNP is just a single nucleotide difference in the genome. Many statistical methods have been proposed to predict the racial classification of individuals based on SNP genetic data. The selection of the right classification method is very important because it will determine the accuracy of the classification results. This research aims to identify the highest average accuracy between two popular classification methods in Machine Learning (ML), including K-Nearest Neighborhood (KNN) and Support Vector Machine (SVM). This study used SNP genetic data for 120 samples from 2 CEU-European races and Yoruba-African races, where for each sample 10 SNPs were selected with the same location identity. The experiment was carried out by testing each classification method with variations in the percentage of test data 10, 20, 30, 40 and 50, which was combined with Euclidean distance for the KNN classification method. Based on the results of the study, the accuracy of the prediction of the classification of individual races based on SNP genetic data, the classification using KNN has an average prediction accuracy that is better than the SVM classification if the SNP location used tests has a high correlation with the sample class. In this case, the highest average accuracy value of KNN is 98.906% and SVM is 98.779%. There is a significant difference between the highest average accuracy of KNN and SVM based on the Wilcoxon statistical test with a significance level of $\alpha = 0.05$. Benefits of this research are to find the right classification method for predictions of individual racial classification based on SNP genetic data.

Keywords Machine learning · K-Nearest Neighborhood · Support vector machine · Single nucleotide polymorphism

P. N. Basuki (✉) · J. P. Sri Yulianto
Faculty of Information Technology, Universitas Kristen Satya Wacana, Salatiga, Indonesia
e-mail: ngesti@uksw.edu

A. Setiawan
Faculty of Science and Mathematics, Universitas Kristen Satya Wacana, Salatiga, Indonesia

T. Triwiyanto et al. (eds.), *Proceeding of the 3rd International Conference on Electronics, Biomedical Engineering, and Health Informatics*, Lecture Notes in Electrical Engineering 1008, https://doi.org/10.1007/978-981-99-0248-4_28

1 Introduction

The characteristics of the human race can be seen from the color of the skin, eye color, hair type, eye shape, face shape and much more. DNA (Deoxyribonucleic acid) Humans consist of about 3×10^9 genetic codes, that are A (Adenine), C (Cytosine), G (Guanine) and T (Thymine) [1]. SNP (Single Nucleotide Polymorphism) is a form of genetic code diversity that is mostly found in human DNA which is around 3×10^6 SNPs. Therefore, SNP is often used as a marker in identifying which genes are responsible for influencing human susceptibility in certain diseases [2]. Likewise, the human race of course is also much influenced by many genes. In medical research, SNPs can be used to predict a person's ethnicity or race, where knowledge of a person's race can minimize the possibility of confounding, which is useful for forensic investigation purposes [3]. In addition, predictions of a person's weight, height, eye color, skin color and even facial structure can be done through the identification of SNP changes [4]. SNPs can also be effectively used to differentiate between individuals with complex disease and healthy individuals [5].

Data mining is data extraction in information processing with the aim of finding important patterns in the database to obtain a knowledge representation. One of the techniques used in data mining is data classification [6]. Classification is a process of grouping data into certain classes based on available classes [7], whereas performance measurements are done using confusion matrix [8]. Classification also makes it possible to easily identify data in categories and groups, so that classifications can predict group members from each data [9]. There are many methods available for data classification, including the KNN and SVM algorithms. The data classification process without much human intervention can be done with Machine Learning. Machine Learning is understood as an automated computational process based on logical operations that learns a task from a series of examples [10]. In terms of classification efficiency, machine learning algorithms are better than port based methods [11]. One of the expected targets in data classification is the achievement of high accuracy for prediction of new data classifications for available classes. Therefore, the selection of the right classification method is very necessary in various fields of research related to data classification.

KNN is a classification method by finding a group of *k* objects from a collection of training data that is most similar to test data, with labeling based on certain class dominance in its environment [12]. The value of *k* in KNN is the number of nearest neighbors whose distance is calculated against test data. In the measurement of closeness between new data and old data (training data), the most commonly used method is the distance of Euclidean [13]. KNN method is often used because it is relatively simple compared to others [14], and is often used for text-based data classification [15]. This method works well in handling classification tasks with multi-category documents. The main disadvantage of the KNN method is that it uses all the features in the distance calculation, and causes the computation to be very intensive, especially when the training set size is increased. In addition, the accuracy of KNN classification is greatly decreased in the presence of irrelevant features [15].

Several studies related to the KNN method are water quality data classification [6], development of a diagnostic system using the KNN method to predict the type of breast cancer [16], identification and classification of skin lesions using KNN [17]. Another study used the KNN method to produce a species-level aboveground forest biomass mapping in Northeast China [18].

SVM is a nonparametric technique used in data classification and image processing. The accuracy of the SVM classification method is based on the choice of parameters and kernel [19]. The idea of SVM is designing the optimal hyperplane that can classify all training data into two classes [20]. The limitations of SVM are the choice of the kernel that must be right, as well as the problem of optimizing the classification in the case of many classes [9]. Research related to SVM is the comparison of polygenic risk values with SVM kernels for predictive modeling of schizophrenia based on genomic data [21].

Many studies on the comparison between the KNN and SVM methods have been carried out in various fields, including finding the right algorithm for cardiovascular disease prediction [22], determining the right method for classifying poverty data in Papua [7], as well as comparing the KNN method and SVM based on neural network architecture to find accurate predictions of plant classification [23]. In addition, there are also studies that compare KNN and SVM to obtain an accurate classification of information on cybercrime [24], also classification for the detection of breast cancer types [25].

In the field of genomics studies, machine learning is widely used for SNP identification and disease risk prediction [26, 27], to solve the SNP classification problem in humans [28], even the development of machine learning has been applied to classify healthy and sick people based on their genomic information [29]. Genetic Algorithms Support Vector Machines (GASVeM) is a machine learning based methodology that uses genetic algorithms and SVM to find a selected set of SNPs from paths that can differentiate between cases and controls [30]. A hybrid feature selection technique based on machine learning called Minimum Redundancy Maximum Relevancy and Particle Swarm Optimization for Gene Selection with SVM (mRMR and PGOGS-SVM) was used to select a significant subset of SNPs that act as markers for disease [31]. The combination of genetic algorithm and KNN known as Genetic KNN (GKNN) is used for early detection of lung cancer symptoms by means of lung CT image classification [32]. Another study combined KNN and multi-dimensional reduction (MDR) methods for the detection of interactions between genes [33]. In addition, there are studies that evaluate machine learning performance in computational gene selection models [1]. Machine learning is also used to measure the prediction accuracy performance of several classification methods. KNN and SVM tend to have better performance in predicting categorical output than numerical output. In addition, these two classification methods can be used to classify many classes with many predictors to get the probability of class membership [34].

Although the average accuracy value between the SVM and KNN classifications shows that SVM has a higher accuracy for high-resolution spatial image data, in studies that compare the two algorithms on post-fire wildland mapping, the accuracy values of the two are still considered high [20]. Several studies in various fields have compared the accuracy of SVM and KNN classifications based on text data. This study conducted tests on text-based data. However, there has not been much comparison between the KNN method and the SVM method in determining the accuracy of classification in SNP genetic data. This study compares the accuracy of the prediction of classification between the KNN method and the SVM method in the racial classification based on SNP genetic data, where this comparison is carried out by testing the percentage of test data that varies and will observe the correlation between the response variable and the independent variable (SNP location data) whether there is an effect on changes in the average value of accuracy.

2 Research Methods

This study aims to compare the prediction accuracy of individual racial groupings based on SNP genetic data. The stages of the research carried out are shown in Fig. 1.

2.1 Research Data

The data source of this study is SNP genetic data from two individual racial groups, CEU (Utah Residence with Northern and Western European Ancestry) or European Race and YRI (Yoruba in Ibadan, Nigeria) or African race. Data is taken

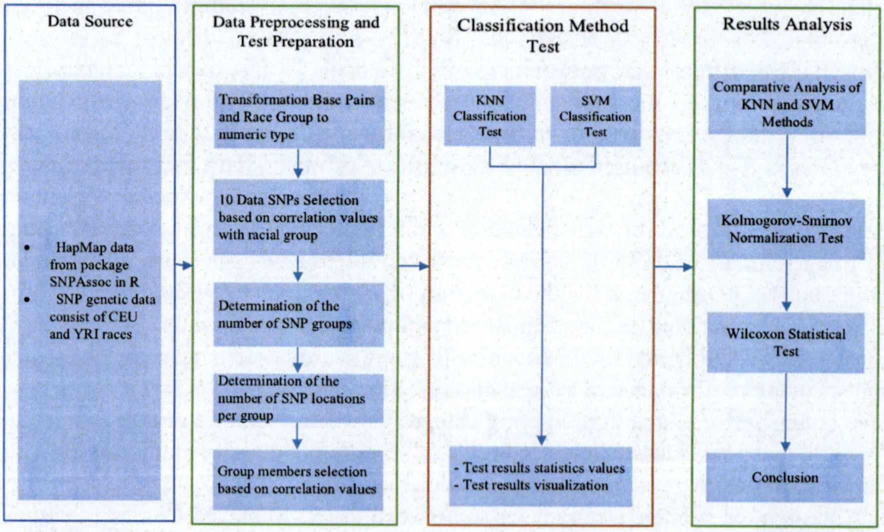

Fig. 1 Stages of comparative research of classification methods on individual races based on genetic data SNP

Table 1 Selected SNP genetic data

Sample	rs12405926	rs7419115	…	rs7833862	rs2370893	Group
1	AA	GG		AA	CC	CEU
2	AA	GG	…	AA	CC	CEU
…	…	…	…	…	…	…
40	AA	AG	…	AA	CC	CEU
…	…	…	…	…	…	…
100	AG	GG	…	AT	TT	YRI
…	…	…	…	…	…	…
120	AA	GG	…	TT	TT	YRI

from HapMap (Haplotype MAP) measuring 120 × 9305 contained in the *SNPAssoc* package in the R application. The number of samples taken from the two races is 120, and CEU and YRI respectively are 60. Each sample is taken from 10 SNPs at the same location from 9305 SNPs available. In each sample, SNPs were taken by considering the correlation value between the class and the location of the SNP. The ten SNPs are two SNPs with correlation values below 0.2, three SNPs between 0.2 and 0.7, and five others above 0.7. Ten SNP locations from each sample used by the test were rs12405926, rs7419115, rs397488, rs4653095, rs1888339, rs11692789, rs12485761, rs13071547, rs7833862 and rs2370893. The location of the SNP is sorted according to its correlation value. Table 1 presents some of the research data used, where the data are still in the form of base pairs consisting of two alleles that must be converted to numeric so that they can be used as input models.

Data Preprocessing. The research activity begins by transforming the base pairs to numerical form so that it can be used as an input model. There are three transformation values, namely 0, 0.5 and 1. The transformation is carried out based on the alphabetical order. Base pairs that have the same allele in an SNP are given a value of 0 or 1. Given a value of 0 if the allele of base pairs contains an alphabetical order that is earlier than other alleles in the same SNP location, on the contrary given a value of 1. Base pairs consisting of two different alleles are given a value of 0.5. For example, the pair of bases AG, GG and AA, each will be transformed to a value of 0.5, 1, and 0. The race group is given a value of 0 for CEU and a value of 1 for YRI. Table 2 presents the results of the transformation of the base pair of each SNP to the numeric value.

Each SNP location is labeled x_1, x_2, and so on. Each SNP is calculated its correlation value r by class using the Pearson correlation coefficient as shown in Eq. (1):

$$r = \frac{\sum(x_i - \overline{x})(y_i - \overline{y})}{\sqrt{\sum(x_i - \overline{x})^2}.\sqrt{(y_i - \overline{y})^2}} \tag{1}$$

Table 2 SNP genetic data converted to numeric

Sample	rs12405926	rs7419115	…	rs7833862	rs2370893	Group
1	0	1	…	0	0	0
2	0	1	…	0	0	0
…	…	…	…	…	…	…
40	0	0.5	…	0	0	0
…	…	…	…	…	…	…
100	0.5	1	…	0.5	1	1
…	…	…	…	…	…	…
120	0	1	…	1	1	1

where $i = 1, \ldots, 120$, x_i is the ith SNP conversion value, and y_i is the ith class conversion value.

Ten SNP locations in Table 2 are labeled ×1, …, ×10 with a Pearson correlation coefficient (as given in (1)) of 0.092, 0.186, 0.341, 0.430, 0.570, 0.708, 0.752, 0.764, 0.810, and 0.904.

2.2 Research Stages

The experimental stage begins with determining the number of SNP locations selected and used for testing individual racial classification predictions. The tests were carried out for three SNP groups. The first group consists of 5 SNPs, namely ×2, ×4, ×5, ×6 and ×8. The second group consists of 5 SNPs belonging to the first group plus one SNP highly correlated, ×10. The third group contains 6 SNP belonging to the second group added with one SNP highly correlated, ×9. Classification testing using Machine Learning. The classification method used is KNN and SVM. The test was carried out with five percentage of test data, namely 10, 20, 30, 40 and 50%. In addition, the random state runs from 1 to 1000 for both classification methods. In the KNN classification, the definition of distance used is the distance of Euclidean. In SVM, linear kernel is used as the kernel type.

3 Results and Discussion

3.1 Results Analysis

KNN Classification Test. In testing, each experiment at a certain k value is calculated as the average accuracy value of 1000 iterations. The $k$value is as much as the amount of training data. Each iteration is calculated as the minimum value, the average accuracy, standard deviation, median and maximum. Table 3 presents the statistical values of the results of the KNN classification test in the 5 SNPs group, where the highest average accuracy value is 93.456%, achieved in the percentage of the 30% test data at $k = 38$ with the required processing time is 34 min 5 s. The graph of the results of the KNN classification test with the highest average accuracy value in Table 3 is presented in Fig. 2, where it appears that the average accuracy value continues to increase from $k = 1$ to $k = 38$, and then decreases until the last k value, which is 88.615%.

Table 4 presents the statistical values of the 6 SNPs group test results. The highest average accuracy value is 98.906% on 30% of test data with $k = 62$ and the processing time is 41 min 9 s. There is an increase in the average accuracy value in the 6 SNPs group compared to the 5 SNPs group, this is probably due to the addition of 1 highly correlated SNP data, namely ×10. In addition, it is also seen in Table 4 that there was an increase in processing time from the previous SNP group. The graph of the highest average accuracy value in Table 4 is presented in Fig. 3, where the value of $k = 1$ achieved an average accuracy of 98.196%. It appears that the average accuracy increases as k increases to a value of $k = 23$, then decreases to a value of $k = 27$. Then it continued to increase until it peaked at the value of $k = 62$, then decreased to the value of 96.028% at the last k. In Table 5 which presents the statistical value of the test results for the 7 SNPs group, it appears that the highest average accuracy

Table 3 Statistical values of KNN classification test for 5 SNPs ×2, ×4, ×5, ×6, ×8

Training data size	Test data size (%)	Min	Avg	StDev	Median	Max	k	Elapsed time
108	10	50	93.330	6.89	91.67	100	44	44 m
96	20	58.33	93.438	4.53	95.83	100	40	24 m 8 s
84	30	63.89	93.456	3.58	94.44	100	38	34 m 5 s
72	40	62.5	93.339	3.06	93.75	100	32	32 m 5 s
60	50	63.33	93.052	2.88	93.33	100	24	27 m 36 s

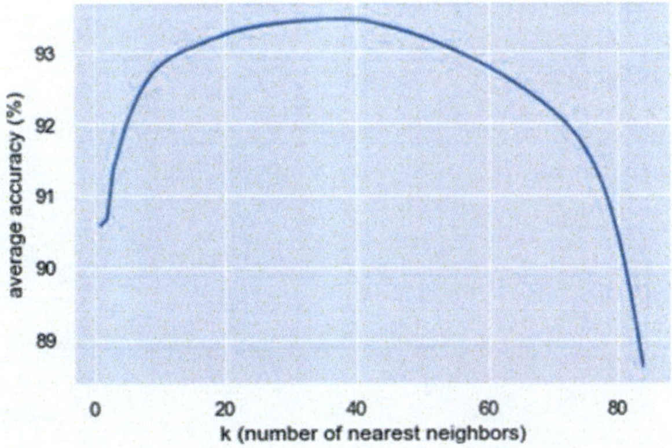

Fig. 2 KNN classification test graphs for 5 SNPs with 30% test data

value in this group is 98.697%, slightly lower than the highest score achieved in the 6 SNPs group, possibly due to the addition of 1 highly correlated SNP data, but still lower than the highest correlation SNP in the group. The highest average accuracy value was achieved by groups of 20 and 30% of test data, and both were at a value of $k = 58$, with the required processing time of 38 min 25 s and 34 min 52 s, respectively. Table 5 also shows that the standard deviation in 30% of the test data is smaller than 20% of the test data. A graphical visualization of the results of the KNN classification test with the highest average accuracy value in Table 5 is presented in Fig. 4, which looks similar to the graph in Fig. 3. The lowest value of the average accuracy in this classification test before reaching the highest value is 97.71% at the $k = 2$, then propagated up to a value of 98.579% at $k = 16$ and fell again to reach 98.55% at $k = 23$. Furthermore, the average accuracy continues to increase and reaches the maximum value at $k = 58$, then decreases to a value of 95.56% at the last k value.

The graphs as shown in Figs. 2, 3 and 4 are visualizations of the highest value of the average accuracy, in a group of 5 SNPs, 6 SNPs and 7SNPs, respectively. The x-axis is the k value (number of nearest neighbors) that runs from 1 to a number of training data according to the percentage of the test data applied and the y-axis represents the average accuracy value in percent. In Fig. 3, it appears that the highest average accuracy was achieved in the group of 6 SNPs (with 20% of the test data). This can be seen in the value of the y-axis which reaches a value of 99%.

Table 4 Statistical values of KNN classification test for 6 SNPs ×2, ×4, ×5, ×6, ×8, ×10

Training data size	Test data size (%)	Min	Avg	StDev	Median	Max	*k*	Elapsed time
108	10	83.33	98.885	2.869	100	100	48	26 m
96	20	87.5	98.906	1.891	100	100	62	38 m 17 s
84	30	88.89	98.884	1.465	100	100	52	44 m 21 s
72	40	91.67	98.815	1.188	97.917	100	16	32 m 1 s
60	50	91.67	98.727	1.130	98.333	100	36	32 m 8 s

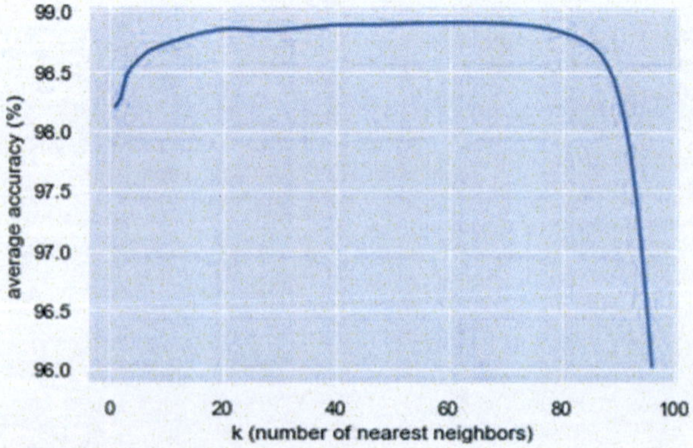

Fig. 3 KNN classification test graphs for 6 SNPs with 20% test data

Table 5 Statistical values of KNN classification test for 7 SNPs ×2, ×4, ×5, ×6, ×8, ×9, ×10

Training data size	Test data size (%)	Min	Avg	StDev	Median	Max	*k*	Elapsed time
108	10	83.33	98.621	3.182	100	100	78	43 m 33 s
96	20	87.5	98.697	2.082	100	100	58	38 m 25 s
84	30	88.89	98.697	1.629	100	100	58	34 m 53 s
72	40	91.67	98.633	1.362	97.917	100	48	30 m 33 s
60	50	91.67	98.613	1.192	98.333	100	40	25 m 25 s

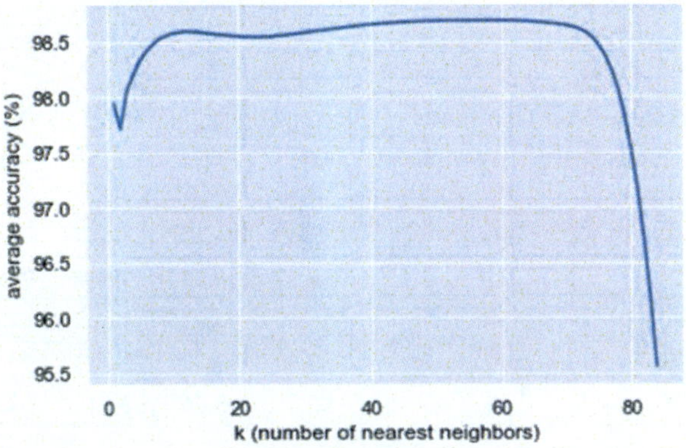

Fig. 4 KNN classification test graphs for 7 SNPs with 30% test data

SVM Classification Test. The configuration of the SVM classification test, in this case, uses linear kernel as the type of kernel. The test was carried out for five different percentages of test data, the same as in the KNN method testing. The results of the SVM classification test for 5 SNPs group are presented in Table 6, where the highest value of the average accuracy in the 5 SNPs group was 94.242%, achieved at 10 and 20% of the test data. The visualization of Table 6 is presented in Fig. 5, where the average accuracy value is above 91%, and the frequency of this accuracy value is above 800.

Table 7 shows the results of the SVM classification test for 6 SNPs group, with the highest value of average accuracy being 98.779%, achieved at 20% of the test data. There is a significant increase in the average accuracy value in this group compared to the 5 SNPs group, which is shown in Table 7 that in all test data percentages, the average accuracy value is above 98%. This is due to the addition of 1 highly correlated SNP to the dataset. Visually, the increase in the average accuracy value is shown in Fig. 6, where the value is close to 100%, this is also reinforced by the median value which reaches 100 in Table 7.

Table 8 shows the results of the SVM classification test for group 7 SNPs. The highest average accuracy is 98.567%, achieved at 50% of the test data. The average accuracy in group 7 SNPs is lower than the group of 6 SNPs, due to the addition of 1 highly correlated SNP which is still lower than the highest correlated SNP in the

Fig. 5 SVM classification test graphs for 5 SNPs with 20% test data

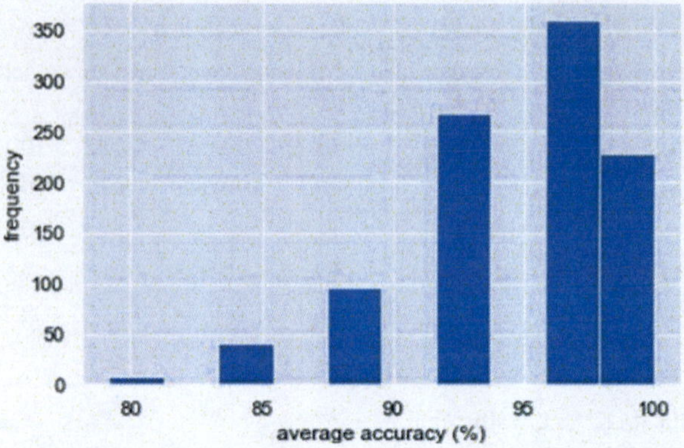

Table 6 Statistical values of SVM classification test for 5 SNPs ×2, ×4, ×5, ×6, ×8

Training data size	Test data size (%)	Min	Avg	StDev	Median	Max	Elapsed time (s)
108	10	58.33	94.242	6.647	91.667	100	7.1
96	20	79.17	94.242	4.586	95.833	100	7.4
84	30	80.56	93.936	3.597	94.444	100	7.7
72	40	83.33	93.888	2.782	93.750	100	7.4
60	50	85	93.76	2.44	93.33	100	7.3

Table 7 Statistical values of SVM classification test for 6 SNPs ×2, ×4,×5, ×6, ×8, ×10

Training data size	Test data size (%)	Min	Avg	StDev	Median	Max	Elapsed time (s)
108	10	83.33	98.650	3.226	100	100	7.8
96	20	91.67	98.779	2.210	100	100	7.4
84	30	91.67	98.764	1.674	100	100	7.3
72	40	91.67	98.694	1.398	97.917	100	7.4
60	50	93.33	98.660	1.223	98.333	100	7.2

Fig. 6 SVM classification test graphs for 6 SNPs with 20% test data

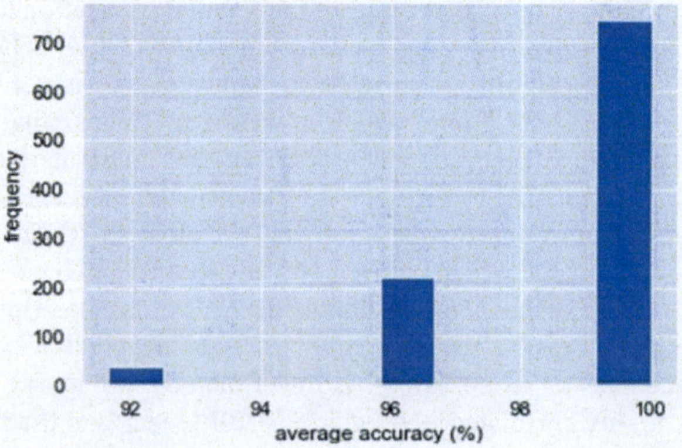

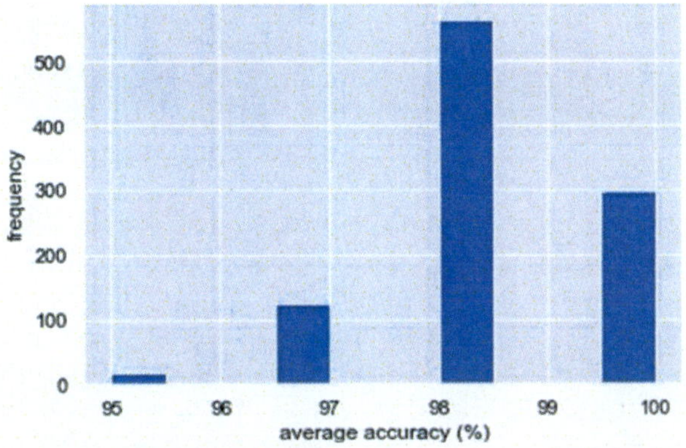

Fig. 7 SVM classification test graphs for 7 SNPs with 50% test data

dataset. However, the average accuracy in group 7 SNPs is still above 98%. Visually, the decrease in the average accuracy value is shown in Fig. 7.

Figures 5, 6 and 7 presents graphs of the SVM classification method testing results with the highest average accuracy value for each SNPs group. The x-axis represents the average of the accuracy values in percent, and the y-axis values represent the frequency values of accuracy with random states from 1 to 1000.

Comparative analysis of classification methods. Based on the results of the KNN and SVM classification testing that has been carried out in the SNP genetic data, a comparison of statistical values of the three SNP groups is presented in Tables 9, 10 and 11. The results presented in the three tables are the highest value of the average accuracy, respectively for group 5 SNPs, 6 SNPs and 7 SNPs. In each table, the left side presents the test results data for the KNN classification method, while the right side of the table presents the test results for the KNN classification method.

In the test results for the 5 SNPs group as presented in Table 9, it was found that in all percentages of SVM, test data had a higher average accuracy than KNN. The result of 6 SNPs group testing in Table 10 also shows that the average deviation of group 6 SNPs is smaller than group 5 SNPs in Table 9, after being added 1 highly correlated SNP (with response variable or class).

Table 11 presents data test results in group 7 SNPs, which is similar to the results in group 6 SNPs, namely KNN has an average accuracy that is higher than SVM in

Table 8 Statistical values of SVM classification test for 7 SNPs ×2, ×4, ×5, ×6, ×8, ×9, ×10

Training data size	Test data size (%)	Min	Avg	StDev	Median	Max	Elapsed time (s)
108	10	83.33	98.400	3.409	100	100	7.6
96	20	91.67	98.475	2.291	100	100	7.6
84	30	94.44	98.547	1.680	100	100	7.4
72	40	93.75	98.563	1.334	97.917	100	7.8
60	50	95	98.567	1.141	98.333	100	7.5

Table 9 The highest accuracy statistical value of KNN and SVM classification for 5 SNPs

Test data (%)	KNN						SVM				
	Min	Avg	Std Dev	Median	Max	*k*	Min	Avg	Std Dev	Median	Max
10	50	93.330	6.893	91.667	100	44	58.333	94.242	6.647	91.667	100
20	58.333	93.438	4.527	95.833	100	40	79.167	94.242	4.586	95.833	100
30	63.889	93.456	3.583	94.444	100	38	80.556	93.936	3.597	94.444	100
40	62.5	93.339	3.063	93.75	100	32	83.333	93.888	2.782	93.750	100
50	63.333	93.052	2.877	93.333	100	24	85	93.76	2.44	93.33	100

Table 10 The highest accuracy statistical value of KNN and SVM classification for 6 SNPs

Data test (%)	KNN						SVM				
	Min	Avg	Std Dev	Median	Max	k	Min	Avg	Std Dev	Median	Max
10	83.333	98.885	2.869	100	100	48	83.333	98.650	3.226	100	100
20	87.5	98.906	1.891	100	100	62	91.667	98.779	2.210	100	100
30	88.889	98.8839	1.465	100	100	52	91.667	98.764	1.674	100	100
40	91.667	98.815	1.188	97.917	100	16	91.667	98.694	1.398	97.917	100
50	91.667	98.7267	1.130	98.333	100	36	93.333	98.660	1.223	98.333	100

Table 11 The highest accuracy statistical value of KNN and SVM classification for 7 SNPs

Data test (%)	KNN						SVM				
	Min	Avg	Std Dev	Median	Max	*k*	Min	Avg	Std Dev	Median	Max
10	83.333	98.621	3.182	100	100	78	83.333	98.400	3.409	100	100
20	87.5	98.697	2.082	100	100	58	91.667	98.475	2.291	100	100
30	88.889	98.697	1.629	100	100	58	94.444	98.547	1.680	100	100
40	91.667	98.633	1.362	97.917	100	48	93.75	98.563	1.334	97.917	100
50	91.667	98.613	1.192	98.333	100	40	95	98.567	1.141	98.333	100

all percentages of test data. In this case, SVM tends to have greater accuracy in the percentage of large test data. Among the three SNP groups, 6 SNPs group have the highest average accuracy in both classification methods than the other two groups. Group 6 SNPs has a small standard deviation, as well as the median value reaches 100 which shows that at least 50% of all accuracy average value reaches a maximum value.

Wilcoxon Statistical Test. Wilcoxon statistical test is used to test the difference in the mean two data groups that are not normally distributed. To find out whether the average prediction accuracy in the KNN classification is different from SVM, take the results of the classification test experiment for 6 SNPs at the percentage of the

20% test data contained in Table 10. Consideration of data selection in the percentage of this test data is because this percentage has achieved the highest accuracy value for both methods.

The next step is to take a complete dataset as much as the random variation of the random state (1000 data) for the KNN classification at the value of $k = 62$ and the complete dataset of the SVM classification which both use the 20% test data. The normality test of Kolmogorov-Smirnov was carried out on both datasets with the null hypothesis (H_0) as a normally distributed dataset at the level of significance $\alpha = 0.05$. The normality test in the two complete dataset results of the KNN and SVM classification gives p-value $= 2.2 \times 10^{-16}$. The p-value is smaller than the value of α, so H_0 is rejected, meaning that the two complete datasets are data that are not normally distributed.

Next, in the two sets of data, the Wilcoxon test was carried out to compare the average two dependent samples that were not normally distributed. The hypothesis test is carried out at the level of significance $\alpha = 0.05$ with the null hypothesis being that there is no mean difference in both sets of data. Based on the Wilcoxon test conducted, obtained p-value $= 8{,}169 \times 10^{-5}$. The p-value is smaller than the value of α, so H_0 is rejected, meaning that there is a difference in mean between the two complete datasets of the KNN class and SVM classification.

3.2 Discussion

Based on the results of testing the accuracy of classification predictions by the KNN and SVM methods in three groups of SNP, there is a patterned tendency. The 5 SNPs group consisting of 1 SNP correlated low with its class, 2 SNPs moderately correlated and 2 SNPs highly correlated, giving the average result of higher prediction accuracy for SVM compared to KNN in all percentages of test data. Inverted behavior occurs from the previous pattern when SNP is added highly correlated to the dataset to be tested, which is obtained the average prediction accuracy in SVM is higher than KNN in all percentage of test data. In this research, the highest average value for the accuracy of KNN was 98.906% and SVM was 98.779%, and both were achieved at 20% of test data. Changes in the percentage of test data in each experiment of the two methods not formed specific patterns at high and low values of classification prediction accuracy.

In a previous study comparing the performance of KNN and SVM for cardiovascular disease classification, the accuracy value of SVM was higher than KNN [22], where the experiment was only carried out with one value of $k = 5$ for KNN and random state using the default value. This study uses many k values as well as random states and varying percentages of test data so that the resulting accuracy value is not only one value and can be traced to the k value with the most optimal accuracy value.

Another previous study conducted a comparison between SVM and KNN in the classification of breast cancer, by classifying cancer malignancies with both methods

[25]. The evaluation techniques used are the percentage split technique and cross-validation. The first technique splits the data into two parts, 80% for training data and 20% for test data. The second technique is k-folder cross-validation ($k = 10$). Both techniques are applied to both methods. In the cross-validation technique, the accuracy value of SVM is 95.7081%, better than KNN. In the percentage split technique, the accuracy of KNN is better than SVM, which is 97.8571%. In this previous study, there was also no random state variation and no variation in the percentage of test data. The current study uses many k values with variations in random states and the percentage of test data, so that the resulting accuracy value is not only one value or has a distribution.

Another previous study, on the comparison and development of Machine Learning for the prediction of chronic obstructive pulmonary disease (COPD) in a Chinese population, involved 393 participants as training data and 240 as test data. The models involved to predict the development of COPD are logistic regression model (LR), Multilayer Perceptron (MLP), Decision Tree (DT), XGboost model, SVM and KNN. It also includes 5 clinical features and 9 SNPs. k-fold cross-validation was used in the training set, and a performance evaluation index was adopted to assess the mean predictive performance of each model [35]. One of the performance measurement results produced in the study [35] was the accuracy values of KNN, LR, SVM, DT, MLP, and XGBoost which were 83, 89, 88, 85, 80 and 94%, respectively. The accuracy of KNN is lower than that of SVM, a result that is very different from the present study. However, this previous research is the same as in previous studies, namely, there is no variation in random state, test data and k values, and also no correlation measurement variable between predictor and response variable. It means that the current research results are better in the case of measuring the average value of accuracy.

The weakness of the current research is that the KNN classification test only uses Euclidean distance. In addition, in the SVM classification only the linear kernel is used, and also the performance that is measured is only the classification prediction accuracy value. There are several parameters that should be varied, but in this case, they are kept constant, such as the definition of distance in KNN which only uses Euclidean distance and also the type of SVM kernel which only uses linear kernel. However, this result will be useful as a consideration and reference for researchers in choosing a classification method if known SNP genetic data or other text-based data.

4 Conclusion

Comparison of the two classification methods has been carried out in this study. The purpose of this study is to identify the highest average accuracy between the two classification methods KNN and SVM based on SNP genetic data using machine learning approach. Based on the results of the study, the accuracy of the prediction of the classification of individual races based on SNP genetic data, the KNN classification has an average prediction accuracy that is better than the SVM classification if the SNP location used tests has a high correlation with the sample class. In this research, the highest average value for the accuracy of KNN was 98.906% and SVM was 98.779%. Regarding the KNN and SVM classification methods, research can be developed with variations in the definition of distance for KNN and variations in kernel types for SVM, a comparison of several classification methods including Artificial Neural Network algorithm.

References

1. Mahendran N, Durai Raj Vincent PM, Srinivasan K, Chang CY (2020) Machine learning based computational gene selection models: a survey, performance evaluation, open issues, and future research directions. Front Genet 11:1–25. https://doi.org/10.3389/fgene.2020.603808
2. Kaur S, Ali A, Ahmad U, Siahbalaei Y, Pandey AK, Singh B (2019) Role of single nucleotide polymorphisms (SNPs) in common migraine. Egypt J Neurol, Psychiatry Neurosurg 55(1). https://doi.org/10.1186/s41983-019-0093-8
3. Sampson J, Kidd KK, Kidd JR, Zhao H (2011) Selecting SNPs to identify ancestry. Nat Inst Health 539–553. https://doi.org/10.1111/j.1469-1809.2011.00656.x
4. Lippert C et al (2017) Identification of individuals by trait prediction using whole-genome sequencing data. Proceed Nat Acad Sci USA 114(38):10166–10171. https://doi.org/10.1073/pnas.1711125114
5. Batnyam N, Gantulga A, Oh S (2013) An efficient classification for single nucleotide polymorphism (SNP) dataset. Stud Comput Intell 493:171–185. https://doi.org/10.1007/978-3-319-00804-2_13
6. Nababan AA, Khairi M, Harahap BS (2022) Implementation of K-Nearest Neighbors (KNN) algorithm in classification of data water quality. J Mantik 6(36):30–35
7. Tiro MA (2022) Comparison of k-Nearest Neighbor (k-NN) and support vector machine (SVM) methods for classification of poverty data in Papua. ARRUS J Math Appl Sci 2(2):83–91. https://doi.org/10.35877/mathscience741
8. Maria Navin JR, Pankaja R (2016) Performance analysis of text classification algorithm using confusion matrix. Int J Eng Tech Res (IJETR) 6(4):75–78
9. Bhavsar H, Panchal MH (2012) A review on support vector machine for data classification. Int J Adv Res Comput Eng Technol (IJARCET) 1(10):185–189
10. Michie D, Speigelhalter DJ, Taylor CC (1994) Machine learning: neural and statistical classification. Overseas Press
11. AlZoman RM, Alenazi MJF (2021) A comparative study of traffic classification techniques for smart city networks. Sens J 21(14):43–63. https://doi.org/10.1007/978-3-319-61313-0
12. Wu X et al (2008) Top 10 algorithms in data mining. Knowl Inf Syst 14(1):1–37. https://doi.org/10.1007/s10115-007-0114-2
13. Bramer M (2013) Principles of data mining, 2nd ed., Springer. https://doi.org/10.1007/978-1-4471-4884-5
14. Ul Hassan CA, Khan MS, Shah MA (2018) Comparison of machine learning algorithms in data classification. In: Proceedings of the 24th international conference on automation & computing 2018, pp 1–6, Newcastle University. https://doi.org/10.23919/IConAC.2018.8748995
15. Khan A, Baharudin B, Lee LH, Khan K (2010) A review of machine learning algorithms for text-documents classification. J Adv Inf Technol 1(1):4–20. https://doi.org/10.4304/jait.1.1.4-20

16. Chawla S, Kumara R, Aggarwal E, Swain S (2018) Breast cancer detection using K-nearest neighbour algorithm. In: Proceedings of international conference on computational intelligence and internet of things 2(4). https://papers.ssrn.com/sol3/papers.cfm?abstract_id=3361553
17. Hatem MQ (2022) Skin lesion classification system using a K-nearest neighbor algorithm. Vis Comput Ind Biomed Art 5(1). https://doi.org/10.1186/s42492-022-00103-6
18. Fu Y, He HS, Hawbaker TJ, Henne PD, Zhu Z, Larsen DR (2019) Evaluating k-nearest neighbor (kNN) imputation models for species-level aboveground forest biomass mapping in Northeast China. Remote Sens J 11(17). https://doi.org/10.3390/rs11172005
19. Ustuner M, Sanli FB, Dixon B (2015) Application of support vector machines for landuse classification using high-resolution rapideye images: a sensitivity analysis. Eur J Remote Sens 48(1):403–422. https://doi.org/10.5721/EuJRS20154823
20. Hamilton D, Pacheco R, Myers B, Peltzer B (2018) kNN vs. SVM: a comparison of algorithms. In: Proceedings of the fire continuum—preparing for the future of wildland fire, Missoula, Montana, United States Department of Agriculture, pp 95–110
21. Vivian-Griffiths T et al (2019) Predictive modeling of schizophrenia from genomic data: Comparison of polygenic risk score with kernel support vector machines approach. Am J Med Gene Part B Neuropsychiatric Gene 180(1):80–85. https://doi.org/10.1002/ajmg.b.32705
22. Lestari W, Sumarlinda S (2022) Implementation of K-nearest neighbor (KNN) and suport vector machine (SVM) for Classification cardiovascular disease. Int J MultiSci 2(10). https://archive.ics.uci.edu/ml/datasets/heart+disease
23. Ghosh S, Singh A, Kavita Z, Jhanjhi NZ, Masud M, Aljahdali S (2022) SVM and KNN based CNN architectures for plant classification. Comput Mater Continua 71(3):4257–4274. https://doi.org/10.32604/cmc.2022.023414
24. Veena K, Meena K, Teekaraman Y, Kuppusamy R, Radhakrishnan A (2022) *C* SVM classification and KNN techniques for cyber crime detection. Hindawi Wirel Commun Mob Comput 2022. https://doi.org/10.1155/2022/3640017
25. Desiani A, Lestari AA, Al-Ariq M, Amran A, Andriani Y (2022) Comparison of support vector machine and K-nearest neighbors in breast cancer classification. Pattimura Int J Mathe (PIJMath) 1(1):33–42. https://doi.org/10.30598/pijmathvol1iss1pp33-42
26. Enoma DO, Bishung J, Abiodun T, Ogunlana O, Osamor VC (2022) Machine learning approaches to genome-wide association studies. J King Saud Univ Sci 34(8). https://doi.org/10.1016/j.jksus.2022.101847
27. Pudjihartono N, Fadason T, Kempa-Liehr AW, O'Sullivan JM (2022) A review of feature selection methods for machine learning-based disease risk prediction. Front Bioinform 2:1–17. https://doi.org/10.3389/fbinf.2022.927312
28. Azizzadeh-Roodpish S, Garzon MH, Mainali S (2021) Classifying single nucleotide polymorphisms in humans. Mol Gene Genomics 296(5):1161–1173. https://doi.org/10.1007/s00438-021-01805-x
29. Romagnoni A et al (2019) Comparative performances of machine learning methods for classifying Crohn Disease patients using genome-wide genotyping data. Sci Rep 9(1):1–18. https://doi.org/10.1038/s41598-019-46649-z
30. Díaz FD, Lasheras FS, Moreno V, Moratalla-Navarro F, de la Torre AJM, Sánchez VM (2021) GASVeM: a new machine learning methodology for multi-SNP analysis of GWAS data based on genetic algorithms and support vector machines. Mathematics 9(6). https://doi.org/10.3390/math9060654
31. Phogat M, Kumar D (2021) Disease single nucleotide polymorphism selection using hybrid feature selection technique. J Phys Conf Ser (ICMAI 2021) 1950(1). https://doi.org/10.1088/1742-6596/1950/1/012079
32. Bhuvaneswari P, Therese AB (2015) Detection of cancer in lung with K-NN classification using genetic algorithm. In: 2nd international conference on nanomaterials and technologies (CNT2014) procedia materials science, vol 10, pp 433–440. https://doi.org/10.1016/j.mspro.2015.06.077
33. Alchamlat SA, Farnir F (2017) KNN-MDR: a learning approach for improving interactions mapping performances in genome wide association studies. BMC Bioinform 18(1):1–12. https://doi.org/10.1186/s12859-017-1599-7

34. Bzdok D, Krzywinski M, Altman N (2018) Machine learning: supervised methods, SVM and kNN. Nat Methods 15(1):1–6. https://doi.org/10.1038/nmeth.4551
35. Ma X et al (2020) Comparison and development of machine learning tools for the prediction of chronic obstructive pulmonary disease in the Chinese population. J Transl Med 18(1):1–14. https://doi.org/10.1186/s12967-020-02312-0

FMCW Radar Signal Processing for Human Activity Recognition with Convolutional Neural Network

Rayhan Rafli, Fiky Y. Suratman, and Istiqomah

Abstract Human Activity Recognition (HAR) is a system for identifying, monitoring, and analyzing a person's behavior. Sensors that are commonly used to be able to identify human activities are cameras or wearable sensors. However, cameras and wearable sensors have several weaknesses, such as the camera cannot capture images in the dark, and the use of wearable sensors has many things to consider for user comfort. So, an alternative way to solve those problems is to use radar as a sensor base for HAR. This study proposes methods by presenting an explanation of signal processing from raw data signals to images containing only the target distance information and then comparing the number of convolutional layers and the number of epochs to determine the best Convolutional Neural Network (CNN) architecture to perform HAR using uRAD Radar Frequency Modulated Continuous Wave by Anteral. These methods separate this study from previous HAR studies using Radar, which is the preprocessing method and comparing of various CNN architectures. Finally, with two convolutional layers and ReLU activation, the final result classification got 99.9% accuracy resulting in a higher classification accuracy than in previous studies. This study obtained high classification accuracy results due to the proposed preprocessing method and conducted experiments on various CNN architectures to obtain the best model for classifying human activities.

Keywords Human Activity Recognition · uRAD radar · Convolutional Neural Network

1 Introduction

HAR (Human Activity Recognition) is a system for identifying, monitoring, and analyzing a person's behavior or in other words concluding human activities [1]. In simple terms, the identification is done by obtaining information from sensors or it could be with a camera that will take videos of human activity for information

R. Rafli (✉) · F. Y. Suratman · Istiqomah
School of Electrical Engineering, Telkom University, Bandung, Indonesia
e-mail: rayhanrafli@student.telkomuniversity.ac.id

T. Triwiyanto et al. (eds.), *Proceeding of the 3rd International Conference on Electronics, Biomedical Engineering, and Health Informatics*, Lecture Notes in Electrical Engineering 1008, https://doi.org/10.1007/978-981-99-0248-4_29

[1, 2]. Research related to HAR has had very good progress and there have also been implementations for HAR such as smart home, autopilot, surveillance, and Fall Detection [2–6]. These studies use cameras or wearable sensors (sensors that are attached to the human body) as the sensor base.

Many studies have used cameras for HAR and yielded very satisfactory results. Cameras are widely used for HAR because the camera can capture images with high resolution [7–11]. However, using a camera for HAR has several disadvantages, such as relying on light to capture images, meaning that it cannot capture images in the dark, and the camera cannot maintain user privacy [12–14]. Wearable sensors for HAR have also been the subject of several studies [15–18]. However, the use of wearable sensors for HAR has many things to consider, such as the possibility of thermal damage to the human body, the appearance of the sensor, the size of the sensor must be easily fit, water resistance, user comfort, and power consumption because it uses batteries to operate [19]. An alternative solution to solve these problems is to use radar as the sensor base for HAR. Radar has advantages such as being able to capture images even in dark conditions and can also maintain privacy because radar uses reflected radio waves to get the information of an object or target [6, 20–24], unlike cameras that capture light to produce images like the human eye. HAR using radar has also been developed in several studies. There is a study that discusses human motion classification based on range information. This study uses ultra-wideband radar to obtain range information and uses Deep Convolutional Neural Network for classification. This study gives a classification result that reaches 95.24% accuracy [21]. However, this study did not go into detail about the process used to obtain range information. Another study discusses the Frequency Modulated Continuous Wave (FMCW) radar for HAR that aims to classify human activities in an unconstrained environment, obtaining an overall accuracy of 91% [23]. However, this study only uses one Convolutional Neural Network (CNN) architecture, and all activities are taken with the human subject always facing the radar. So, the purpose of this study is to be able to develop HAR using FMCW radar by presenting an explanation of signal processing from raw data signals to images containing only the target distance information and comparing the number of convolutional layers and the number of epochs to determine the best CNN architecture to perform HAR, hoping to achieve classification accuracy above 95%.

In order to detect human activity, this study makes use of the uRAD Radar FMCW by Anteral. This radar has several features, one of which can get raw data in the form of I and Q signals. These signals will be used to obtain distance information. These I and Q signals will continue to be captured for 150 s for each activity and then turn them into a dataset of I and Q signals over time. This dataset will then go through preprocessing, where at this stage, the dataset will be processed so that it gets the target (human) distance information, then it will be cropped into many images and extracted for each time slot. These images will later be used as input for training using CNN.

This paper is divided into five sections. Section 1 describes the introduction to this paper. Section 2 describes the materials and methods used in this research. Section 3 shows the results of the proposed method. Section 4 describes the results that have

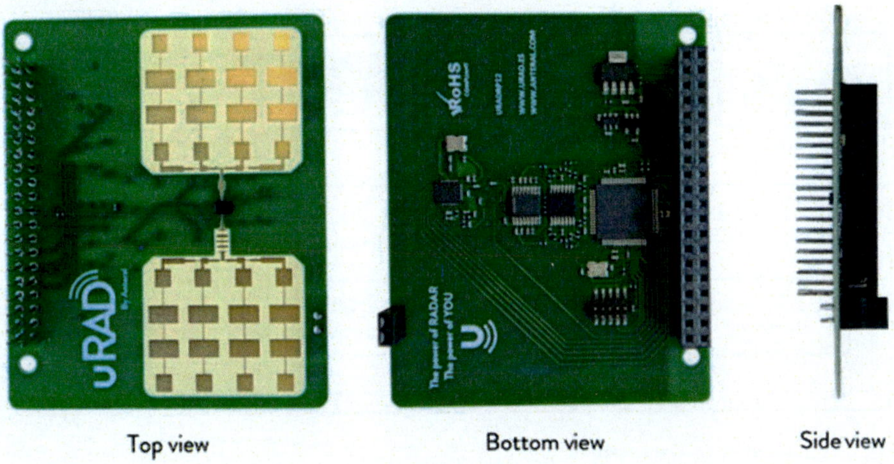

Fig. 1 uRAD Raspberry Pi v1.2

been obtained, compared with other studies, the weaknesses of the proposed method, and the implications of this study. And lastly, Sect. 5 concludes the results of this study and the proposed method.

2 Materials and Method

2.1 *Material*

This study uses uRAD Raspberry Pi v1.2 by Anteral as the basis sensor for the FMCW Radar to detect human activities and can be installed on the Raspberry Pi easily. The radar has dimensions of 70 × 56 × 18 mm and a weight of 13 g [25]. Radar with this small size makes it easy to carry anywhere. This radar has several features, one of which can get raw data in the form of I (In-Phase) and Q (Quadrature) signals. This raw data will be used for classification purposes. Figure 1 shows the component of uRAD Raspberry Pi v1.2.

2.2 *Experimental Procedures*

This study uses a dataset containing IQ signals accumulated over time as input for the proposed method. This dataset will then go through preprocessing before being used as input for training using CNN. This study will also compare three CNN architectures by comparing the number of convolutional layers and the number of different epochs. We compare several CNN architectures to get the best architecture

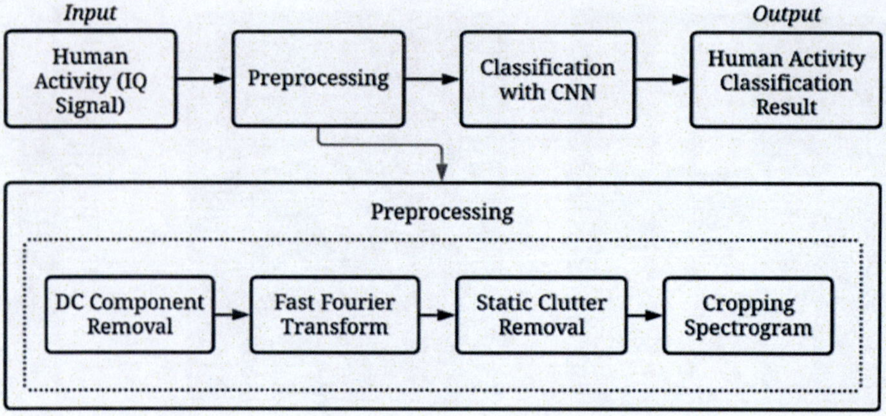

Fig. 2 Proposed method diagram block

for HAR classification in order to get the best classification results. The process of the proposed method can be seen in Fig. 2.

Data Collection. As we can see in Fig. 3, data collection is done by installing the uRAD radar with a height of one meter from the ground and the target (Human) being three meters from the radar. This paper classifies four activities, such as crawling, sitting, standing, and walking. The configuration on uRAD used for data retrieval is using f0 (starting frequency) = 24.005 GHz, Bandwidth = 240 MHz, using sawtooth signal, and Ns = 50 (Ns is the number of samples in one capture/period). Data collection for each class or each type of activity is carried out for 150 s or 3000 periods (one period takes 50 ms). Data collection for walking and crawling activities were carried out by walking or crawling around three meters and continued for up to 150 s. Then the data collection for standing and sitting activities were carried out by standing or sitting with radar distance to the subject of three meters with several different points of view of the human subject and continued for up to 150 s.

Preprocessing. The data obtained from uRAD is raw data which is the total reflected signal decomposed in two arrays with components I (In-phase) and Q (Quadrature). To get the total received signal, these I and Q signals can be made into a complex signal I + jQ. That way, we can extract the magnitude of the reflected signal. Figure 4 is a form of magnitude I and Q for each type of activity that indicate Ns and the columns indicate one period (frame). Because one period takes 50 ms, the column displayed can be converted to seconds by assuming a column of 0.05 s.

It can be seen that the raw data results have different image patterns for each type of activity. However, the results are still unclear because there are no visible human objects and no other static objects. Therefore, it is necessary to do FFT to obtain information about the distance from the radar to the detected object [23]. Nevertheless, before doing FFT, this raw data needs to be converted into a voltage with maximum GPIO voltage in Raspberry Pi 3.3V because this raw data has arbitrary units from 0 to 4095 [26]. Then we need to remove the DC component by applying

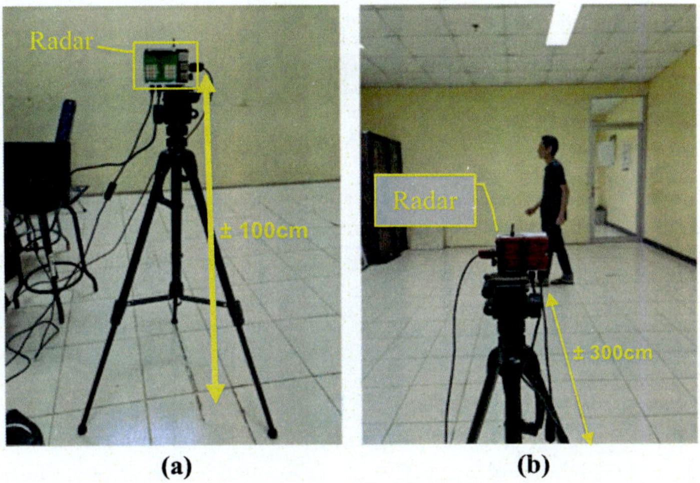

Fig. 3 Data collection: **a** Radar height, **b** Distance between radar and target

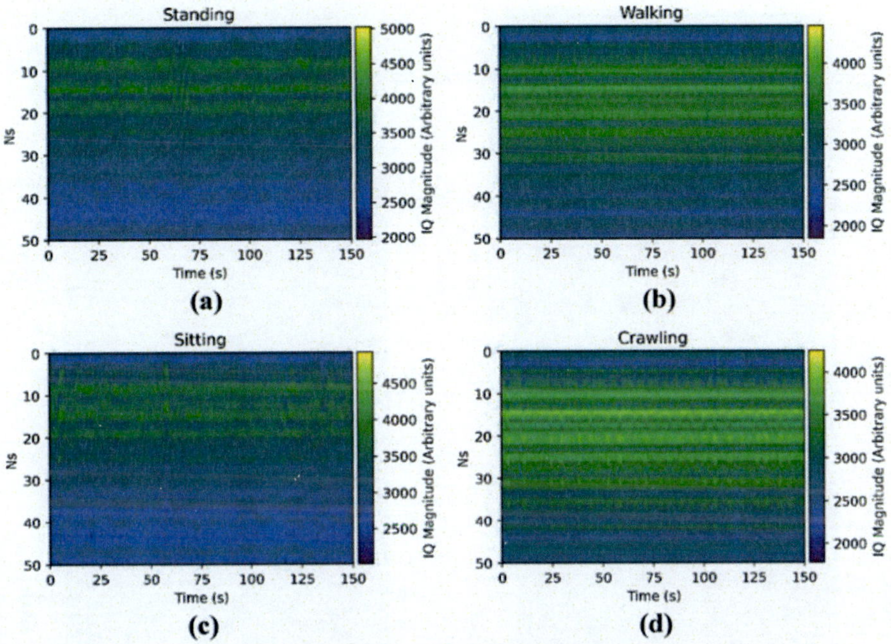

Fig. 4 Raw data in form of 2D: **a** Standing, **b** Walking, **c** Sitting, **d** Crawling

I and Q to Eq. 1.

$$\boldsymbol{x} = x_{N_s} - \frac{1}{N_s} \sum_{n=0}^{N_s-1} x_{N_s}[n] \tag{1}$$

where $x_{N_s} = [x[0], x[1], x[2], \ldots, x[N_s - 1]]$ and N_s is the number of samples. DC component removal is needed to reduce noise at 0 Hz frequency. After that, this data will go through the FFT process, where the I and Q signals will be applied to Eq. 2.

$$X[k] = \sum_{n=0}^{N_p-1} \boldsymbol{x}[n] e^{-2\pi j \frac{nk}{N_p}} \tag{2}$$

where $k = (0, 1, \ldots, K - 1)$ is the frequency index, N_p is the number of periods.

The column part of the spectrogram Fig. 5 are frequency indexes, but this figure has been converted to a distance with a maximum distance of 15.625 m. This maximum distance is obtained from calculating Eq. 3 for the maximum distance in uRAD [26].

$$\text{Maximum Distance} = 75 \times \frac{N_s}{BW} \tag{3}$$

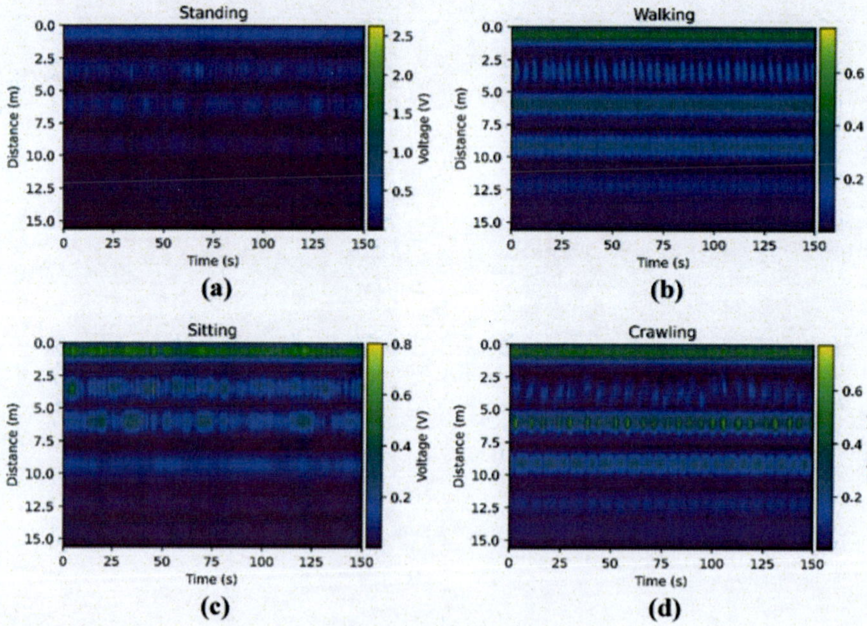

Fig. 5 Spectrograms: **a** Standing, **b** Walking, **c** Sitting, **d** Crawling

where N_s is the number of samples and BW is Bandwidth, because the N_s that we use is 50 and bandwidth 240, so we will get a maximum radar distance of 15.625 m. Furthermore, the row part in the spectrogram Fig. 5 is the same as the figure before going through the FFT process, namely N_p (number of periods) or time in seconds. The spectrogram figure accumulated over N_p can be written as $\mathbb{X}^{(N_p)} = \left[\boldsymbol{X}^{(0)}, \boldsymbol{X}^{(1)}, \ldots, \boldsymbol{X}^{(N_p-1)}\right]$, where $\boldsymbol{X}^{(i)} = \left[X^{(i)}[0], X^{(i)}[1], \ldots, X^{(i)}[K-1]\right]$, K is the number of frequency indexes, and i is the frequency index per one period. It can also be seen in the spectrogram in Fig. 5 that there is a static clutter. The static clutter in this figure are walls and other static objects. Therefore, this static clutter needs to be removed. The equation for static clutter removal can be expressed in Eq. 4.

$$\mathbb{Y}^{(N_p)} = \mathbb{X}^{(N_p)} - \frac{1}{N_p}\left[\sum_{i=0}^{N_p} X^{(i)}[0], \sum_{i=0}^{N_p} X^{(i)}[1], \ldots, \sum_{i=0}^{N_p} X^{(i)}[K-1]\right] \times J_{1,N_p} \tag{4}$$

where J_{1,N_p} is a matrix $1 \times N_p$ which contains all its elements are 1 [20].

Figure 6 is the result of the spectrograms after static clutter removal. The spectrogram has distance information from 0 to 15,625 m. However, the distance information needed is only for the target object (human) to make datasets for CNN training. Therefore, unnecessary distance information needs to be removed. To do this, we calculate the average of each row and then collect them into an array so that the spectrogram images become one-dimensional images.

To find the target object (human), we first determine the minimum peak to be searched for (green line in Fig. 7). Then if there are two or more peaks, the peak taken is the first peak because the first object captured by the radar is a human. After getting the target peak (orange "x" symbol in Fig. 7), the frequency index range to be taken is 440 (two red lines in Fig. 7), because the target distance range information is spread up to 440 frequency indexes.

After knowing the frequency index range for each type of activity, then applying the frequency index range to the spectrograms so as to produce a spectrogram that contains information about the target (humans) only. Furthermore, the spectrogram in Fig. 8 will go through the cropping process. In this process, the spectrogram will be cropped to form a rectangle of distance over time with a time of 2 s. Distance is an index of frequency and time is periods (one period is equal to 50 ms), so in this case, the spectrogram is cropped to form a rectangle or 440×40 matrix. This matrix is then extracted every time slot (50 ms), resulting in many rectangular images and this image will be used as a dataset for Deep Learning. With the dataset that has been collected and the dataset has gone through the preprocessing stage, the final dataset obtained is 2961 data for each type of activity and the total data is 11844 data.

Convolutional Neural Network. One of the algorithms of Deep Learning is CNN or Convolutional Neural Network and is a development of MPL (Multilayer Perceptron). CNN is designed to process data in two-dimensional form [27]. CNN combines several layers by adding several input layers in order to obtain the pattern value of a measurement with maximum results [28]. In general, CNN is divided

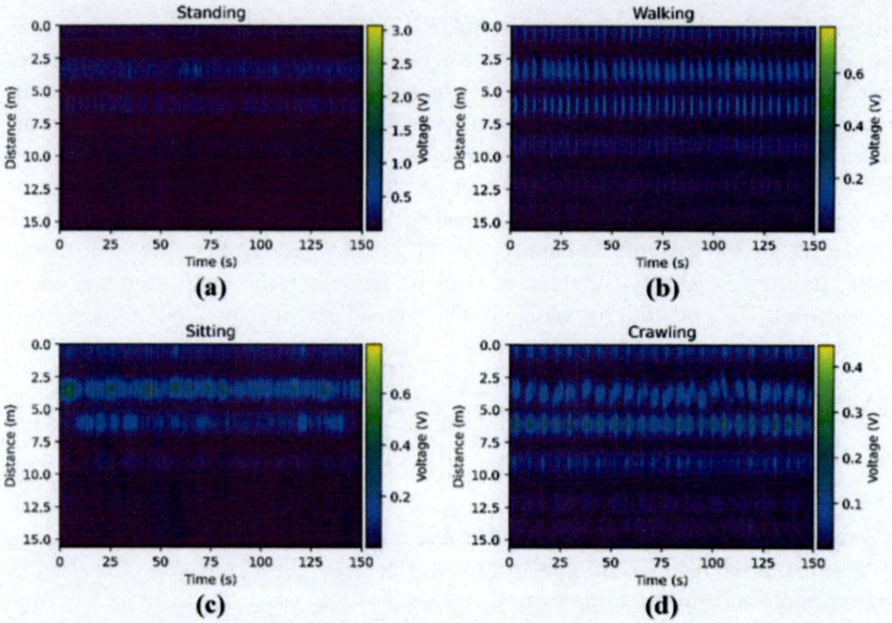

Fig. 6 Spectrograms after static clutter removal: **a** Standing, **b** Walking, **c** Sitting, **d** Crawling

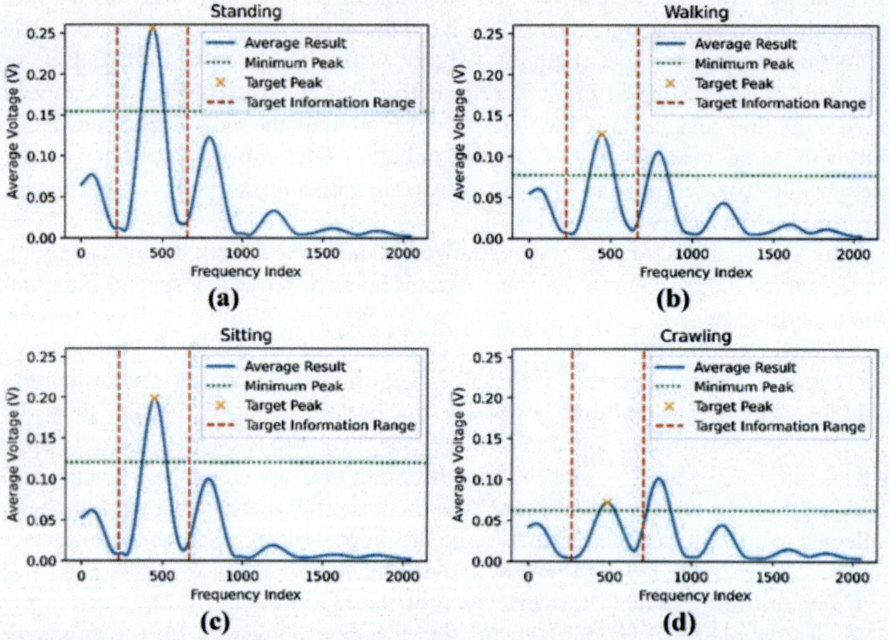

Fig. 7 The average result of the spectrograms becomes 1D: **a** Standing, **b** Walking, **c** Sitting, **d** Crawling

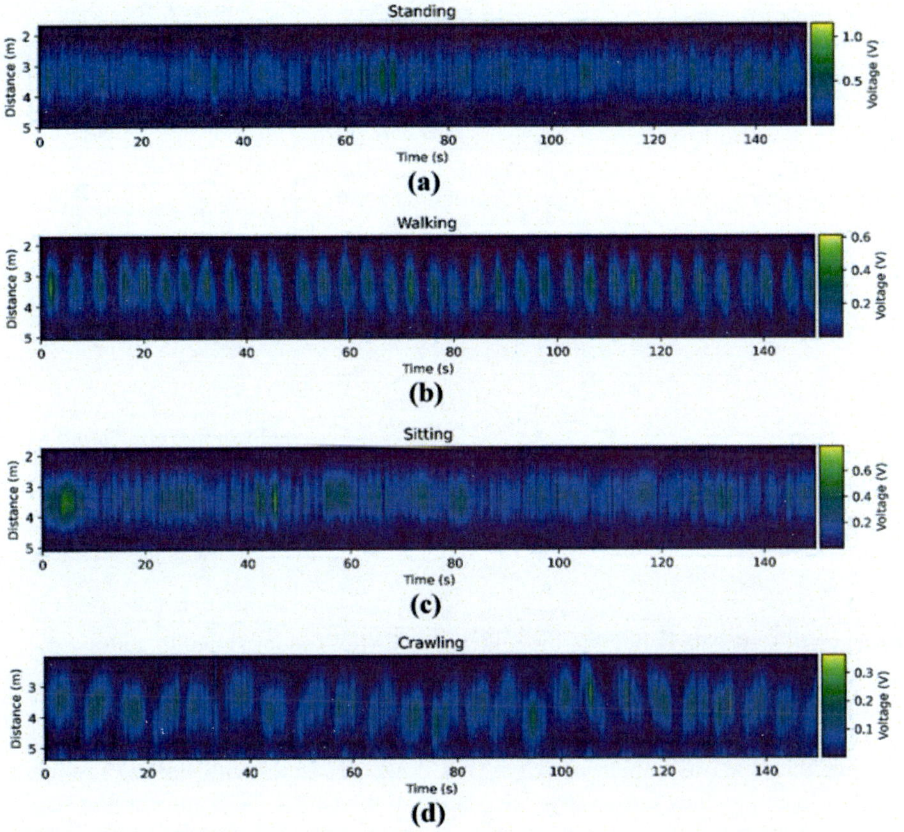

Fig. 8 Spectrograms contains target information only: **a** Standing, **b** Walking, **c** Sitting, **d** Crawling

into two types of layers, the first layer is the Feature Learning/Feature Extraction Layer and the second layer is the Classification Layer. Layers of the first type are Convolutional Layer and Pooling Layer. Then the second type of layer is a Fully Connected Layer. Convolutional layer, Pooling layer, and Full Connected layer are the three main layers in CNN [27, 29].

2.3 *Flowchart*

Flowchart Data Collection. Figure 9 is a flowchart for collecting datasets. The flowchart begins by entering the time limit for data collection, meaning that this input will be the determination of when the data collection ends. Then the Raspberry Pi will connect to uRAD, if the uRAD error occurs at that time then the Raspberry Pi will try to reconnect it. If the Raspberry Pi is already connected to uRAD, then

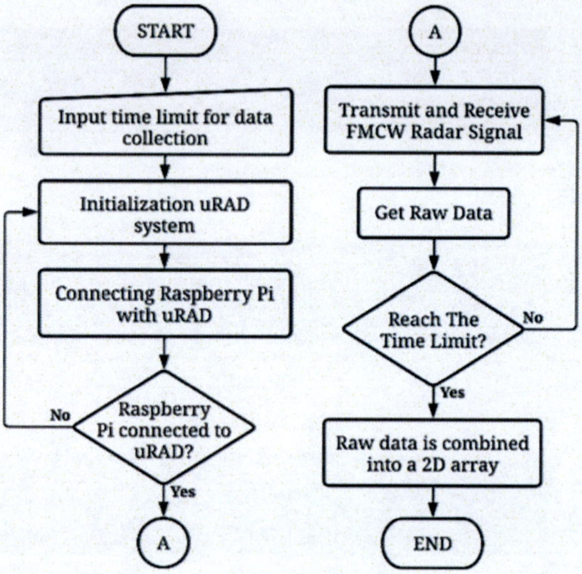

Fig. 9 Flowchart data collection

uRAD will start data collection by emitting an FMCW radar signal to get raw data. This raw data collection will continue until the specified time limit. If the time limit is reached, the raw data will be collected in one 2D array.

Flowchart Training. Figure 10 is a flowchart training so that the system can classify the types of human activity. This flowchart starts with the 2D raw data that has been obtained previously. This data will then enter the preprocessing stage, where this stage performs data processing so that it gets good data for training. This preprocessing stage includes removing DC components, FFT, static clutter removal, and cropping spectrograms. Data that has passed preprocessing will be divided into two data with a percentage of 75% train data and 25% test data. With the data that has been collected, the train data will be 8883 data and the test data will be 2961 data. The train data will then be trained according to the CNN architecture that has been determined and validated with test data to get good classification accuracy.

3 Result

3.1 CNN Architecture

This study has two parameters to determine the best architecture for designing CNN architecture. The parameters are the number of convolutional layers and the number of epochs. In this experiment, we train the dataset with different tests depending on the built CNN architecture. The results of the experiments for each architecture can

Fig. 10 Flowchart training

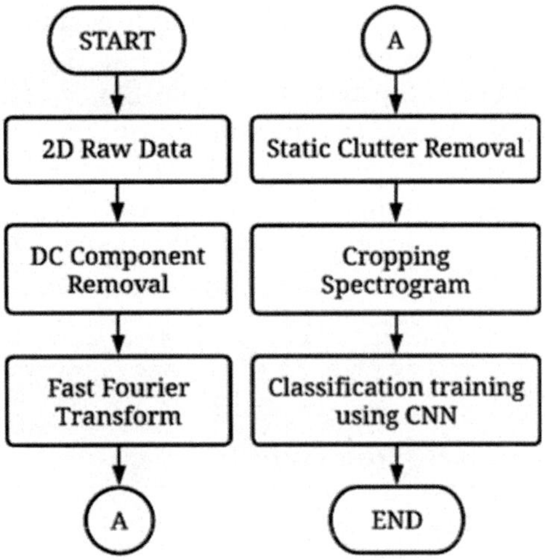

be seen in Table 1. It can be proven that the CNN architecture, with two convolution layers and 300 epochs, has the highest validation accuracy with 99.9% accuracy and the lowest validation loss which is 0.0067, as seen in Table 1. Therefore, the CNN architecture with two convolutional layers and 300 epochs is the best architecture for this study, and we will continue to use this architecture for further analysis.

The best CNN architecture for this study is shown in Fig. 11, which is the CNN architecture with two convolutional layers and 300 epochs. The input image is a spectrogram with dimensions of 440 × 40. First of all, this study uses 2 × 2 zero padding so that no information is wasted when entering the first convolution layer. Then it will enter the convolution process with each convolution using a 3 × 3 filter size except the first one, which is a 5 × 5 filter size. Each convolution uses ReLU activation. ReLU works on the threshold values at 0, i.e. $f(x) = \max(0, x)$. It simply produces 0 when $x < 0$, and vice versa will produce a linear function when

Table 1 Results of all CNN architecture experiments

Convolutional layer	Epoch	Validation accuracy (%)	Validation loss (cross entropy value)
1	100	97.16	0.0759
	200	98.95	0.0349
	300	99.59	0.0139
2	100	98.24	0.054
	200	99.73	0.0172
	300	99.9	0.0067
3	100	95.84	0.1072
	200	99.12	0.0331
	300	99.62	0.0137

$x \geq 0$ [30]. This study also uses max pooling method after every convolution. Then the next process is the fully connected layer which is part of an artificial neural network consisting of several neurons connected by connecting weights [31]. This layer serves to transform the dimensions of the data so that the data can be classified linearly [29]. Finally, the last process in this CNN model is the activation of the softmax function. Softmax activation is useful for converting the output of the last layer to its basic probability distribution. The advantage of softmax activation is that the output probability ranges from 0 to 1, and the sum of the probabilities is equal to 1 [32].

3.2 Training Results

Figure 12 is a CNN performance evaluation using the CNN architecture in Fig. 11. The accuracy of the classification is nearly 1 with the loss value almost reaching 0, more precisely the classification accuracy is 99.9% and the loss value is 0.0067 with 300 epochs. The graph also looks stable between training and validation. This means that the CNN Architecture created works very well for the classification of human activities.

3.3 Testing Results

The testing process uses 2961 test data and randomly selects different types of activities to be able to determine CNN's performance in predicting data that has never been trained. The prediction results are shown in Fig. 13 which is a confusion matrix.

As shown in Fig. 13, the CNN architecture that has been designed shows that the model can classify the types of activities well. However, the activity of standing and sitting had three inaccurate predictions. This happens because the activities of standing and sitting have similar spectrograms. If analyzed, the two activities have similar spectrograms because they do not have much movement change. Even so, this model is suitable for classifying human activities. Table 2 shows the quality of predictions of the CNN architecture that has been made.

Table 2 shows precision, recall, and F1 score for each activity. The data shows that the precision, recall, and F1 score value is 1, which is the highest value for each activity. This data also shows that the CNN architecture created has excellent predictions for HAR. Therefore, this CNN architecture can classify HAR with a low classification error rate for each activity.

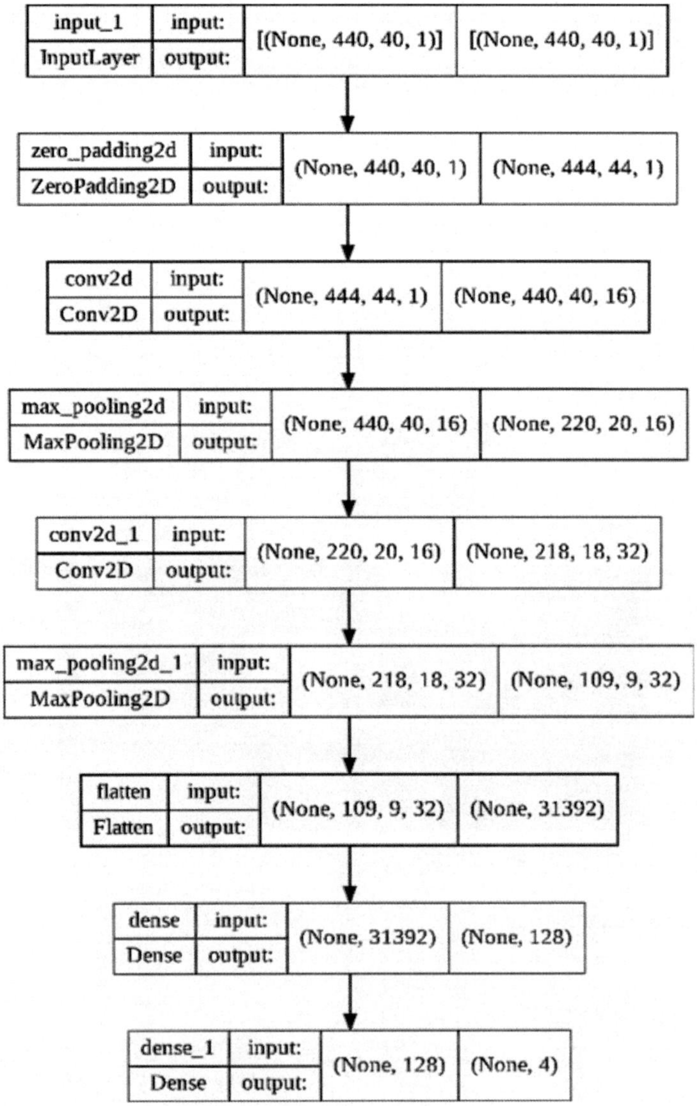

Fig. 11 CNN Architecture with two convolutional layers

4 Discussion

This study succeeded in obtaining high classification results. The preprocessing stage supports this result because this stage also determines the classification accuracy results. This preprocessing stage contains DC components removal, FFT, static clutter removal, and cropping spectrograms to obtain CNN input data which only

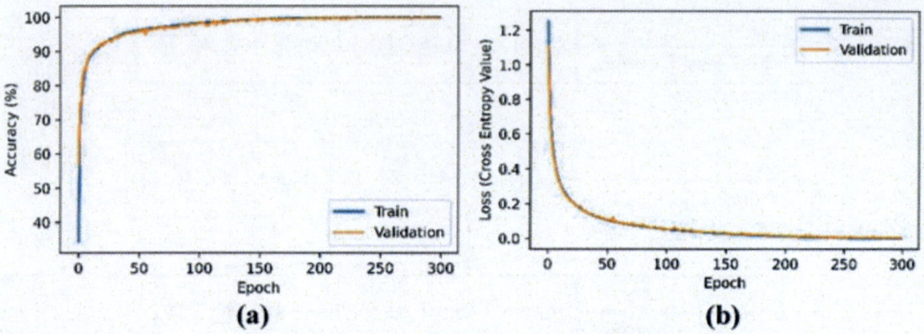

Fig. 12 CNN performance evaluation: **a** Classification accuracy, **b** Loss value

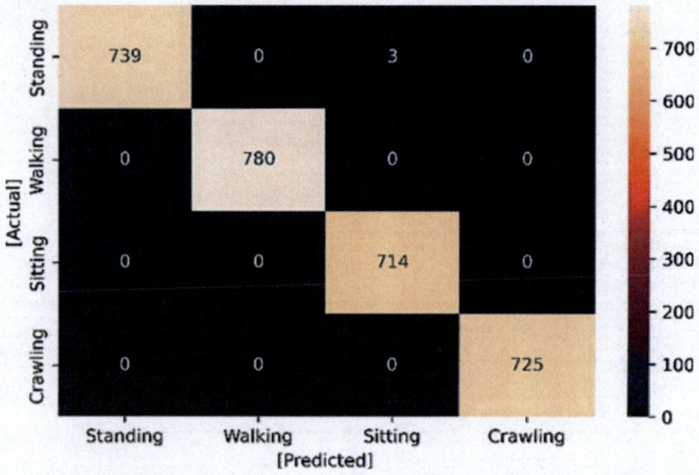

Fig. 13 Test data confusion matrix

Table 2 Quality of predictions

Activity	Precision	Recall	F1-score	Support
Standing	1.00	1.00	1.00	742
Walking	1.00	1.00	1.00	780
Sitting	1.00	1.00	1.00	714
Crawling	1.00	1.00	1.00	725

contains information on the radar distance to the target. This research then compares the different CNN architectures by comparing the number of convolutional layers and the number of different epochs to get the best architecture for classifying human activities. Finally, the CNN architecture with two convolution layers, ReLU activation, max pooling, and softmax, has the best accuracy classification result and can classify four activities (Standing, Walking, Sitting, and Crawling) with 99.9% accuracy.

This study can solve problems related to HAR from previous studies, such as using this Radar to classify even though the surroundings are dark, maintain privacy, and is contactless. This study also explains how the preprocessing is carried out to obtain proper data to be trained using CNN and conduct experiments with various CNN architectures to obtain the best model for the classification of human activities and high classification accuracy. This method is what separates this study from previous HAR studies using Radar. The classification accuracy results in this study also got 99.9% accuracy, which also has a higher classification accuracy than previous studies. This study is more specific in using uRAD by Anteral as the radar sensor. uRAD is easy to use, portable and has many built-in features that can be used easily, one of which can obtain raw data for advanced signal processing. Because of that, we can usc the raw data to classify human activities.

Although it has a high classification accuracy, this study still has weaknesses. The weakness is in the uRAD component, where uRAD has a distance resolution between object of 1.5 m. This means that if there are two objects that are close together and the distance between the objects is less than 1.5 m, the information about the two objects will be mixed. However, this system will still be able to classify human activities but with the condition that the target must not be close to other objects with a limit of 1.5 m including walls. A study discusses this weakness with a distance between targets as far as 15 m, where the distance between targets is much further compared to this study [22]. Moreover, other studies do not discuss this weakness [20, 21, 23, 24].

The implication of this research is that this study obtains HAR classification results with a high level of accuracy due to the preprocessing method and the determination of the CNN architecture. The preprocessing method gives CNN training a higher classification accuracy compared to previous studies. This high accuracy is also obtained because we choose the best CNN architecture for classifying human activities.

5 Conclusion

This study intends to explain signal processing from raw data signals to images containing only target distance information so that it becomes appropriate data for training in order to be able to develop HAR using FMCW radar. In order to find the optimum CNN architecture for HAR, this study will also compare the number of convolutional layers and the number of epochs. The objective is to reach classification accuracy above 95%. This study uses uRAD by Anteral and Raspberry Pi to be able to operate it. The output of uRAD is raw data which later be combined to form a 2D number of samples over time. The collected data will then enter the preprocessing stage, where this stage will remove the DC component, perform FFT to convert it into a time frequency domain (spectrogram), static clutter removal, taking spectrogram images that contain information about the target (humans) only, and finally cropping to get matrix data or a 440 × 40 spectrogram image. After going through the process, this data will be the input to be trained using CNN. The best CNN architecture for HAR classification was then determined by comparison of the three CNN architectures. The results of the training gave very good results, which is 99.9%. This study experimented in a room which caused the data that had been collected to have information about the distance of the walls although we removed the information regarding the existing wall. We aim to work in different environments, such as outdoors and can identify many activities with multiple targets for future work.

References

1. Bouchabou D, Lohr C, Kanellos I, Nguyen SM (2021) Human Activity Recognition (HAR) in smart homes
2. Jatkar DD, Surve AR (2021) Human activity recognition and fall detection
3. Wan Q, Li Y, Li C, Pal R (2014) Gesture recognition for smart home applications using portable radar sensors. In: 2014 36th annual international conference of the IEEE Engineering in Medicine and Biology Society, EMBC 2014. Institute of Electrical and Electronics Engineers Inc., pp 6414–6417. https://doi.org/10.1109/EMBC.2014.6945096
4. Molchanov P, Gupta S, Kim K, Kautz J (2015) Hand gesture recognition with 3D convolutional neural networks
5. Cristani M, Raghavendra R, del Bue A, Murino V (2013) Human behavior analysis in video surveillance: a social signal processing perspective. Neurocomputing 100:86–97. https://doi.org/10.1016/j.neucom.2011.12.038
6. Li X, He Y, Jing X (2019) A survey of deep learning-based human activity recognition in radar. https://doi.org/10.3390/rs11091068
7. Jalal A, Kim YH, Kim YJ, Kamal S, Kim D (2017) Robust human activity recognition from depth video using spatiotemporal multi-fused features. Pattern Recognit 61:295–308. https://doi.org/10.1016/j.patcog.2016.08.003
8. Jalal A, Kamal S, Kim D (2017) A depth video-based human detection and activity recognition using multi-features and embedded hidden Markov models for health care monitoring systems. Int J Interact Multimedia Artif Intell 4:54. https://doi.org/10.9781/ijimai.2017.447
9. Yang X, Tian YL (2017) Super normal vector for human activity recognition with depth cameras. IEEE Trans Pattern Anal Mach Intell 39:1028–1039. https://doi.org/10.1109/TPAMI.2016.2565479
10. Simonyan K, Zisserman A (2014) Two-stream convolutional networks for action recognition in videos
11. Wang L, Xiong Y, Wang Z, Qiao Y, Lin D, Tang X, van Gool L (2016) Temporal segment networks: towards good practices for deep action recognition. https://doi.org/10.1007/978-3-319-46484-8
12. Ren Y, Zhu C, Xiao S (2018) Deformable faster R-CNN with aggregating multi-layer features for partially occluded object detection in optical remote sensing images. Remote Sens 10:1470. https://doi.org/10.3390/RS10091470
13. Markman A, Shen X, Javidi B (2017) Three-dimensional object visualization and detection in low light illumination using integral imaging. Optics Lett 42(16):3068–3071. https://doi.org/10.1364/OL.42.003068
14. Bouachir W, Gouiaa R, Li B, Noumeir R (2018) Intelligent video surveillance for real-time detection of suicide attempts. Pattern Recognit Lett 110:1–7. https://doi.org/10.1016/J.PATREC.2018.03.018

15. Reyes-Ortiz JL, Oneto L, Samà A, Parra X, Anguita D (2016) Transition-aware human activity recognition using smartphones. Neurocomputing 171:754–767. https://doi.org/10.1016/J.NEUCOM.2015.07.085
16. Liu Y, Nie L, Liu L, Rosenblum DS (2016) From action to activity: sensor-based activity recognition. Neurocomputing 181:108–115. https://doi.org/10.1016/J.NEUCOM.2015.08.096
17. Ronao CA, Cho SB (2016) Human activity recognition with smartphone sensors using deep learning neural networks. Expert Syst Appl 59:235–244. https://doi.org/10.1016/J.ESWA.2016.04.032
18. Shoaib M, Bosch S, Incel OD, Scholten H, Havinga PJM (2016) Complex human activity recognition using smartphone and wrist-worn motion sensors. Sensors 16:426. https://doi.org/10.3390/S16040426
19. Serpush F, Menhaj MB, Masoumi B, Karasfi B (2022) Wearable sensor-based human activity recognition in the smart healthcare system. Comput Intell Neurosci 2022. https://doi.org/10.1155/2022/1391906
20. Kang SW, Jang MH, Lee S (2021) Identification of human motion using radar sensor in an indoor environment. Sensors 21. https://doi.org/10.3390/s21072305
21. Shao Y, Guo S, Sun L, Chen W (2017) Human motion classification based on range information with deep convolutional neural network 1519–1523. https://doi.org/10.1109/ICISCE.2017.317
22. Chen Z, Li G, Fioranelli F, Griffiths H (2018) Personnel recognition and gait classification based on multistatic micro-doppler signatures using deep convolutional neural networks. IEEE Geosci Remote Sens Lett 15:669–673. https://doi.org/10.1109/LGRS.2018.2806940
23. Ahmed S, Park J, Cho SH (2022) FMCW radar sensor based human activity recognition using deep learning. In: 2022 international conference on electronics, information, and communication, ICEIC 2022. Institute of Electrical and Electronics Engineers Inc. https://doi.org/10.1109/ICEIC54506.2022.9748776
24. Gurbuz SZ, Amin MG (2019) Radar-based human-motion recognition with deep learning: promising applications for indoor monitoring. IEEE Signal Process Mag 36:16–28. https://doi.org/10.1109/MSP.2018.2890128
25. Anteral (2018) uRAD—Datasheet—Raspberry Pi v1.2—EN
26. Anteral, uRAD: user manual Raspberry Pi version Software SDK v1.1
27. Sharma S, Pham VH, Boscoboinik JA, Rebeggiani S, Wagner M, Mazal J, Ayu Anjani I, Rizky Pratiwi Y, Bagas Nurhuda NS (2021) Implementation of deep learning using convolutional neural network algorithm for classification rose flower. J Phys Conf Ser 1842:012002. https://doi.org/10.1088/1742-6596/1842/1/012002
28. Rasyid R, Ibrahim A (2021) Implementation of machine learning using the convolution neural network method for Aglaonema interest classification. Jurnal E-Komtek (Elektro-Komputer-Teknik) 5:21–30. https://doi.org/10.37339/e-komtek.v5i1.434
29. Anton A, Nissa NF, Janiati A, Cahya N, Astuti P (2021) Application of deep learning using Convolutional Neural Network (CNN) method for women's skin classification. Sci J Inf 8:144–153. https://doi.org/10.15294/sji.v8i1.26888
30. Agarap AF (2018) Deep learning using Rectified Linear Units (ReLU)
31. Hijazi S, Kumar R, Rowen C (2015) Using convolutional neural networks for image recognition
32. Fu'Adah YN, Wijayanto I, Pratiwi NKC, Taliningsih FF, Rizal S, Pramudito MA (2021) Automated classification of Alzheimer's disease based on MRI image processing using Convolutional Neural Network (CNN) with AlexNet architecture. In: Journal of physics: conference series. IOP Publishing Ltd. https://doi.org/10.1088/1742-6596/1844/1/012020.

Classification of Alphabets and Numbers Indonesian Sign System Using uRAD Radar Based on FMCW Radar and Deep Learning Techniques

Fasya Abhirama Kausar, Fiky Y. Suratman, and Istiqomah

Abstract The difficulty of society, especially in Indonesia, for interacting with people who are deaf and speech impaired is the Indonesian Language Sign System (SIBI). Technology is needed to translate the SIBI language to make it easier for Indonesian people to interact with deaf and speech-impaired people. This research proposal uses uRAD radar based on FMCW radar to detect the SIBI language used to collect datasets with the addition of Deep Learning Convolutional Neural Network (CNN) techniques for classification algorithms. The designed system can classify Alphabet Letters and Numbers into five classes, namely Letters C, F, and T, and Numbers 3 and 6. The classification results using six layers of Convolutional Neural Network (CNN), and ReLu activation obtained an accuracy of more than 92%. The proposed system's results can help translate and understand the SIBI Alphabet and Numbers.

Keywords uRAD Radar · Alphabet dan Number SIBI · CNN

1 Introduction

Some people with disabilities, especially the deaf and speech impaired in Indonesia, have difficulty interacting with the public verbally and physically. Skills in understanding sign language in communicating with deaf and speech-impaired persons are critical because deaf and speech-impaired persons communicate with each other using sign language [1]. When interacting with normal society, they have difficulty. Deaf and speech-impaired people generally use Indonesian Sign Language (BISINDO). However, the Indonesian government has established the Indonesian Sign Language System (SIBI), and it is used in school curricula in Indonesia [2].

Many studies on Hand Gesture Recognition have been carried out [3–15], both in gesture detection and in translating Sign Language, such as translating the Indonesian Sign System (SIBI). The SIBI translation system has been carried out using a

F. A. Kausar (✉) · F. Y. Suratman · Istiqomah
School of Electrical Engineering, Telkom University, Bandung, Indonesia
e-mail: fasyakausar@student.telkomuniversity.ac.id

T. Triwiyanto et al. (eds.), *Proceeding of the 3rd International Conference on Electronics, Biomedical Engineering, and Health Informatics*, Lecture Notes in Electrical Engineering 1008, https://doi.org/10.1007/978-981-99-0248-4_30

WebCam sensor to detect the letters of the alphabet "A" to "Z" and the numbers "0" to "9". This system is supported using the Artificial Neural Network (ANN) method in classifying hand motion images, with 100 images per movement, and detection accuracy reaches 90% [16]. Another study discusses hand gesture recognition for human–computer interaction (HCI). This journal uses FMCW radar, which has specifications of 60 GHz with a detection distance of 10–15 cm. In the classification, we used 8 types of hand gestures with the 2D FFT method on the radar output. This journal performs hand gesture recognition using CNN with an additional adaptive domain, which is used to deduce whether the target domain is labelled or not labelled and compares results for 3D-CNN model accuracy, 2D-CNN, and RNN. The biggest advantage of this system is that it increases performance maximally from little training data [17]. The use of radar in sign language recognition has been carried out using Doppler radar and American sign language for vigilance purposes using DCNN with an accuracy of 87.5% and the VGG-16 algorithm with an accuracy of 95%, other studies related to sign language recognition using multi-antenna radar and American sign language with CNN's deep learning method [18]. In addition to the two types of radar above, research using millimetre wave radar has been carried out, which applies American sign language using the CNN method in 18 movement classes to get an accuracy of 95% [19].

Using uRAD radar based on FMCW radar is important for providing solutions to the above problems. This study uses several methods to handle, such as uRAD radar, data preprocessing, and deep learning Convolutional Neural Network (CNN) methods. The advantage of using uRAD radar compared to the use of WebCam is that uRAD radar does not need to be concerned with light intensity, maintains privacy, and is not affected by weather [10, 11]. Research on sign language recognition using uRAD radar has never been done, especially in Indonesia, especially in the application to the SIBI movement of letters and numbers. In this study, it is hoped that the uRAD radar can be applied directly in public places such as buying tickets, ordering food, etc. uRAD radar focuses on obtaining data on letters of the alphabet and SIBI numbers, which uses three letters and 2 SIBI numbers, namely "Letter C", "Letter F", "Letter H", "Number 3", and "Number 6", then preprocessing the data using the cropping image method in multiplying the dataset and the FFT method in converting the data structure into frequency and distance domains. After that, there will be a dataset classification process that has been processed using the Deep Learning CNN method, and there are three classification scenarios.

This paper is structured as follows. Section 2 provides information related to data collection. Section 3 provides research results that have been processed through the stages of data processing to classification. Section 4 explains the results and comparisons. Finally, Sect. 5 summarizes the study's results and provides conclusions and suggestions for further research.

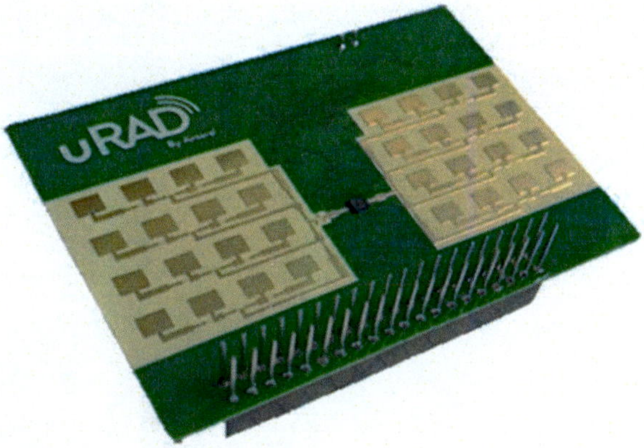

Fig. 1 URAD radar as a tool for detecting the movement of SIBI letters and numbers

2 Materials and Method

2.1 *Materials*

This study uses a radar sensor called uRAD radar (see Fig. 1). *uRAD radar* is a radar-based FMCW radar integrated with the Raspberry Pi 4. This type of uRAD radar can be used as a portable radar where there are various modes in this radar. Frequency Modulated Continuous Wave (FMCW) is a radar that emits continuous waves by modulating the frequency within a specific time range and period. [20].

2.2 *Experimental Procedures*

The dataset was collected in this study using the uRAD radar sensor, which has been integrated with the Raspberry Pi 4. The uRAD radar and Raspberry Pi 4 are combined using a shield and mounted on a camera tripod as high as 100 cm (see Fig. 2).

The camera tripod and uRAD radar are then aligned with the object to be detected. In this study, the distance between the uRAD radar and the object is 1.2 m (see Fig. 3).

Dataset retrieval is done by recording using uRAD radar for 180 seconds with specifications Ns = 50, namely the number of samples in one data frame (Ns). The maximum sample in one data frame is 200. Only 50 is used BW = 240 MHz radar and used to work in the 24 GHz frequency with a bandwidth of 240 MHz, uRAD mode = Mode 2, which mode is only for detecting distances in the form of a sawtooth signal [21]. After getting the desired dataset then, enter the data preprocessing process. The dataset will be processed to get a large number of datasets (see Fig. 4).

Removes DC Component. The 5-class raw dataset generated by the radar is still in the form of an I (in-phase) Q (Quadrature) signal. The 5-class dataset that has been collected has dimensions of 1 data class (3600, 50), meaning that 1 dataset

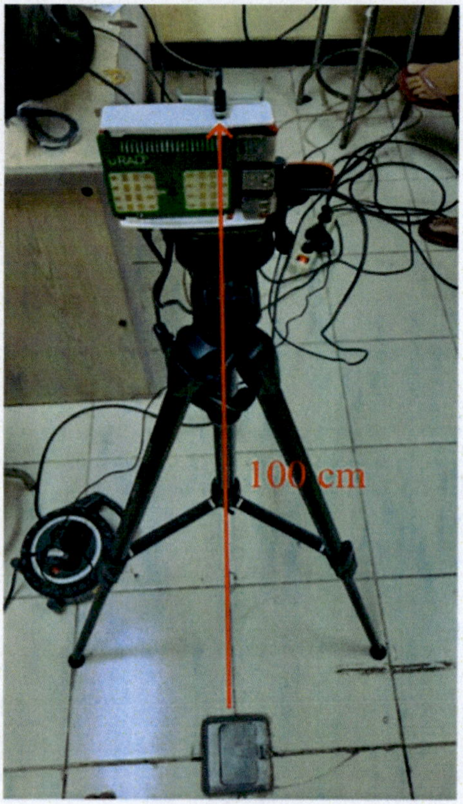

Fig. 2 Form the foundation of uRAD radar using a tripod

class has 50 samples in 1 data frame and 180 s in length in 1 data class. The author converts the form of the I/Q signal contained in the dataset so that the data can be converted into voltage because this raw data has arbitrary units from 0 to 4095. The signal conversion calculates the maximum voltage GPIO on the Raspberry Pi 4 3.3 V divided by ADC Intervals from uRAD. Components I and Q have a DC Component. Therefore, the removal of the DC Component is necessary [14], the removal of the DC Component by applying I and Q with the following Eq. (1):

$$\mathrm{x} = \mathrm{x}_{\mathrm{N_s}} - \frac{1}{\mathrm{N_s}} \sum_{\mathrm{n}=0}^{\mathrm{N_s}-1} \mathrm{x}_{\mathrm{N_s}}[\mathrm{n}] \quad (1)$$

where $x_{N_s} = [x[0], x[1], x[2], \ldots, x[N_s - 1]]$ and N_s It is the number of samples.

In one data frame, the deletion of the DC Component is the value of each sample. (n_{column}) on the data, the frame is reduced by the average of the sample ($\text{avg}_{\text{column}}$).

Fast Fourier Transform. Suppose you look at the output images of the I and Q signals (see Fig. 5). In that case, the data still has an unclear pattern because there is no visible object of movement of the letters of the alphabet and SIBI numbers

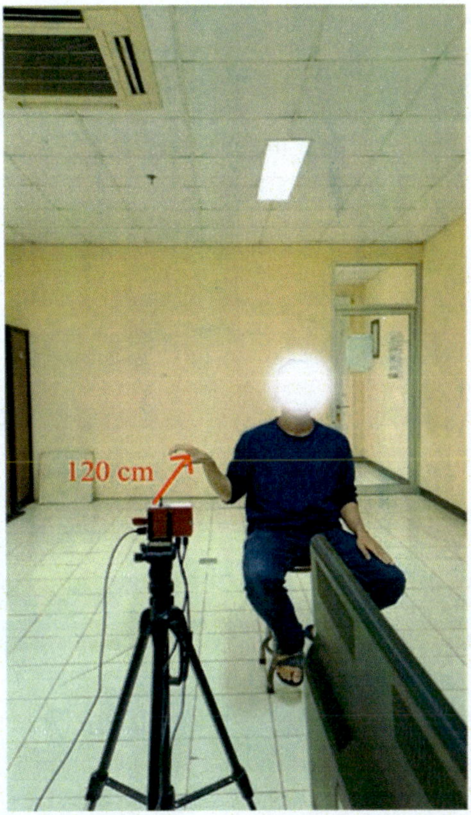

Fig. 3 The position of dataset retrieval before entering the machine learning process

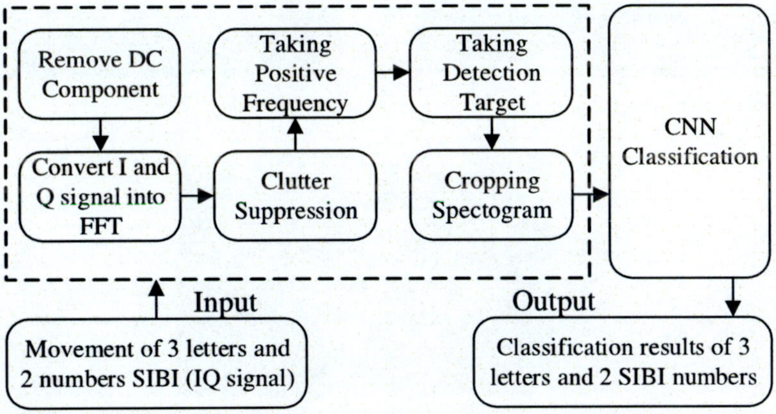

Fig. 4 Block diagram system of each process that works in this research

and no other static objects are visible. To be able to find out information about the distance from the radar to the object movement of the letters of the alphabet and SIBI numbers, the Fast Fourier Transform method is needed [22, 23]. The I and Q signal data converted into voltage will then be entered into the FFT process with a frequency index of 4096. The FFT method can be calculated using the following Eq. (2).

$$X[k] = \sum_{n=0}^{N-1} x[n]e^{-j2\pi \frac{n}{N}k} \tag{2}$$

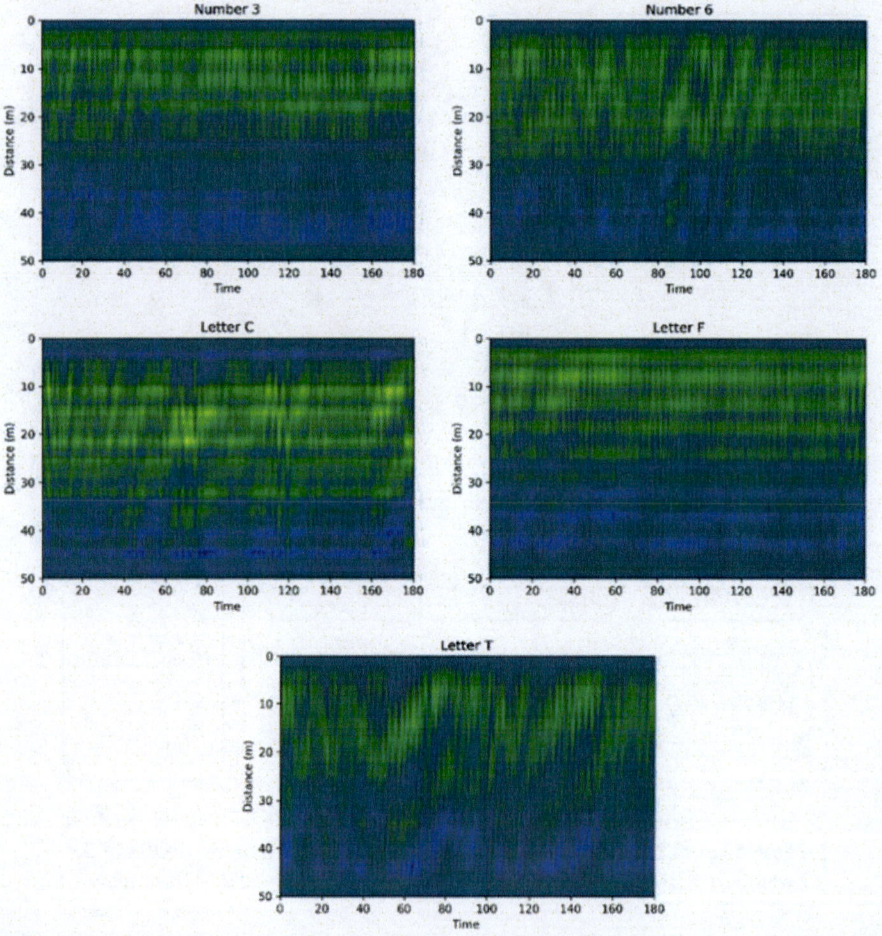

Fig. 5 Form the IQ signal (raw data) in 2 dimensions before going through the preprocessing stage

where $k = 0, \ldots, N{-}1$ and $x[n]$ is a number of samples.

There are two different frequencies, namely positive and negative frequencies (see Fig. 6), so if you want to have information about the distance between the radar and the target frequency index, only the index from the range 2048 to 4096 is used because the range is part of the positive frequency and has information, regarding the distance between the radar and the target (Fig. 7).

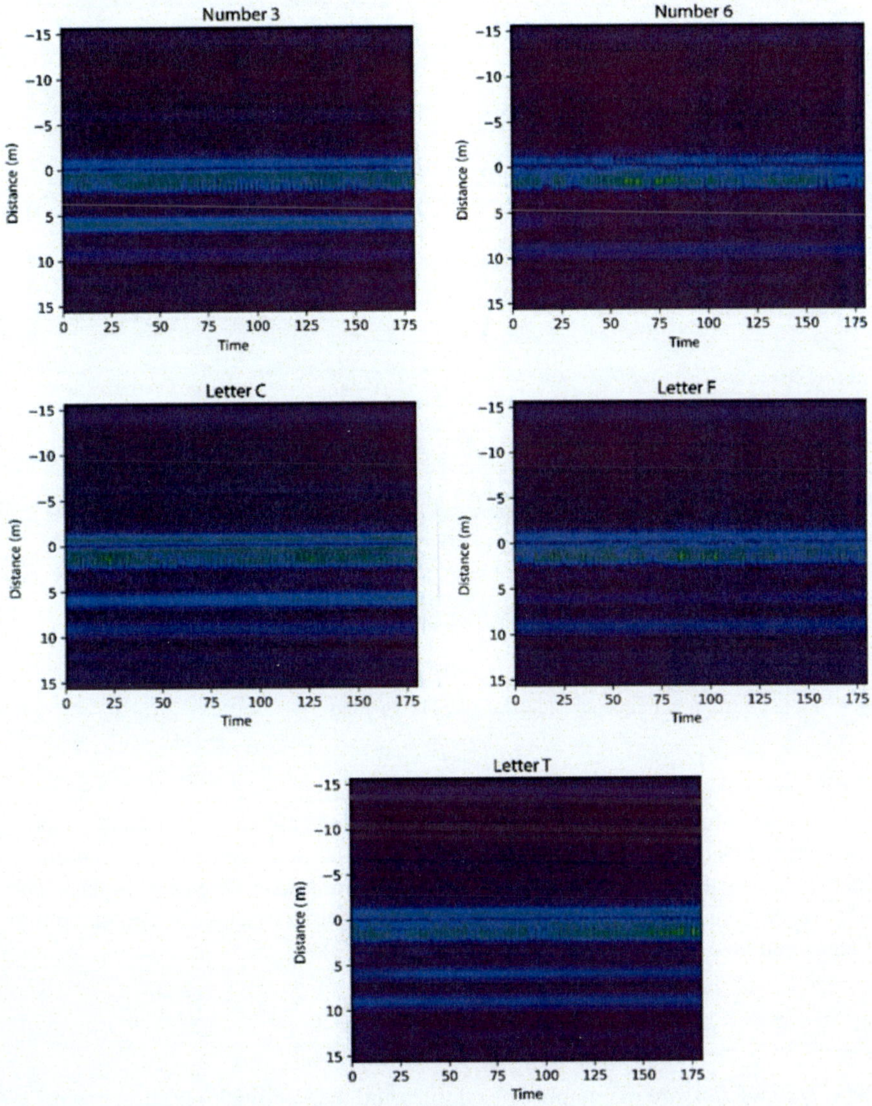

Fig. 6 Spectrogram form of raw data IQ signal which has been converted into frequency domain

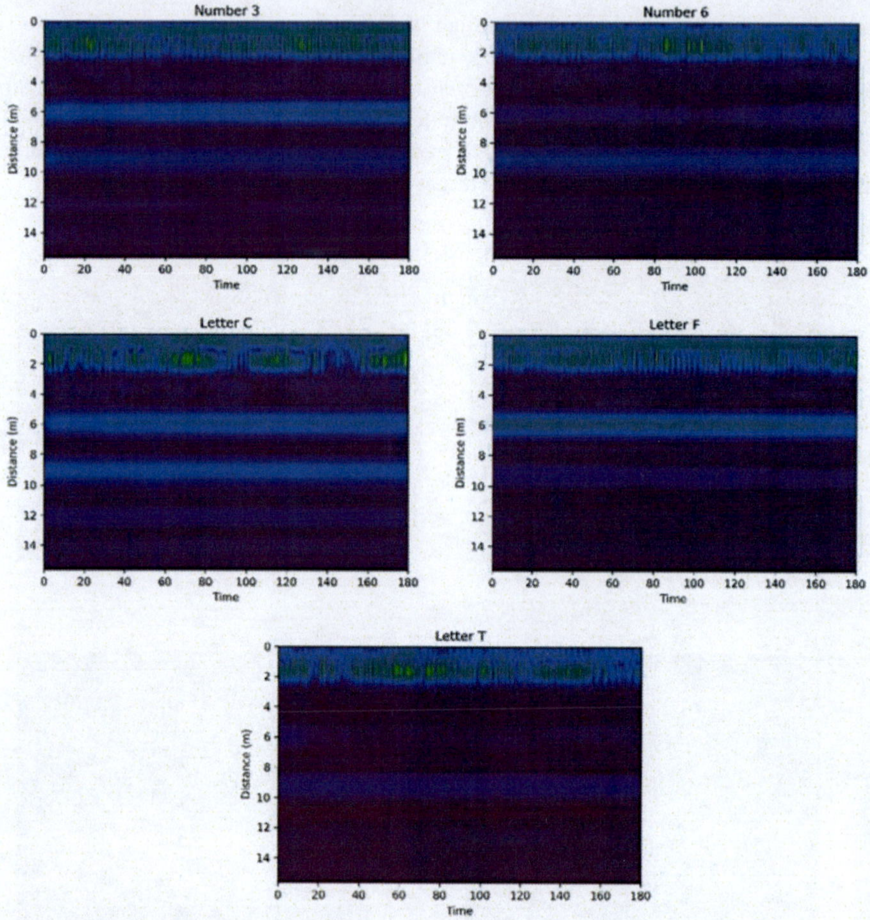

Fig. 7 Plot spectrogram frequency index range 2048 To 4096

If we see the spectrogram above is the data accumulated during N_p (number of frames). The column part (y) in the spectrogram image above is a frequency index. However, the frequency index has been converted into a distance with a maximum distance achieved by uRAD 15.625 m with calculations according to formula 3. The row (x) section in the spectrogram image above is the time in seconds. The maximum distance can be calculated using the following Eq. (3):

$$\text{DistanceMax} = 75x\frac{Ns}{BW} \tag{3}$$

where Ns and BW are the number of samples and the bandwidth used by radar.

Removes Clutter. The I and Q signal data that have been converted into voltage and frequency domains still have static objects (interference). So we need a method to dampen the static object so that the movement can be seen more clearly [24, 25]. In reducing the disturbance of the static object, it can be eliminated mathematically, which can be written as the following Eq. (4) and (5):

$$\mathbb{Y}^{(N_p)} = \mathbb{X}^{(N_p)} - \frac{1}{N_p}\left[\sum_{i=0}^{N_p} X^{(i)}[0], \sum_{k=0}^{N_p} X^{(i)}[1], \ldots, \sum_{k=0}^{N_p} X^{(i)}[K-1]\right] \times J_{1,N_p} \tag{3}$$

where $\mathbb{X}^{(N_p)} = \left[X^{(0)}, X^{(1)}, \ldots, X^{(N_p-1)}\right] J_{1,N_p}$ is a $1 \times N_p$ matrix where all elements contain 1, which means that the way to reduce Clutter is the value of each row (n_{row}) in the data frame is reduced by the average of each row (avg_{row}). Where $X^{(i)} = \left[X^{(i)}[0], X^{(i)}[1], \ldots, X^{(i)}[K-1]\right]$, , and K is the number of frequency indices, and i is the frequency index per one frame. The results of clutter suppression can be shown in the images below (see Fig. 8).

Cropping Spectrogram. Before being included in the training model, the authors first cut back, which only trimmed the targets detected by the uRAD radar. The authors wanted to remove features from unused data into the Deep Learning Convolutional Neural Network method.

After trimming the target detected by uRAD (see Fig. 9), the data will be cropped 45 frames to the right by forming a rectangle following the time series (time) or with a time of 2.25 s. The cropping aims to increase the number of datasets. Hence, there is no need to take manual data periodically, and the number of cropping is 45 frames or 2.25 s because if you use a small cropping value, the resulting data results are not good, and the more cropping values, the better the data will be.

Classification Deep Learning Convolutional Neural Network (CNN). Convolutional Neural Network (CNN) is the first Deep Learning architecture with a sequence of layers.[26]. CNN is an algorithm developed from MLP (Multilayer Perceptron), designed to process 2D data [27–29]. The CNN algorithm has been widely applied to image data and classified as a Deep Neural Network. The difference between MLP and CNN is only in the size of the neurons; MLP adopts neurons with only one dimension, while in CNN, each neuron is described in two dimensions[30, 31]. This study uses 3 CNN scenarios where each layer is different in number, which aims to find the best model. CNN will classify five classes (see Fig. 10) which use 3 Letters and 2 Numbers SIBI movement. The detection system is processed from the radar, and a programming algorithm is designed in the system flowchart (see Fig. 11).

3 Result

The dataset that has been completed in the data preprocessing process will then enter the classification stage, which is divided into three scenarios (see Table 1).

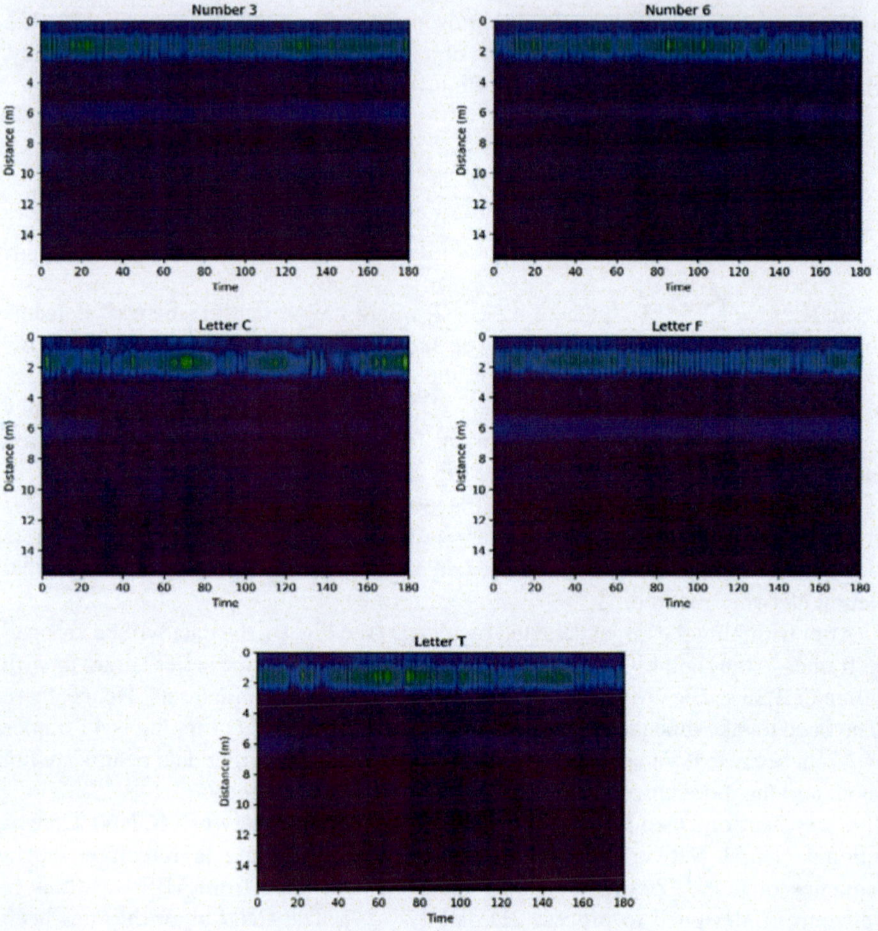

Fig. 8 Plot of Removes Clutter Spectrogram Results

Not only from testing through the model but to testing performance from a model to classifying, it can be seen through. The results of the confusion matrix and classification report used in testing based on the max pooling layer and average pooling layer are shown following the analysis results in obtaining the best model. In (see Fig. 12) below is a picture of the confusion matrix in calculating the factors in the classification performance.

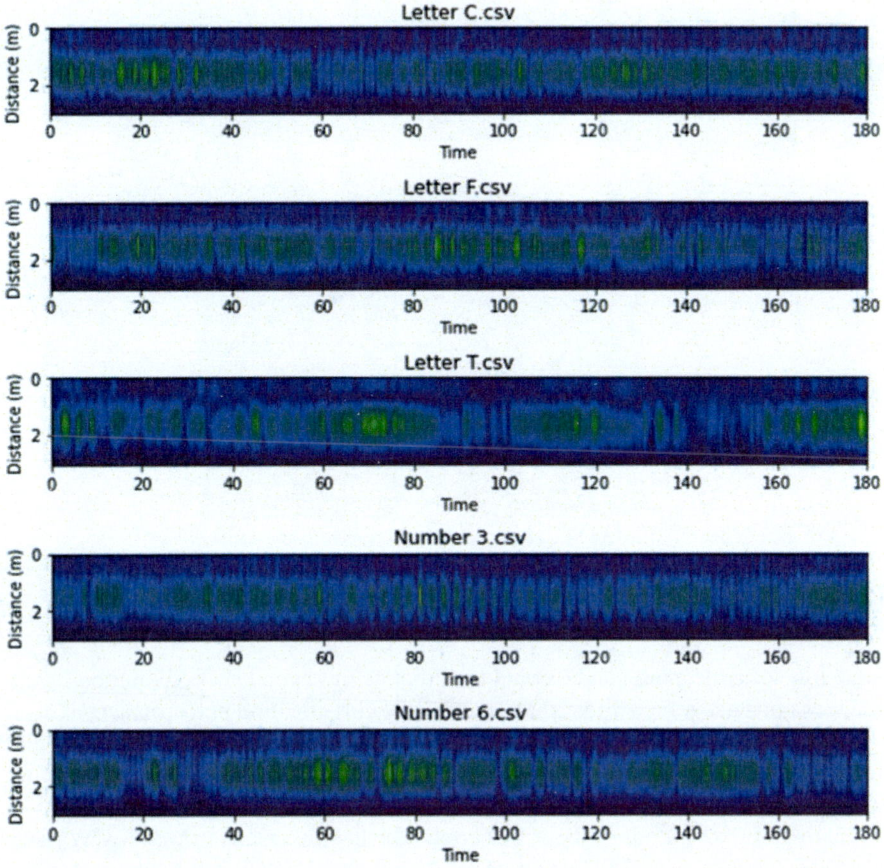

Fig. 9 Signal Cropping by only picking up targets detected by radar

4 Discussion

Testing on this classification system uses various parameters, including the number of convolution layers and the number of epochs. The use of 1 to 6 convolution layers, but each layer produces a different classification performance. Processing using a confusion matrix will show the performance of each layer and the number of epochs tested. When using a simple number of layers, namely 1, 2 and 3, convolution layers produce good accuracy but not on the classification results. Where the classification results occur, there are many misclassifications in the movement of the letters of the alphabet and SIBI numbers. To improve the performance of the classification, the test adds the number of convolution layers in which the layers become more complex. The use of 4, 5, and 6 layers of convolution resulted in perfect accuracy, but the number of epochs of 70 in the number of 4 layers experienced a decrease in accuracy. When using several six convolution layers, excellent accuracy is obtained, namely 100%

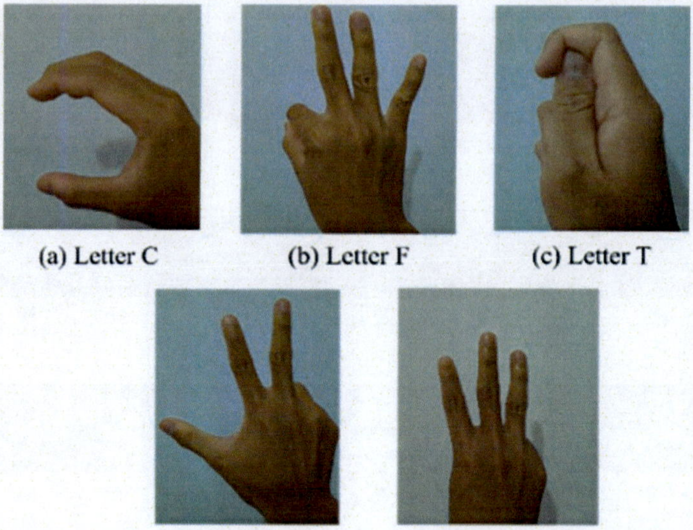

(a) Letter C (b) Letter F (c) Letter T

(d) Number 3 (e) Number 6

Fig. 10 Five classes of movement of letters and numbers SIBI used in this study

with a low loss rate, so it can be concluded that using several six convolution layers produces good accuracy validation and excellent classification performance, as seen in Fig. 12. In previous studies, the results obtained 90% accuracy using WebCam and machine learning Artificial Neural Network, and the use of Doppler radar in detecting American sign language with the DCNN algorithm obtained an accuracy of 95%. Comparing previous studies, it can be concluded that the results using FMCW radar and CNN algorithms get 100% accurate results which are better than previous studies. In the future, it is expected that when taking datasets, the room for recording must be transparent because if there are many objects around the radar, the radar will reflect all objects so that movement is disrupted, and do not use the remote desktop method which will result in interference with the data generated.

5 Conclusion

The main objective of this research has been achieved, which is to classify the letters of the alphabet and SIBI numbers successfully. The CNN deep learning method is also helpful in this classification. Compared to other convolution layer tests using six convolution layers with 70 epochs resulted in a good accuracy of 100% and an excellent movement classification performance. With this accuracy, this study succeeded in comparing previous studies which used WebCam and Doppler radar. The CNN deep learning method is also helpful in this classification. The weakness in this research is that there is no real-time system to detect the letters of the alphabet

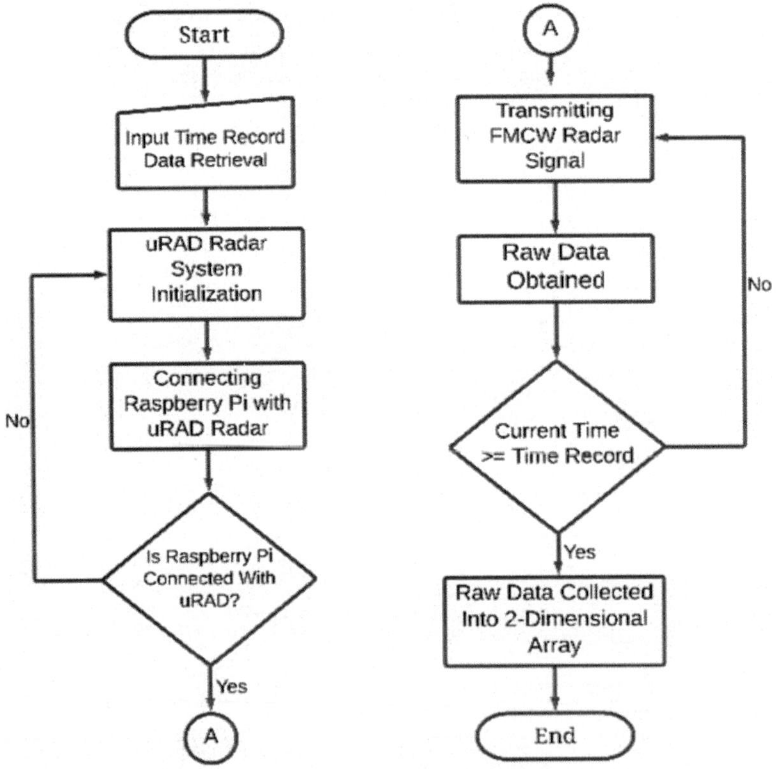

Fig. 11 Flowchart system in the process of collecting SIBI movement datasets

and the SIBI numbers, and the radar resolution is not yet high. For further research, it is hoped that they can create a real-time system to prove that movement classification can be detected or use other types of radar with higher resolution, and add movement classes for more classification.

Table 1 Classification table for testing the number of convolution layers and epoch

Convolution layer	Epoch	Accuracy (%)	Loss (%)	Validation accuracy (%)	Validation loss (%)
1	30	95.68	11.99	93.36	17.29
	50	99.51	2.36	95.95	12.11
	70	99.50	1.99	96.72	12.04
2	30	97.44	7.28	96.58	9.29
	50	99.77	1.55	98.88	3.16
	70	100	0.016	99.35	1.73
3	30	97.06	8.11	96.13	9.68
	50	99.08	3.19	95.91	9.65
	70	100	0.091	99.89	0.51
4	30	98.51	4.53	95.88	11.58
	50	99.21	2.80	99.73	1.53
	70	99.90	0.032	96.36	11.01
5	30	97.37	7.02	96.15	9.88
	50	99.88	0.67	96.20	11.13
	70	99.12	3.17	98.54	3.51
6	30	98.21	5.29	99.19	2.42
	50	100	0.045	99.91	0.36
	70	100	0.064	100	0.098

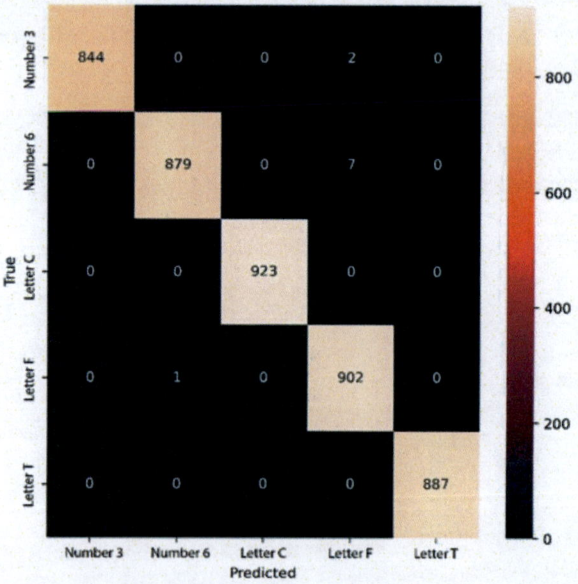

Fig. 12 The results of the confusion matrix from the best classification test model

References

1. Bantupalli K, Xie Y (2019) American sign language recognition using deep learning and computer vision. In: Proceedings of the 2018 IEEE international conference on big data. Big Data 2018, pp 4896–4899. https://doi.org/10.1109/BigData.2018.8622141
2. Aditama PW, Putra PSU, Yusa IMM, Putra INTA (2021) Designing augmented reality sibi sign language as a learning media. J Phys Conf Ser 1810. https://doi.org/10.1088/1742-6596/1810/1/012038
3. Abid MR, Petriu EM, Amjadian E (2015) Dynamic sign language recognition for smart home interactive application using stochastic linear formal grammar. IEEE Trans Instrum Meas 64:596–605. https://doi.org/10.1109/TIM.2014.2351331
4. Zhang Z, Tian Z, Zhou M (2018) Latern: dynamic continuous hand gesture recognition using FMCW radar sensor. IEEE Sens J 18:3278–3289. https://doi.org/10.1109/JSEN.2018.2808688
5. Naguri CR, Bunescu RC (2017) Recognition of dynamic hand gestures from 3D motion data using LSTM and CNN architectures. In: Proceedings of the 16th IEEE international conference on machine learning and applications. ICMLA 2017, pp 1130–1133. https://doi.org/10.1109/ICMLA.2017.00013
6. Islam MR, Mitu UK, Bhuiyan RA, Shin J (2018) Hand gesture feature extraction using deep convolutional neural network for recognizing American sign language. In: 2018 4th International Conference on Frontiers of Signal Processing. ICFSP 2018, pp 115–119. https://doi.org/10.1109/ICFSP.2018.8552044
7. Dong X, Xu Y, Xu Z, Huang J, Lu J, Zhang C, Lu L (2018) A static hand gesture recognition model based on the improved centroid watershed algorithm and a dual-channel CNN. In: ICAC 2018—2018 24th IEEE international conference automation and computing Improv. Product. through Automation and Computing. https://doi.org/10.23919/IConAC.2018.8749063
8. Devineau G, Moutarde F, Xi W, Yang J (2018) Deep learning for hand gesture recognition on skeletal data. In: Proceedings of the—13th IEEE international conference on automation face gesture recognition. FG 2018, pp 106–113. https://doi.org/10.1109/FG.2018.00025
9. Lin HI, Hsu MH, Chen WK (2014) Human hand gesture recognition using a convolution neural network. In: IEEE international conference on automation science and engineering, pp 1038–1043. https://doi.org/10.1109/CoASE.2014.6899454
10. Pyo J, Ji S, You S, Kuc T (2016) Depth-based hand gesture recognition using convolutional neural networks. In: 2016 13th international conference ubiquitous robots and ambient intelligence. URAI 2016, pp 225–227. https://doi.org/10.1109/URAI.2016.7625742
11. Jani AB, Kotak NA, Roy AK (2018) Sensor based hand gesture recognition system for English alphabets used in sign language of deaf-mute people. In: Proceedings of the IEEE Sensors, pp 1–4. https://doi.org/10.1109/ICSENS.2018.8589574
12. Berru-Novoa B, Gonzalez-Valenzuela R, Shiguihara-Juarez P (2018) Peruvian sign language recognition using low resolution cameras. In: Proceedings of the 2018 IEEE 25th international conference on electronics, electrical and engineering and computing. INTERCON 2018. https://doi.org/10.1109/INTERCON.2018.8526408
13. Hazra S, Santra A (2018) Robust gesture recognition using millimetric-wave radar system. IEEE Sensors Lett 2:1–4. https://doi.org/10.1109/lsens.2018.2882642
14. Institute of Electrical and Electronics Engineers. In: IEEE communications society: 2018 10th international conference on wireless communications and signal processing (WCSP), Hangzhou, China
15. Peng Z, Li C, Muñoz-Ferreras JM, Gómez-García R (2017) An FMCW radar sensor for human gesture recognition in the presence of multiple targets. In: 2017 1st IEEE MTT-S international microwave bio conference (IMBioC) 2017, pp 7–9. https://doi.org/10.1109/IMBIOC.2017.7965798
16. Yusnita L, Roestam R, Wahyu RB (2017) Implementation of real-time static hand. CommIT (Commun Inf Technol) 11:85–91

17. Lee HR, Park J, Suh YJ (2020) Improving classification accuracy of hand gesture recognition based on 60 GHz FMCW radar with deep learning domain adaptation. Electron 9:1–24. https://doi.org/10.3390/electronics9122140
18. Kulhandjian H, Sharma P, Kulhandjian M, D'Amours C (2019) Sign language gesture recognition using doppler radar and deep learning. In: 2019 IEEE Globecom Workshops. GC Wkshps 2019—Proc. (2019). https://doi.org/10.1109/GCWkshps45667.2019.9024607
19. Adeoluwa O, Kearney SJ, Kurtoglu E, Connors C, Gurbuz SZ (2021) Near real-time ASL recognition using a millimeter wave radar. Radar Sensor 43. https://doi.org/10.1117/12.2588616
20. Pal S (2019) FMCW—radar design. https://doi.org/10.1080/03772063.2019.1615392
21. Analysis A, Manual U (2012) User manual. Data Base 3304:1–148
22. Ahmed S, Park J, Cho SH (2022) FMCW radar sensor based human activity recognition using deep learning. In: 2022 international conference on electronics and information, communications. ICEIC 2022. https://doi.org/10.1109/ICEIC54506.2022.9748776
23. Pratiwi H, Hidayat MR, Pramudita AA, Suratman FY (2019) Improved FMCW radar system for multi-target detection of human respiration vital sign. J Elektron dan Telekomun 19:38. https://doi.org/10.14203/jet.v19.38-44
24. Kang SW, Jang MH, Lee S (2021) Identification of human motion using radar sensor in an indoor environment. https://doi.org/10.3390/s21072305
25. Verma PK, Gaikwad AN, Singh D, Nigam MJ (2009) Analysis of clutter reduction techniques for through wall imaging in UWB range. Prog Electromagn Res B 29–48. https://doi.org/10.2528/PIERB09060903
26. Li X, He Y, Jing X (2019) A survey of deep learning-based human activity recognition in radar. Remote Sens 11. https://doi.org/10.3390/rs11091068
27. Albawi S, Mohammed TAM, Alzawi S (2017) Layers of a convolutional neural network. Icet 2017:1–6
28. O'Shea K, Nash R (2015) An introduction to convolutional neural networks. 1–11
29. Gonzalez TF (2007) Handbook of approximation algorithms and metaheuristics. Handb Approx Algorithms Metaheuristics 1–1432. https://doi.org/10.1201/9781420010749
30. Fu'adah YN, Pratiwi NC, Pramudito MA, Ibrahim N (2020) Convolutional neural network (CNN) for automatic skin cancer classification system. In: IOP conference series materials science and engineering, p 982. https://doi.org/10.1088/1757-899X/982/1/012005
31. Yang XZ (2020) Hand gesture recognition based-on three-branch CNN with fine-tuning using MIMO radar. In: IET international radar conference (IET IRC 2020), pp 1650–1655. https://doi.org/10.1049/icp.2021.0509

Heart Rate Variability of Photoplethysmography for Hypertension Detection Using Support Vector Machine

Aulia Octaviani, Nuryani Nuryani, Umi Salamah, and Trio Pambudi Utomo

Abstract Early detection of hypertension is essential as it is a common chronic age-related disease often associated with debilitating cardiovascular complications. The aim of this article is to find the best accuracy performance in detecting hypertension. This article introduced a method for hypertension detection without a cuff using parameters of photoplethysmography (PPG) and support vector machine (SVM). The parameters were heart rate variability (HRV) of PPG. Both the time domain and frequency domain of HRV were utilized. The HRV was obtained from the respiratory rate (RR) interval of PPG, which was the time interval between two consecutive peaks of PPG. An SVM with a radial basis function (RBF) was used. SVM parameters were tuned to find the optimal one. Furthermore, a feature selection of PPG-HRV was conducted to find appropriate features. Experiments using clinical data showed that SVM with HRV of PPG resulted in a good performance for hypertension detection. The performance of hypertension detection with different values of SVM parameters and different features of HRV was presented. This method found accuracies of 98.89 and 80.68% for training and testing, respectively. Based on the results, the use of HRV from PPG is quite effective and can contribute to medical development to detect hypertension.

Keywords Hypertension detection · Heart rate variability (HRV) · Support vector machine (SVM) · Photoplethysmography

A. Octaviani (✉) · N. Nuryani · T. P. Utomo
Department of Physics, Universitas Sebelas Maret, Jl. Ir. Sutami No. 36, Kentingan, Kec., Jebres, Surakarta, Central Java 57126, Indonesia
e-mail: auliaoctaviani77@student.uns.ac.id

U. Salamah
Department of Informatics, Universitas Sebelas Maret, Jl. Ir. Sutami No. 36, Kentingan, Kec., Jebres, Surakarta, Central Java 57126, Indonesia

T. Triwiyanto et al. (eds.), *Proceeding of the 3rd International Conference on Electronics, Biomedical Engineering, and Health Informatics*, Lecture Notes in Electrical Engineering 1008, https://doi.org/10.1007/978-981-99-0248-4_31

1 Introduction

Hypertension is diagnosed when a person's systolic blood pressure (SBP) in the office or clinic is ≥120 mm Hg and/or their diastolic blood pressure (DBP) is ≥90 mm Hg [1]. Chronic hypertension (HT) can inflict damage on various vital organs of the body, such as the lungs, brain, heart, and kidneys [2]. One of the World Health Organization's (WHO) global targets is to reduce prevalence by 33% between 2010 and 2030.

In a clinical environment, blood pressure measurement has always been the gold standard for diagnosing hypertension. There are a variety of simple home sphygmomanometers that the general public can use to measure blood pressure. The user should follow each instruction with the right gestures at the right time and act calmly.

Aletta and his team investigated blood pressure and its variability using classic and novel measurement techniques, with the conclusion that BP recording without a cuff can improve prediction and treatment beyond conventional capabilities [3]. Several articles have reported research on the detection of hypertension using PPG, and some studies have been conducted without cuffs. PPG signals contain information about the arterial and venous circulation systems. PPG uses a low-intensity infrared (IR) light sensor to detect the amount of light absorbed or reflected by tissue supplied by blood vessels. It produces a transmissive or reflective photoelectric signal that reflects the pulsatile volume of blood within the area covered by the sensor [4, 5]. PPG has been correlated and applied with measurements of heart rate, blood pressure, and blood oxygenation, providing clinically useful information for physiological monitoring [4, 5]. Dual-wavelength PPGs are routinely used in hospitals to derive oxygen saturation, usually using fingertip sensors. Recently, the pulse interval of PPG has also been used to estimate HRV [6].

HRV monitoring is a new alternative treatment for hypertension that enables users to keep an unobtrusive eye on their health, like when they naturally sleep [7]. HRV is the change in the time interval between beats. It is produced by the autonomic nervous system, including the sympathetic nervous system (SNS) and the parasympathetic nervous system (PNS) [8]. HRV includes both the time domain and frequency domain methods. Because it is based on widely used statistical metrics, the time-domain technique of HRV is the simplest to utilize. In contrast to the time-domain method, the frequency content of the signal is quantified using spectral analysis for the frequency-domain method of HRV calculation [9].

A significant and independent predictor of patients' hypertension is a reduction in HRV. Despite the paucity of research, this review indicates that employing relaxation techniques regarded as healthy habits may reduce blood pressure and boost HRV and parasympathetic activity [8].

Time-domain measures of HRV quantify the amount of variability in measures of interbeat interval (IBI), the length of time between successive heartbeats [10]. The time domain analysis allows extracting many measurements from the raw RR interval signal. The simplest variables derived directly from the RR interval signal are time-domain parameters [11].

Frequency domain measurements estimate the absolute or relative power distribution in four frequency bands. Heart rate (HR) vibrations in ultra-low frequency (ULF), very low frequency (VLF), low frequency (LF), and high frequency (HF) bands are the four frequency bands [12].

More than 30 HRV parameters were used in the research by Christoph and his team. They used PPG signals to investigate the accuracy of heart rate variability [1] but have not been as specific in testing the algorithm. This article presents a new method to identify hypertension using both the time domain and frequency domain of HRV using PPG. This article also introduces a support vector machine (SVM) as a classifier for hypertension detection with more specific variations on gamma and SVM-C. Different mapping functions of SVM are investigated as well. The hope of this article is that it can help in the medical field in detecting hypertension.

2 Method

The method for hypertension detection using PPG and SVM is shown in Fig. 1. The basic basis of this research is the extracted ppg signal to obtain the HRV value followed by feature selection to obtain significant features. The selected features will be classified using SVM, and the output of the SVM is the classification between hypertension and normal.

2.1 PPG Database

Materials, in this study is PPG records, were taken from the MIMIC database [13]. At the time of data acquisition, there were several recordings of anomalies and noise, such as missing peaks and pulse buffering. Records are outside the scope of this study. In this study, data from MIMIC database parsing was used with a total of 264 hypertension data and 172 normal data with 30-s segments with an 80% data distribution of training data and 20% of testing data.

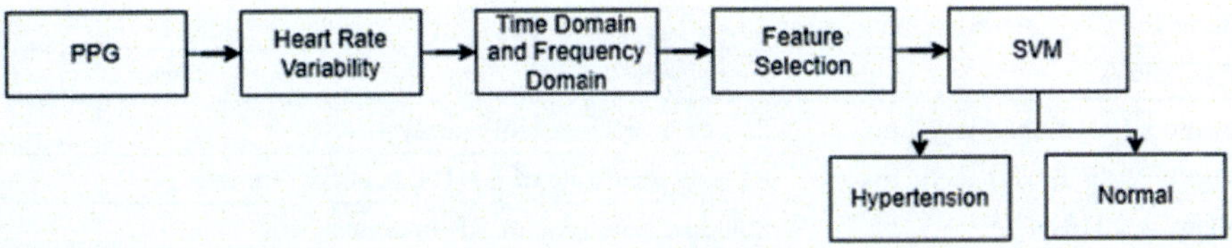

Fig. 1 General structure of hypertension detection using SVM

2.2 Heart Rate Variability

The HRV consists of two parts, namely the time domain and the frequency domain. In this study, the time domain of the HR, RR, SDNN, and RMSSD sections was used. The frequency domains used are LF and HF.

The time domain method is derived from the RR interval value between beats in the time domain. Some variables related to HR kubios, HR beats, SD RR, RMSSD, SD RR, and SDNN were calculated. Table 1 shows the description of these variables.

Next, the average RR interval (RR) and average heart rate (HR) are defined as follows:

$$\mathrm{RR} = \frac{1}{N}\sum_{n=1}^{N} \mathrm{RR}_n \tag{1}$$

$$\mathrm{HR} = \frac{60}{\mathrm{RR}} \tag{2}$$

RR_n indicates the value of the nth RR interval. There are several heart rate variability parameters that measure variability within the RR time interval in the time domain. The standard deviation (SDNN) of the RR interval is defined as follows [14]:

$$\mathrm{SDNN} = \sqrt{\frac{1}{N-1}\sum_{n=1}^{N} \left(\mathrm{RR}_n - \overline{\mathrm{RR}}\right)^2} \tag{3}$$

Variations in RR interval time series as a whole can be reflected by SDNN, where the standard deviation is SDSD which can be written as follows:

$$\mathrm{SDSD} = \sqrt{E\{\Delta \mathrm{RR}_n^2\} - E\{\Delta RR_n\}^2} \tag{4}$$

For a stationary series on the RR series $E\{\Delta \mathrm{RR}_n\} = E\{\mathrm{RR}_{(n+1)}\} - E\{\mathrm{RR}_n\} = 0$ and SDSD is equal to the square root of the mean of the sequential differences

Table 1 HRV time-domain measures [12]

Parameters	Unit	Description
Fiture 1 (HR Kubios)	ms	Part of heart variability analysis
Fiture 2 (HR Beats)	ms	Resting heart rate of 60–100 beats per minute
Fiture 4 (SDRR)	ms	Standard deviation of RR intervals
Fiture 3 (RMSSD)	ms	Root mean square of successive RR interval differences
Fiture 5 (SD HR)	ms	Standard deviation of RR intervals
Fiture 6 (SDNN)	ms	Standard deviation of NN intervals

Table 2 HRV frequency-domain measures [12]

Parameters	Unit	Description
Fiture 1 (VLF)	ms^2	Absolute power of the very-low-frequency band (0.0033–0.04 Hz)
Fiture 2 (VLF)	Hz	Low-frequency band (0.04–0.15 Hz)
Fiture 3 (LF)	ms^2	Low-frequency band (0.04–0.15 Hz)
Fiture 4 (LF)	nu	Low-frequency band (0.04–0.15 Hz)
Fiture 5 (HF)	Hz	High-frequency band (0.15–0.4 Hz)
Fiture 6 (HF)	ms^2	High-frequency band (0.15–0.4 Hz)
Fiture 7 (HF)	nu	High-frequency band (0.15–0.4 Hz)
Fiture 8 (LF/HF)	%	Relative power of the high-frequency band (0.15–0.4 Hz)

(RMSSD) which can be written,

$$\text{RMSSD} = \sqrt{\frac{1}{n-1}\sum_{j=1}^{n} \Delta NNI_j^2} \tag{5}$$

Frequency domain measurements estimate the absolute or relative power distribution in four frequency bands. Table 2 shows the description of these variables of frequency domains.

Common Frequency Domain HRV metrics include High-Frequency power (HF), Low-Frequency power (LF), and LF/HF Ratio. The frequency domain parameters used are equations [15].

$$n\text{LF} = \frac{\text{LF}}{(\text{Total Power} - \text{VLF})} \times 100 \tag{6}$$

$$n\text{HF} = \frac{\text{HF}}{(\text{Total Power} - \text{VLF})} \times 100 \tag{7}$$

$$\frac{\text{LF}}{\text{HF}}\text{ratio} = \frac{\text{LF}}{\text{HF}} \tag{8}$$

2.3 Support Vector Machines

SVM is a popular machine-learning algorithm widely used in pattern recognition, object identification, character recognition, image segmentation, and classification [16]. The SVM classification used in this study is used specifically during the training and testing phases. In this study, the data distribution was 80% training and 20% testing. The function used is the radial basis function. The SVM-C value is 100, and the gamma for this study is 50,000. The performance of this variation is measured by comparing the drawing accuracy with different characteristics and the best test accuracy.

3 Results

A discussion of the results of the correlation between features is presented in Table 3 with the highest result at 0.1482 and the lowest at 0.0372.

Based on Table 3, if the Pearson Significance table [17] is used with the amount of data more than 280 then 0.085 is used, so the features that can be used for the next step are std hr, hr beats, and so on. The next step is to correlate between features, and obtained as in Table 4.

Table 4 shows that the correlation between features after the feature significance selection has the highest value of 1 and the lowest value of 0.0032. In the table using T-test [18] with an alpha value of 0.5, then 6 features are obtained. The 6 selected feature is HR Kubios, HR Beats, RMSSD, STD RR, VLF (Hz) dan VLF (ms2).

Table 5 presents the comparison results between linear, RBF and sigmoid kernels. The results of the comparison of the three kernels have the highest accuracy in the RBF kernel, while the linear and sigmoid kernels produce the same accuracy. By using the RBF kernel, the SVM-C value is varied from 10 to 100,000 and does not produce a significant increase or decrease in accuracy. It can be concluded that the

Table 3 Correlation between features

Feature	Correlation
STD HR	0.1482
HR BEATS	0.1445
HR KUBIOS	0.1390
VLF (ms2)	0.1310
VLF (HZ)	0.1298
RMSSD	0.1012
STD RR	0.0998
HF (NU)	0.0920
LF (NU)	0.0919
LF (HZ)	0.0734
STD RR	0.0725
HF (HZ)	0.0715
TOTAL (ms2)	0.0610
LF/HF	0.0460
LF (ms2)	0.0372

Table 4 Correlation between features

	STD HR	HR BEATS	HR KUBIOS	VLF (ms2)	VLF (HZ)	RMSSD	STD RR	HF (NU)	LF (NU)
STD HR	1	0.67	0.46	0.14	0.92	0.65	0.58	0.09	0.09
HR BEATS	0.67	1	0.96	0.12	0.16	0.21	0.13	0.1	0.1
HR KUBIOS	0.46	0.96	1	0.15	0.14	0.06	0.0032	0.08	0.08
VLF (ms2)	0.14	0.12	0.15	1	0.21	0.24	0.35	0.12	0.12
VLF (HZ)	0.092	0.16	0.14	0.21	1	0.07	0.11	0.12	0.12
RMSSD	0.65	0.21	0.061	0.24	0.079	1	0.98	0.14	0.14
STD RR	0.58	0.13	0.0032	0.35	0.11	0.98	1	0.09	0.09
HF(NU)	0.095	0.1	0.087	0.12	0.12	0.14	0.09	1	1
LF (NU)	0.095	0.1	0.087	0.12	0.12	0.14	0.09	1	1

Table 5 Comparison of SVM Ker Kernels

Kernel	Training accuracy (%)	Testing accuracy (%)
Linear	60.63	60.23
RBF	98.85	79.55
Sigmoid	60.63	60.23

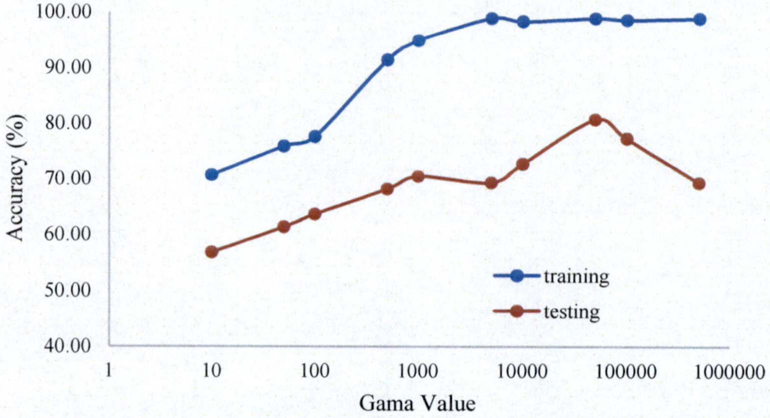

Fig. 2 Accuracy of detecting hypertension with gamma variation of 10–100,000

value of SVM-C is not very influential in this study. As for the varied gamma values, it can be seen as shown in the image below:

From Fig. 2, it can be seen that the accuracy value of the training data continues to increase but reaches a gamma of 50,000 the graph is flat, which means that the value is the same. For testing data, the graph increases up to gamma 50,000 the value drops significantly, which means that the best testing value is at gamma 50,000. At gamma 50,000, the accuracy of the training data is 98.85%, while the accuracy of the testing data is 80.68%, which is the highest value.

Figure 3 is the result of gamma variation in more detail, producing a graph for training data that is flat or constant at 98.85%. As for the test data graph, it increases and decreases with a flat end and has the highest value at 80.68% with a gamma of 50,000 and 60,000.

4 Discussion

In this paper, the 30-s segment length in PPG is used. The use of this length is not discussed, but Baek HJ and his team varied the 30-s segment length, resulting in segments less than 5 min suitable for HRV calculations [19]. The 30-s segment allows for HRV data retrieval.

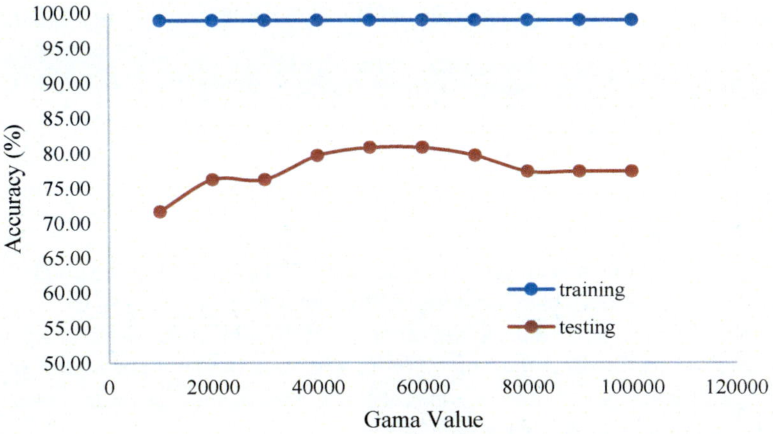

Fig. 3 Accuracy of detecting hypertension with gamma variation of 10,000–100,000

The features used in this study were previously 15 in number, but after selection, they were reduced to 6. These features include HR kubios, HR beats, RMSSD, STD HR, VLF (ms2), and VLF (Hz) based on the results of feature selection using the Pearson correlation t-test. Soku Chen used Pearson's correlation and t-test to verify the research data [20].

Time-domain and frequency-domain HRV were used to improve accuracy on training data but were suboptimal on test data. As Christoph and his team have shown in their work, the LH and HF parameters should be used with caution and can be influenced by other parameters [21].

In this paper, the SVM algorithm with the RBF kernel is used. There are some articles using RBF as a kernel for SVM. One of them is written by Harun Al-Aziz and RBF. He says the kernel is the kernel with the best performance [22]. In an article written by Venkatesan [23] entitled ECG Signal Preprocessing and SVM Classifier-Based Abnormality Detection in Remote Healthcare Applications, SVM gives the best accuracy.

Accuracy results before using feature selection and after using feature selection have significant results. Before using feature selection, 15 parameters were used and had the results of accuracy training 99.85% and accuracy testing 63.64%. The use of feature selection is 6 as explained in Table 4, and it was able to increase accuracy with training at 98.89% and testing at 80.68% like the graph in Fig. 3, in the paper Christoph and the team in his research it was explained that some parameters should be used with caution because it has a significant effect [21]. The limitation of this study is the use of PPG signals only, but these limitations provide more specificity that PPG signals are able to predict hypertension and this is very useful in the health sector for early detection.

This paper uses six parameters from the HRV time domain and the frequency domain of the PPG signal, which are more specific than previous studies. The methods used are SVM kernel RBF, gamma 50,000 to 60,000, and SVM-C 100, which produce the best accuracy at training accuracy values of 98.89% and testing accuracy of 80.68%.

5 Conclusion

The aim of this article is to find the best accuracy performance in detecting hypertension. In this paper, the best classification uses the SVM kernel RBF from HRV time domain data and the frequency domain of PPG recordings, producing the best accuracy on SVM-C 100 and gamma 50,000 and 60,000 with training accuracy values of 98.89% and testing accuracy of 80.68%. The results of research with training data and testing data show quite a high accuracy. This allows for future research by exploring other algorithms that produce better accuracy.

References

1. Unger T et al (2020) Clinical practice guidelines. Hypertension 75:1334–1357
2. Soh DCK et al (2020) A computational intelligence tool for the detection of hypertension using empirical mode decomposition. Comput Biol Med 118:103630
3. Schutte AE, Kollias A, Stergiou GS (2022) Blood pressure and its variability: classic and novel measurement techniques. Nat Rev Cardiol 1–12
4. Elgendi M et al (2019) The use of photoplethysmography for assessing hypertension. NPJ Digit Med 2(1):1–11
5. Liang Y et al (2018) Hypertension assessment using photoplethysmography: a risk stratification approach. J Clin Med 8(1):12
6. Kinnunen H et al (2020) Feasible assessment of recovery and cardiovascular health: accuracy of nocturnal HR and HRV assessed via ring PPG in comparison to medical grade ECG. Physiol Meas 41(4):04NT01
7. Ni H et al (2019) Multiscale fine-grained heart rate variability analysis for recognizing the severity of hypertension. Comput Math Methods Med
8. Terathongkum S, Pickler RH (2004) Relationships among heart rate variability, hypertension, and relaxation techniques. J Vasc Nurs 22(3):78–82
9. Aydin SG, Kaya T, Guler H (2016) Heart rate variability (HRV) based feature extraction for congestive heart failure. Int J Comput Electr Eng 8(4):275
10. Tarvainen MP, Niskanen JP, Lipponen JA, Ranta-Aho PO, Karjalainen PA (2014) Kubios HRV–heart rate variability analysis software. Comput Methods Programs Biomed 113(1):210–220
11. Djermanova N, Marinov M, Ganev B, Tabakov S, Nikolov G (2016) LabVIEW based ECG signal acquisition and analysis. In: 2016 XXV international scientific conference electronics (ET), September. IEEE, pp 1–4
12. Shaffer F, Jay P (2017) Ginsberg. An overview of heart rate variability metrics and norms. Front Public Health 258
13. Physionet homepage. https://archive.physionet.org/physiobank/database/mimicdb/. Last accessed 1 June 2022
14. Electrophysiology TFOTESOCTNASOP (1996) Heart rate variability: standards of measurement, physiological interpretation, and clinical use. Circulation 93(5):1043–1065
15. Van Dongen HPA et al (1999) Searching for biological rhythms: peak detection in the periodogram of unequally spaced data. J Biol Rhythms 14(6):617–620

16. Wang CC, Chang CD (2010, July) SVD and SVM based approach for congestive heart failure detection from ECG signal. In: The 40th international conference on computers & industrial engineering. IEEE, pp 1–5
17. Pearson ES (1947) The choice of statistical tests illustrated on the interpretation of data classed in a 2× 2 table. Biometrika 34(1/2):139–167
18. Semenick D (1990) Tests and measurements: the T-test. Strength Condition J 12(1):36–37
19. Baek HJ et al (2015) Reliability of ultra-short-term analysis as a surrogate of standard 5-min analysis of heart rate variability. Telemed e-Health 21(5):404–414
20. Chen S et al (2020) Linear and nonlinear analyses of normal and fatigue heart rate variability signals for miners in high-altitude and cold areas. Comput Methods Programs Biomed 196:105667
21. Hoog Antink C et al (2021) Accuracy of heart rate variability estimated with reflective wrist-PPG in elderly vascular patients. Sci Rep 11(1):1–12
22. Al Azies H, Trishnanti D, Elvira Mustikawati PH (2019) Comparison of kernel support vector machine (SVM) in classification of human development index (HDI). IPTEK J Proc Ser 6:53–57
23. Venkatesan C et al (2018) ECG signal preprocessing and SVM classifier-based abnormality detection in remote healthcare applications. IEEE Access 6:9767–9773

Enhancing the Diagnosis of Skin Neglected Tropical Diseases by Artificial Neural Networks Using Evolutionary Algorithms: Implementation on Raspberry Pi

Steyve Nyatte, Steve Perabi, Gregoire Abessolo, Salomé Ndjakomo Essiane, and Pierre Ele

Abstract Neglected TROPICAL diseases related to the skin with similar manifestations in their early phase persist in remote areas and are characterized by the prevailing poverty of populations. If not detected early, they very often lead to severe ulcerations and permanent disabilities. We present an approach to optimize the early detection of neglected tropical skin diseases (NTDs) by automatic identification of skin lesions. As contributions, we propose a web-mobile AI-powered automatic skin lesion recognition system optimized by a new hybrid Whale-Shark optimization algorithm (WOA-SSO-ANN) that can help frontline health workers without state-of-the-art equipment to detect NTDs in their beginning stage. We extract the relevant regions features of the lesions. The dataset resulting from this preprocessing is classified by artificial neural networks optimized by a new hybrid Whale-Shark optimization algorithm to develop an improved artificial neural network in terms of processing time and/or accuracy. The best result was obtained with an overall classification accuracy of 93% and a processing time reduced by almost half compared to other optimizers. The proposed application is able to recognize cases of Buruli ulcer, leprosy, and leishmaniasis in our database (nodule and plaque) and classify new patients, thus reducing the cost of management of these diseases when they are detected late. The AI models implemented in this work have satisfactory accuracy

---

S. Nyatte (✉) · S. Perabi · S. Ndjakomo Essiane · P. Ele
Laboratory of Technology and Applied Sciences, University of Douala, Douala, Cameroon
e-mail: ssteyve@gmail.com

S. Ndjakomo Essiane
Signal, Image and Systems Laboratory, University of Yaounde 1, Yaoundé, Cameroon

P. Ele
Laboratory of Electrical Engineering, Mechatronic and Signal Treatment, National Advanced School of Engineering, University of Yaoundé 1, Yaoundé, Cameroon

G. Abessolo
Oceanography Department, Institute of Fisheries and Aquatic Sciences, University of Douala, Douala, Cameroon

T. Triwiyanto et al. (eds.), *Proceeding of the 3rd International Conference on Electronics, Biomedical Engineering, and Health Informatics*, Lecture Notes in Electrical Engineering 1008, https://doi.org/10.1007/978-981-99-0248-4_32

and could be a complementary diagnostic tool, especially in remote areas where medical specialists are scarce.

Keywords Artificial neural network · Metaheuristic optimization · Image processing · Skin neglect tropical diseases

1 Introduction

Of the more than 20 neglected tropical diseases (NTDs), over half have skin manifestations and are often associated with long-term disability, stigma, and mental health problems. Yet the early diagnosis of these disabling diseases is key to successful treatment to avoid irreversible consequences [1]. NTDs affect more than 1,000 million people in tropical and subtropical countries, with a very high financial cost for these poor countries [2]. These diseases are spread over almost all continents as shown in Table 1 [3]. The predominance of these diseases can be seen in Africa. As can be seen in this table, the three most prevalent diseases are represented by two + signs and are present in almost all continents. The World Health Organization (WHO) reported about 130,500 new leprosy (LEP) cases in 2020, with around 9000 children under the age of 15 afflicted and roughly 8000 suffering from grade 2 impairments (G2D). In the same year, around 1 million new leishmaniasis (LEI) cases were recorded internationally, while approximately 5000 suspected Buruli (BU) ulcer cases were reported globally in one year, with the majority of patients under the age of 15. Current diagnostic procedures are unluckily costly, unsuitable for endemic locations, and occasionally ineffective. WHO intends to stop the neglect of tropical skin diseases (NTDs) by 2030, according to SDG Target 3.3.

In order to achieve this objective, tools need to be developed that are adapted to areas where these diseases are prevalent. The current methods are not appropriate in terms of feasibility and reliability, as shown in Table 2 [3]. For example, diagnosing these diseases frequently necessitates a highly sophisticated technological platform that is not available in these endemic locations. Various ways are utilized, each with its own set of pros and limitations.

Antibiotics can easily control NTDs if they are detected early. However, poverty, in combination with the precarious situation of the endemic-infected areas where they live, makes early diagnosis of these diseases difficult. Therefore, it is important

Table 1 Regional distribution of targeted cutaneous NTDs

NTDs	Africa	Asia	America	Europe	Mediterranean Eastern	Pacific Western
BU	**	*	*	–	–	*
LEI	**	*	**	*	**	–
LEP	**	*	*	–	*	*

Note Legend: ** = current; * = present but not common; – = absent;

Table 2 Current diagnostic methods' limitations and advantages

Test	Limitation
Smear testing	– No more than 60% sensitivity – Requires skilled physician – Strict quality control
In vitro culture	– Modern laboratory expected – Requires a modern laboratory – Qualified personnel are requested–long time to results – Limited sensitivity (20–60%) – Unsuitable for immediate patient care – Not suitable for emergency patient treatment – Extensive quality control is required
Polymerase chain reaction	– Modern laboratory expected – Expensive – Skilled physician – Strict quality control – Impossible to differentiate viable and non-viable organisms
Histopathology	– Modern laboratory expected – Expensive – Highly skilled physician – Invasive method

to equip frontline staff with a tool that can quickly identify a neglected skin-related disease just by taking a picture with a computer-aided diagnosis (CAD). With the fast growth of artificial intelligence in recent years, computer-aided diagnosis (CAD) has also experienced a number of breakthroughs, notably in the field of medical imaging [4–6]. The latter has played a very positive role in improving diagnostic accuracy and reducing false diagnosis. However, one of the most widely used artificial intelligence algorithms is neural networks, whose back-propagation technique has shown high performance in very large datasets but often has a number of drawbacks such as solutions often local and not global [7, 8]. The actual performance of backpropagation on a specific problem depends on the input data [9], the objective function must be differentiable [10], backpropagation can be very sensitive to noisy data often derived from analogue images [11]. Given the variable nature of the images to be processed by our CAD, it is therefore important to find a better-performing algorithm that is not sensitive to noise and data variations.

Several studies have been done in the academic field on the optimization of artificial neural networks in the identification of skin disorders such as skin malignancies [12–14], but there has also been some work on skin-related NTDs. This subsection focuses on current work on machine learning-based automated skin lesion detection systems for neglected tropical diseases.

Hu et al. [15–18] has studied, through several papers and scientific articles, the possibility of identifying cutaneous lesions of UB. The author has studied dermoscopic images in the ulcer phase for diagnostic purposes. We can also mention the work of Bamoravat et al., who developed a diagnostic approach for leishmaniasis with a machine-learning algorithm [19]. The best result was obtained by a multilayer perceptron with an accuracy of 88%. Zare et al. [20] developed a neural network-based model to detect and recognize leishmaniasis parasites through microscopy images. An accuracy of 50% was obtained. Using cognitive computing data, the authors of [21] created a leishmaniasis diagnosis system based on a feedforward neural network. After normalization, the experimental findings of the multilayer feedforward perceptron model showed an accuracy of 85.71%, indicating an outstanding fit of the model to the process. The works of [19, 20], and [21] are based on a microscopic image of parasites rather than actual skin lesions. This does not address the root cause of the problem in the afflicted areas: a lack of material to identify the microorganisms. Márcio Lus Moreira De Souza et al. created an artificial intelligence-based cross-platform program for leprosy screening (AI). The Random Forest algorithm-based model has sensitivity and specificity of 93.97 and 87.09%, respectively [22]. The authors of [23] set out to develop an AI-powered diagnostic assistance for leprosy based on skin pictures, or a mix of the two. During the initial part of the project, an AI-powered leprosy diagnosis aid was created, which was based on a combination of skin pictures and clinical data acquired in a standardized method. For the diagnosis of leprosy, 1229 skin pictures gathered with 585 pieces of information led in a high classification accuracy (90%) and an area under the curve (AUC) of 96.46%. As previously said, the correctness of these numerous works is not always as great as we would have hoped.

Given the commonality of neglected tropical illnesses, which typically begin as a nodule or plaque, no author has created a technique capable of identifying many diseases at once in this literature study. There has never been a diagnostic application based on neural networks that have been tuned for the demands of the case. As a result, the goal is to create a system for real-time diagnosis of three neglected illnesses.

To make our diagnosis stable and fast, we will test some metaheuristics with our data set to improve the classification indices. Because, according to the authors of [8–10], it is possible to make the learning process of neural networks stable and efficient by introducing metaheuristics. The hypotheses that this work would like to verify are as follows: The optimization of a feedforward neural network by a metaheuristic can increase the accuracy and the speed and stability of a computer-aided diagnosis (CAD), and it is possible to implement this CAD on a Raspberry PI4. The primary goal of this article is to provide a suggestion for an intelligent knowledge-based architecture to identify, extract, and classify the different skin lesions characterizing some neglected tropical diseases prevailing in tropical areas in general and in Cameroon in particular. As contributions, we propose a web-mobile AI-powered automatic skin lesion recognition system optimized by a metaheuristic that can help frontline health workers without state-of-the-art equipment to quickly detect illnesses in their early stages. To achieve this goal, we first present in Sect. 2 the hardware and methods used, the third section discusses the different data acquired in this investigation, and lastly, following a brief discussion of the topics raised in this study, a conclusion is suggested.

2 Materials and Method

2.1 Theoretical Background (Math Modeling)

Feedforward Neural Network. A feedforward neural network model is the most basic type of ANN. The layers are made up of neurons. The nodes in each layer are fully linked to all the nodes in the adjacent layer via interconnections or weighted linkages. The multilayer perceptron (MLP) is a well-known FNN model that is mostly used for data classification. Consider the MLP in Fig. 1 with two neurons in the hidden layer.

Forward propagation is the first phase of the learning process of a neural network. Mathematically, it consists of calculating the successive outputs of each neuron by applying an activation function, which can be either the logistic function, the hyperbolic tangent function, or the ReLu function. We take into account these metrics:

$\boldsymbol{w_{ij}}$: Parameters associated with the neuron $\boldsymbol{i}$ and coming from the $\boldsymbol{j}$; $\boldsymbol{b_i}$: neuron bias $\boldsymbol{i}$; $\boldsymbol{a_i}$: activation of the neuron $\boldsymbol{i}$; z_i: weighting of neuron inputs $\boldsymbol{i}$. The weighting equation for each neuron is given by Eq. 1 below.

$$z_i = \left(\sum w_{ij} x_i\right) + b_i \tag{1}$$

And the activation of the neuron can be done by a sigmoid function represented by Eq. 2, which introduces the notion of probability into the neuronal calculation.

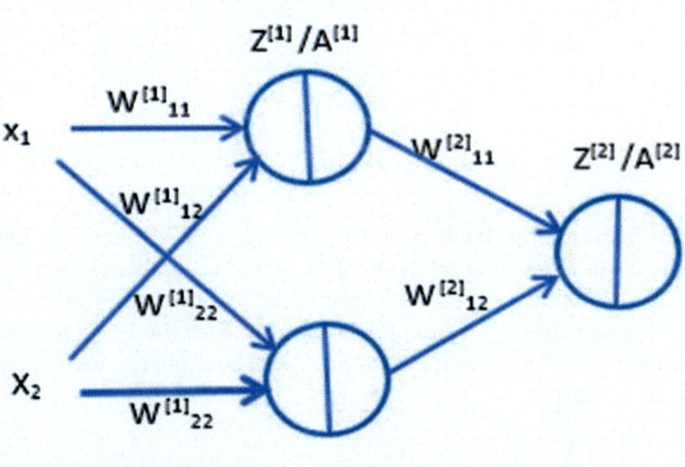

Fig. 1 Multilayer perceptron model

$$\boldsymbol{a}_i = \frac{1}{1 + \boldsymbol{e}^{-z_i}} \tag{2}$$

Considering $\boldsymbol{w}_{ij}$ the Parameter associated with the neuron $\boldsymbol{i}$ and coming from the neuron $\boldsymbol{j}$, $.^{[c]}$ the number of the C layer being worked on $z^{[1]}$, $z^{[2]}$, for layers 1 and 2. To ensure propagation to the next layer neuron, we will calculate the z-values of a layer $.^{[c]}$ using activations $\boldsymbol{a}$ of the layer $.^{[c-1]}\cdot$ according to the following Eqs. 3 and 4 below:

$$z_i^{[c]} = \sum \boldsymbol{w}_{ij}^{[c]} \boldsymbol{a}_i^{[c-1]} + \boldsymbol{b}_i^{[c]} \tag{3}$$

$$\boldsymbol{A}^{[c]} = \frac{1}{1 + \boldsymbol{e}^{-z^{[c]}}} \tag{4}$$

The most commonly used cost function is the log loss function (Eq. 5), which reduces the error between the calculated and desired output.

$$\boldsymbol{l} = -\frac{1}{\boldsymbol{m}} \sum \boldsymbol{y} * \log\left(\boldsymbol{A}^{[c]}\right) + (1 - \boldsymbol{y})\log(1 - \boldsymbol{A}^{[c]}) \tag{5}$$

This back-propagation method, although very reliable, seems cumbersome and often requires a high computation time and powerful hardware resources. Metaheuristics are serious alternatives to gradient descent. In this respect, we combine the formidable exploitation capacity of the grey wolf with the exploratory capabilities of the shark to build a new metaheuristic. The objective is to find the weights that minimize the mean square error given by Eq. (6)

$$\text{MSE} = \frac{1}{N} \sum_{i=1}^{N} (f_i - y_i)^2 \tag{6}$$

with $f_i = \left(\sum w_{ij} x_i\right) + b_i$.

2.2 *Hybrid Whale Shark Algorithm.*

Whale Optimization Algorithm (WOA). Developed by Mirjalili and Lewis [24], the WOA algorithm is inspired by the hunting technic used by a humpback whale. Humpbacks create bubble nets to catch their prey. This method is called the bubble net method; the cycle consists of two phases: the search for food until it is surrounded (the exploration phase) and the exploitation phase. These phases are mathematically modeled by Eqs. 7 to 13:

Exploration Phase:

$$D = |C * X_{rand}(t) - X(t)| \tag{7}$$

$$X(t+1) = (X_{rand}(t) - A * D) \tag{8}$$

$$a = 2 - \frac{2t}{t_{\max}} \tag{9}$$

$$A = 2 * a * r - a \tag{10}$$

$$C = 2 * r \tag{11}$$

Exploitation Phase:

$$X(t+1) = \begin{cases} D' * e^{bl} * \cos(2\pi l) + X^*(t), & p \geq 0.5 \\ X^*(t) - A * D, & p < 0.5 \end{cases} \tag{12}$$

$$D^{'} = \left|X^*(t) - X(t)\right| \tag{13}$$

In this study, we want to give this ability to trap prey in a ball to a hunting shark troop. The paragraph below presents the Shark Optimization Algorithm.

Shark Smell optimization Algorithm. Develop by par Mohammad-Azari et al. [25], the Shark Smell optimization Algorithm is a population-based metaheuristic that is inspired by shark Food forging behavior characterize by his sense of smell. His strategy is based on forward movement and rotational movement with à certain velocity. The modeling of the two behavior is done in Eqs. 14 and 15 below.

$$Y_i^{k+1} = X_i^k + V_i^k \Delta t_k \tag{14}$$

This equation calculates the position based on the forward motion of the shark. Then another equation models the ability to turn around the prey, with k as the current iteration, V as the velocity; X as the position; i as the individual shark and Y as the Forward position; Here we consider $\Delta t_k = 1$ and R = random number the new position taking into account the rotational behavior is given by Eq. 15 below.

$$Z_i^{k+1} = Y_i^{k+1} + R * Y_i^{k+1} \tag{15}$$

In the literature this algorithm has been used successfully in areas such as the identification of "the optimal parameters of the proton exchange membrane fuel cell model" [26]; "Optimal placement of capacitors in radial distribution system" [27].

Hybridization of Shark Smell Algorithm and Whale Optimization Algorithm to train weights of Neural Networks. The hybridization here is to combine the trapping ability of the whale in creating a giant bubble net with the speed and precision of the shark in its forward propagation phase. This is mathematically modeled by merging Eqs. 12 and 13 in the exploitation phase as follows.

$$X(t+1) = \begin{cases} D' * e^{bl} * \cos(2\pi l) + X^*(t), & p \geq 0.5 \\ X^*(t) - A * D, & p < 0.5 \end{cases} \tag{16}$$

with

$$\begin{aligned} \boldsymbol{D}_{i}^{'k} &= \left|\boldsymbol{X}^*(\boldsymbol{t}) - \boldsymbol{Y}_i^k(\boldsymbol{t})\right| \\ &= \left|\boldsymbol{X}^*(\boldsymbol{t}) - X_i^k(t) V_i^k(t) \Delta t_k\right| \end{aligned} \tag{17}$$

2.3 Dataset

We gathered skin lesions from the three principal illnesses in Cameroon, leprosy, leishmaniasis, and Buruli ulcer, in order to detect neglected tropical diseases in their early stages [3]. Figure 2 depicts the number of photos per ailment. We have 25% leishmaniasis lesions, 40% UB lesions, and 35% leprosy lesions. We separated the data into test and training sets. For the test data we have 234 images distributed as follows: 26% are Leishmaniosis lesions, 43% are UB lesions, and 26% are leprosy lesions. For training data, 24% are Leishmaniasis lesions, 39% are BU lesions, and 37% are leprosy lesions. As indicated in Fig. 2, there are a maximum of 1054 photos to be processed. This dataset was obtained from Akonolinga and Ayos hospitals in Cameroon and from the internet (DermNet website and https://doi.org/10.35078/1PSIEL). The International Skin Imaging Collaboration's (ISIC) fundamental requirements for background color, brightness, area of view, emphasis or depth of field, resolution, scaling, and color calibration were satisfied by all pictures.

2.4 Experimental Procedure

The experimental procedure will be done according to the following synoptic. This experimental procedure is presented in Fig. 3. The first step is to transform the RGB image taken by the smartphone into a grey image. The second step consists of the automatic thresholding of the image in order to binarize it. The third step is the morphological transformation of the image, and then we proceed to the extraction of characteristic parameters that serve as a database for the classification and the development of a diagnostic model.

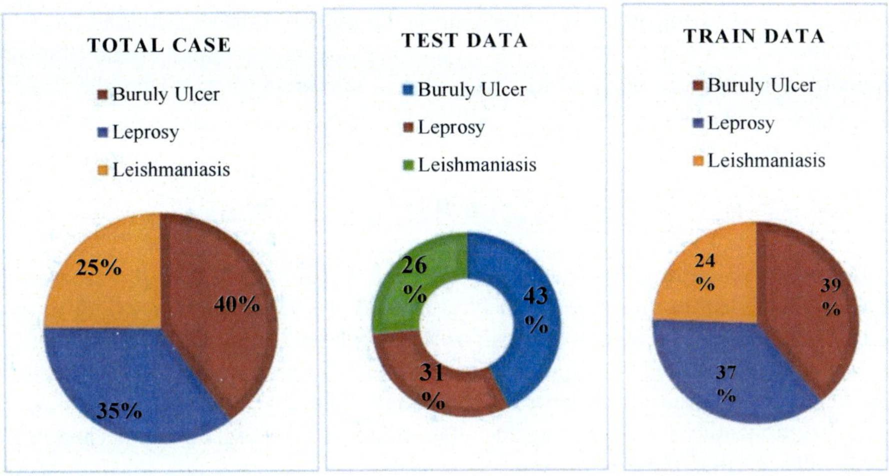

Fig. 2 Composition of the dataset

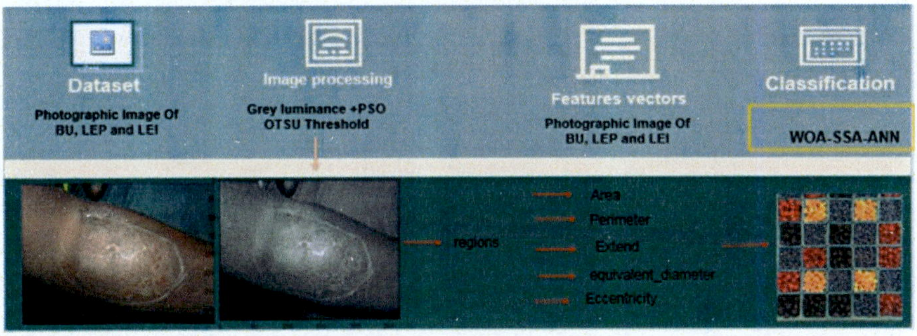

Fig. 3 Synopsis of our classification methodology

2.5 Data Processing

This stage consists of standardizing the pictures in order to get the best parametric characteristics of each lesion. This phase takes place in three stages.

Grey level transformation. To avoid severe compression on high contrast images and thus avoid destroying the subtle details and textures that are an important part of the original image characteristics, a gamma expansion compression to calculate the luminance in grey levels was sized according to the luminance levels of our source images. Equation 18 was obtained [3].

$$C_{\text{linear}} = \begin{cases} \frac{C_{srgb}}{12.92}, C_{srb} \leq 0.04045 \\ \left(\frac{C_{srgb}+0.055}{1.055}\right)^{2.4}, C_{srgb} > 0.04045 \end{cases} \tag{18}$$

where C_{srgb} represents one of the three gamma-compressed sRGB primaries (R_{srgb}, G_{srgb} and B_{srgb}, each in the range [0, 1]) and C_{linear} is the corresponding linear intensity value (R_{linear}, G_{linear}, and B_{linear}, also in the range [0, 1]). Then the linear luminance is calculated as a weighted sum of the three linear intensity values which is given by Eq. 19 [17].

$$Y_{\text{linear}} = 0.2126R_{\text{linear}} + 0.7152G_{\text{linear}} + 0.0722B_{\text{linear}} \tag{19}$$

Image thresholding. To binarize our database we apply adaptive thresholding. The OTSU algorithm optimized by a PSO is used. To obtain an image with more feature details the Otsu thresholding algorithm has been used a lot in the literature to avoid losing features, this algorithm has often been optimized by metaheuristics [28–32] and very good results have been obtained. Figure 4 depicts a strategy based on PSO optimization for generating an enhanced image with higher contrast and less entropy change than the original image.

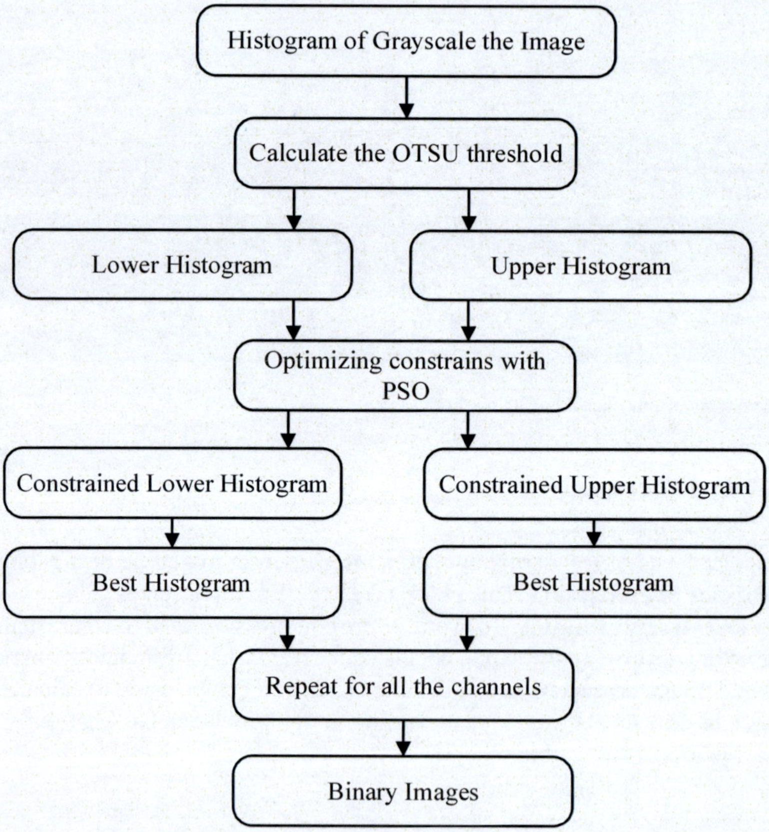

Fig. 4 Otsu PSO flowchart

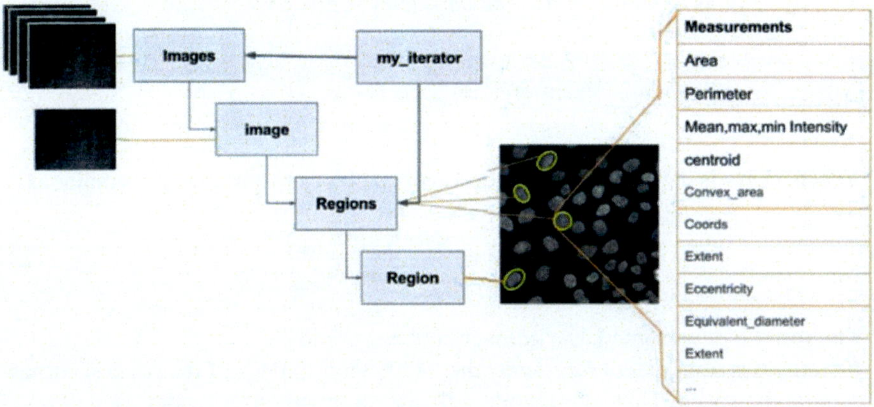

Fig. 5 Feature extraction process

Image after morphological transformation. After the automatic thresholding of the image we apply some morphological transformations to transform our binary images obtained by thresholding. This will allow us to standardize our raster structures. These treatments will be of two natures:

- Dilation: which will allow us to print pixels
- Erosion: erase pixels to uniformize contours

Feature extraction. The extraction process is as follows in Fig. 5. The goal of image analysis is to extract quantitative features from images. The goal of this research is to measure and define the shape of structures. In this study we will extract six features which are: The area, The perimeter, Extent, Equivalent diameter, and Eccentricity. All these features are dimensionless as described below.

Area: The number of pixels of a form represents the area. We can compute it easily with a Matlab function bwarea (). It is a non-dimensional number. Consider a binary object noted $O_i(x)$ with N points along the boundary of the feature.

$$x = [x_1 y_1 x_2 \dots x_N y_N] \tag{20}$$

the area of the i-th object, measured in pixels, is given by:

$$\boldsymbol{A_i} = \sum_{x=0}^{M-1} \sum_{y=0}^{N-1} \boldsymbol{O_i(x, y)} \tag{21}$$

The perimeter feature is defined as the total number of pixels within the object's boundaries.

If $x_1, \ldots, x_N$ is a boundary list, the perimeter is given by

$$\textbf{Perimeter} = \sum_{i=1}^{N-1} |\boldsymbol{x}_i - \boldsymbol{x}_{i+1}| \tag{22}$$

Eccentricity is defined as the proportion of an object's short axis to its major axis:

$$\textbf{Eccentrity} = \frac{\textbf{axis length}_{\textbf{short}}}{\textbf{axis length}_{\textbf{long}}} \tag{23}$$

The result is represented as a number between 0 and 1.

Extent: A spatial extent represents the "X, Y" coordinates of the raster's corners in geographic space. This information tells how to position or render each pixel in two dimensions.

$$\text{Extent} = \frac{\text{Total Area}}{\text{Area Bounding Rectangle}} \tag{24}$$

Data analysis. In our literature review it has been shown that metaheuristics contribute to improving the performance of artificial neural networks [29]. We are inspired by this to build a hybrid WOA-Shark-ANN Algorithm to analyze our dataset presented in Fig. 6.

1. Initialize the whale and shark populations at random.
2. Determine the optimum search agent X* by evaluating the fitness values of whales and sharks.
3. **while** $t < t_{max}$
4. compute the value of a Using Equation 9, $\boldsymbol{a} = \mathbf{2} - \frac{\mathbf{2t}}{\boldsymbol{t_{max}}}$
5. **for** each search agent
6. **if** $p < 0.5$ then
7. **if** $|A| < \mathbf{1}$ **then** $X_i^k(t+1) = X_i^{\,*}(t) - A * |\boldsymbol{X_i}^*(\boldsymbol{t}) - X_i^k(t) + V_i^k(t)\Delta t_k|$
8. **if** $|A| \geq \mathbf{1}$ **then** $X_i^k(\boldsymbol{t}+\mathbf{1}) = \boldsymbol{X_{rand}}(\boldsymbol{t}) - A * |\boldsymbol{X_i}^*(\boldsymbol{t}) - X_i^k(t) + V_i^k(t)\Delta t_k|$
9. **end if**
10. **else if** $p \geq 0.5$ then
11. $X_i^k(\boldsymbol{t}+\mathbf{1}) =' |\boldsymbol{X}^*(\boldsymbol{t}) - X_i^k(t) + V_i^k(t)\Delta t_k| * e^{bl} * \cos(2\pi l) + X^*(t)$
12. **end if**
13. **end for**
14. evaluate the fitness of $X_i^k(\boldsymbol{t}+\mathbf{1})$// *for one whale* $i = 1$ and k number of iterations
15. Update $\boldsymbol{X}^*$

16 **end while**

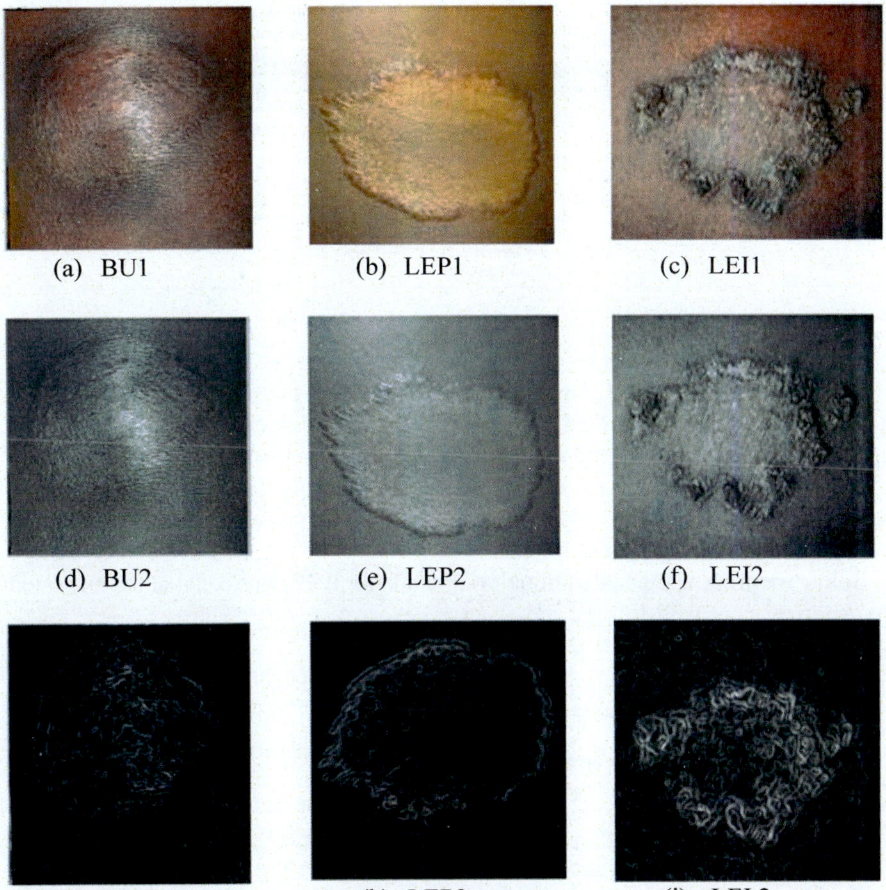

(a) BU1 (b) LEP1 (c) LEI1

(d) BU2 (e) LEP2 (f) LEI2

(g) BU3 (h) LEP3 (i) LEI 2

Fig. 6 Pre-processing Skin lesions images (BU1, LEP1, LEI1: Buruli ulcer, Leprosy and *leishmaniasis Original image* BU2, LEP2, LEI2: Buruli ulcer, Leprosy and *leishmaniasis Greyscale image*; BU3, LEP3, LEI3: Buruli ulcer, Leprosy and *leishmaniasis OTSU image*

3 Results

3.1 Image Pre-processing and Processing

Figure 6 consists of three columns, each describing a disease during the treatment phase. The first column represents Buruli Ulcer (BU), the second column represents reshmaniasis between leprosy and leprosy and the last column represents leishmaniasis in their different phases of processing from the real image to the binary image.

Table 3 Dataset head

ID_image	Area	Perimeter	Extend	Equivalent_diameter	Eccentricity	Class_name
UB0	17	17.4353467	0.456	7.9898	0.77845	0
UB1	21	33.5657979	0.675	11.5656	0.76676	0
UB2	32	24.7684543	0.986	9.56576	0.99994	0
UB3	25	28.8686554	0.767	12.78679	0.89005	0
UB4	42	17.9086567	0.988	8.65676	0.99875	0
…	…	…	…	…	…	…

The resulting dataset has 6 columns and 6000 records, so 5 will be the input data and one will be the output class. Here we have three possible outputs which are positive for Buruli Ulcer noted 0 and positive for leishmaniasis noted 1 and 2 for leprosy. Table 3 present ahead of the dataset obtained with Matlab code according to Eqs. 19 to 22. As said before all features are dimensionless. This table presents the results of the extractions of the five characteristics that will serve as the learning base (dataset) considered in this work.

Below we present a visualization of our database. It can be seen that the extracted characteristics are well-limited and observable.

3.2 *Data Analysis*

We have analyzed our data with several configurations of neural networks optimized by metaheuristics and compared them with our own hybrid WOA-SSO-ANN model. The obtained error minimization results are presented in Fig. 7.

This figure shows the learning process by the different algorithms. We can see that the minimization time by gradient descent of the non-optimized ANN represented by the blue curve is large compared to the other ANNs optimized by different metaheuristics. In order of performance, we observe that WOA moves from third place to first place when it is optimized by SSO represented by the green curve. The result in terms of MSE and accuracy can be seen in Table 4.

The results of testing the neglected tropical skin disease dataset using a single neural network's hidden layer are presented in Table 4. The WOA-SS0-MLP hybrid achieves the greatest results in terms of error reduction and accuracy. This information can be visualized in Fig. 9. It shows us a histogram of the accuracies, the highest bar of which is that of the hybrid of the Hawk-WOA (Fig. 8).

To validate the results, we will simulate various neural networks ranging from one layer to three hidden layers with a fixed number of neurons in each layer. The number of neurons in the hidden layers will be fixed for each configuration. Table 5 shows the various results in terms of accuracy and errors (MSE). We have rounded the accuracies to the nearest integer values.

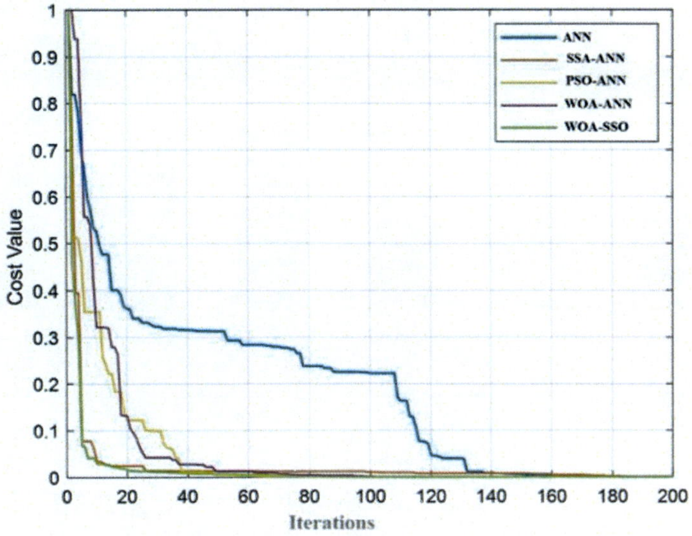

Fig. 7 Learning process

Table 4 Performance of the various algorithms on a single-layer neural network

Algorithm	Structure of ANN						
	1 hidden layer with 10 neurons						
	MSE * 10^{-9}				Accuracy (%)		
	Best	Worst	Mean	STD	Best	Worst	Mean
ANN	0.0017	0.0036	0.04606	0.0552	72.84	71.05	70.66
WOA-ANN	0.0015	0.0033	0.04605	0.0482	**81.84**	66.10	76.89
GA-ANN	0.0045	0.0064	0.0472	0.0650	77.56	70.11	68.13
SSA-ANN	0.0061	0.0106	0.04335	0.0423	77.88	69.33	69.03
PSO-MLP	0.0054	0.0055	0.0587	0.0551	74.1	66.56	70.73
WOA-SSO-ANN	0.00008	0.00032	0.0072	0.0090	**87.45**	**80.34**	72.25

This study just validates the results obtained with a single layer of neurons that the WOA-SSO hybridization has better results and will be used in the implementation on Raspberry pi. The various experiments done on our own NTD dataset allow us to show the effectiveness of metaheuristics in general and WOA-SSO on learning and training ANNs and to draw significant conclusions. As summarized in Figs. 9 and 10.

We note that the performance improves as the number of hidden layers and neurons rises. On the other hand, as the number of concealed layers increases, so does the mistake. This is due to the population number of our metaheuristics which

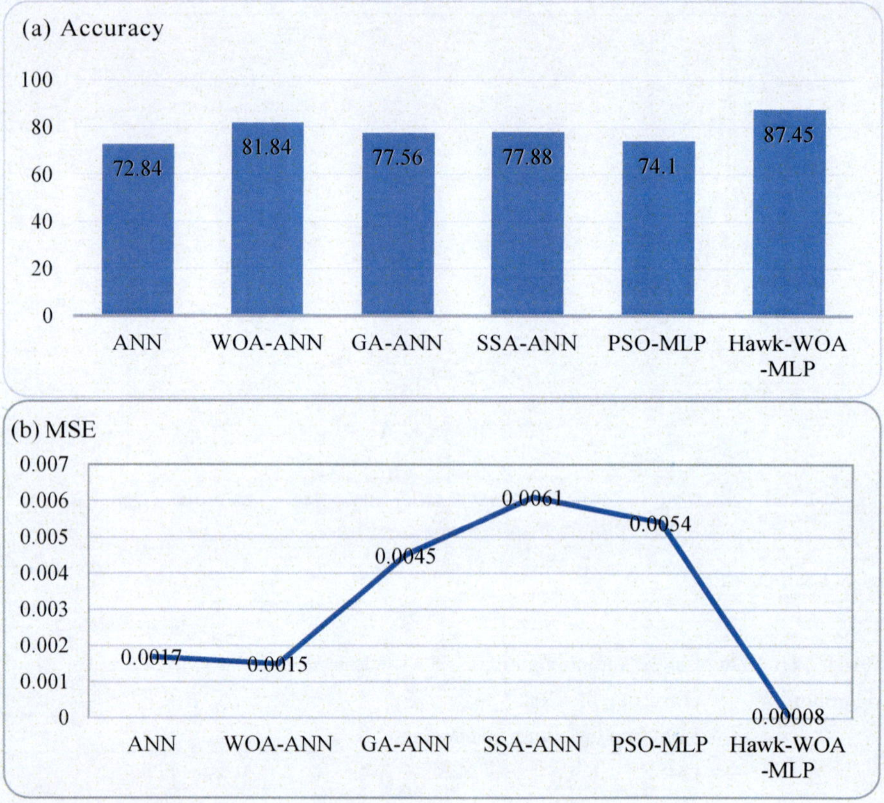

Fig. 8 Comparison of **a** accuracies and **b** errors

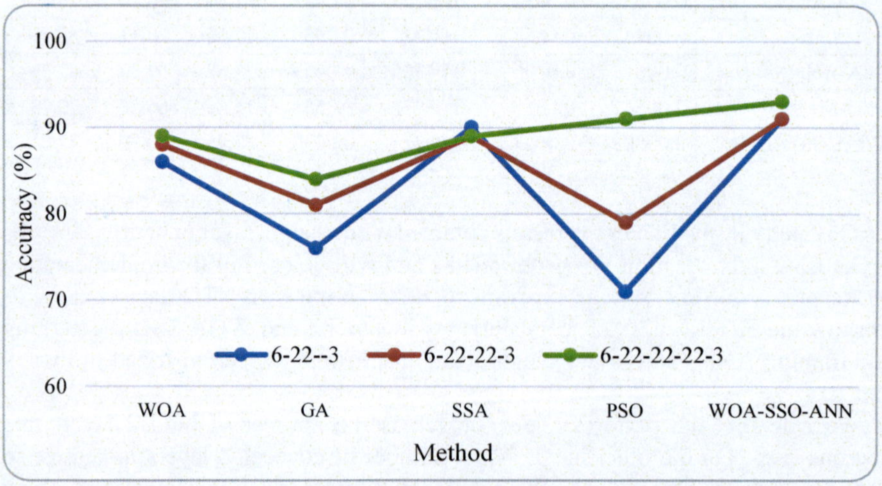

Fig. 9 Graphs of accuracy performance for each configuration utilizing various approaches

Table 5 Performance of various algorithms on various neural network structures (skin NTDS diseases) (MSE is mean square error, and Ac is accuracy)

ANN architecture	WOA-ANN		GA-ANN		SSA-ANN		PSO-ANN		WOA-SSO-ANN	
	MSE	Ac	MSE	Ac	MSE	Ac	MSE	Ac	MSE	Ac
6-22-3	0.0012	86	0.0132	76	0.0009	90	0.0007	71	0.0005	91
6-22-22-3	0.0009	88	0.0014	81	0.0021	89	0.0011	79	0.0008	91
6-22-22-22-3	0.0002	89	0.0021	84	0.0088	89	0.0002	91	0.0007	93

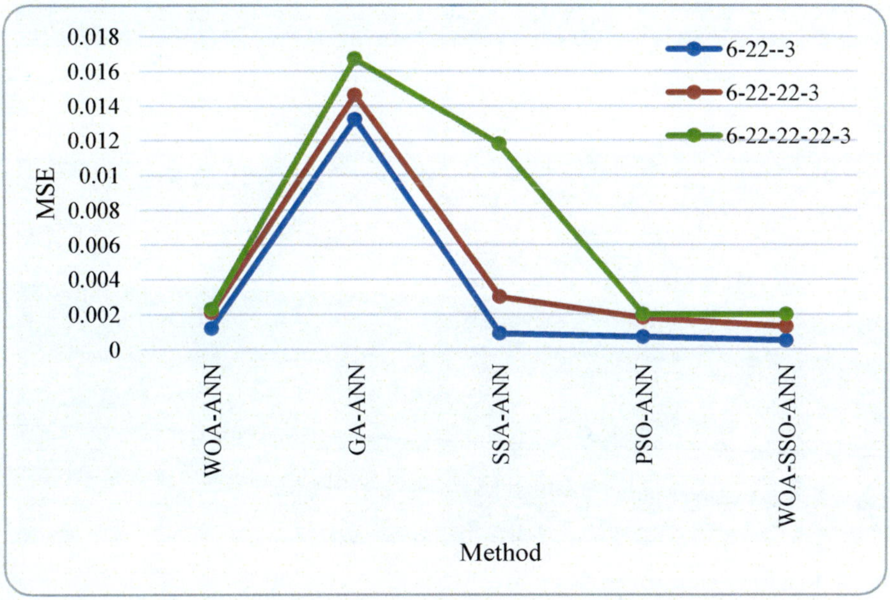

Fig. 10 MSE performance graphs for each configuration using different methods

has remained fixed. The classification accuracy increases with the structure of the neural network as shown in Fig. 10.

3.3 Deployment Result

Figure 11 shows the simple user interface. The user simply enters the image or the link to the image. Very simple to use, this application is hosted on a Raspberry pi4 board. The interface is built on HTML, CSS, JavaScript, and Flask. Once the application is opened, the user presses the UPLOAD button to upload a suspected skin lesion image. Once the image is uploaded, he clicks on the PROCEED button and the whole process of preprocessing, extraction of parameters, and classification

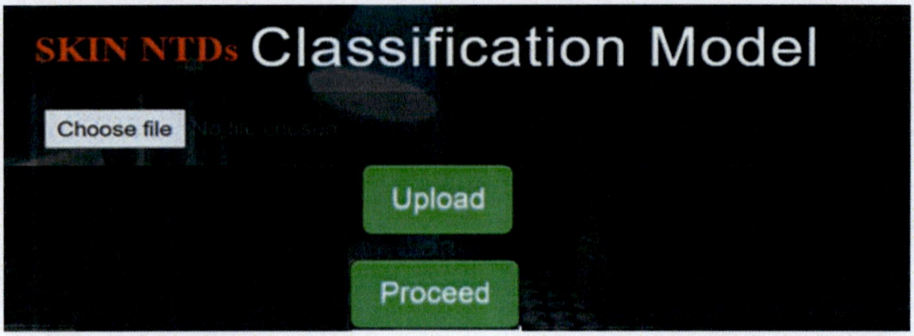

Fig. 11 User-friendly interface

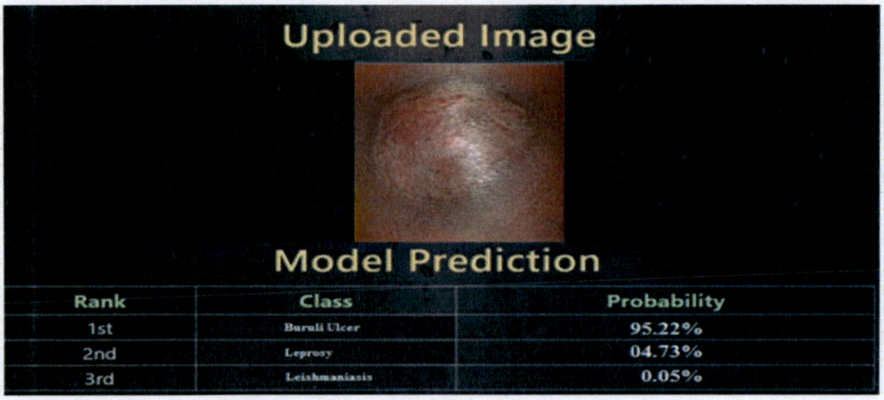

Fig. 12 Result of a diagnosis on flask

is done at the back end. The result, as shown in Fig. 12, consists of the classification of the diseases from highest to lowest probability.

Figure 12 shows a good prediction of Buruli ulcer from the image of the plaque lesion. The result confirmed a Buruli ulcer lesion with a probability of 95.22%. The probabilities of other diseases being very low, and they can be excluded from the final diagnosis. This is the ideal early phase for initiating treatment with guaranteed low-cost healing.

4 Discussion

This study analyzed the database of skin lesion images of three neglected tropical diseases regardless of the epidemiological and clinical background of patients diagnosed with leprosy, Buruli ulcer, and leishmaniasis (Table 3). By analyzing the extracted features through the appropriate image processing, we observed that although the diseases develop almost identically at their onset, there is a visible difference in the pixel distribution of each lesion. Therefore, we were able to extract a database that could be used as a diagnostic tool for neglected tropical diseases using machine learning. After observing the work in the literature concerning the classification of NTDs whose accuracy results were always lower than 91%, we therefore improved these results by proposing a new method of optimization of artificial neural networks. In response to the query, what share of forecasted positives are actually positives? The 93% solution is superb and ranks first in the literature for similar issues. The web application we have developed allows frontline staff, without necessarily being experts in these diseases, to not only perform initial tests on the spot just from the image of the lesion but also to refer online to an expert.

Some authors have focused on categorizing NTDs in the literature in order to develop diagnostic tools for neglected tropical diseases. To our knowledge, no author has yet tried to classify a set of several tropical diseases, although they are very similar in their onset because they develop as nodules or plaques. We have done so successfully. For example, Hu et al. [15] used SVM on dermoscopic images to diagnose Buruli ulcers in the ulcer phase but achieved less than 90% accuracy. Souza et al. [21] used a random forest algorithm on a database of leishmaniasis patients and obtained an accuracy of 87.09%, and Barbier et al. [22] used a CNN algorithm on a set of photographic images of leprosy lesions. Table 6 depicts a comparison of the outcomes in terms of technique and amount.

The differences in results can be seen graphically in the following figure.

The comparison of the various algorithms with our own on our dataset shows that it is the best method in terms of accuracy, as shown in Fig. 13. We believe that the number of images is not yet optimal. Therefore, we will continue to collect images in the field and we also plan to use data augmentation methods to expand our data base and thus add reliability to our study. However, we must also provide information such as socio-geographical and clinical features of the illnesses in concern. The high accuracy (93.21%) of this application provides a multi-platform method to support the characterization and classification of many neglected diseases in isolated communities in Cameroon and worldwide. In this way, we are responding at our level to the WHO's goal of eradicating NTDs by 2030.

Table 6 Performance of various algorithms on various neural network structures

References	NTDs	Data		
		Images	Clinical data	Accuracy (%)
[15]	Buruli ulcer	26	No	85.70
[21]	Leishmaniasis	300	No	50
[22]	Leprosy	1229	587	90
*Nyatte et al.	Buruli ulcer Leishmaniasis Leprosy	1054	No	93

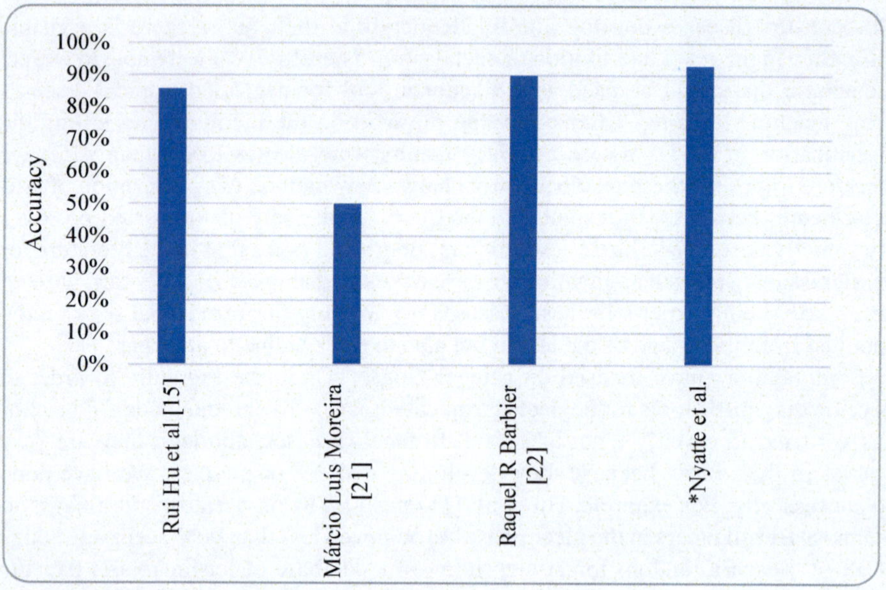

Fig. 13 Comparison of the result

5 Conclusion

The primary goal of this research is to demonstrate that it is possible to optimize the classification (diagnose) of neglected tropical diseases such as Buruli Ulcer, leprosy, and leishmaniasis by optimizing ANN through metaheuristic algorithms using a web application on a Raspberry pi4 module. The computational power and price of this tool allow us to combine a low-cost system and performance. The experimental results demonstrated the exceptional performance of the hybridization of two metaheuristics, whale optimization and shark smell optimization (WOA-SSO), in most of the evaluation cases. When differentiate from other optimization strategies, the acquired accuracy of 93% validates the efficacy of the suggested methodology for FNN training, namely WOA, PSO, GA, SSA. In the future work you are going to use data augmentation et feature selection techniques to improve our results.

References

1. Casulli A (2021) New global targets for NTDs in the WHO roadmap 2021–2030. PLoS Negl Trop Dis 15:e0009373. https://doi.org/10.1371/journal.pntd.0009373
2. Carrion C, Robles N, Sola-Morales O, Aymerich M, Ruiz Postigo JA (2020) Mobile health strategies to tackle skin neglected tropical diseases with recommendations from innovative experiences: systematic review. JMIR MHealth UHealth 8:e22478. https://doi.org/10.2196/22478

3. Steyve N, Steve P, Ghislain M, Ndjakomo S, pierre E (2022) Optimized real-time diagnosis of neglected tropical diseases by automatic recognition of skin lesions. Inform Med Unlocked 33:101078. https://doi.org/10.1016/j.imu.2022.101078
4. Chan H-P, Hadjiiski LM, Samala RK (2020) Computer-aided diagnosis in the era of deep learning. Med Phys 47:e218–e227. https://doi.org/10.1002/mp.13764
5. Fujita H (2020) AI-based computer-aided diagnosis (AI-CAD): the latest review to read first. Radiol Phys Technol 13:6–19. https://doi.org/10.1007/s12194-019-00552-4
6. Suzuki K (2013) Machine learning in computer-aided diagnosis of the thorax and colon in CT: a survey. IEICE Trans Inf Syst E96-D:772–783. https://doi.org/10.1587/transinf.E96.D.772
7. Gori M, Tesi A (1992) On the problem of local minima in backpropagation. IEEE Trans Pattern Anal Mach Intell 14:76–86. https://doi.org/10.1109/34.107014
8. Agustyawan A, Laksana TG, Athiyah U (2022) Combination of backpropagation neural network and particle swarm optimization for water production prediction in municipal waterworks. Sci J Inform 9:84–94. https://doi.org/10.15294/sji.v9i1.29849
9. Singh A, Kushwaha S, Alarfaj M, Singh M (2022) Comprehensive overview of backpropagation algorithm for digital image denoising. Electronics 11:1590. https://doi.org/10.3390/electronics11101590
10. Wright LG, Onodera T, Stein MM, Wang T, Schachter DT, Hu Z, McMahon PL (2022) Deep physical neural networks trained with backpropagation. Nature 601:549–555. https://doi.org/10.1038/s41586-021-04223-6
11. Mouloodi S, Rahmanpanah H, Gohari S, Burvill C, Davies HMS (2022) Feedforward backpropagation artificial neural networks for predicting mechanical responses in complex nonlinear structures: a study on a long bone. J Mech Behav Biomed Mater 128:105079. https://doi.org/10.1016/j.jmbbm.2022.105079
12. Xu L, Si Y, Guo Z, Bokov D (2022) Optimal skin cancer detection by a combined ENN and fractional order coot optimization algorithm. Proc Inst Mech Eng [H]. 9544119221113180. https://doi.org/10.1177/09544119221113180
13. Tan T, Zhang L, Neoh S, Lim C (2018) Intelligent skin cancer detection using enhanced particle swarm optimization. Knowl-Based Syst 158. https://doi.org/10.1016/j.knosys.2018.05.042
14. Dildar M, Akram S, Irfan M, Khan HU, Ramzan M, Mahmood AR, Alsaiari SA, Saeed AHM, Alraddadi MO, Mahnashi MH (2021) Skin cancer detection: a review using deep learning techniques. Int J Environ Res Public Health 18:5479. https://doi.org/10.3390/ijerph18105479
15. Hu R, Queen CM, Zouridakis G (2013) Detection of Buruli ulcer disease: preliminary results with dermoscopic images on smart handheld devices. In: 2013 IEEE point-of-care healthcare technologies (PHT), pp 168–171. https://doi.org/10.1109/PHT.2013.6461311
16. Hu R, Queen CM, Zouridakis G (2012) Lesion border detection in Buruli ulcer images. Annu Int Conf IEEE Eng Med Biol Soc. IEEE Eng Med Biol Soc Annu Int Conf 2012:5380–5383. https://doi.org/10.1109/EMBC.2012.6347210
17. Hu R (2013) 1984 Automatic recognition of Buruli ulcer images on smart handheld devices. https://uh-ir.tdl.org/handle/10657/3396
18. Hu R, Queen CM, Zouridakis G (2014) A novel tool for detecting Buruli ulcer disease based on multispectral image analysis on handheld devices. In: IEEE-EMBS international conference on biomedical and health informatics (BHI), pp 37–40. https://doi.org/10.1109/BHI.2014.6864298
19. Bamorovat M, Sharifi I, Rashedi E, Shafiian A, Sharifi F, Khosravi A, Tahmouresi A (2021) A novel diagnostic and prognostic approach for unresponsive patients with anthroponotic cutaneous leishmaniasis using artificial neural networks. PLoS ONE 16:e0250904. https://doi.org/10.1371/journal.pone.0250904
20. Zare M, Akbarialiabad H, Parsaei H, Asgari Q, Alinejad A, Bahreini MS, Hosseini SH, Ghofrani-Jahromi M, Shahriarirad R, Amirmoezzi Y, Shahriarirad S, Zeighami A, Abdollahifard G (2022) A machine learning-based system for detecting leishmaniasis in microscopic images. BMC Infect Dis 22:48. https://doi.org/10.1186/s12879-022-07029-7
21. Souza MLMD, Lopes GA, Branco AC, Fairley JK, Fraga LADO (2021) Leprosy screening based on artificial intelligence: development of a cross-platform app. JMIR MHealth UHealth 9:e23718. https://doi.org/10.2196/23718

22. Barbieri RR, Xu Y, Setian L, Souza-Santos PT, Trivedi A, Cristofono J, Bhering R, White K, Sales AM, Miller G, Nery JAC, Sharman M, Bumann R, Zhang S, Goldust M, Sarno EN, Mirza F, Cavaliero A, Timmer S, Bonfiglioli E, Smith C, Scollard D, Navarini AA, Aerts A, Ferres JL, Moraes MO (2022) Reimagining leprosy elimination with AI analysis of a combination of skin lesion images with demographic and clinical data. Lancet Reg Health—Am 9. https://doi.org/10.1016/j.lana.2022.100192
23. Bhandari A, Meena A (2018) Social spider optimization based optimally weighted Otsu thresholding for image enhancement. IEEE J Sel Top Appl Earth Obs Remote Sens 1–13. https://doi.org/10.1109/JSTARS.2018.2870157
24. Mirjalili S, Lewis A (2016) The whale optimization algorithm. Adv Eng Softw 95:51–67. https://doi.org/10.1016/j.advengsoft.2016.01.008
25. Mohammad-Azari S, Bozorg-Haddad O, Chu X (2018) Shark Smell Optimization (SSO) algorithm. In: Bozorg-Haddad O (ed) Advanced optimization by nature-inspired algorithms. Springer, Singapore, pp 93–103. https://doi.org/10.1007/978-981-10-5221-7_10
26. Rao Y, Shao Z, Ahangarnejad AH, Gholamalizadeh E, Sobhani B (2019) Shark Smell Optimizer applied to identify the optimal parameters of the proton exchange membrane fuel cell model. Energy Convers Manag 182:1–8. https://doi.org/10.1016/j.enconman.2018.12.057
27. Gnanasekaran N, Chandramohan S, Kumar PS, Mohamed Imran A (2016) Optimal placement of capacitors in radial distribution system using shark smell optimization algorithm. Ain Shams Eng J 7:907–916. https://doi.org/10.1016/j.asej.2016.01.006
28. Kumar S, Kumar P, Sharma TK, Pant M (2013) Bi-level thresholding using PSO, Artificial Bee Colony and MRLDE embedded with Otsu method. Memetic Comput 4:323–334. https://doi.org/10.1007/s12293-013-0123-5
29. Raja NSM, Sukanya SA, Nikita Y (2015) Improved PSO based multi-level thresholding for cancer infected breast thermal images using Otsu. Procedia Comput Sci Complete 524–529. https://doi.org/10.1016/j.procs.2015.04.130
30. Helen R, Kamaraj N, Selvi K, Raja Raman V (2011) Segmentation of pulmonary parenchyma in CT lung images based on 2D Otsu optimized by PSO. In: 2011 international conference on emerging trends in electrical and computer technology, pp 536–541. https://doi.org/10.1109/ICETECT.2011.5760176
31. Lokhande NM, Pujeri RV (2018) Novel image segmentation using particle swarm optimization. In: Proceedings of the 2018 8th international conference on biomedical engineering and technology. Association for Computing Machinery, New York, NY, USA, pp 46–50. https://doi.org/10.1145/3208955.3208962
32. Zhao Y, Yu X, Wu H, Zhou Y, Sun X, Yu S, Yu S, Liu H (2021) A Fast 2-D Otsu lung tissue image segmentation algorithm based on improved PSO. Microprocess Microsyst 80:103527. https://doi.org/10.1016/j.micpro.2020.103527

Small Displacement Detection System of Landslide Using FMCW Radar with Phase-Detection and Change Point Detection Method

Wilma Christy Natalia, Fiky Yosef Suratman, and Aloysius Adya Pramudita

Abstract The threat of landslides often occurs during the rainy season in mountainous and hilly areas. Small displacement from the slope that occurs landslides will move slowly on a millimeter scale. To minimize the impact of material losses and fatalities, a landslide monitoring system was developed using uRAD based on FMCW (Frequency Modulated Continuous Wave) radar with landslide miniatures used in the simulation to prove the concept of the phase-detection method in small displacement detection and the self-designed CPD (Change Point Detection) method. The system designed is able to detect when the movement of the miniature landslide is detected by radar. The result shows that the phase-detection method used is suitable for detecting small displacement of the object and the self-designed CPD method can determine the change point of time is good and accurate, which is CPD time detected above the 3rd second this is in accordance with the experiments carried out at the time of data collection. Based on the results, the proposed system can help to detect landslides in simulations carried out with miniature landslides as an object.

Keywords Small Displacement · uRAD Radar · Phase-Detection · Change Point Detection

1 Introduction

Small displacement detection is a system for detecting the displacement of an object where the shift can be on a millimeter scale. Small displacement can be applied to several detection cases, such as health monitoring, medical, and natural disaster monitoring [1–6]. In this research, small displacement detection will be applied to landslide disaster simulation using landslide miniature. Landslides are one of the natural occurrences that often occur during the rainy season in Indonesia, especially in hilly and mountainous areas. This landslide occurs due to the movement of rock or soil mass, where there are driving and triggering factors [7, 8]. Therefore, landslides

W. C. Natalia (✉) · F. Y. Suratman · A. A. Pramudita
School of Electrical Engineering, Telkom University, Bandung, Indonesia
e-mail: wilmachristyna@gmail.com

T. Triwiyanto et al. (eds.), *Proceeding of the 3rd International Conference on Electronics, Biomedical Engineering, and Health Informatics*, Lecture Notes in Electrical Engineering 1008, https://doi.org/10.1007/978-981-99-0248-4_33

harm humans. Slope shift from landslide is very small; it takes millimeters to meters to shift per year [9].

Several studies have used the Synthetic Aperture Radar (SAR) system to detect landslides [10–12]. SAR can detect a large enough area and surface deformation in the range of millimeters to a distance, so it is widely used in remote sensing techniques such as uniting the earth's surface and humans [13–16]. SAR is one of the radar systems that work by making patterns from data records that produce a radar image with a high resolution [17–19], which inflicts the use of SAR requires infrastructure investment and considerable computing resources in monitoring erosion-prone areas. From the research results obtained, SAR can monitor erosion but does not provide real-time information about the speed of movement of slope erosion due to the time difference when the radar emits a signal, and the object reflecting on the ground surface until the receiver receives it [20]. SAR can also cause slant range distortion; it causes the target object in the close range to appear compressed compared to the area at the far range [21].

The development of uRAD radar can be used as an alternative to the use of SAR, allowing it to monitor a large area with infrastructure that requires a lower investment than SAR. uRAD is a Frequency Modulated Continuous Wave (FMCW) radar with a frequency of 24 GHz and integrated with Raspberry Pi. Detecting small displacement objects such as slope shifts can be detected with uRAD by processing the signal received by the radar using the phase-detection method, in which the phase values can indicate a small displacement detected by the radar [22]. Hence, it is possible to use uRAD radar to detect a small displacement from landslide miniature. Change Point Detection (CPD) is used to determine the pattern change of the phase data obtained from the phase-detection method, where there is a change in the pattern of the phase data, it is indicated that there is a small displacement from the landslide miniature.

This paper is divided into five sections. Section 1 describes the introduction to this paper. Section 2 describes the materials and methods used in this research. Section 3 shows the results of the proposed method. Section 4 describes the results that have been obtained, compared with other studies, the weaknesses of the proposed method, and the implications of this study. And lastly, Sect. 5 concludes the results of this study and the proposed method.

2 Materials and Method

2.1 Material

uRAD v.1.2. uRAD is an FMCW radar with a simple but high-performance device, and the specifications are at the same level as professional radars [23]. The frequency of this radar is 24 GHz with a bandwidth of 240 MHz and the maximum number of samples in one frame (Ns) is 200, whereas in this experiment, the author only uses

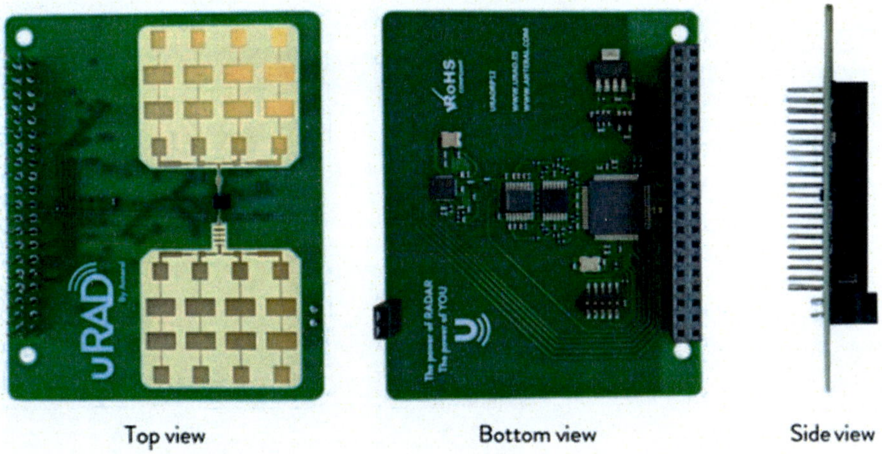

Fig. 1 URAD Raspberry Pi v1.2

50 Ns. In data collection, the author uses uRAD on mode 2 where the mode is only to detect distance with sawtooth waveform, and MTI (Moving Target Indication) mode is OFF. uRAD is already integrated with Raspberry Pi, so as to run programming from uRAD can only be processed by the Raspberry Pi. The output of uRAD is raw data form of I (In-phase) and Q (Quadrature) signals, where this output comes from the results of signal processing in uRAD which has been filtered by LPF (Low Pass Filter) and has Arbitrary units from 0 to 4095 (Fig. 1).

Landslide Miniature. This landslide miniature is conducted as a simulation of landslide incidents so that the small displacement of the sand and gravel can be seen as a detected object. Landslide miniature is made using a plywood board with a thickness of 2 cm and arranged into a block with dimensions of 1.26 × 2.5 × 1.2 m. The beam has an open top and front and is filled with sand and gravel, and it can be manually adjusted to form a slope so that it resembles a slope. A sack is buried under the sand, and on both sides is connected with a long wire, later used to pull the sack so that the sand and gravel above it will slowly move down. The datasets used in this study are three wire-pulling methods, wire-pulling as far as 1 cm, 3 cm, and 5 cm. This wire pulling is related to the distance of the landslide slope shift (Fig. 2).

2.2 *Experimental Procedures*

Diagram Block System. In the research conducted, the IQ data obtained from the uRAD output will be processed by the FFT method and eliminate DC components and clutter. The data is cropped according to the distance that there is movement and is detected by radar. Then look for the magnitude to get the location of the index where the peak of the spectrum is. Because the location of the spectrum peak index

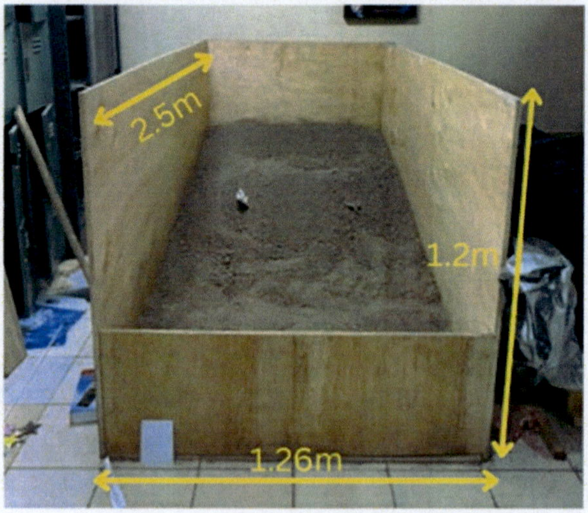

Fig. 2 Landslide miniature

is not in the same place, it is necessary to find the mode of the spectrum peak index that has been found. After getting the spectrum peak index mode, the cropped IQ data is reprocessed by searching for the phase value in the index mode that has been previously set and getting the phase value from the data. The phase value will be stable when no movement is detected, and the value will change significantly when a small movement is detected. To determine the point of significant phase change, the CPD method is used to get the time when the change occurs in the phase pattern. This indicates there is a movement time obtained by the CPD method (Fig. 3).

Data Collection. The dataset collection process in this study uses uRAD v1.2. It is connected to a Raspberry Pi 4, paired on a tripod with a height of 67 cm, and placed 2 cm in front of the landslide miniature. The height of the tripod is adjusted to the height of the slope that is made. There are several procedures carried out in data collection, namely by pulling the wire connected to the sack buried by sand and gravel as far as 1, 3, and 5 cm. Each procedure is performed ten times with a radar record time of 8 s and a pulling time starting on the 3rd second. The configuration on uRAD

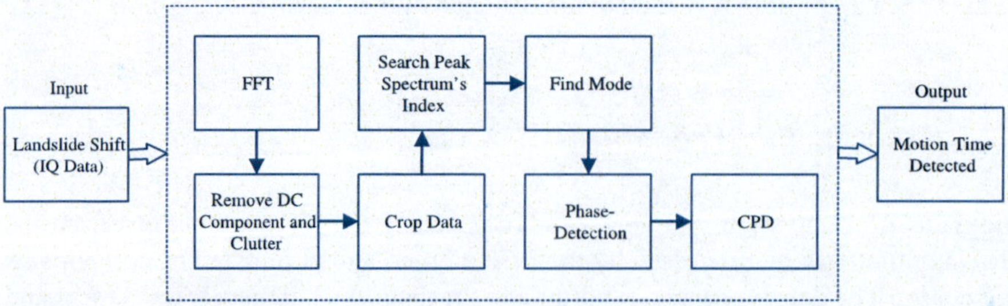

Fig. 3 Diagram block system

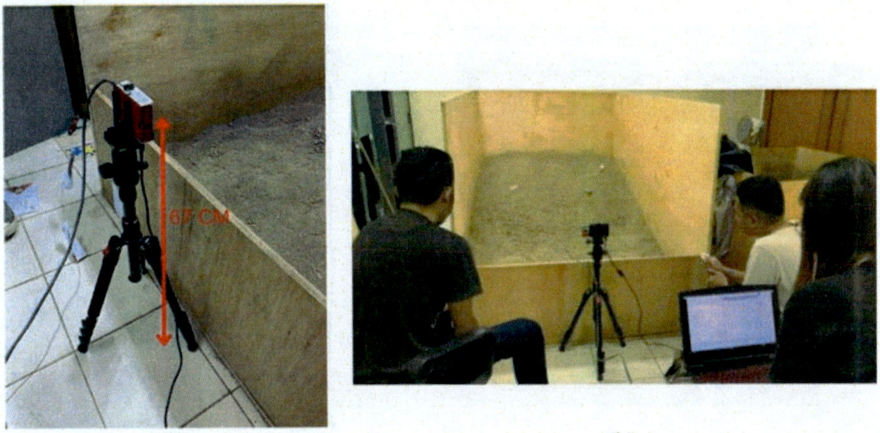

(a) (b)

Fig. 4 **a** Radar height, **b** method to collect dataset

used for data retrieval is using f0 = 24.005 GHz, Bandwidth = 240 MHz, using a sawtooth signal, and Ns = 50 (Ns is the number of samples in one capture/period), which one period takes 50 ms (Fig. 4).

2.3 *Pre-Processing*

Fast Fourier Transform. After getting IQ data from the results recorded by uRAD, the data is processed by the FFT method to convert IQ data into a frequency domain. IQ data which initially has 50 samples in one frame is changed to 4096 samples in one frame by FFT on uRAD because FFT uRAD has an N_FFT (FFT index) of 4096. Where the index consists of real and imaginary parts spread from $-\pi$ to π, and the data needed for processing is only the real part (Fig. 5).

The FFT index is the beat frequency index, where the beat frequency has distance information. The equation of the maximum distance of uRAD can be expressed in the formula (1) [23, 24]. The brighter the index color in the data plot results, the greater the power possessed by the index. Where this indicates the detected movement of the object, the systematic equation of the FFT method can be expressed in formula (2) [25].

$$\text{Maximum Distance} = 75 \times \frac{N_s}{BW} \quad (1)$$

where N_s is the number of samples and BW is the Bandwidth, because the N_s that author use is 50 and the bandwidth is 240, so we will get a maximum radar distance of 15.625 m.

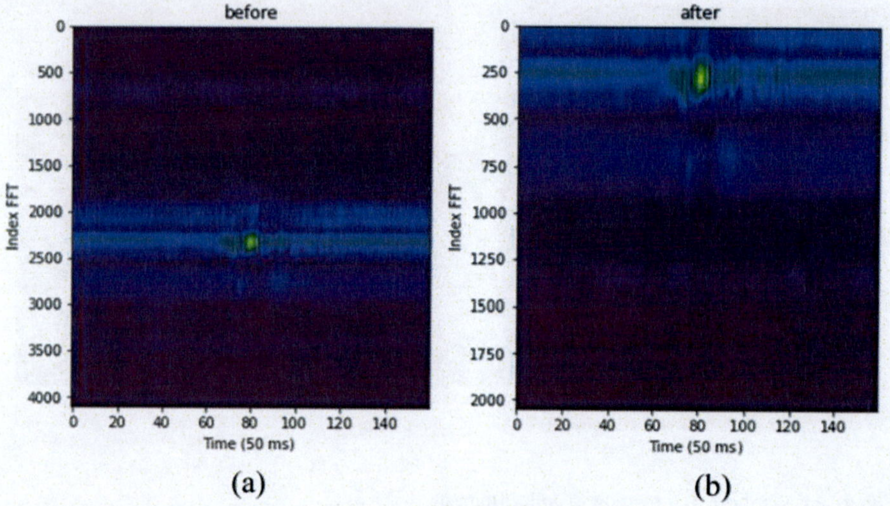

Fig. 5 **a** Spectrogram real and imaginary, **b** spectrogram real only

$$X[k] = \sum_{n=0}^{N_p-1} x[n]e^{-2\pi j \frac{nk}{N_p}} \tag{2}$$

where $k = (0, 1, \ldots, K - 1)$ is the frequency index, N_p is the number of periods.

Remove DC Component and Clutter. Remove DC component and clutter method are used to remove noise signals caused by electronic interference from the uRAD radar or other signals that can interfere, such as signals obtained from static objects during experiments. The formula for removing the DC component is explained in Eq. (3) and removing clutter in Eq. (4).

$$\text{Remove DC component} = n_{\text{row}} - \text{avg}_{\text{row}} \tag{3}$$

In one data frame, the remove DC component is the value of each row (n_{row}) minus the average of each row (avg_{row}).

$$\text{Remove DC clutter} = n_{\text{column}} - \text{avg}_{\text{column}} \tag{4}$$

The removed clutter is the value of each column (n_{column}) minus the average of each column ($\text{avg}_{\text{column}}$).

Cropping Data. The FFT process makes one data frame has 2048 indexes, which not all indexes are used because all that is needed is the index where there is movement. Therefore, it is necessary to do a data crop method which is done manually by the author (Fig. 6).

Mode Of Peak Spectrum's Index. After cropping the data, the search for the location of the peak spectrum for each index is carried out. Because the location of

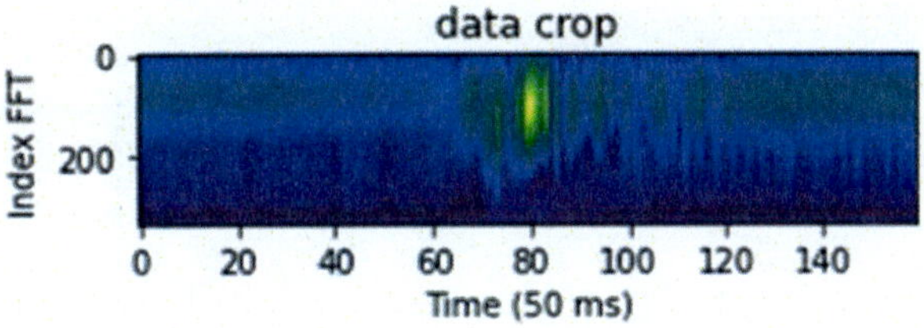

Fig. 6 Cropped spectrogram

the peak spectrum index for each frame is different, a search of mode is carried out to find the location of the most detected index.

Phase-Detection. Phase-Detection is a method to determine the presence of small displacements that occur in data collection results. The trick is to change the data that has been cropped into a phase value and the only phase value taken is the phase value in the predetermined index mode. This method is suitable for finding small displacements from the object. The phase value is stable when there is no movement and will change significantly when there is a small movement of the detected data. The phase value can be found in Eq. (5).

$$\theta = \tan^{-1}\frac{Q}{I} \tag{5}$$

Q is the real number, and I is the imaginary number of IQ from raw data.

As shown in Fig. 7, from the 0th second to the 3.25th second, the phase value did not change significantly or was in a stable position. Because the pulling to move the slope is carried out in the 3rd second, the movement will be detected after 3 s. Movement is detected at 3.25 s to 6 s and returns to steady or no motion detected from 6 to 8 s (finished).

Change Point Detection. Change Point Detection is a method to find abrupt changes in data when a property of the time series changes [26–31]. The Change Point Detection method used by the author is a method for finding the point of change from phase data. As described in the phase-detection method, the phase value will change significantly when there is movement and will be stable when no movement

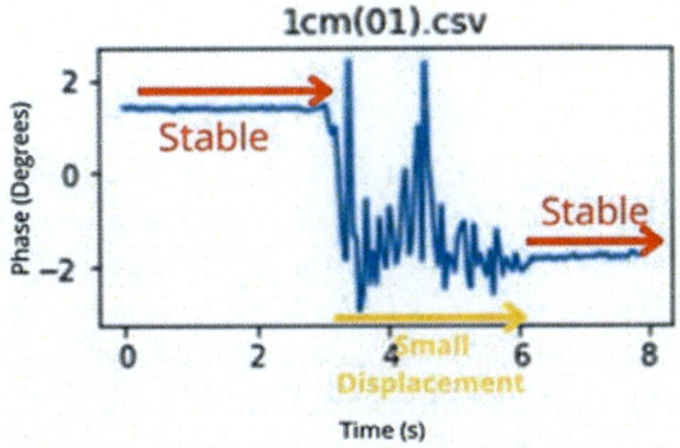

Fig. 7 Phase-detection in one data

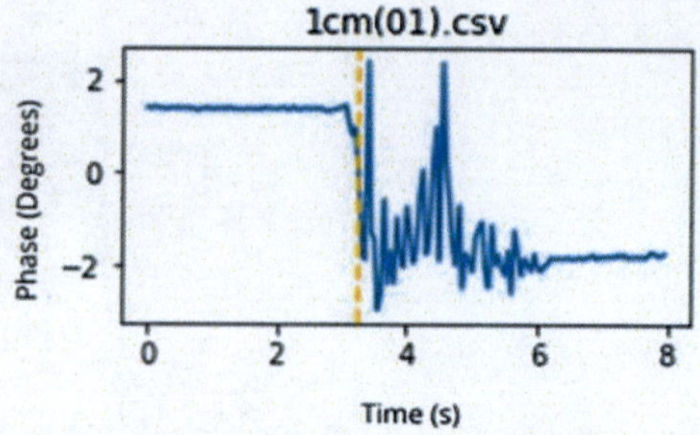

Fig. 8 Phase-detection graph with CPD

is detected. With this concept, the authors make the CPD method with the following working principles:

1. Find x (difference) from the phase value at the i-time index minus the phase value at the (i–1) time index.
2. Observed from the pattern of phase values, the authors set a threshold of the difference of 1.
3. Because the phase pattern when there is a change can change significantly, namely the phase value can go up or down, the author makes a threshold $x > 1$ or $x < 1$.
4. When x (difference) is detected in accordance with the threshold, then look for where the position of the time index is located to find the point of change (change point). The author will only take one x value that is found first.
5. After finding the change point (change point) is located, combine it with the phase data to see a graph of the detection.

The CPD formula made by the author is explained in Eq. (6).

$$x = |\text{phaseindex}[i] - \text{phaseindex}[i-1]|, x < 1 \text{ or } x > 1 \tag{6}$$

In Fig. 8, the yellow line represents CPD. The change point value is 3.25, which means that the data pattern changes at 3.25 s. The change point value is obtained with a threshold of 1 which has been set by the author.

2.4 Flowchart

The system starts by entering the time limit for data collection; this input will determine when data collection ends. Raspberry Pi will connect to the uRAD radar and get data IQ. If an error occurs, the Raspberry Pi will reconnect to the radar. If successful, the radar transmits FMCW radar signals and receives raw data from I/Q signals. Data collection continues for the specified period. If the time limit is not reached, the radar will continue to transmit FMCW signals. The resulting raw data is collected in a 2D array which will later be processed in the data preprocessing data section (Fig. 9).

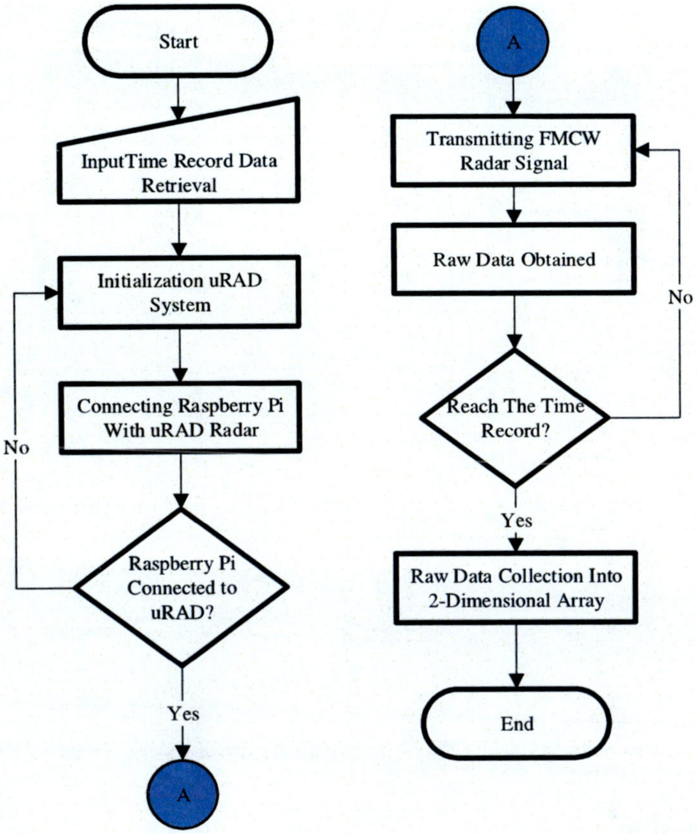

Fig. 9 Flowchart system

3 Result

In the experiments, the results obtained from the system output are graphs of the self-designed CPD method. For each wire-pulling experiment, shown in Figs. 10, 11, and 12, the blue line is the value of the phase, and the yellow line is the time-change point data. The *x*-axis is Time (s), and the *y*-axis is the Phase value (degrees). The time-change point data is obtained from self-designed CPD. The results of the time-change point data obtained from the self-designed CPD for each experiment are described in Tables 1, 2, and 3.

As in the data attached in Tables 1, 2, and 3, the time of movement detected by the system using the CPD method is always above the 3rd second, which is true because the author tested the slope pullout at the 3rd second so that the movement will occur after the 3rd second.

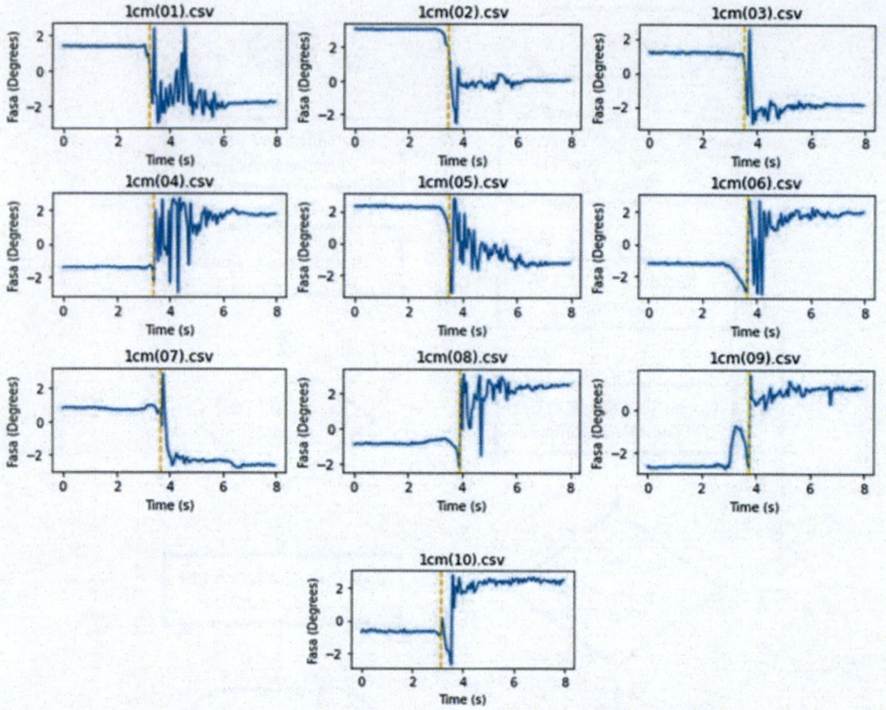

Fig. 10 Phase-detection graph with CPD for 1 cm pullout experiment

4 Discussion

This research purposed to create a landslide detection system by utilizing a miniature landslide to perform simulations. It proves that phase-detected is suitable for detecting small displacements in landslide shifts. This study utilizes the FFT method, phase-detection, and self-designed CPD, so the result gets the detection time by the system above the 3rd second, in accordance with data collection where the wire-pulling is carried out in the 3rd second; this is related to the movement of the sand and the gravel in the miniature landslide will move after the wire-pulling is done. In testing the movement detection system with a miniature landslide object, the result of the system can detect small movements of the object using the phase detection method. To achieve detection success, several methods are used in processing the signal received from the radar, namely, the FFT method, removing DC components and clutter, cropping data, finding the peak spectrum's index and mode, phase detection, and CPD. System testing can detect the object's movement by getting the system detection time with the change point obtained.

This research compares the detection results from the self-designed CPD method with the CPD method using Probability Density Function (PDF) to find false alarms. PDF results can't determine when there is a small displacement from the object, so

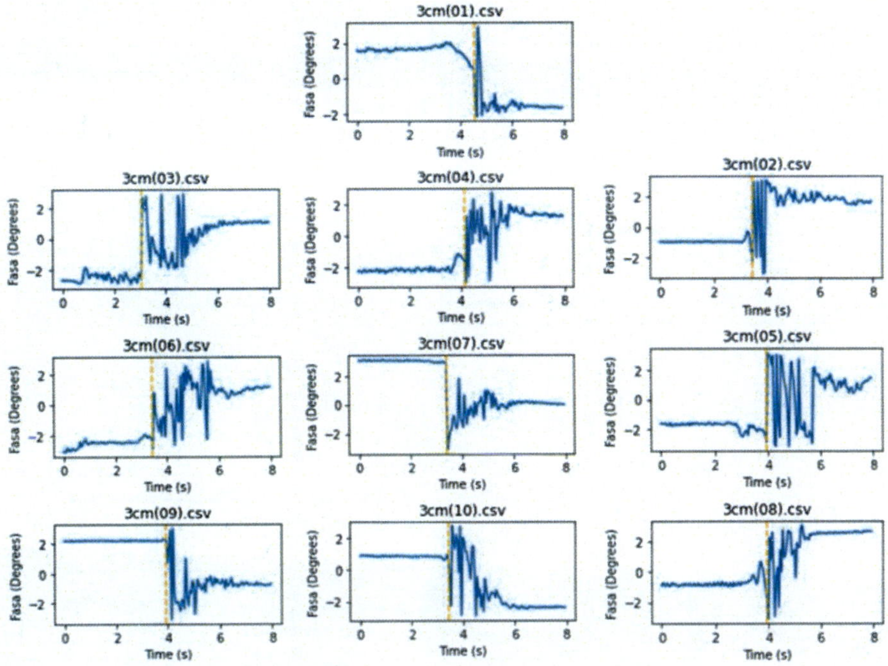

Fig. 11 Phase-detection graph with CPD for 3 cm pullout experiment

this is not good enough compared to the self-designed CPD method. Many factors cause the PDF method for false detection cannot be used on phase-detection data, including fluctuating phase-detection data, and when taking data with slope draws, it is not certain when the object movement occurs to what seconds because the movement of the object is very high. Which cannot be controlled and observed manually by the author. Therefore, by using the phase-detection method, it can show whether the object is moving or not. And the self-designed CPD method is sufficient to find the time when the object is moving.

The weakness of this study is that it is not possible to determine how far the displacement of the sand or gravel is; because of a large amount of sand and gravel that cannot be identified, it cannot be ascertained which target is moving. The uRAD system that has been created has not been able to implement real-time landslide monitoring.

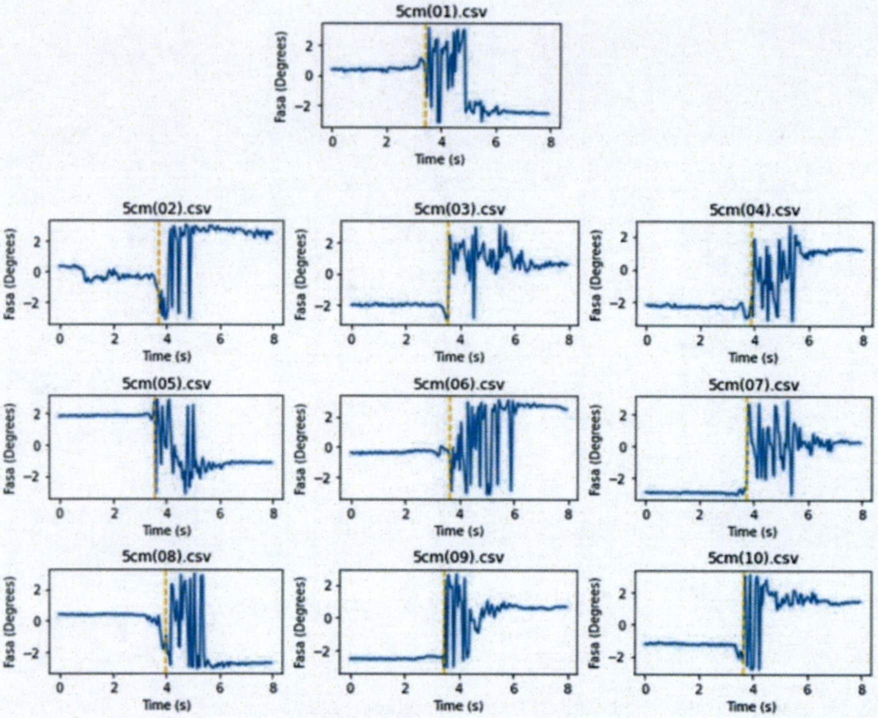

Fig. 12 Phase-detection graph with CPD for 5 cm pullout experiment

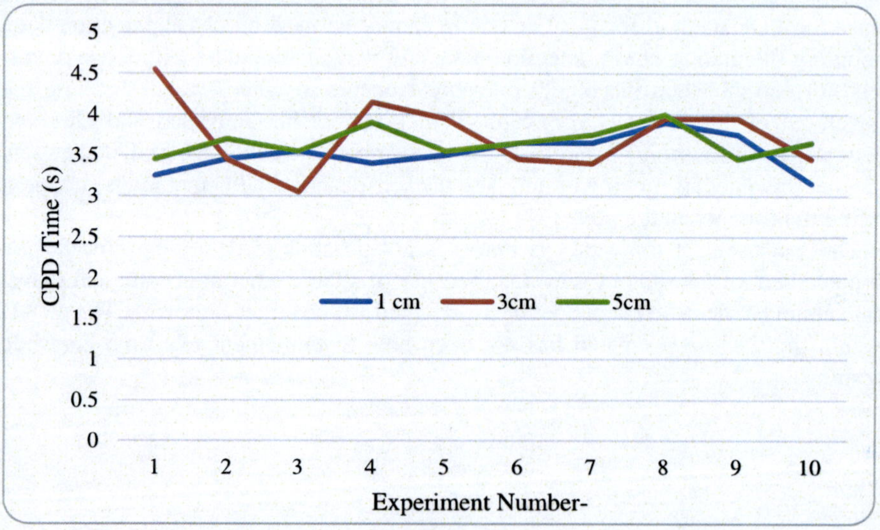

Fig. 13 Graphic result from data Tables 1, 2, and 3

Table 1 Result of detection time for pullout experiment 1 cm

Pullout procedure	CPD time (s)
1 cm (01)	3.25
1 cm (02)	3.45
1 cm (03)	3.55
1 cm (04)	3.4
1 cm (05)	3.5
1 cm (06)	3.65
1 cm (07)	3.65
1 cm (08)	3.9
1 cm (09)	3.75
1 cm (10)	3.15

Table 2 Result of detection time for pullout experiment 3 cm

Pullout procedure	CPD time (s)
3 cm (01)	4.55
3 cm (02)	3.45
3 cm (03)	3.05
3 cm (04)	4.15
3 cm (05)	3.95
3 cm (06)	3.45
3 cm (07)	3.4
3 cm (08)	3.95
3 cm (09)	3.95
3 cm (10)	3.45

Table 3 Result of detection time for pullout experiment 5 cm

Pullout procedure	CPD time (s)
5 cm (01)	3.45
5 cm (02)	3.7
5 cm (03)	3.55
5 cm (04)	3.9
5 cm (05)	3.55
5 cm (06)	3.65
5 cm (07)	3.75
5 cm (08)	4
5 cm (09)	3.45
5 cm (10)	3.65

5 Conclusion

The purpose of this study is to prove the concept of detection using uRAD radar with the Phase-detection method to detect small displacements of miniature landslides that have been made. Using the CPD method to find the time of detection when the target movement occurs gets a fairly good result, which is the result of the system is CPD time detected above the 3rd second this is in accordance with the experiments carried out at the time of data collection, where the wire-pulling is carried out in the 3rd second; this is related to the movement of the sand and the gravel in the miniature landslide will move after the wire-pulling is done. For further research, it is expected to be able to monitor landslides in real-time and find out the distance of the shift from the detection target so that the system can be realized as an erosion early warning system.

References

1. de Macedo KAC, Ramos FLG, Gaboardi C, Moreira JR, Vissirini F, da Costa MS (2017) A compact ground-based interferometric radar for landslide monitoring: the xerém experiment. IEEE J Selected Top Appl Earth Observ Remote Sens 10(3):975–986
2. Pramudita AA, Suratman FY, Arseno D, Ali E (2018) FMCW radar post processing method for small displacement detection. In: 2018 IEEE international conference on aerospace electronics and remote sensing technology (ICARES), pp 1–5
3. Pramudita AA, Suratman FY, Arseno D (2020) Modified FMCW system for non-contact sensing of human respiration. J Med Eng Technol 44(3):114–124
4. Dzvonkovskaya A, Petersen L, Insua TL (2017) Real-time capability of meteotsunami detection by WERA ocean radar system. In: 2017 18th international radar symposium (IRS), pp 1–10
5. Pisa S, Pittella E, Piuzzi E (2016) A survey of radar systems for medical applications. IEEE Aerosp Electron Syst Mag 31(11):64–81
6. Pramudita AA, Suratman FY (2021) Low-power radar system for noncontact human respiration sensor. IEEE Trans Instrum Meas 70:1–15
7. Thein TL, Sein MM, Mutara KT, Tungpimolrut K (2020) Real-time monitoring and early warning system for landslide preventing in Myanmar. In: 2020 IEEE 9th global conference on consumer electronics (GCCE)
8. Bhosale A, Nimbore P, Shitole S, Govindwar O (2017) Landslides monitoring system using IoT. Imperial J Interdisc Res (UIR) 3(4)
9. Lacroix P, Handwerger AL, Bièvre G (2020) Life and death of slow-moving landslides. Nat Rev Earth Environ 1–16
10. Tien-Hao L, Seung-Bum K, Alexander LH, Eric FJ (2021) Soil moisture retrieval using L-band SAR over landslide regions in northern California grasslands. In: IEEE 2000 international geoscience and remote sensing symposium, Brussels, Belgium, pp 2153–6996
11. Amitrano D, Costantini M, Dell'Aglio D, Iodice A, Malvarosa F, Minati F, Riccio D, Ruello G (2018) Landslide monitoring using Sar sub-pixel offset tracking. In: 2018 IEEE 4th international forum on research and technology for society and industry (RTSI), Palermo, Italy, pp 1–5
12. Yuta I, Motoyuki S (2021) Temporal H/alpha target decomposition for landslide monitoring using Ku-band GB-SAR time series. IEEE J Select Top Appl Earth Observ Remote Sens, pp 3318–3329

13. Sabrian PG, Saepuloh A, Koike K (2019) Detection of surface displacement from large baseline data pairs by multi-temporal D-insar with application to Bandung Basin, Indonesia. In: IEEE international geoscience and remote sensing symposium, pp 2153–6996
14. Zhang C, Wang C, Zhang H, Zhang B, Tian S (2017) An efficient object-oriented method of azimuth ambiguities removal for ship detection in SAR images. In: IEEE international geoscience and remote sensing symposium (IGARSS), pp 2153–7003
15. Berardino P, Fornaro G, Lanari R, Sansosti E (2002) A new algorithm for surface deformation monitoring based on small baseline differential SAR interferograms. IEEE Trans Geosci Remote Sens 40:2375–2383
16. Belloni V, Tullio MD, Ravanelli R, Fratarcangeli F, Nascetti A, Crespi M (2021) COSMO-Skymed range measurements for displacement monitoring using amplitude persistent scatterers. In: IEEE international geoscience and remote sensing symposium, pp 2153–6996
17. Schwegmann CP, Kleynhans W, Engelbrecht J, Mdakane LW, Meyer RGV (2017) Subsidence feature discrimination using deep convolutional neural networks in synthetic aperture radar imagery. In: IEEE international geoscience and remote sensing symposium (IGARSS), pp 2153–7003
18. Theron A, Engelbrecht J, Kemp J, Kleynhans W, Turnbull T (2016) Detection of sinkhole precursors through SAR interferometry: first results from South Africa. In: IEEE international geoscience and remote sensing symposium (IGARSS), pp 5398–5401
19. Dell'Amore L, Villano M, Krieger G, Moreira A (2019) Waveform-encoded synthetic aperture radar: image quality assessment using satellite data. In: IEEE transactions on geoscience and remote sensing, 2019 Kleinheubach conference
20. Thomas Z, Jan P, van Adriaan N, Roderik L (2021) Integrated monitoring of a slowly moving landslide based on total station measurements, multi-temporal terrestrial laser scanning and space-borne interferometric synthetic aperture radar. In: IEEE 2000 international geoscience and remote sensing symposium, Brussels, Belgium, pp 2153–6996
21. Xiong X, Li G, Ma Y, Chu L (2021) New slant range model and azimuth perturbation resampling based high-squint maneuvering platform SAR imaging. J Syst Eng Electron 545–558
22. Pramudita AA, Suratman FY, Arseno D (2021) Radar application for small displacement detection. In: 2021 IEEE Asia-Pacific conference on applied electromagnetics
23. uRAD by Anteral. User manual raspberry Pi version Software SDK v1.1
24. Anteral (2018) uRAD - Datasheet - RaspberryPi v1.2 - EN
25. Bucci OM, Migliore MD (2017) A novel nonuniform fast Fourier transform algorithm and its application to aperiodic arrays. In: 2017 IEEE antennas and wireless propagation letters, vol 16, pp 1472–1475
26. Truong C, Oudre L, Vayatis N (2020) Selective review of offline change point detection methods. Signal Process 167:107299
27. Militino AF, Moradi M, Ugarte MD (2020) On the performances of trend and change-point detection methods for remote sensing data. Remote Sens 12(6):1008
28. An RQ, Yang CJ, Pan YJ (2019) Unsupervised change point detection using a weight graph method for process monitoring. Ind Eng Chem Res 58(4):1624–1634
29. Chen H (2019) Sequential change-point detection based on nearest neighbors. Ann Stat 47(3):1381–1407
30. Eriksson M, Olofsson T (2019) Computationally efficient off-line joint change point detection in multiple time series. IEEE Trans Signal Process 67(1):149–163
31. Chu L, Chen H (2019) Asymptotic distribution-free change-point detection for multivariate and non-Euclidean data. Ann Stat 47(1):382–414

Machine Learning Performance Analysis for Classification of Medical Specialties

Dimas Chaerul Ekty Saputra, Yusuf Maulana, Evvin Faristasari, Alfian Ma'arif, and Iswanto Suwarno

Abstract Recently supervised machine learning studies have become increasingly significant due to the increasing availability of electronic documents from different sources. Text classification can be defined as a task that automatically categorizes a group of documents into one or more predefined classes according to the subject. The main purpose of text classification is to assist users in extracting information from textual sources and dealing with processes such as retrieval, classification, and machine learning techniques together to classify different patterns. Based on machine learning algorithms, the text classification system includes four processes, that is text preprocessing, text representation, classification, and evaluation. In this paper, a text classification system model for medical specialties is designed. This research aims to assist nurses in diagnosing patients more quickly through the text of the patient's medical record so that it can be recommended to a more appropriate medical specialty. In the classification section, we separately select and compare five different methods, that is multi-layer Perceptron, Logistic Regression, Random Forest, K-Nearest Neighbor, and Support Vector Machine as our classification algorithm. The best method for 4,998 data and 40 classes is Random Forest and Multi-Layer Perceptron with an accuracy of 47.53%. Then, we tested and analyzed the classifier model to conclude. The experimental conclusion shows that the medical

D. C. E. Saputra (✉)
Department of Computer Science and Information Technology, College of Computing, Khon Kaen University, Khon Kaen, Thailand
e-mail: dimaschaerulekty.s@kkumail.com

Y. Maulana · E. Faristasari
Department of Biomedical Engineering, Graduate School, Universitas Gadjah Mada, Yogyakarta, Indonesia

A. Ma'arif
Department of Electrical Engineering, Faculty of Industrial Technology, Universitas Ahmad Dahlan, Yogyakarta, Indonesia

I. Suwarno
Department of Electrical Engineering, Faculty of Engineering, Universitas Muhammadiyah Yogyakarta, Yogyakarta, Indonesia

T. Triwiyanto et al. (eds.), *Proceeding of the 3rd International Conference on Electronics, Biomedical Engineering, and Health Informatics*, Lecture Notes in Electrical Engineering 1008, https://doi.org/10.1007/978-981-99-0248-4_34

specialization text classification system still obtains results that are not optimal based on machine learning algorithms.

Keywords Text classification · Text representation · Medical specialization · Machine learning · Evaluation

1 Introduction

The health sector has its own challenges in classifying various types of patient diagnoses that are useful for the integration of the health care system, this is also discussed in research [1] which explains that scientific collaboration with various health workers plays an important role in improving the quality of patient health by considering examination according to the patient's condition. Tracking patient health requires a process that starts from reading patient complaints upon arrival to treatment obtained while in the hospital from medical records to retrieve information needed when as an ongoing evaluation [2]. The classification system in the health sector can assist the performance of medical personnel in classifying types of treatment, therapy, and diagnosis [3]. Text classification has an approach to grouping various documents based on certain goals so that it takes a technique using machine learning in processing the process which is collected from a large amount of data that continues to grow every day using Natural Language Processing (NLP) which is one of the contributions of Artificial Intelligence (AI) [4, 5].

A medical record is any written or recorded information about an individual's identity, medical history, physical examination, laboratory results, and diagnosis of all medical services and actions provided to patients and treatment, including inpatients, outpatients, and those receiving emergency services [6]. Medical records have a far broader meaning than just tracking activities [7]. However, it is recognized as a medical record management system [8]. While the recording activity is simply one component of medical record management [9].

Organizing medical records is a procedure that begins when the patient is admitted to the hospital and continues as long as the patient gets medical care at the hospital [10]. And then proceed with the processing of medical record files, which includes the storage and release of files from the storage area to service requests/borrows from patients or for other purposes [11]. This paper is compiled by coding using the python programming language in classifying text based on patient data.

Medical records have much important information that can be processed to make patient decisions. Currently, medical records only function when the patient wants to seek treatment or the doctor wants to provide further action when the patient is seeking treatment. In fact, with the very diverse medical record information, it can be used as a form of recommendation for health facilities for patients who need immediate treatment. The development of the world of machine learning is growing significantly, so it is possible to apply this technology to medical record data. This aims to increase the acceleration of patient handling in health facilities to reduce greater risks.

There are many studies that have been done in medical classification, such as [12] using the ensemble meta-learning method with baseline deep learning using two levels of meta-classifier can improve performance than the state of art ensemble method [13] using Naive Bayes, SVM, Logistic Regression, and Random Forest, XLNet, BERT, RoBERTa, ALBERT, DistillBERT, FastText, Logit, CNN-LSTM, Ordered Logit, BiLSTM, CNN, LSTM, MNB, XGBoost, FNN, AdaBoost, KNN, Decision Tree explains that the selection of methods should be based on the purpose of prediction. While the research conducted by [14] using a combination of multilayer perceptron (MLP) neural network and Markov chain (MC) to predict the number of patients discharged and death from the number of hospitalized patients with better accuracy. This study aims to facilitate medical personnel in classifying texts related to specific diseases based on the medical records of each patient so that they can provide appropriate medical specialty recommendations.

2 Methods

2.1 Dataset

The dataset contains medical specification information and patient medical transcriptions that describe the patient's condition and correct referrals. Data is crawled from https://www.kaggle.com/code/ritheshsreenivasan/clinical-text-classification/data. The dataset consists of 40 classes with five attributes used for processing classification text using five different machine learning methods, that is Multi-Layer Perceptron, Logistic Regression, Random Forest, k-Nearest Neighbor, and Support Vector Machine. Table 1 is the dataset used in this study. There are 4.998 patient medical records with 40 different classes. Consider Fig. 1 regarding the amount of data in each dataset class.

Table 1 Confusion matrix [28]

Prediction	True values	
	True	False
True	TP	FP
False	FN	TN

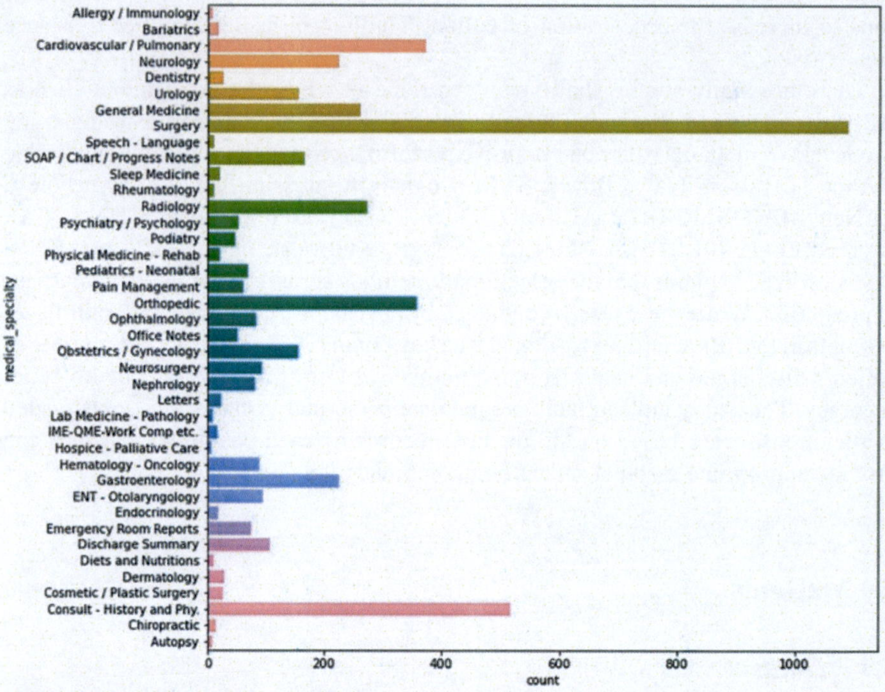

Fig. 1 Dataset recapitulation for each class

2.2 *Multi-layer Perceptron*

Perceptron, known as part of a neural network introduced in the 1950s, is a simple algorithm to perform a binary classification that is to predict whether an input is in the yes or no category or in binary (-1 and 1) [15, 16]. A perceptron is classified as linear in the sense that it is used to separate categories with a straight line. The input is usually a vector x which is then multiplied by the weight w and added to the bias or y. Where y is the bias equation, w is the weight, x is the input vector, b is the bias, and π is the non-linear activation function [17] Eq. (1).

$$y = \varphi\left(\sum_{i=1}^{n} w_i x_i + b\right) = \varphi(W^T X + b) \tag{1}$$

Each layer is represented as $y = f(WxT + b)$. Where f is the activation function (covered below), W is the set of parameters, or weights, in the layer, x is the input vector, which can also be the previous layer's output, and b is the bias vector.

In a Multilayer perceptron, there can be more than one linear layer (a combination of neurons) (Fig. 2). MLP consists of three layers; namely, the first layer is the input layer. The middle layer is the hidden layer, and the last layer is the output layer. The

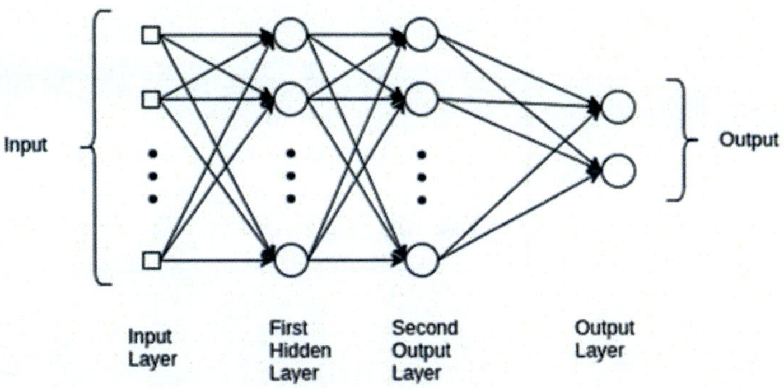

Fig. 2 Multi-layer perceptron architecture [19]

input data will be entered first into the input layer to find the output, then into the output layer. In the hidden layer, we can add as much data as we want to make the model more complex as we wish [18].

2.3 *Logistic Regression*

Logistics Regression (LR) is machine learning with probability modeling on data with discrete results given input variables [20]. The model most often used in this method uses binary results, which have only two values: true/false, yes/no, and so on [21]. Meanwhile, multinomial LR is used to model scenarios where there are more than two possible discrete outcomes. LR is an analytical machine learning method used to perform classification, where the user will determine whether the new sample entered best fits which category [22]. For example, in the cybersecurity aspect, which is one of the classification problems, such as attack detection, LR is the most frequently used analysis method. LR is very suitable to be used for binary classification problems. LR uses the logistic function defined below to model binary output variables [23] (Eq. 2)

$$LF = \frac{1}{1 + e^{-x}} \tag{2}$$

where LF is defined as the net input.

$$z = w_0x_0 + w_1x_1 + \cdots + w_mx_m = \sum_{j=0}^{m} w_jx_j = w^Tx$$

The net input is in turn based on the logit function.

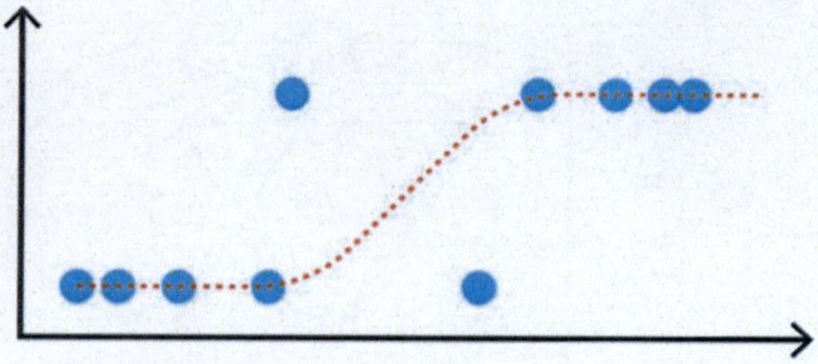

Fig. 3 Logistic regression architecture

$$logit(p(y = 1|x)) = z$$

Here, $p(y = 1|x) p(y = 1|x)$ is conditional probability indicating that a particular sample belongs to class 1, which has the feature. This logit function will later take input with a range of [0, 1] and convert it back into a value above the range of natural numbers. Meanwhile, in contrast to the logistic function, it will take the input value above the actual number range and then convert it to a value with the range [0, 1]. From the above, it can be concluded that the logistic function is the inverse of the logit function. This will allow us to predict the conditional probability that a particular sample belongs to class 1 (or class 0) (Fig. 3).

2.4 Random Forest

Random Forest (RF) is a machine learning method that consists of a collection of unprotected classification or regression trees caused by training data samples that use random feature selection in the tree induction process [24]. Predictions using RF are made by combining the form of the most votes for classification or the average regression value of the ensemble predictions. RF generally shows substantial performance improvements (such as f-1 score and accuracy) compared to single tree classifiers such as the C4.5 Algorithm. Of concern, RF can also fail or fail when the training data set makes the tree unbalanced (Eq. 3). RF is built to minimize the error rate in the overall data, which is more focused on the prediction accuracy level of the majority class, thus producing poorer accuracy for the minority class [25, 26] (Fig. 4).

$$\text{Entropy} = \sum_{j=1} -p_j \cdot log_2 \cdot p_j \tag{3}$$

where p_j is the probability of class j.

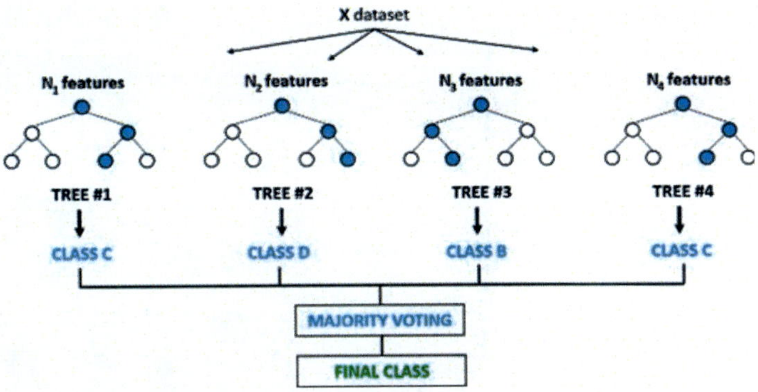

Fig. 4 Random forest visualization [27]

Pseudo-Code Random Forest:

```
clf = RandomForestClassifier(n_estimators=100,
criterion = 'entropy', random_state = 0)
```

Pseudo-Code Entropy Random Forest:

```
for each branch in split:
    Calculate percent branch represents #Used for
    weighting
    for each class in branch:
        Calculate probability of class in the given
        branch.
                Multiply probability times
                log(Probability,base=2)
                Multiply that product by -1
                Sum the calculated probabilities.
                Weight each branch based on the
                baseline probability.
                Sum the weighted entropy for each
                split.
```

2.5 K-nearest Neighbor

K-Nearest Neighbor (KNN) is an algorithm used for classifying data [28]. The data obtained must go through the *Euclidean Distance* search process to find the nearest neighbor [29] (Eq. 4). The grade of K data used in KNN is known. The value of K is an *integer* number. KNN visualization can be seen in Fig. 5.

Fig. 5 KNN visualization [28]

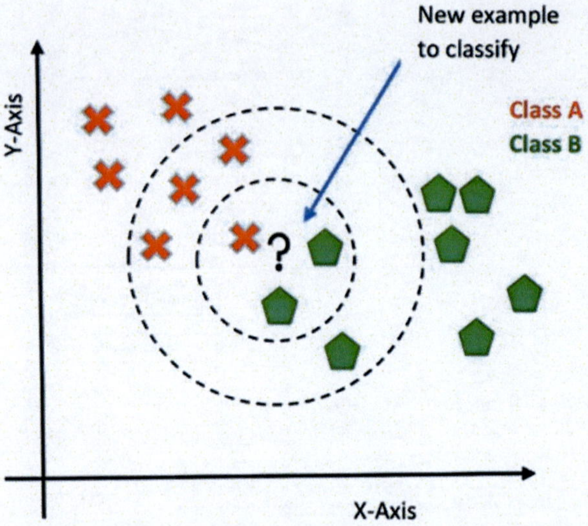

$$d(x, y) = \sqrt{\sum_{i=1}^{n} (x_i - y_i)^2} \tag{4}$$

where d indicates dissimilarity degree, n is the number of vectors, x shows the input image vector, and y indicates comparison image vector/output.

If there are 2 data whose class is known, then we can determine the class of a data X by looking at the K closest neighbors. For example, K = 3, then the class of the 3 nearest neighbors of X data is red, green, and green. Because 80% of the nearest neighbors are green, the data class X prediction is green. Meanwhile, if K = 7, then the classes of the 2 closest neighbors from data X are red, red, red, red, green, green, and green. So, the prediction result from data X is red. So, it can be concluded that the KNN algorithm is an algorithm to perform a classification based on the data of the most dominant class based on a predetermined K value.

2.6 Support Vector Machine

Support Vector Machine (SVM) is an algorithm that uses non-linear mapping that is used to convert training data into training data that has higher dimensions [30]. In this method, each data item will be plotted as a point in n-dimensional space (n is the number of features) with the value contained in each feature which then becomes a certain coordinate value. The next step, classification, will be done by finding the best hyperplane that is able to distinguish the two classes so that each input data from each category will be separated by a gap in the hyperplane. The new sample results or output from the classification will be mapped into the same space and predicted to

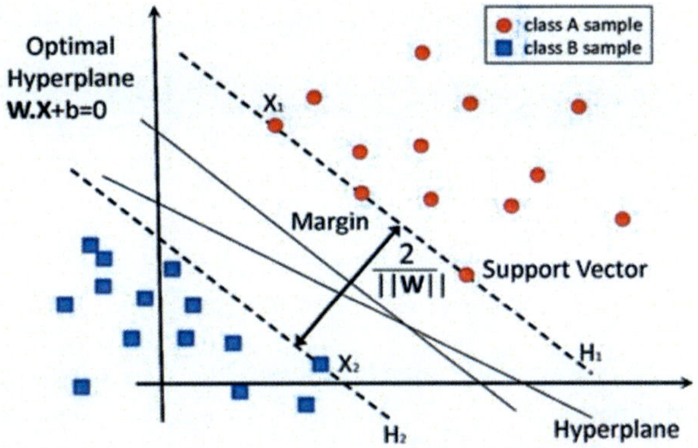

Fig. 6 SVM visualization [32]

fall into categories based on the side gap fit. A hyperplane H in n-dimensional space is a set of points $(x_1, x_2, \ldots, x_n)$ that satisfy a linear equation [31] (Eq. 5).

$$a_1x_1 + a_2x_2 + \cdots + a_nx_n \tag{5}$$

where a is slack variables, x is set of points

For SVM, there can be an infinite number of separate hyper fields (Fig. 6). The best one should be found which will have minimum misclassification on previously unseen tuples.

2.7 *Confusion Matrix*

The confusion matrix aims to assess the performance of machine learning in performing the classification used and to describe the performance of the classification model on the test data the actual value is known. Confusion matrices are usually very easy to reach, but the terminology can be astounding [28, 29].

From Table 1, it can be explained that:

1. TP, namely True Positive, is the number of positive data that is classified correctly by the system.
2. TN, which is True Negative, is the number of negative data correctly classified by the system.
3. FN, namely False Negative, is the number of negative data but is classified incorrectly by the system.
4. FP, which is False Positive, is the number of positive data but is classified as wrong by the system.

Based on the values above, it can produce values of accuracy, precision, recall/sensitivity, and F1-Measure. The formulas for calculating the value can be explained as follows.

Accuracy is shown in Eq. (6)

$$\frac{\text{TP} + \text{TN}}{\text{TP} + \text{TN} + \text{FP} + \text{FN}} \tag{6}$$

Precision is shown in Eq. (7)

$$\frac{\text{TP}}{\text{FP} + \text{FN}} \tag{7}$$

Precision is the match between the part of the data taken with the required information.

Recall is shown in Eq. (8)

$$\frac{\text{TP}}{\text{FP} + \text{FN}} \tag{8}$$

The recall is a return of information—the system's success rate in finding the Accuracy obtained against the actual value.

F1-Measure is shown in Eq. (9)

$$2 \times \frac{\text{Recall} \times \text{Precision}}{\text{Recall} + \text{Precision}} \tag{9}$$

F-1 score is the Harmonic Mean value of Precision and Recall. If the F1-Score scores, our classification model has good precision and recall.

3 Result and Discussion

3.1 Pre-processing

In this study, the dataset went through a preprocessing stage by adding a number of features to the data set, namely the number of words, characters, and punctuation marks in the data description, medical specialization, sample name, transcription, and keywords. Then clean and sort the data into certain patterns to get a clean dataset and process it to the next stage (Fig. 7).

Fig. 7 Text preprocessing

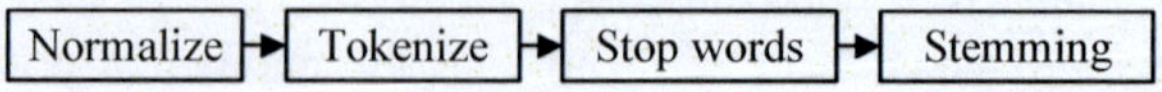

3.2 Text Representation

Text Representation used in this study using Bag of Word (BoW). Bag of Word is a basic technique in Natural Language Processing (NLP) to convert words in vector form and is used in NLP applications. In simple terms, BoW itself is a representation of words into vectors whose values are zero (0) and one (1). These words can come from various sentences and paragraphs (Eq. 10).

$$W_{x,y} = tf_{x,y} \times \log\left(\frac{N}{df_x}\right) \tag{10}$$

where $\boldsymbol{tf_{x,y}}$ is the frequency of $\boldsymbol{x}$ in $\boldsymbol{y}$, $\boldsymbol{df_x}$ is the number of documents containing $\boldsymbol{x}$, and N is a total number of documents

3.3 Classification

The model used to perform the classification uses:

1. SVMs
   Supervised machine learning algorithm that can be used for classification and regression. SVM works based on SRM or Structural Risk Minimization, which is designed to process data into a Hyperplane that classifies the input space into two classes. SVM theory begins with linear grouping cases that can be separated by hyperplane and divided according to their class. The kernel used in this method uses the RBF kernel.
2. Logistic Regression
   Logistic regression is a classification machine learning algorithm that is commonly used to find the relationship between one feature and another discrete/continuous (input) feature with a certain discrete output probability. In this method, various penalties are used based on the algorithms in Logistic Regression, such as lbfgs, saga, and sag.
3. K-Nearest Neighbor
   An algorithm that functions to classify data based on learning data (train data sets) is taken from k closest neighbors (nearest neighbors). Where k is the number of nearest neighbors. K-nearest neighbors perform classification by projecting learning data on a multidimensional space. This space is divided into sections that represent the learning data criteria. Each learning data is defined as point c in a multidimensional space. Two algorithms are used in K-NN, namely, the K-d tree and the Ball Tree.
4. Random Forest
   A random forest is machine learning that consists of a combination of each tree which is then combined into a single model for classification. Random Forest is highly dependent on an arbitrary vector value with the same distribution in all

Table 2 Performance evaluation of each method

Method	Algorithm	Accuracy (%)
SVMs	–	42.61
MLP	**Adam**	**47.53**
KNN	K-d Tree	47.51
KNN	Ball Tree	47.51
Random forest	**n_estimators: 100 Criterion: Entropy**	**47.53**
Logistic regression	Saga Penalty: None	46.38
Logistic regression	Lbfgs Penalty: None	47.25
Logistic regression	Newton-cg Penalty: l2	47.25
Logistic regression	Liblinear Penalty: l2	47.11
Logistic regression	Saga Penalty: None	47.49
Logistic regression	Sag Penalty: None	47.51
Logistic regression	Sag Penalty: l2	47.29

trees; each decision tree in the model has a maximum depth. In this method, the number of estimators (n_estimator) used in this method is 100.

5. Multi-Layer Perceptron
   Multi-layer perceptron (MLP) is one of the models in artificial neural network (ANN) technology with a better weight value than other models, resulting in more accurate classification. In this study using the following parameters: Hidden layer: 5000. Solver: adam. Learning rate: adaptive. Activation: relu.

3.4 Evaluation

Table 2 is the results of the comparison of each method and algorithm used in this study.

3.5 Discussion

Based on all the methods used, the Multilayer Perceptron and Random Forest methods are the methods with the highest accuracy, which is only 47.53%. Of course, this is a fairly low accuracy rate, this is due to several possibilities, including the occurrence of imbalanced datasets between medical specialty classed as surgery, totaling 1.103 data, while Hospice—Palliative Care only had 6 data and some classes only had less than 20 data. This causes the data training process to be not good, so it has consequences in testing the data will have a decreased accuracy. In addition, another thing that causes low accuracy is the detail of the transcription of patients with doctors. This makes it possible when a patient consults with a doctor, the information conveyed is not detailed and specific, so keywords in the medical specialty class will be affected, causing the accuracy value to decrease.

Support Vector Machine (SVM) is a classifier to find the best hyperplane by maximizing the distance between classes. The hyperplane is a function that can be used to separate between classes. This algorithm generates an optimal hyperplane that categorizes the new example. This model provides an accuracy of 42.61%. Multilayer perceptron (MLP) is a class of feedforward artificial neural networks. An artificial neural network (ANN) is a computational model based on the structure and function of a biological neural network. Information flowing through the network affects the structure of the ANN because the network changes to input and output. This model provides the highest accuracy of the various configurations tested at 47.53%. The K-Nearest Neighbor Algorithm (k-NN or KNN) is a method for classifying objects based on the learning data closest to the object. Learning data is projected onto a multidimensional space, each dimension representing a data feature. This model provides the highest accuracy of the various configurations tested at 47.51%. Random Forest Classifier This model provides the highest and most stable accuracy in each configuration tested, which is 47.53%. Therefore, this model can be the best for predicting the predictive results of this study. Logistic regression is used to predict the probability of the occurrence of an event by matching the data to the logit function of the logistics curve. This method is a general linear model commonly used for binomial regression. This model provides the highest accuracy of the configurations tried at 47.51%. Research with other NLP techniques, especially on health topics, uses datasets such as CT, MRI corpus medic, Ohsumed, and medical notes. The average research carried out has the highest accuracy value of 86.32%. While research on the classification of medical specialties is still little done, this paper's highest accuracy is still 47.53%. This is because many classes are used in the dataset, and there is an imbalanced dataset.

Limitations in this study, due to the many diseases experienced by patients, affect the medical specialty recommendations on machine learning systems. To improve accuracy, future research can be done by adding medical record data from patients with more specific diseases, for example, common diseases that occur in the community. This makes it possible to obtain a higher classification accuracy of common illnesses so that treatment can be carried out more quickly. This research aims to assist nurses in diagnosing patients more quickly through the text of the patient's medical record so that it can be recommended to a more appropriate medical specialty. This research is the first step to help health workers in health facilities so that in the future, it is expected to help diagnose patients' illnesses more quickly based on medical records. In the end, it is also necessary to add a medical record database so that the results of the recommendations are to the expected results. This research has implications for preliminary research to apply patient medical record data in helping patients find specialist doctor recommendations according to the condition of their medical records to reduce the risk of death or severity.

4 Conclusion

This paper is compiling a transcription of patient complaints with a classification system model using machine learning algorithms. This paper describes K nearest neighbors, Multi-layer Perceptron algorithm, Logistic Regression algorithm, Random Forest algorithm, Support Vector Machine algorithm with linear kernel and RBF, and describes every aspect of the system model in detail, providing evaluation metrics. The results show that the Logistic Regression classifier with the tf-idf feature achieves the highest accuracy and is the most stable in large-scale datasets. However, there are many problems with text classifiers on datasets such as that small classes yield better results than large classes, and that there is insufficient semantic information on text features. Thus, how to make classification more effective is the next main content of the study.

References

1. Kocher KE, Arora R, Bassin BS, Benjamin LS, Bolton M, Dennis BJ, Ham JJ, Krupp SS, Levasseur KA, Macy ML, O'Neil BJ, Pribble JM, Sherwin RL, Sroufe NS, Uren BJ, Nypaver MM (2020) Baseline performance of real-world clinical practice within a statewide emergency medicine quality network: the Michigan Emergency Department Improvement Collaborative (MEDIC). Ann Emerg Med 75:192–205. https://doi.org/10.1016/j.annemergmed.2019.04.033
2. Collins S, Klinkenberg-Ramirez S, Tsivkin K, Mar PL, Iskhakova D, Nandigam H, Samal L, Rocha RA (2017) Next generation terminology infrastructure to support interprofessional care planning. J Biomed Inform 75:22–34. https://doi.org/10.1016/j.jbi.2017.09.007
3. Duarte J, Castro S, Santos M, Abelha A, Machado J (2014) Improving quality of electronic health records with SNOMED. Procedia Technol 16:1342–1350. https://doi.org/10.1016/j.protcy.2014.10.151
4. Luo X (2021) Efficient English text classification using selected machine learning techniques. Alex Eng J 60:3401–3409. https://doi.org/10.1016/j.aej.2021.02.009
5. Cheng MY, Kusoemo D, Gosno RA (2020) Text mining-based construction site accident classification using hybrid supervised machine learning. Autom Constr 118:103265. https://doi.org/10.1016/j.autcon.2020.103265
6. Sun Y, Liu J, Yu K, Alazab M, Lin K (2022) PMRSS: privacy-preserving medical record searching scheme for intelligent diagnosis in IoT healthcare. IEEE Trans Ind Inf 18:1981–1990. https://doi.org/10.1109/TII.2021.3070544
7. DesRoches CM, Leveille S, Bell SK, Dong ZJ, Elmore JG, Fernandez L, Harcourt K, Fitzgerald P, Payne TH, Stametz R, Delbanco T, Walker J (2020) The views and experiences of clinicians sharing medical record notes with patients. JAMA Netw Open 3:e201753. https://doi.org/10.1001/jamanetworkopen.2020.1753

8. Subahi AF (2019) Edge-based IoT Medical record system: requirements, recommendations and conceptual design. IEEE Access 7:94150–94159. https://doi.org/10.1109/ACCESS.2019.2927958
9. Barlow C (2020) Oncology research: clinical trial management systems, electronic medical record, and artificial intelligence. Semin Oncol Nurs 36:151005. https://doi.org/10.1016/j.soncn.2020.151005
10. Chushig-Muzo D, Soguero-Ruiz C, Engelbrecht AP, De Miguel Bohoyo P, Mora-Jimenez I (2020) Data-driven visual characterization of patient health-status using electronic health records and self-organizing maps. IEEE Access 8:137019–137031. https://doi.org/10.1109/ACCESS.2020.3012082
11. Sun W, Cai Z, Li Y, Liu F, Fang S, Wang G (2018) Data processing and text mining technologies on electronic medical records: a review. J Healthcare Eng 2018:1–9. https://doi.org/10.1155/2018/4302425
12. Mohammed A, Kora R (2021) A novel effective ensemble deep learning framework for text classification. J King Saud Univ—Comput Inf Sci. https://doi.org/10.1016/j.jksuci.2021.11.001
13. Alantari HJ, Currim IS, Deng Y, Singh S (2021) An empirical comparison of machine learning methods for text-based sentiment analysis of online consumer reviews. Int J Res Mark. https://doi.org/10.1016/j.ijresmar.2021.10.011
14. Haghighat F (2021) Predicting the trend of indicators related to Covid-19 using the combined MLP-MC model. Chaos Solitons Fractals 152:111399. https://doi.org/10.1016/j.chaos.2021.111399
15. Chitore S, Phalke DAM (2017) Sentiment analysis with multilayer perceptron using emoticon space model. Int J Adv Eng Res Dev 4:410–419
16. Pamiela GA, Azhari A (2021) Deep learning on EEG study concentration in pandemic. Jurnal Ilmiah Ilmu Komputer 16:10. https://doi.org/10.30872/jim.v16i2.6474
17. Akhtar MS, Kumar A, Ghosal D, Ekbal A, Bhattacharyya P (2017) A multilayer perceptron based ensemble technique for fine-grained financial sentiment analysis. In: EMNLP 2017—conference on empirical methods in natural language processing, proceedings, pp 540–546. https://doi.org/10.18653/v1/d17-1057
18. Gururangan S, Dang T, Card D, Smith NA (2019) Variational pretraining for semi-supervised text classification. https://doi.org/10.48550/ARXIV.1906.02242
19. Wang Y, Li X, Zhang LL, Mo D (2021) Configuring products with natural language: a simple yet effective approach based on text embeddings and multilayer perceptron. Int J Prod Res 1–13. https://doi.org/10.1080/00207543.2021.1957508
20. Padurariu C, Breaban ME (2019) Dealing with data imbalance in text classification. Procedia Comput Sci 159:736–745. https://doi.org/10.1016/j.procs.2019.09.229
21. Pranckevičius T, Marcinkevičius V (2017) Comparison of naive bayes, random forest, decision tree, support vector machines, and logistic regression classifiers for text reviews classification. Baltic J Modern Comput 5:221–232. https://doi.org/10.22364/bjmc.2017.5.2.05
22. Vimal B (2020) Application of logistic regression in natural language processing. Int J Eng Res 9. https://doi.org/10.17577/ijertv9is060095
23. Tolles J, Meurer WJ (2016) Logistic regression: Relating patient characteristics to outcomes. JAMA—J Am Med Assoc 316:533–534. https://doi.org/10.1001/jama.2016.7653
24. Salles T, Gonçalves M, Rodrigues V, Rocha L (2018) Improving random forests by neighborhood projection for effective text classification. Inf Syst 77:1–21. https://doi.org/10.1016/j.is.2018.05.006
25. Tong Y, Lu K, Yang Y, Li J, Lin Y, Wu D, Yang A, Li Y, Yu S, Qian J (2020) Can natural language processing help differentiate inflammatory intestinal diseases in China? Models applying random forest and convolutional neural network approaches. BMC Med Inform Decis Mak 20:248. https://doi.org/10.1186/s12911-020-01277-w
26. Antony Vijay J, Anwar Basha H, Arun Nehru J (2021) A dynamic approach for detecting the fake news using random forest classifier and NLP. In: Singh V, Asari VK, Kumar S, Patel RB (eds) Computational methods and data engineering. Springer Singapore, Singapore, pp 331–341. https://doi.org/10.1007/978-981-15-7907-3_25

27. Abilash R, Applying random forest (classification)—machine learning algorithm from scratch with real datasets. https://medium.com/@ar.ingenious/applying-random-forest-classification-machine-learning-algorithm-from-scratch-with-real-24ff198a1c57. Last accessed 29 May 2022
28. Saputra DCE, Azhari A, Ma'arif A (2022) K-nearest neighbor of beta signal brainwave to accelerate detection of concentration on student learning outcomes. Eng Lett 30:234–318. http://www.engineeringletters.com/issues_v30/issue_1/EL_30_1_38.pdf
29. Chen Z, Zhou LJ, Li XD, Zhang JN, Huo WJ (2020) The Lao text classification method based on KNN. Procedia Comput Sci 166:523–528. https://doi.org/10.1016/j.procs.2020.02.053
30. Goudjil M, Koudil M, Bedda M, Ghoggali N (2018) A novel active learning method using SVM for text classification. Int J Autom Comput 15:290–298. https://doi.org/10.1007/s11633-015-0912-z
31. Abu Taher S, Afsana Akhter K, Azharul Hasan KM (2018) N-gram based sentiment mining for Bangla text using support vector machine. In: 2018 international conference on Bangla speech and language processing, ICBSLP 2018, pp 21–22. https://doi.org/10.1109/ICBSLP.2018.8554716
32. García-Gonzalo E, Fernández-Muñiz Z, Nieto PJG, Sánchez AB, Fernández MM (2016) Hard-rock stability analysis for span design in entry-type excavations with learning classifiers. Materials 9:1–19. https://doi.org/10.3390/ma9070531

Controlling the Temperature of PID System-Based Baby Incubator to Reduction Overshoot

Bambang Guruh Irianto, Anita Miftahul Maghfiroh, Moh Sofie, Abd. Kholiq, Syevana Dita Musvika, and Dzulhij Aulia Akbar

Abstract According to estimates, there are 15 million preterm births each year and 1 million fatalities as a result of the viability gap between high-income and low-income nations. Lack of basic medical care and adequate equipment, such as an incubator, contributes to a large number of newborn fatalities that might have been prevented. An incubator is medical equipment for premature infant treatment functioning to give warmth, moisture, and oxygen as required for newborn babies in a controlled condition. Therefore, this study aimed at making a correct control system for controlling the temperature of the baby incubator to meet the predetermined standard value. The advantage of this study was that selecting the correct control system could help minimize the overshoot value at room temperature in a baby incubator. Furthermore, for keeping the temperature stability of a heater, it was controlled by the PID control system to prevent the oscillation of the predetermined maximum overshoot value from exceeding 5%. From the measurement result between the reading of the AHT10 sensor and INCU Analyzer, the error at different temperature settings, namely 33, 34, 35, 36, and 37 °C, was less than 5% respectively. Meanwhile, the t-test obtained a p-value greater than 0.05. Besides, the overshoot value and steady-state error were less than 5%. This study is expected to be able to better control and produce temperature stability faster as well as reduce the overshoot at a low temperature.

Keywords Baby incubator PID · System · Temperature

B. G. Irianto · A. M. Maghfiroh (✉) · Abd. Kholiq · S. D. Musvika · D. A. Akbar
Department of Electromedical Engineering, Politeknik Kesehatan Kemenkes Surabaya, Surabaya, Indonesia
e-mail: anitamiftah@poltekkesdepkes-sby.ac.id

M. Sofie
Akademi Teknik Elektromedik, Sekolah Tinggi Kesehatan Semarang, Semarang, Indonesia

T. Triwiyanto et al. (eds.), *Proceeding of the 3rd International Conference on Electronics, Biomedical Engineering, and Health Informatics*, Lecture Notes in Electrical Engineering 1008, https://doi.org/10.1007/978-981-99-0248-4_35

1 Introduction

It is estimated around 15 million premature infants and one million deaths annually [1] because of the disparity in viability between high- and low-income countries. Preterm births typically happen before 34 weeks of pregnancy [2, 3]. According to UNICEF, Indonesia's premature birth rate on January 18th, 2018, ranked sixth with a total of 13,370 premature infants [4]. Many premature infant deaths are caused by the factor of lacking simple treatment and sufficient medical equipment, such as an incubator [5–7]. An incubator is medical equipment for premature infant treatment functioning to give warmth, moisture, and oxygen as required for newborn babies in a controlled condition [8–10]. Even congenital heart disease can result in a fetus being born prematurely since it puts them at risk for cardiac issues[11, 12]. Premature children are housed in an area known as the Neonatal Intensive Care Unit (NICU), where they are kept warm like they were in the womb by a baby incubator. Therefore, a correct control system is needed to set the temperature of a baby incubator to give warmth according to the predetermined standard [13]. Some researchers had developed a control system for baby incubators [6, 13–15], Hitu Bansal et al. created and used a closed-loop control system to regulate the temperature, moisture, light level, and oxygen in a neonatal incubator [16]. This system is quite effective for maintaining the threshold temperature. However, the threshold value is still set manually using a potentiometer. Ary Virgiawan Zaelani et al., the natural convection and natural circulation method were used in a baby incubator; the main component is a lamp as a heater and digital thermostat as a temperature controller [17, 18]. If the baby incubator is merely operating at ambient temperature, this technology is highly effective and steady. Fuzzy-PI control adaptive was implemented for a baby incubator by Sumardi et al.; DHT11 was used as a temperature sensor and a fluorescent light was used as a control method [19]. This system is considered to be able to stabilize and restore the system response to the desired reference temperature. Nevertheless, the computation in this system is quite difficult. The baby incubator made by Megha Koli et al. was equipped with an IoT system to monitor the temperature in the baby [20, 21], however, the temperature control used here was the Arduino program. So, this system tended to have a higher overshoot value. The temperature stability was controlled using the Fuzzy-PID system by Satryo Budi Utomo et al.; this system was measured using a DHT22 sensor and the heating system was measured using a fluorescent light [4]. The weakness when the heating system using a fluorescent light was that the temperature stability based on the temperature setting needed a longer time. Muslim Ali et al. used Arduino to control the temperature in the baby incubator [22] by using 2 temperature sensors for measuring the stability of DHT11 temperature. This system can control the temperature automatically. However, the overshoot value in this system is unidentified.

Some researchers developed a control system in a baby incubator, and some other researchers also developed the automatic control and used the PID control system [23]. Nonetheless, as far as the author knows, some authors did not investigate the overshoot value of each control system that was developed and the heating system still used a fluorescent light. Therefore, this study aimed at making a correct control system to prevent the overshoot value from exceeding the predetermined standard value. The contribution obtained in this study is that other researchers can use references in designing baby incubators by paying attention to the level of overshoot so that the monitored room temperature remains at standard limits. The PID control system used in this study was the AHT10 sensor for measuring the temperature in the baby incubator; then, for the heating system, the researcher used the 350 W-dry heater. This study is expected to be able to better control the temperature and produce temperature stability faster as well as reduce the overshoot at a low temperature. The next chapters in this paper following this chapter were arranged in the following order: Sect. 2 discusses the subject, data acquisition, data collection, data processing, and statistical analysis, while Sect. 3 explains the result and research findings. Subsequently, Sect. 4 discusses the result of the study and compares it with other studies and the implication. Further, Sect. 5 concludes the study entirely.

2 Research Method

2.1 Data Acquisition

This study used the AHT10 sensor to monitor the temperature in a baby incubator and a 350 W-dry heater. Next, the heater was controlled using the PID control system for maintaining the temperature stability and the oscillation of a predetermined maximum overshoot value of 5% [12]. The process of data collection for temperature was done using the INCU 2 type Incu Analyzer from the Fluke brand. In this study, the measurement was taken for 7 h to know the temperature stability in each temperature setting, namely 33, 34, 35, 36, and 37 °C, and the overshoot value of each temperature. The design of the PID control system is explained in Fig. 2. The temperature setting was compared with the temperature reading in the AHT10 sensor to obtain the difference in error value as the input in a microcontroller; the PID system was implanted in the microcontroller with a K_p value of 10; K_i of 0.04 and K_d of 0.8 as the output values for moving the driver heater; so, the room temperature in the baby incubator was controlled. For testing the endurance of PID, an input disturbance (interruption) was applied. In this experiment, the interruption was given by opening the baby incubator door for some minutes when the temperature was stable at a set temperature. This experiment was conducted to test the endurance of the PID control system explained in Fig. 1.

In this study, the researchers used the closed-loop PID system that experienced an interruption; the interruption in a baby incubator was detected when the temperature of the baby incubator was stable; in this case, the nurse can put a baby inside so that the door of the baby incubator opens for some minutes and it causes an interruption in temperature reading. For solving the problem, the PID system uses an equation as shown in Eqs. 1 and 2 [24]:

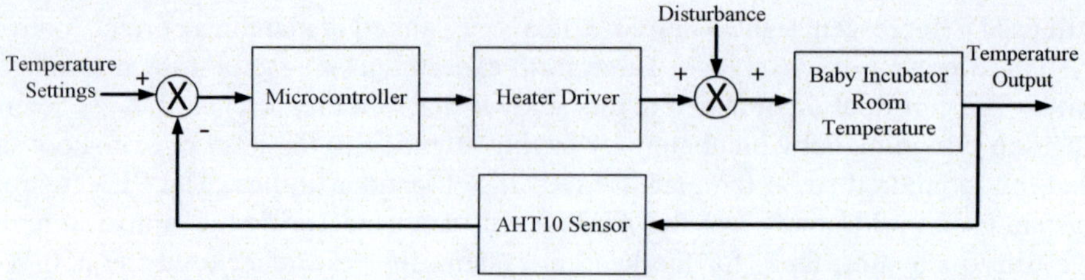

Fig. 1 The design of PID Control System, In the description of the image setting the temperature as a microcontroller input with a PID embedded system to control the heater, then after the temperature is stable, it is tested by providing interference to test the PID system

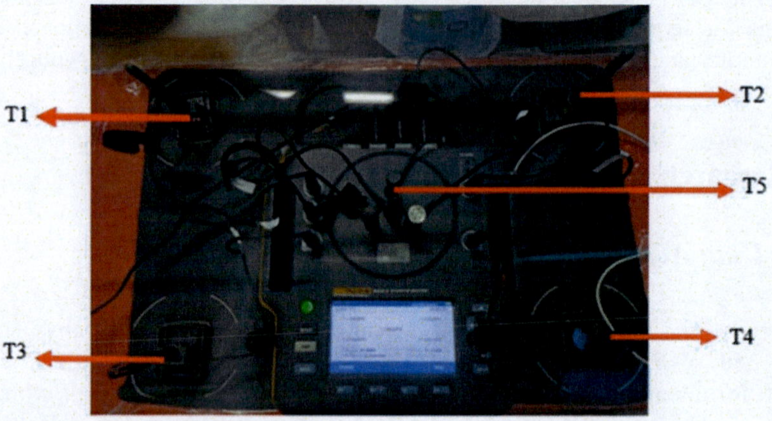

Fig. 2 Temperature data collection utilizing the Fluke INCU 2 type Incu Analyzer with temperature parameters T1, T2, T3, T4, and T5

$$G(s) = K_P + K_I \frac{1}{s} + K_D s \tag{1}$$

$$= K_P + \left(1 + \frac{1}{T_I s} + T_D s\right) \tag{2}$$

where T_i is the integral time constant, T_d is the derivative time constant, K_i is the integral gain, K_d is the derivative gain, and K_p is the proportional gain.

For a PID system that has the disturbances from Eq. 3 [25]

$$\frac{C_D(s)}{D(s)} = \frac{G_2(s)}{1 + G_1(s)G_2(s)H(s)} \tag{3}$$

where the interference effect test is $D(s)$ and $CD(s)$ is the reaction to disturbance test.

It is anticipated that there would be no disturbance in response to the reference input $R(s)$. Then, using Eq. 4, the response $CR(s)$ to the reference input $R(s)$ is obtained [25].

$$\frac{C_R(s)}{R(s)} = \frac{G_1(s)G_2(s)}{1 + G_1(s)G_2(s)H(s)} \tag{4}$$

The two individual replies are added together to give the simultaneous application of the reference and perturbation input responses. It is generated using Eq. 5 by applying the simultaneous $C(s)$ response of the reference input $R(s)$ and the disturbance $D(s)$ [25].

$$\begin{aligned} C(s) &= CR(s) + CD(s) \\ &= \frac{G_2(s)}{1 + G_1(s)G_2(s)H(s)}[G_1(s)R(s) + D(s)] \end{aligned} \tag{5}$$

To achieve satisfactory closed-loop performance in the PID system, the control system control procedure utilizes the right selection of K_p, $_{Ki}$, and K_d. These characteristics, including the response time and the appropriate amount of overshoot, must be carefully selected in order for the system's stability to be good. The system's transfer function is based on Eq. 6 [26].

$$\begin{aligned} G_{PID}(s) &= K_p + \frac{K_P}{S} + K_D S \\ &= \frac{K_D S^2 + K_p + K_I}{S} \end{aligned} \tag{6}$$

where the appropriate control for closed-loop performance is applied using the selection of K_p, K_i, and K_d.

2.2 Data Collection

In this study, the measurement was taken for 7 h to know the temperature stability in each temperature setting, namely 33, 34, 35, 36, and 37 °C. Each temperature setting was taken for 6 measurement times to know the average temperature, error, and standard deviation. The overshoot of each measurement was observed. At a temperature setting of 36 °C, when the temperature was stable, the interruption was applied by opening the baby incubator door for some seconds to know the endurance of the PID performance. This measurement uses the INCU 2 type Incu Analyzer from the Fluke brand with five points of measurement temperature at T1, T2, T3, T4, and T5 as explained in Fig. 2.

2.3 Data Processing

To achieve satisfactory closed-loop performance in the PID system, the control system method employed the right selection of K_p, K_i, and K_d. To achieve satisfactory system stability, this parameter should be properly chosen, including the appropriate response speed and overshoot level.

A system's transfer function is based on Eq. 7 [26].

$$G_{PID}(s) = K_p + \frac{K_p}{S} + K_D S = \frac{K_D S^2 + K_p + K_I}{S} \tag{7}$$

After completing the data collection process, to get the error value and the accuracy of each measurement it is necessary to calculate it based on Eq. (8) [27]:

$$\text{Mean} = \frac{\sum_{i=1}^{n} Xi}{n} = \frac{X1 + X2 + X3 \ldots Xn}{n} \tag{8}$$

where x represents the data retrieval and n is the number of data retrievals.

2.4 Statistical Analysis

In this study, the system performance was calculated based on the temperature control capability displayed on the baby incubator LCD using the PID system. The performance measurement was done in each temperature setting parameter, namely 33, 34, 35, 36, and 37 °C; the data collection was done 6 times for each temperature setting. Moreover, the interruption test was conducted at 36 °C to test the PID responses. The accuracy of the temperature reading system was measured using the standard calibration tool for the baby incubator, namely INCU Analyzer. Then, the t-test was conducted to know if there was a significant difference between the temperature reading on the AHT10 sensor and the temperature reading on INCU Analyzer. The alpha value of 0.05 was used in this study. So, a p-value greater than 0.05 indicates that there is no significant difference between the two groups. On the other hand, a p-value of less than 0.05 indicates a significant difference between the two groups.

3 Results Discussion

This study aimed at identifying the temperature stability using the PID control system by measuring the performance at various temperature parameters, namely 33, 34, 35, 36, and 37 °C; the interruption was then applied two times by opening the baby incubator door. The first interruption was tested for 5 min and the second interruption was tested for 5 min at 36 °C.

3.1 *Test Results of Temperature Control Based on PID Control System*

Table 1 explains the result of the temperature measurement read by the AHT10 sensor at a displayed temperature with the temperature reading on the INCU Analyzer in 5 points of measurement temperature, namely 5 T1, T2, T3, T4, and T5 shown in Fig. 3.

Based on the measurement result explained in Table 1 at 33 °C, the average temperature at temperature display of 33.7 °C is obtained, while the temperature reading on INCU analyzer in different points is as follows: T1 = the average temperature of 33.7 °C with an error value of 0 °C, T2 = the average temperature of 33.3 °C with an error value of 0.4 °C, T3 = the average temperature of 33.6 °C with an error value of 0.1 °C, T4 = the average temperature of 33.2 °C with an error value of 0.5 °C, and T5 = the average temperature of 34.15 °C with an error value of −0.45 °C. At a temperature setting of 34 °C, the average temperature at a temperature display is 34.7 °C, while the temperature reading on the INCU analyzer in different points is as

Table 1 The result of the temperature measurement read by AHT10 sensor at a displayed temperature with the temperature reading on INCU analyzer

Temperature setting (°C)			33	34	35	36	37
Temperature on INCU analyzer (°C)	T1	Mean	33.7	34.8	35.4	36.5	37.6
		Error (±)	0	−0.1	0.3	0.1	0.1
	T2	Mean	33.3	34.7	35	35.9	37.8
		Error (±)	0.4	0	0.7	0.7	−0.1
	T3	Mean	33.6	34.6	35.3	36.4	37
		Error (±)	0.1	0.1	0.4	0.2	0.7
	T4	Mean	33.2	34.2	35.1	36	37.2
		Error (±)	0.5	0.5	0.6	0.6	0.5
	T5	Mean	34.15	35	35.5	36.7	37.5
		Error (±)	−0.45	−0.2	−0.1	−0.2	0.1

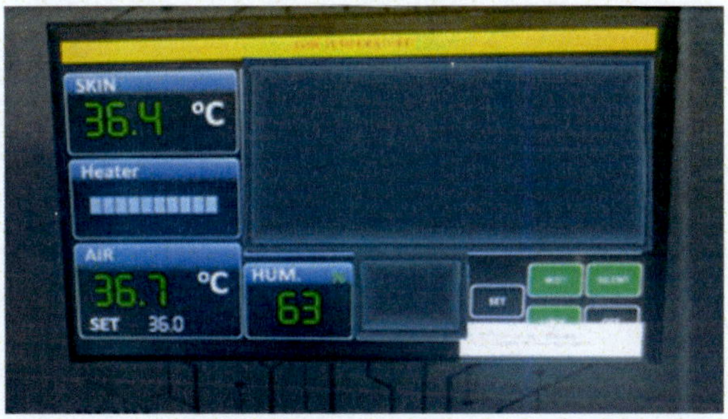

Fig. 3 Temperature on a baby incubator display. On the display there are temperature settings, display room temperature, skin temperature, humidity and display heater performance

follows: T1 = the average temperature of 34.8 °C with an error value of −0.1 °C, T2 = the average temperature of 34.7 °C with an error value of 0 °C, T3 = the average temperature of 34.6 °C with an error value of 0.1 °C, T4 = the average temperature of 34.2 °C with an error value of 0.5 °C, and T5 = the average temperature of 35 °C with an error value of −0.2 °C. At a temperature setting of 35 °C, the average temperature at a temperature display is 35.7 °C, while the temperature reading on the INCU analyzer in different points is as follows: T1 = the average temperature of 35.4 °C with an error value of 0.3 °C, T2 = the average temperature of 35 °C with an error value of 0.7 °C, T3 = the average temperature of 35.3 °C with an error value of 0.4 °C, T4 = the average temperature of 35.1 °C with an error value of 0.6 °C, and T5 = the average temperature of 35.5 °C with an error value of −0.1 °C. At a temperature setting of 36 °C, the average temperature at a temperature display is 36.6 °C, while the temperature reading on the INCU analyzer in different points is as follows: T1 = the average temperature of 36.5 °C with an error value of 0.1 °C, T2 = the average temperature of 35.9 °C with an error value of 0.7 °C, T3 = the average temperature of 36.4 °C with an error value of 0.2 °C, T4 = the average temperature of 36 °C with an error value of 0.6 °C, and T5 = the average temperature of 36.7 °C with an error value of −0.2 °C. At a temperature setting 37 °C, the average temperature at a temperature display is 37.7 °C, while the temperature reading on the INCU analyzer in different points is as follows: T1 = the average temperature of 37.6 °C with error value of −0.1 °C, T2 = the average temperature of 37.8 °C with an error value of −0.1 °C, T3 = the average temperature of 37 °C with an error value of 0.7 °C, T4 = the average temperature of 37.2 °C with an error value of 0.5 °C, and T5 = the average temperature of 37.5 °C with an error value of 0.1 °C. From the information, it can be inferred that the average error value is less than 5% [28], so the tool is fit to be used. The following is Fig. 4 which is the average and error obtained from each temperature measurement and is read at 5 measurement points.

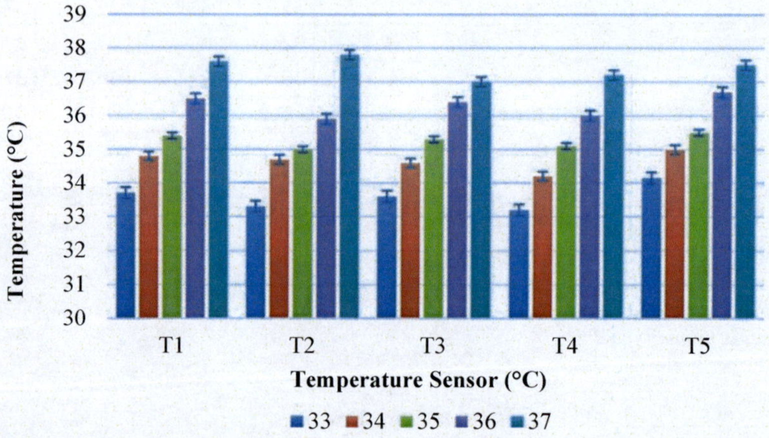

Fig. 4 Which is the average and error obtained from each temperature measurement and is read at 5 measurement points

Table 2 T-Test for the reading of the AHT10 sensor and INCU analyzer

Temperature setting (°C)	P-value
33	0.07114539
34	0.299301243
35	0.310109983
36	0.469996494
37	0.404487384

After obtaining the error value of each temperature setting, the t-test was conducted to see if there was a difference in the significance value between the reading of the AHT10 sensor and the reading of the INCU Analyzer explained in Table 2.

Based on the table shown above, the p-value of each temperature setting is obtained in the reading of the AHT10 sensor that appears on the baby incubator display and the reading of the INCU Analyzer is the standard tool. At 33 °C, a p-value of 0.07114539 was obtained, while at 34 °C, a p-value of 0.299301243 was obtained. At 35 °C, it obtained a p-value of 0.310109983. At 36 °C, it obtained a p-value of 0.469996494, while at 37 °C, it obtained a p-value of 0.404487384.

3.2 *Testing the PID System by Giving an Interruption*

In this study, the process of data collection was conducted in a room with an ambient temperature of 25 °C with a relative humidity of 60 RH. The overshoot value and the testing for the PID system when giving an interruption are shown in Fig. 5. In this test, the temperature was set to 36 °C. The data were taken using the INCU Analyzer in different temperature points, namely T1, T2, T3, T4, and T5.

In Fig. 5 T1, an overshoot value of 1.8 °C is obtained in 17 min and the steady-state error is 3% in 63 min or 3,800 s; it was given an interruption by opening the baby incubator door for 5 min, and the temperature decreased to 32.5 °C. After the door closed in 70 min, the temperature started to be stable. In Fig. 5 T2, an overshoot value of 1.8 °C is obtained in 17 min and the steady-state error is 3% in 63 min or 3,800 s; it was given an interruption by opening the baby incubator door for 5 min, and the temperature decreased to 32.5 °C. After the door closed in 70 min, the temperature started to be stable. In Fig. 5 T3, an overshoot value of 0.8 °C is obtained in 17 min and the steady-state error is 2% in 63 min or around 3,800 s; it was given an interruption by opening the baby incubator door for 5 min, and the temperature decreased to 31.5 °C. After the door closed in 70 min, the temperature started to be stable. In Fig. 5 T4, an overshoot value of 2.1 °C is obtained in 17 min and the steady-state error is 3% in 63 min or around 3,800 s; it was given an interruption by opening the baby incubator door for 5 min, and the temperature decreased to 30.5 °C. After the door closed in 70 min, the temperature started to be stable. In Fig. 5 T5, an overshoot value of 0.9 °C is obtained in 17 min and the steady-state error is 3% in 63 min or

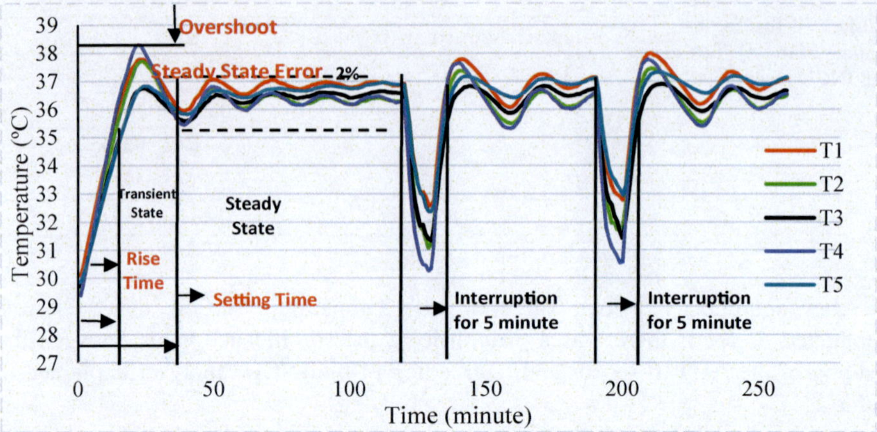

Fig. 5 Overall test of temperature reading: temperature 1, temperature 2, temperature 3, temperature 4, and temperature 5. In the picture above, 2 times interference is carried out within 5 min to test the PID system

around 3,800 s; it was given an interruption by opening the baby incubator door for 5 min, and the temperature decreased to 32.5 °C. After the door closed in 70 min, the temperature started to be stable.

4 Discussion

From the temperature data that has been calibrated using the INCU Analyzer, a significant value is obtained, it can be concluded that the average P-Value is greater than 0.05, indicating that there is no significant difference between the two groups. On the contrary, if the p-value is less than 0.05, it indicates that there is a significant difference between the two groups. From Fig. 4 it is explained that it takes 7 min after the simulation to apply the interrupt to get a stable temperature value. The steady-state value is still within the permissible tolerance limit of 5% [29].

This study's findings were contrasted with those of previous studies. Adhi ksatria theopaga and colleagues also created a PID control system with the following K_p, K_i, and K_d values: 13,828, 0,576, and 82.962. With a temperature setting of 32 C, the numbers produced a rise time of 200.47 s and a setting time of 306.16 s. Although the explanation indicates that it takes only a little time to attain the desired temperature, the steady-state error percentage, or 29.16%, is extremely high [30, 31].

Furthermore, the weakness of this study is that the overshoot value of each measurement point, namely T1, T2, T3, T4, and T5, is different. It is caused by the location of the AHT10 sensor that does not reach all points in the baby incubator. So, an advanced evaluation of the correct location of the sensor is needed. The product of this study was expected to be applied in selecting the correct temperature control system for a baby incubator to decrease the mortality risk in premature infants.

5 Conclusion

This study aims to make a temperature control system for a baby incubator by using PID and analyze the overshoot level as well as the PID responses when there is an interruption. From the result of the measurement conducted between the reading of the AHT10 sensor and INCU Analyzer, the respective error of less than 5% is obtained at different temperature settings, namely 33, 34, 35, 36, and 37 °C. Meanwhile, the t-test obtains a p-value of greater than 0.05, an overshoot value, and a steady-state error of less than 5% respectively. As a development of the study, several things can be developed in the next study. In this study, the control system only controls the temperature. It is suggested to control the moisture in the baby incubator and add a telemedicine-based remote control in the next study.

Acknowledgements Appreciation is addressed to the Department of Electromedical Engineering and Research Management & Innovation Centre, Poltekkes Kemenkes Surabaya for supporting this research.

References

1. Lawn JE et al (2013) Preterm baby survival and care round the world born too soon: care for the preterm baby. Reprod Health 10(10), 5 [Online]. http://www.reproductive-health-journal.com/content/10/S1/S5
2. Kvalvik LG, Wilcox AJ, Skjærven R, Østbye T, Harmon QE (2020) Term complications and subsequent risk of preterm birth: registry based study. BMJ 369. https://doi.org/10.1136/bmj.m1007
3. Frischer R, Penhaker M, Krejcar O, Kacerovsky M, Selamat A (2014) Precise temperature measurement for increasing the survival of newborn babies in incubator environments. Sensors (Switzerland) 14(12):23563–23580. https://doi.org/10.3390/s141223563
4. Utomo SB, Irawan JF, Mujibtamala A, Nari MI, Amalia R (2021) Automatic baby incubator system with fuzzy-PID controller. IOP Conf Ser Mater Sci Eng 1034(1):012023. https://doi.org/10.1088/1757-899x/1034/1/012023
5. Shaib M, Hamawy L, El Majzoub I (2017) Advanced portable preterm baby incubator, October. https://doi.org/10.1109/ICABME.2017.8167522
6. Vyas DD (2017) System for remote monitoring and control of baby incubator and warmer, May 2016
7. Kristya F, Luthfiyah S, Hari Wisana IDG, Thaseen M (2021) Baby incubator monitoring center for temperature and humidity using WiFi network. J Electron Electromed Eng Med Inf 3(1):8–13. https://doi.org/10.35882/jeeemi.v3i1.2
8. Janney JB, KrishnaKumar S, AnuShree PB, Rayshma V, Suresh S (2018) Design of mobile infant incubator with comforting pillow. Int J Eng Technol 7(2):6–9. https://doi.org/10.14419/ijet.v7i2.25.12353

9. Latif A, Arfianto AZ, Poetro JE, Phong TN, Helmy ET (2021) Temperature monitoring system for baby incubator based on visual basic. J Robot Control 2(1):47–50. https://doi.org/10.18196/jrc.2151
10. Rahman ZSA, Hussain FSA (2017) Smart incubator based on PID controller. Int Res J Eng Technol 4(3):2501–2509. https://doi.org/10.13140/RG.2.2.21917.77282
11. Kanáliková K (1990) Diagnosis of congenital heart defects in childhood. Bratisl Lek Listy 91(12):868–873
12. Widhiada W, Nindhia TGT, Gantara IN, Budarsa IN, Suarndwipa IN (2019) Temperature stability and humidity on infant incubator based on fuzzy logic control. ACM Int Conf Proceeding Ser April:155–159. https://doi.org/10.1145/3330482.3330527
13. Widhiada W, Antara ING, Budiarsa IN, Karohika IMG (2019) The robust PID control system of temperature stability and humidity on infant incubator based on Arduino at mega 2560. IOP Conf Ser Earth Environ Sci 248(1). https://doi.org/10.1088/1755-1315/248/1/012046
14. Suruthi M, Suma S (2015) Microcontroller based baby incubator using sensors, pp 12037–12044. https://doi.org/10.15680/IJIRSET.2015.0412050
15. Widhiada W (2017) Temperature distribution control for baby incubator system using Arduino AT Mega 2560. World Acad Eng Technol Conf Proc. Bali Int Sch Sci Res Innov 10(1):XV [Online]. https://simdos.unud.ac.id/uploads/file_penelitian_1_dir/d8cee6e73f739dc11ac9590012345664.pdf
16. Mathew BDL, Gupta A (2015) Controlling of temperature and humidity for an infant incubator using microcontroller. Int J Adv Res Electr Electron Instrum Eng 4(6):4975–4982. https://doi.org/10.15662/ijareeie.2015.0406012
17. Zaelani AV, Koestoer RA, Roihan I, Harinaldi (2019) Analysis of temperature stabilization in grashof incubator with environment variations based on Indonesian national standard (SNI). AIP Conf Proc 2062. https://doi.org/10.1063/1.5086550
18. Irsyad A, Isnawaty, Saputra RA (2017) Implementasi Sistem Navigasi Dengan Metode Proportional Integral Derivative (Pid) pada robot wall follower. semanTIK 3(2):9–12
19. Sinuraya EW, Pamungkas RJ (2019) Design of temperature control system for infant incubator using auto tuning fuzzy-PI controller. Int J Eng Inf Syst 3(1):33–41
20. Koli M, Ladge P, Prasad B, Boria R, Balur NJ (2018) Intelligent baby incubator. In: Proc 2nd Int Conf Electron Commun Aerosp Technol ICECA 2018 Iceca:1036–1042. https://doi.org/10.1109/ICECA.2018.8474763
21. Febriyanti AZ, Nugraha PC, Syaifudin (2020) Temperature calibrator using thermocouple based on microcontroller. Indones J Electron Electromed Eng Med Inf 2(1):13–20. https://doi.org/10.35882/ijeeemi.v2i1.3
22. Ali M, Abdelwahab M, Awadekreim S, Abdalla S (2018) Development of a monitoring and control system of infant incubator. In: 2018 Int Conf Comput Control Electr Electron Eng ICCCEEE 2018 Lcd:1–4. https://doi.org/10.1109/ICCCEEE.2018.8515785
23. Hidayati NF, Yulianto E, Kholiq A (2019) Baby incubator based on PID control with kangaroo mode (kangaroo mode and humidity). J Electron Electromed Eng Med Inf 1(2):13–17. https://doi.org/10.35882/jeeemi.v1i2.3
24. Ang KH, Chong G, Li Y (2005) PID control system analysis, design, and technology. IEEE Trans Control Syst Technol 13(4):559–576. https://doi.org/10.1109/TCST.2005.847331
25. Ogata K (2005) Mathematical modelling of control systems. Mod Control Eng 13–62
26. Nayak A, Singh M (2015) Study of tuning of PID controller by using particle swarm optimization. Int J Adv Eng Res Stud IV(Jan.-March), 346–350
27. Duvernoy J (2015) Guidance on the computation of calibration uncertainties. World Meteorol Organ 119 [Online]. http://www.wmo.int/pages/prog/www/IMOP/publications-IOM-series.html%0D
28. Prinyakupt J, Roongprasert K (2019) Verification device for temperature and relative humidity inside the infant incubator via IoT. BMEiCON 2019—12th Biomed Eng Int Conf 1–6. https://doi.org/10.1109/BMEiCON47515.2019.8990351

29. Ambitiously E (2020) PID theory explained—NI, pp 1–7 [Online]. http://www.idc-online.com/technical_references/pdfs/electrical_engineering/Introduction_to_Second_Order_Systems.pdf%0A http://engineering.electrical-equipment.org/panel-building/introduction-to-second-order-systems.html
30. Theopaga AK, Rizal A, Susanto E (2014) Design and implementation of PID control based baby incubator. J Theor Appl Inf Technol 70(1):19–24
31. Mccall EM, Alderdice F, Halliday HL, Vohra S, Johnston L (2018) Interventions to prevent hypothermia at birth in preterm and/or low birth weight infants. Cochrane Database Syst Rev 2:2018. https://doi.org/10.1002/14651858.CD004210.pub5

Improving the Myoelectric Feature Linearity to Enhance the Elbow Motion Estimation Using Kalman Filter

Triwiyanto Triwiyanto, Riky Tri Yunardi, Abdussalam Ali Ahmed, V. H. Abdullayev, Vishwajeet Shankhwar, Levana Forra Wakidi, Lusiana, Bedjo Utomo, and A. T. P. Moch Prastawa

Abstract Myoelectric signal exhibits non-linear and non-stationary characteristics in nature. These phenomena could be a major problem in estimating an elbow motion based on myoelectric. Therefore, the goal of this study was to improve the linearity of the myoelectric features to improve the performance of myoelectric-based elbow motion estimation using the Kalman filter (KF). The contribution of this study was to obtain the linearity improvement of the myoelectric feature in estimating the elbow motion in flexion and extension (FE) motion. The linearity was improved by evaluating the number of time-domain (TD) features. Additionally, the myoelectric feature was filtered using the KF. Ten participants were involved in this study to perform the experiment. The myoelectric collected from the biceps was extracted using TD features. The twelve TD features were further investigated to select the most linear feature in estimating the elbow motion. KF was applied to enhance the linearity of the features so that the performance also increased. In this case, the WAMP and MYOP features showed better performance after the KF process than the others. Additionally, the average of the slope, correlation coefficient, and determination constant were 1.025 ± 0.085, 0.974 ± 0.012, and 0.950 ± 0.024

T. Triwiyanto (✉) · L. F. Wakidi · Lusiana · B. Utomo · A. T. P. Moch Prastawa
Department of Medical Electronics Technology, Poltekkes Kemenkes Surabaya, Surabaya, Indonesia
e-mail: Triwi@poltekkesdepkes-sby.ac.id

T. Triwiyanto
Intelligent Medical Rehabilitation Devices Research Group, Department of Medical Electronics Technology, Poltekkes Kemenkes Surabaya, Surabaya, Indonesia

R. T. Yunardi
Department of Engineering, Faculty of Vocational, Universitas Airlangga, Surabaya, Indonesia

A. A. Ahmed
Mechanical and Industrial Engineering Department, Bani Waleed University, Bani Waleed, Libya

V. H. Abdullayev
Azerbaijan State Oil and Industry University, Baku, Azerbaijan

V. Shankhwar
Space Lab, Mohammed Bin Rashid University, Dubai, United Arab Emirates

T. Triwiyanto et al. (eds.), *Proceeding of the 3rd International Conference on Electronics, Biomedical Engineering, and Health Informatics*, Lecture Notes in Electrical Engineering 1008, https://doi.org/10.1007/978-981-99-0248-4_36

respectively for the WAMP feature and 1.003 ± 0.066, 0.973 ± 0.016, and 0.947 ± 0.031, respectively for MYOP feature. This research has shown the Kalman filter's effectiveness to improve performance. In the practical system, this proposed method can be applied to the design of the upper or lower limb exoskeleton to help post-stroke patients or elderly people.

Keywords Myoelectric · Kalman filter · Time-domain features · Estimation

1 Introduction

The myoelectric signal is widely used in many studies such as sports activities, ergonomic, and biomedical engineering since the myoelectric is related to the movement of the human limb [1]. In biomedical engineering, myoelectric is often used as a control signal for prosthetic and robotic exoskeleton devices [2–6]. Estimation of the elbow motion is important in the development of myoelectric control devices such as robotic exoskeleton for the upper or lower limb because it determines the model's effectiveness. Several studies used mechanical sensors such as force sensors and accelerometers and gyroscope sensors to detect the limb position. However, the main problem for the mechanical sensor is that there was a delay time in response. On the other side, the EMG signal was also used a lot in the robotic exoskeleton design. The advantage of using the EMG signal is that the signal had a better response compared to the mechanical sensors. However, a pre-processing stage should be applied when we used the EMG signal as a control signal such as feature extraction and filtering.

Several studies estimated the elbow motion by applying the pattern recognition method such as a multilayer perceptron with backpropagation algorithm, combination of fuzzy and neural network, and support vector machine (SVM) [7–9]. Tang et al. proposed an artificial neural network (ANN) to model a myoelectric angle with a backpropagation algorithm [10]. In the model, they extracted the myoelectric from four muscle groups (biceps, triceps, ancones, and brachioradialis) using root mean square (RMS). Additionally, the features were also used as inputs for the ANN classifier. Even though their results showed a good performance in estimating the elbow-motion but the method was only able to apply to a single user and needs a re-training for the ANN to recognize a new user or variable. This was due to the variability of myoelectric that depends on subjects. Pau et al. proposed a model to estimate elbow motion based on myoelectric using a Hill model [11]. In the model, two muscle groups (biceps and triceps) were used to estimate elbow motion. Their results show high accuracy in estimating elbow motion. However, in optimizing using the model used a Genetic Algorithm (GA), they reported that GA is a time-consuming method to optimize the model. Furthermore, Li predicted the elbow joint force based on the EMG signal by using linear discriminant analysis (LDA) [12]. However, in order to increase the prediction, several pre-processing was applied including the band-pass filter and Kalman filter. In the experiment, Li obtained the highest accuracy of 95%. Moreover, previously, authors have proposed elbow joint angle prediction by using an EMG signal based on a combination of zero crossing feature and Kalman filter. However, zero crossing feature has a parameter that needed to be adjusted for better prediction.

Due to this fact, a new approach had to be implemented to minimize the problem and limitation in the previous works. In this study, a non-pattern recognition method was presented which means no classifier or machine learning was needed in estimating the elbow motion. In order to perform the estimation, the myoelectric was extracted using time domain (TD) features. Linear Kalman filter (KF) was used to optimize the TD features so that estimated performance could be improved. For this purpose, the twelve (TD) features (RMS, IEMG, VAR, MAV, LOG, WL, AAC, DASDV, ZC, SSC, WAMP, and MYOP) were investigated and evaluated to determine the feature that resulted in the best performance. As well as improving the performance, the KF was also suggested to improve the linearity of the estimation. Therefore, in order to validate the linearity, several linearity parameters were calculated such as slope, correlation coefficient, and determination constant (R^2). The contribution of this study is written as follows:

1. The proposed method, a combination of KF and feature extraction, is able to estimate the elbow joint angle without any learning or training stage.
2. The proposed method is able to estimate the joint angle using single-channel EMG.

2 Materials and Methods

2.1 *Participants*

Ten healthy male participants with no previous injury and muscle disorder were involved in this study. Before the experimental procedures were performed, participants were given the informed consent form. In addition, the ethics committee of Health Polytechnic of Surabaya, Ministry of Health, Indonesia had decided on the experimental protocols in this research.

2.2 *Equipment*

Electromyography system. The system for data acquisition consisted of the bio-amplifier package, D/A (digital to analog converter), and a computer unit (Intel Core i3-3217U CPU at 1.80 GHz, 8 GB of RAM, Windows 8). The bio-amplifier was designed with an AD620 preamplifier, a 20 to 500 Hz band-pass filter, and a summing amplifier. In this analysis, the myoelectric was recorded only from the biceps muscle using two disabled electrodes (Ag/AgCl, size: 57 × 48 mm, Ambu, Blue sensor R,

Malaysia). Because the experiment was conducted in a sagittal plane motion, the myoelectric generated from the triceps showed insignificant activities. The electrode placement was in accordance to SENIAM (Surface Electromyography for the Non-Invasive Assessment of Muscle) rules [13]. The dominant frequency of myoelectric covered between 20 and 150. The sampling frequency in the data collection was therefore 1,000 Hz. This was to qualify the Nyquist rule whose minimum sampling frequency was twice of the maximum frequency of the signal [14–16].

Exoskeleton unit. The exoskeleton unit consisted of two aluminum frames whose length was in accordance with the human arm and forearm. In the elbow joint of the exoskeleton, a potentiometer was placed to detect the elbow motion which was used to compare the measured angle and the estimated angle. A holder and one kg of load were placed at the forearm frame. This exoskeleton was used for the synchronization of elbow movement in FE.

Data Collection. In the data collection process, the participants were in a standing position with holding the exoskeleton unit (Fig. 1). The myoelectric and elbow motion were recorded simultaneously, while the elbow was moved in FE motion, ranging from 0° to 145°. In each trial, the participants performed FE motion for 8 cycles. In this work, the period of motion was performed in 2 s periods. An application program built using Python programming was used to acquire the myoelectric and measured angle.

Data Processing. Myoelectric was extracted using twelve (TD) features with a window length of 200 samples (200 ms) [17]. The twelve TD features (RMS, IEMG, VAR, MAV, LOG, WL, AAC, DASDV, ZC, SSC, WAMP, and MYOP) [18, 19] were evaluated. Each cycle for a total of eight cycles was processed using TD features. In addition, the features were filtered with the KF. In this work, the KF output can be assumed as an estimated angle. The materials related to the Kalman filter can be found in many sources [20–22]. The flowchart of data processing is shown in Fig. 2. The flowchart shows that several values such as threshold, window length (N), process

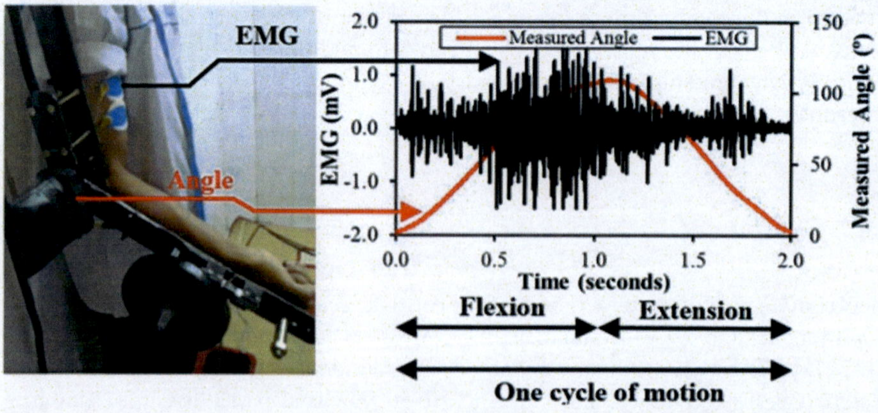

Fig. 1 A typical of MYELECTRIC and angle measurement in one cycle of FE motion

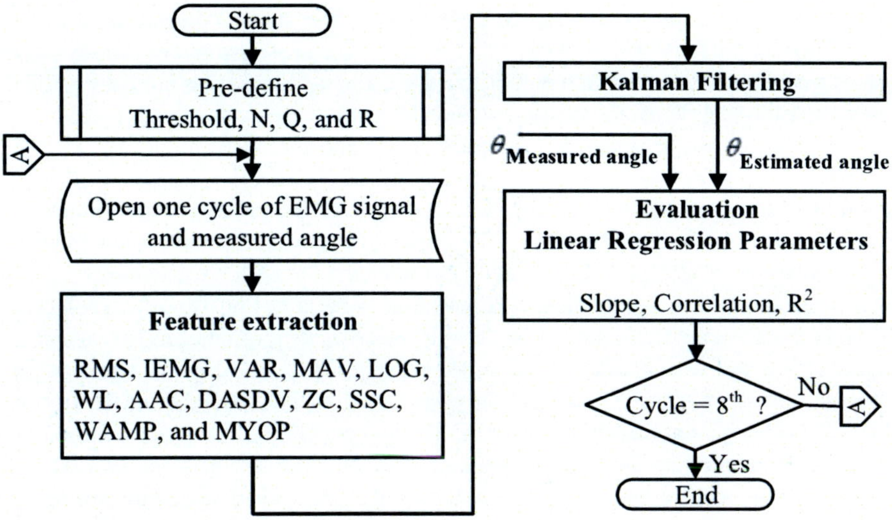

Fig. 2 Flowchart of elbow-motion estimation

Q, and measurement noise R covariance needed to be defined first before the data processing. A complete tutorial discussing Q and R Kalman filter can be found in some materials [20, 23].

Data Analysis. After the myoelectric data processing, the estimated angle was evaluated using regression linear parameters. The regression linear parameters were calculated to describe the linearity of the myoelectric features. These were slope, correlation coefficient, and determination constant (R^2). The myoelectric dataset was obtained from four participants and each participant performed eight cycles of motion. Each cycle was extracted using twelve TD features. The variance of linear regression parameters was described in the boxplot diagrams for both pre and post KF. The significant difference of slope, correlation, and R^2 between pre and single factor ANOVA was used for post KF results. The significance test was performed at a 95% confidence level (alpha = 0.05). The p-value shows whether the parameters reflect a major difference or not.

3 Results and Discussion

The linearity of the twelve TD features was calculated based on the parameter of slope, correlation, and determination constant. In this work, the Kalman filter has demonstrated the effectiveness to enhance the linearity and performance of the features. After the KF process, the WAMP and MYOP features showed better linearity in all parameters than that showed the other features. The slope, correlation, and R2 for the WAMP feature were 1.025 ± 0.085, 1.025 ± 0.085, and 0.950 ± 0.024, respectively. Additionally, for the MYOP feature, the slope, correlation, and R2 were 1.003 ± 0.066, 0.973 ± 0.016, and 0.947 ± 0.031, respectively. Those slope values were equal to ~1.0 which means that the estimated angle was almost identical to the measured angle. Both correlation and R2 showed high values which indicated that the relationship between the estimated angle and measured angle was closely related.

Figure 3 shows how the TD features reacted to the elbow movement in FE motion. As shown in Fig. 3, the trajectory of FE motion was different for each feature. Furthermore, the trajectory of the feature could characterize that the features were a non-linear function. This characteristic was due to the non-linearity of myoelectric [18] and the myoelectric features [24]. In this analysis, the output of the myoelectric function was fed to KF after the feature extraction process. Figure 4 shows the estimated response to the direction of the elbow motion. The trajectory of FE motion showed more adjacent than that before the KF process (Fig. 3). As shown in Fig. 4l, MYOP feature showed the best performance and linearity (with slope = 1.003 ± 0.066, correlation coefficient = 0.973 ± 0.016, R2 = 0.947 ± 0.031) in estimating the elbow motion.

Figure 5 shows the comparison of slope variance before and after the KF process for twelve TD features. As shown in Fig. 4a, b, the variance of slope values varies for all TD features. After the KF process, the slope mean of all the features increased significantly (p-value < 0.05) (Fig. 4b). As shown in Fig. 5b, WAMP and MYOP features showed a higher mean slope value (~1.00) than the other features. This showed that the predicted angle and the measured angle were equivalent in volume. Figure 5c, d showed the comparison of correlation variance between pre and post KF. It was noticeable that the correlation values were increased and the variance was decreased for all the features after the KF process. Figure 5e, f show the comparison of R2 variance between pre and post KF. It was also obvious that all mean values increased significantly after the KF process. Table 1 shows the linear-regression parameters before the KF. It was obvious that WAMP and MYOP features had better values in parameters than the other features. Table 2 shows the summary of the linear-regression parameters after the KF. It was also noticeable that the estimated angle based on WAMP and MYOP features showed better performance than the other features.

This study has proved the effectiveness of KF to improve the linearity and performance of the estimation. The improvement of slope, correlation, and R2 after the KF process was 54.98, 42.94, and 101.21% respectively. In the related work, the results were comparable to the previous works. Tang et al. developed a MYELECTRIC to angle to control an upper limb exoskeleton using a BP ANN. In the experiment, they obtained the R2 between 0.79 and 0.87. Lee at el. presented a method to estimate the elbow motion in lifting tasks using linear regression [25]. They found the correlation between the calculated and measured angle was on average around 0.82.

This work had several limitations that needed to be addressed in the future research. It was the number degree of freedom (DOF) which in this study was limited to one DOF for elbow-joint motion in FE motion. Also, in the proposed method, the causes of muscle fatigue had not yet been understood. Even though, muscle fatigue

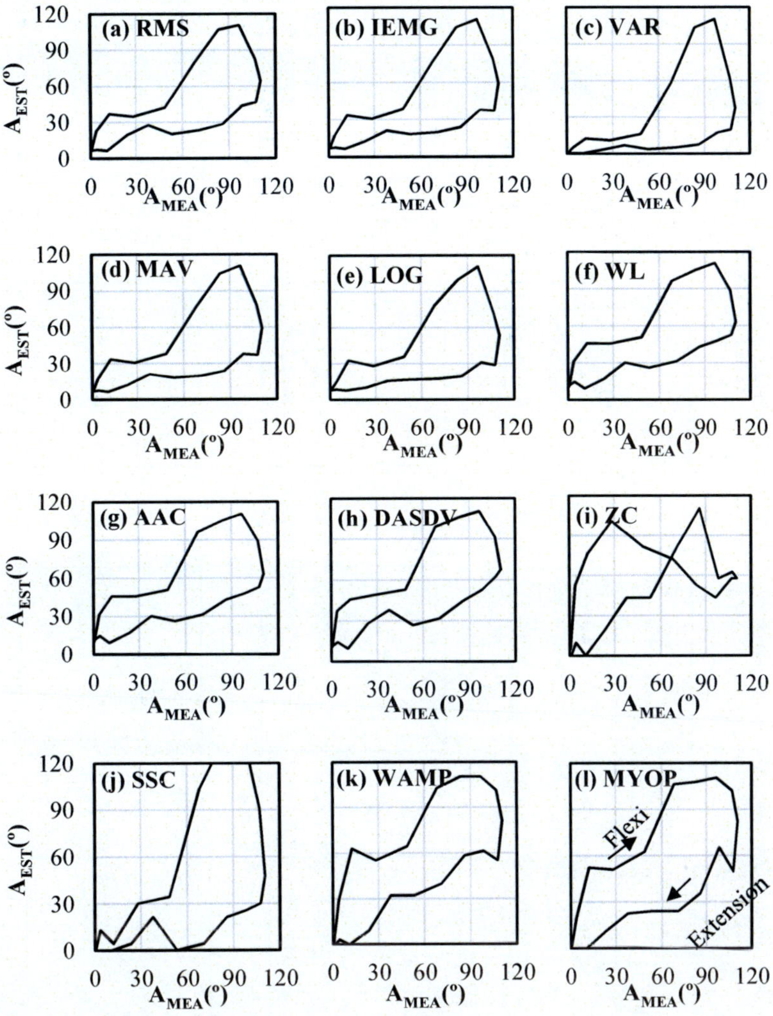

Fig. 3 Response of features to elbow motion in FE motion. X-axis is the measured angle and y-axis is the estimated angle

had proven that it affected the spectral parameters of myoelectric as reported by the previous study [26, 27].

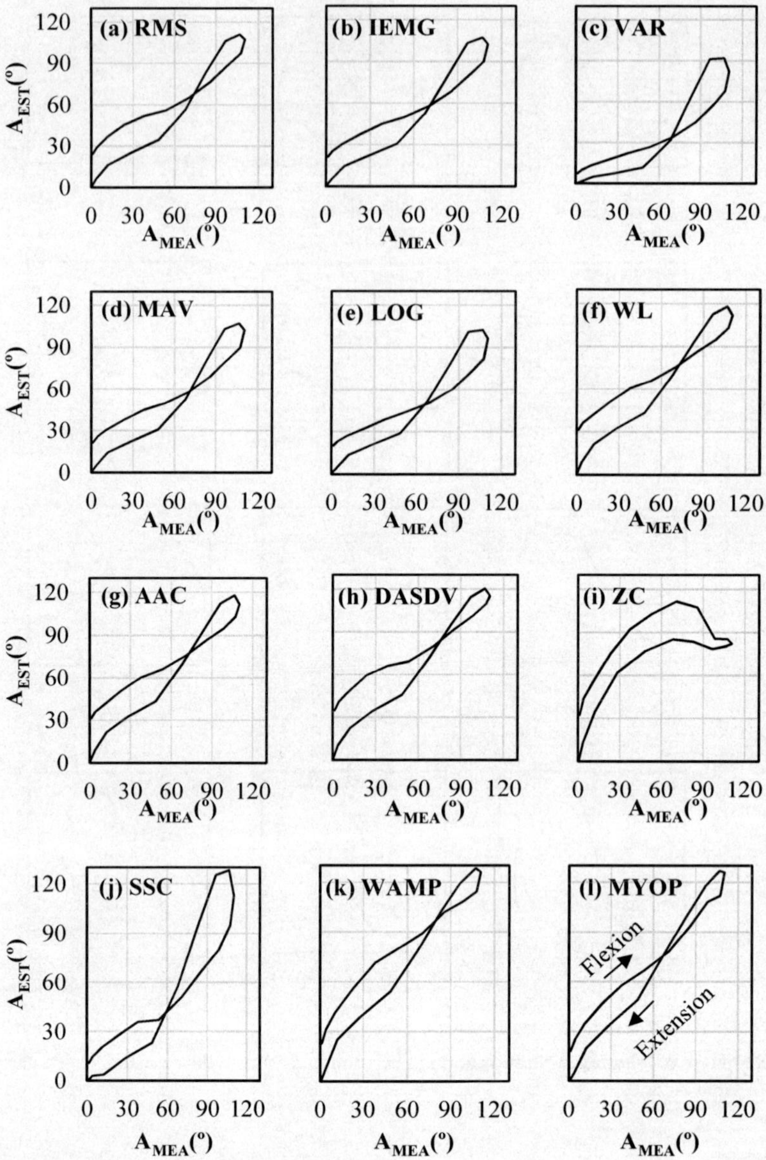

Fig. 4 Response of Kalman filtered features to elbow motion in FE motion. The x-axis is the measured angle and the y-axis is the estimated angle

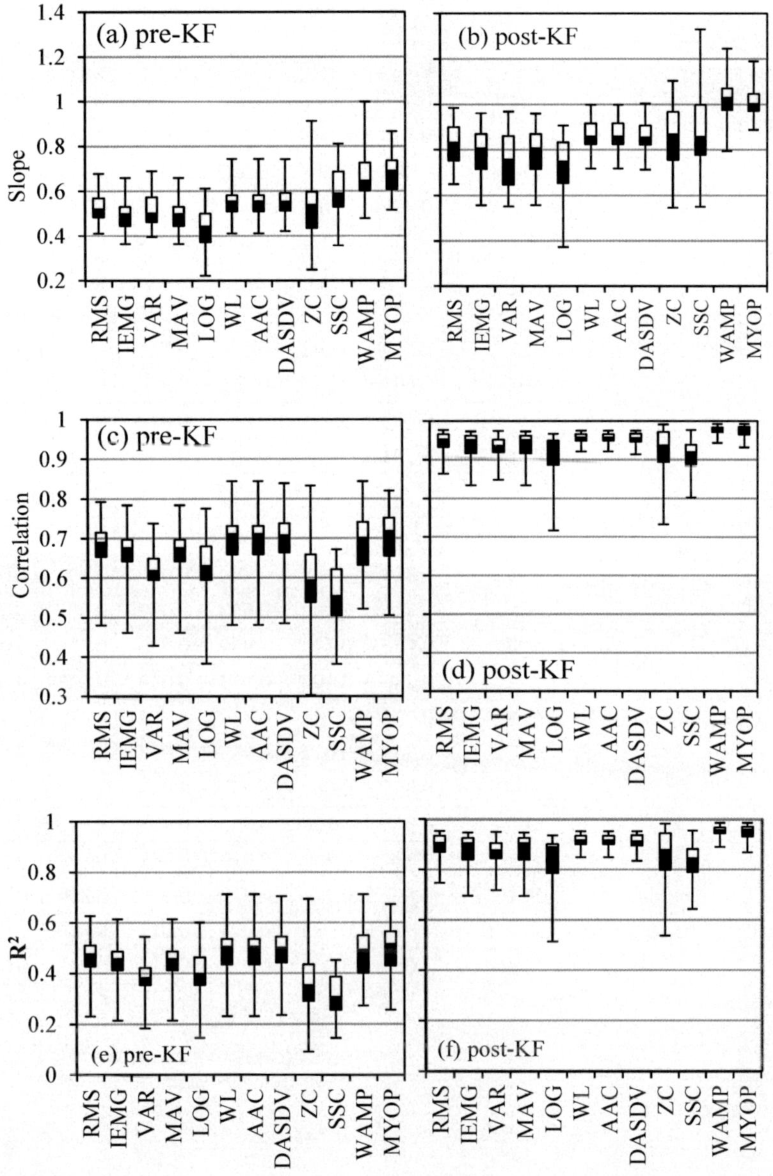

Fig. 5 Boxplot diagram of slope (**a**, **b**), correlation (**c**, **d**), and R2 (**e**, **f**) before and after the KF process, respectively

Table 1 Summary of linear regression parameters for the features before the KF process (mean ± standard deviation)

Features	Slope	Correlation	R2
RMS	0.526 ± 0.056	0.682 ± 0.061	0.468 ± 0.079
IEMG	0.494 ± 0.068	0.665 ± 0.061	0.447 ± 0.078
VAR	0.518 ± 0.073	0.619 ± 0.057	0.386 ± 0.069
MAV	0.494 ± 0.068	0.665 ± 0.085	0.447 ± 0.078
LOG	0.431 ± 0.104	0.623 ± 0.085	0.396 ± 0.100
WL	0.551 ± 0.074	0.697 ± 0.068	0.490 ± 0.093
AAC	0.551 ± 0.074	0.697 ± 0.068	0.490 ± 0.095
DASDV	0.551 ± 0.075	0.699 ± 0.070	0.494 ± 0.093
ZC	0.529 ± 0.142	0.589 ± 0.115	0.360 ± 0.134
SSC	0.605 ± 0.144	0.556 ± 0.078	0.315 ± 0.085
WAMP	0.672 ± 0.105	0.692 ± 0.072	0.485 ± 0.099
MYOP	0.683 ± 0.087	0.706 ± 0.073	0.505 ± 0.101

Table 2 Summary of linear regression parameter of the features after the KF process (mean ± standard deviation)

Features	Slope	Correlation	R2
RMS	0.824 ± 0.093	0.944 ± 0.029	0.892 ± 0.054
IEMG	0.786 ± 0.107	0.933 ± 0.039	0.872 ± 0.072
VAR	0.756 ± 0.120	0.930 ± 0.030	0.866 ± 0.056
MAV	0.786 ± 0.107	0.933 ± 0.039	0.873 ± 0.072
LOG	0.721 ± 0.145	0.899 ± 0.075	0.815 ± 0.127
WL	0.865 ± 0.072	0.955 ± 0.013	0.913 ± 0.026
AAC	0.865 ± 0.067	0.955 ± 0.013	0.913 ± 0.026
DASDV	0.865 ± 0.156	0.953 ± 0.015	0.910 ± 0.030
ZC	0.844 ± 0.156	0.919 ± 0.067	0.849 ± 0.118
SSC	0.897 ± 0.174	0.910 ± 0.041	0.830 ± 0.074
WAMP	1.025 ± 0.085	0.974 ± 0.012	0.950 ± 0.024
MYOP	1.003 ± 0.066	0.973 ± 0.016	0.947 ± 0.031

4 Conclusion

This study develops a method to linearize the non-linear myoelectric feature in estimating elbow motion based on myoelectric. We find that the Kalman filter effectively improves the linearity of the myoelectric features, specifically WAMP and MYOP features. In summary, the achievement of this study is as follows. After the KF process, the linear parameters of the estimated angle are increased. The slope, correlation, and R^2 parameters are 54.98, 42.94, and 101.21%, respectively. Furthermore, the results also prove that all of the linear regression parameters are improved and the WAMP and MYOP features are better in linearity and performance than the other features after the KF process. In the future work, several disturbances such as the shift in electrode location, sweat, and muscle fatigue need to be considered to improve the performance of estimation.

References

1. Sousa ASP, Tavares JMR (2012) Surface electromyographic amplitude normalization methods: a review. Electromyogr New Dev Proced Appl 85–101
2. Asghari Oskoei M, Hu H (2007) Myoelectric control systems—a survey. Biomed Signal Process Control 2:275–294. https://doi.org/10.1016/j.bspc.2007.07.009
3. Tavares R, Abreu P, Quintas MR (2016) Data acquisition glove for hand movement impairment rehabilitation. Int J Online Eng 12:52–54. https://doi.org/10.3991/ijoe.v12i04.5141
4. Triwiyanto T, Wahyunggoro O, Nugroho HA, Herianto H (2017) String actuated upper limb exoskeleton based on surface electromyography control. In: Proceedings—2016 6th international annual engineering seminar, InAES. https://doi.org/10.1109/INAES.2016.7821929
5. Triwiyanto T, Caesarendra W, Purnomo MH, Sułowicz M (2022) Embedded machine learning using a multi-thread algorithm on a Raspberry Pi platform to improve prosthetic hand performance
6. Triwiyanto T, Rahmawati T, Pawana IPA, Lamidi L, Hamzah T, Pudji A, Ridha Mak'ruf M, Luthfiyahtorib S (2021) State-of-the-art method in prosthetic hand design: a review. J Biomim Biomater Biomed Eng 50:15–24
7. Yang D, Jiang L, Huang Q, Liu R, Liu H (2014) Experimental study of an EMG-controlled 5-DOF anthropomorphic prosthetic hand for motion restoration. J Intell Robot Syst Theory Appl 76:427–441. https://doi.org/10.1007/s10846-014-0037-6
8. Tsai AC, Luh JJ, Lin TT (2015) A novel STFT-ranking feature of multi-channel EMG for motion pattern recognition. https://doi.org/10.1016/j.eswa.2014.11.044
9. Gini G, Arvetti M, Somlai I, Folgheraiter M (2012) Acquisition and analysis of EMG signals to recognize multiple hand movements for prosthetic applications. Appl Bionics Biomech 9:145–155. https://doi.org/10.3233/ABB-2011-0024
10. Tang Z, Zhang K, Sun S, Gao Z, Zhang L, Yang Z (2014) An upper-limb power-assist exoskeleton using proportional myoelectric control. Sensors 14:6677–6694. https://doi.org/10.3390/s140406677
11. Pau JWL, Xie SSQ, Pullan AJ (2012) Neuromuscular interfacing: establishing an EMG-driven model for the human elbow joint. IEEE Trans Biomed Eng 59:2586–2593. https://doi.org/10.1109/TBME.2012.2206389
12. Li Z, Wang B, Sun F, Yang C, Xie Q, Zhang W (2014) SEMG-based joint force control for an upper-limb power-assist exoskeleton robot. IEEE J Biomed Heal Inform 18:1043–1050. https://doi.org/10.1109/JBHI.2013.2286455

13. Hermens HJ, Freriks B (2017) SENIAM project. http://www.seniam.org/. Last accessed 16 June 2017
14. Tan L, Jiang J (2008) Digital signal processing: fundamental and applications. Elsevier, California (2008). https://doi.org/10.1088/1751-8113/44/8/085201
15. Suboh MZ, Jaafar R, Nayan NA, Harun NH (2019) ECG-based detection and prediction models of sudden cardiac death: current performances and new perspectives on signal processing techniques. Int J Online Biomed Eng 15:110–126. https://doi.org/10.3991/ijoe.v15i15.11688
16. Ali H, Villanueva BE, Yaqub R (2019) Design and implementation of a low cost wireless ambulatory ECG monitoring system for deployment in rural communities. Int J Online Biomed Eng 15:57–79. https://doi.org/10.3991/ijoe.v15i15.11860
17. Triwiyanto T, Wahyunggoro O, Nugroho HA, Herianto H (2017) Effect of window length on performance of the elbow-joint angle prediction based on electromyography. In: Journal of physics: conference series, p 012014. https://doi.org/10.1088/1742-6596/853/1/012014
18. Triwiyanto T, Wahyunggoro O, Nugroho HA, Herianto H (2017) An investigation into time domain features of surface electromyography to estimate the elbow joint angle. Adv Electr Electron Eng 15:448–458. https://doi.org/10.15598/aeee.v15i3.2177
19. Phinyomark A, Phukpattaranont P, Limsakul C (2012) Feature reduction and selection for EMG signal classification. Expert Syst Appl 39:7420–7431. https://doi.org/10.1016/j.eswa.2012.01.102
20. Triwiyanto T, Wahyunggoro O, Nugroho HA, Herianto H (2017) Evaluating the performance of Kalman filter on elbow joint angle prediction based on electromyography. Int J Precis Eng Manuf 18:1739–1748. https://doi.org/10.1007/s12541-017-0202-5
21. Tao Z, Jin-Xin PEI, Yu-guang SONG, Peng LUO (2015) The attitude signal processing of four rotor aircraft based on a kalman filter. Int J Online Eng 11:8–12. https://doi.org/10.3991/ijoe.v11i8.4883
22. Jin Y, Xia K (2014) Channel aware cooperative FEC/ARQ mechanism based on Kalman filter prediction for wireless sensor networks. Int J Online Eng 10:22–28. https://doi.org/10.3991/ijoe.v10i1.3164
23. Ribeiro MI (2004) Kalman and extended Kalman filters: concept, derivation and properties. Inst Syst Robot Lisboa Port 42. https://doi.org/10.1.1.2.5088
24. Fukuda O, Tsuji T, Kaneko M, Otsuka A (2003) A human-assisting manipulator teleoperated by EMG signals and arm motions. IEEE Trans Robot Autom 19:210–222. https://doi.org/10.1109/TRA.2003.808873
25. Lee S, Kim H, Jeong H, Kim J (2015) Analysis of musculoskeletal system of human during lifting task with arm using electromyography. Int J Precis Eng Manuf 16:393–398. https://doi.org/10.1007/s12541-015-0052-y
26. Triwiyanto T, Wahyunggoro O, Nugroho HA, Herianto H (2016) DWT analysis of sEMG for muscle fatigue assessment of dynamic motion flexion-extension of elbow joint. In: 2016 8th international conference on information technology and electrical engineering (ICITEE). IEEE Conference Publications, Yogyakarta, pp 1–6. https://doi.org/10.1109/ICITEED.2016.7863300
27. Triwiyanto T, Wahyunggoro O, Nugroho HA, Herianto H (2017) DWT analysis of sEMG for muscle fatigue assessment of dynamic motion flexion-extension of elbow joint. In: Proceedings of 2016 8th international conference on information technology and electrical engineering: empowering technology for better future, ICITEE 2016. https://doi.org/10.1109/ICITEED.2016.7863300

State of the Art Methods of Machine Learning for Prosthetic Hand Development: A Review

Triwiyanto Triwiyanto, Anita Miftahul Maghfiroh, Syevana Dita Musvika, Farid Amrinsani, Syaifudin, Ridha Mak'ruf, Nur Rachmat, Wahyu Caesarendra, and Maciej Sulowicz

Abstract In developing countries, a number of upper limb incidence that leads to trauma and amputation is increasing. The development of prosthetic hands has been carried out by several researchers in the past, but research related to prosthetic hands that are light, low battery consumption and high accuracy are still a challenge for researchers. Therefore, this study aims to review papers related to the EMG pattern recognition, analog part, feature extraction and classifier methods to get the best prosthetic hand design recommendations. This review paper collects articles from the Scopus and PUBMED databases from 2012 to 2022. The keywords used are EMG AND pattern recognition AND prosthetic hand. Based on the analysis of the VOSviewer application with these keywords, this topic is grouped into five network clusters. Based on the literature study related to the embedded system platforms used, it was found that 27.7% used microcontroller platforms, 11.11% FPGA platforms, 27.7% Raspberry Pi platforms and 33.5% used computer platforms. Furthermore, conventional supervised machine learning is more widely used as a classifier including decision trees, random forests, K-NN, and support vector machines than

T. Triwiyanto (✉) · A. M. Maghfiroh · S. D. Musvika · F. Amrinsani · Syaifudin · R. Mak'ruf
Department of Medical Electronics Technology, Poltekkes Kemenkes Surabaya, Surabaya, Indonesia
e-mail: Triwi@poltekkesdepkes-sby.ac.id

T. Triwiyanto
Intelligent Medical Rehabilitation Devices Research Group, Department of Medical Electronics Technology, Poltekkes Kemenkes Surabaya, Surabaya, Indonesia

S. D. Musvika
Biomedical Engineering Master Degree, Department of Physics, Faculty of Science and Technology, Universitas Airlangga, Surabaya, Indonesia

N. Rachmat
Department of Orthotic Prosthetic, Poltekkes Kemenkes Surakarta, Surakarta, Indonesia

W. Caesarendra
Universiti Brunei Darussalam, Bandar Seri Begawan, Brunei Darussalam

M. Sulowicz
Poland Cracow University of Technology, Kraków, Poland

T. Triwiyanto et al. (eds.), *Proceeding of the 3rd International Conference on Electronics, Biomedical Engineering, and Health Informatics*, Lecture Notes in Electrical Engineering 1008, https://doi.org/10.1007/978-981-99-0248-4_37

deep learning. This review paper can provide an overview of the state-of-the-art methods used in the development of machine learning-based smart prosthetic hands.

Keywords Prosthetic hand · Machine learning · Pattern recognition · EMG

1 Introduction

Amputation of the hand can be caused by various things, including work accidents, cancer, diabetes, and birth defects [1]. Amputation can cause decreasing productivity due to the impact on physical, physio-social, and decreasing confidence. Based on the location of the amputation, the upper limb amputation is grouped into five categories, transradial (below elbow), trans-humeral (above elbow), forequarter, shoulder disarticulation, and wrist disarticulation [2, 3]. According to these categories, several researchers have developed prosthetic hands that are either cosmetic or functional [4, 5]. Prosthetic cosmetic hands only have complementary properties but cannot function like normal human hands. However, functional prosthetic hands can be used for daily activities as a replacement for the missing hand. The development of a functional prosthetic hand has a high complexity because it involves the process of data acquisition, digital signal processing, pattern recognition, motor activation and prosthetic hand design. So, in general, the price of functional prosthetic hands is very expensive for people in developing countries, which is in the range of 8,000 US$ to 30,000 US$. Commercial prosthetic hand products include the Touch Bionic I-limb hand and Otto bock's. Therefore, research related to the development of functional prosthetic hands is still an attraction for researchers (Fig. 1).

Several researchers have developed prosthetic hands with a focus on prosthetic hand designs using 3D printing technology. In this design, the author generally researches in terms of finger design (anthropomorphic) resembling a real human hand and the use of motors as prosthetic hand propulsion. In addition to the prosthetic hand design, several researchers evaluate feature extraction and classifier to recognize EMG signal-based gestures. Research related to prosthetic hands can be grouped into four, namely control using electroencephalography (EEG) signals, electrooculography (EOG), voice commands, and surface electromyography (sEMG) [6–9]. These four sources will go through a feature extraction process to obtain information related to the desired prosthetic hand gesture. The conventional feature extraction that is commonly used in the implementation of prosthetic hands for both control and analysis purposes is grouped into the time domain, frequency domain, and time–frequency domain features [10]. The time domain feature is still a favorite feature that is often used by researchers related to its light computing time and ease application to various platforms. However, the time-domain features are unable to reveal the frequency component that is hidden in the signal. Therefore, some researchers apply the frequency-domain features to perform signal frequency analysis [11, 12]. Furthermore, for the purposes of analysis of dynamic motions, several authors apply time-domain features to analyze signals against time and frequency

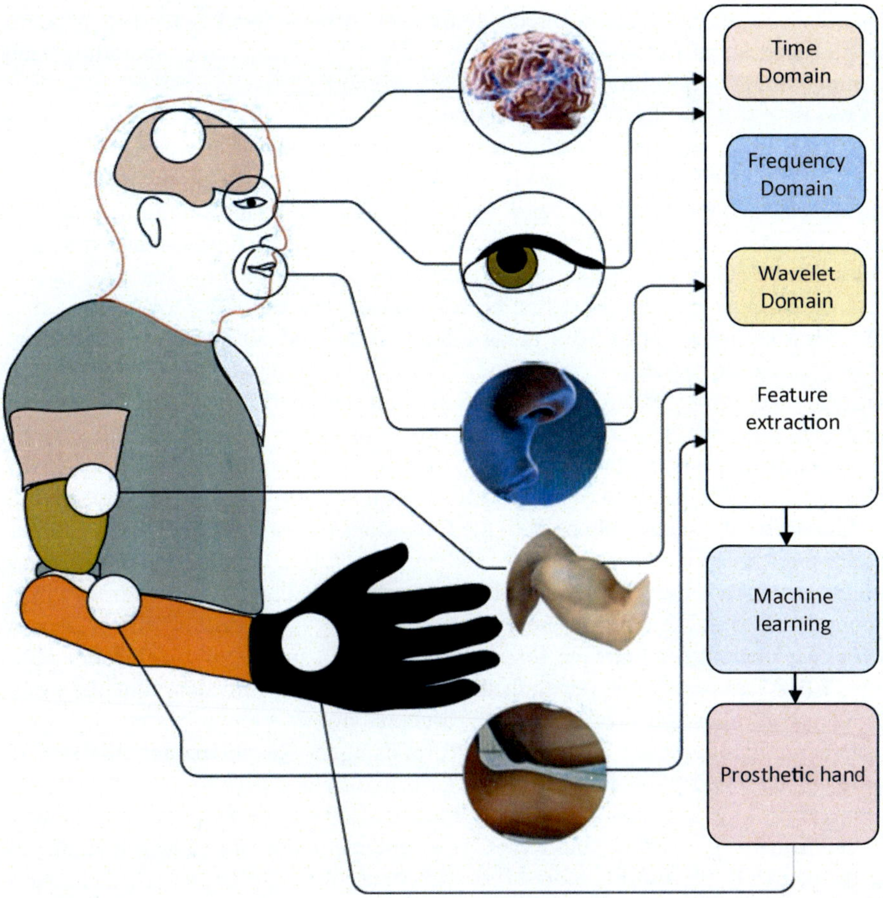

Fig. 1 Prosthetic hand control based on EMG/EOG, EEG and voice pattern recognition which consist of data acquisition, feature extraction (time, frequency, and time–frequency domain)

[11]. Several mother wavelets are applied to get the best features for gesture movements. However, the process of convolution mother wavelet with the signal takes a long time. Therefore, this feature extraction is only suitable for signal complexity analysis purposes.

Several review papers show that time-domain feature extraction is still the favorite feature for signal extraction. Additionally, after the feature extraction process, the next process is the classification process using machine learning. Various types of machine learning have been applied by previous researchers to classify hand gestures, both conventional and modern. Supervised machine learning conventional which is often used for classifier purposes includes decision tree (DT), k-nearest neighbor (k-NN), Random Forest, Ada-Boost, Gradient Boosting, linear discriminant analysis (LDA), quadratic discriminant analysis (QDA), support vector machine (SVM),

Gaussian Naïve Bayes and artificial neural network (ANN) [4, 13–19]. Modern machine learning is also applied by several researchers as a classifier, including deep learning with the convolution neural network method.

Overall prosthetic hand control system based on EMG pattern recognition is shown in Fig. 2 which consists of a prosthetic hand, motor driver, EMG signal data acquisition, feature extraction process and motion classification. Data acquisition consists of a pre-amplifier, band-pass filter, notch filter, and summing amplifier. Sensors used to record muscle signal activity are electrodes. Furthermore, the electrodes can be either disposable or dry electrodes. Before machine learning can be used, the training process must first be carried out. The training process is carried out with a composition of 80% dataset for training and 20% dataset for testing. After the training process is completed, the classifier is then applied to the system platform used. Some researchers use a microcontroller platform to obtain a portable system. In this case, feature extraction and machine learning are embedded in the microcontroller system. However, this system has a general drawback in terms of memory, so the development of machine learning is only appropriate for conventional machine learning. In accordance with the limitations of available memory resources and libraries, in general the classifier implementation is using the Python programming base which is then converted to the C++ programming language format which is compatible with the Arduino programming language. Tensor flow lite is also an alternative method for machine learning developers using a microcontroller platform [20]. As an alternative, due to the limitations of the machine learning library on the microcontroller platform, several researchers have developed machine learning implementations using the Raspberry platform using the Raspbian operating system with Python programming [21, 22]. This platform is open source so many developers are involved. Machine learning libraries that are often used in Python programming are Scikit-learn, Tensorflow, and Keras. The implementation of machine learning on the Raspberry Pi platform is more efficient because the training, testing and evaluation processes can be done online on the system used. However, the weakness of the Raspberry is that it is not equipped with an analog to digital converter (A/D) device, so users must add an additional MCP3008 A/D converter component. Based on the state-of-the-art method in the prosthetic hand development, this study aims to review papers that discussed any related prosthetic hand development based on pattern recognition. The contribution of this paper is:

1. This paper provides an overview and recommendations related to the design of prosthetic hands with a focus on the implementation of feature extraction and machine learning to various platforms.
2. Various kinds of feature extraction and machine learning models, both modern and conventional, are presented in this paper to provide a clear picture of the advantages and disadvantages of previous researchers.
3. Furthermore, exploration related to analog parts and actuators is also discussed in this paper to provide an overview of the proper use of motors in prosthetic hand designs.

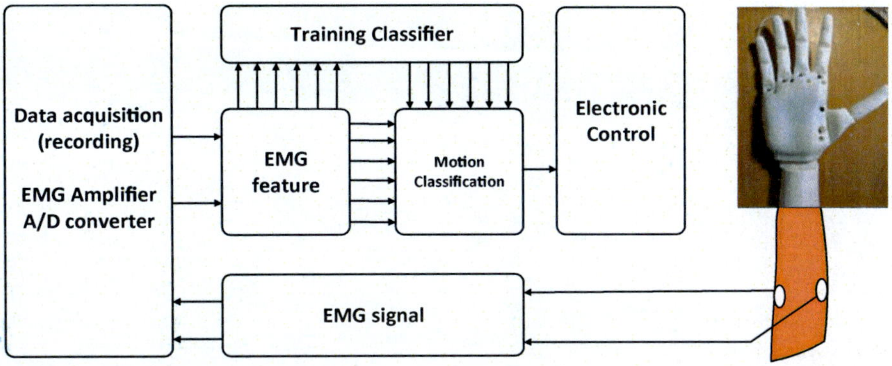

Fig. 2 Basic concept of prosthetics hand based on EMG pattern recognition. This diagram block can be implemented on any platform including, microcontroller, Raspberry Pi, field programmable gate array, and computer system

2 Materials and Method

2.1 Article Publication Trend

This review paper utilizes the article database from Scopus and PUBMED by using a search engine with a filter from 2012 to 2022. In the Scopus database, researchers obtained a total of 258 articles for article prosthetic hands using EMG pattern recognition as a basis. Furthermore, the PUBMED database found 168 articles on the theme of prosthetic hands based on machine learning. Based on the keywords prosthetic AND machine learning AND EMG, there was an increasing trend in the number of articles for the period 2012 to 2022 for both Scopus and PUBMED databases is presented in Fig. 3. The two lines in Fig. 3 show an increasing trend for a number of published papers, especially from 2018 to 2020. The decrease in the number of articles after 2021 is due to data is not completed for the whole year 2022.

2.2 Keyword Network Visualization

Research on prosthetic hands using the basis of EMG pattern recognition is influenced by several main keywords, namely machine learning, prosthetic hands, pattern recognition, signal processing, and rehabilitation. Furthermore, the keywords are grouped into five clusters as shown in Fig. 4. Cluster machine learning (cluster 1) shows the strongest network compared to other clusters. Cluster 1 is closely related to the keywords deep learning, prosthetic hand, prosthesis, EMG signal and myocontrol. Cluster prosthetic hand (cluster 2) is related to the research topic of gesture recognition, surface electromyography, neural network and EMG signal. Another

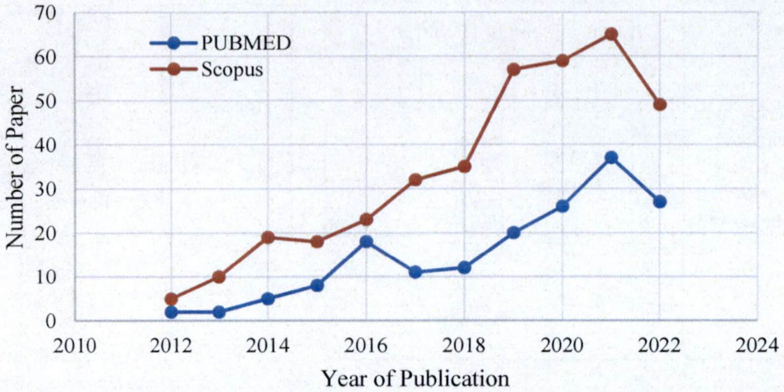

Fig. 3 The trend of increasing the number of articles with the keywords prosthetic hand, EMG pattern recognition and machine learning for the search period from 2012 to 2022. The red line shows an upward trend in the number of articles based on the Scopus and blue databases

network involved in the discussion of prosthetic hands based on EMG pattern recognition is the myoelectric control cluster (cluster 3). Myoelectric control is closely related to keyword pattern recognition, surface electromyography and support vector machines. Signal processing is a major part of the study of prosthetic hands based on EMG pattern recognition and this is shown in cluster 4 (feature extraction) which is part of signal processing. Furthermore, another small cluster that supports the topic of prosthetic hands is rehabilitation (cluster 5) which is supported by several keywords including EEG and prosthetics.

3 Result

Prosthetic hands that are driven using EMG signals generally use 1-to-4-point leads using either dry electrodes or Ag (AgCl) disposable electrodes. The EMG signal will be processed with several analog signal processing methods, including pre-amplifier, band-pass filter (20–500 Hz), notch filter (50 Hz), and summing amplifier [23, 24]. The next step is the digitalization process, which is converting from analog to digital (A/D converter). This conversion process is conducted using the built-in A/D in the microcontroller. The microcontroller records an EMG signal with a sampling frequency of 2000 Hz [25]. This sampling frequency is selected according to the Nyquist rule, which is twice the maximum recorded frequency. Furthermore, the prosthetic hand which is controlled using the basis of EMG pattern recognition will follow the windowing, feature extraction and pattern classification stages. The windowing process is carried out by cutting the recorded EMG signal into several parts. The window length that is often used for classification purposes in real time is 100–200 ms [26]. The feature extraction process must be carried out to reduce

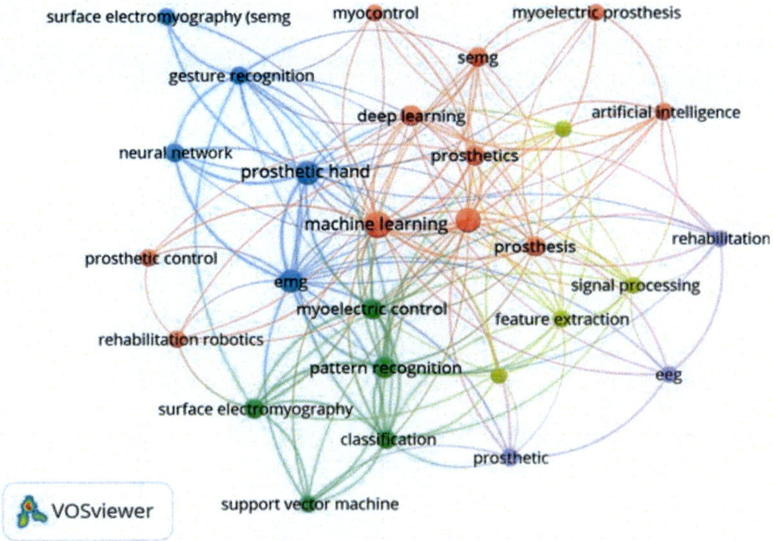

Fig. 4 The networking of the keywords for prosthetic hand based on EMG pattern recognition. This network was created using keyword analysis VOS viewer

the complexity of the EMG signal. The feature extraction process that is commonly used to evaluate an EMG signal is to use time-domain features, frequency-domain features, and time–frequency domain features (wavelets). The time-domain feature is a feature that is often used in the development of prosthetic hands for EMG signal extraction. These features include root mean square (RMS), variance (VAR), mean absolute value (MAV), integrated EMG (IEMG), zero crossing (ZC), sign slope change (SSC), Wilson amplitude (WAMP), window length (WL) [27, 28]. The equations related to the time domain feature extraction are shown in Eqs. (1)–(15).

The Root Mean Square (RMS) value denotes the average signal strength over an EMG sample window length. The following mathematical formula can be used to describe this property:

$$RMS = \sqrt{\frac{1}{N}\sum_{i=1}^{N} x_i^2} \tag{1}$$

where x_i indicates the i-th EMG signal and N indicates the length of the EMG signal.

An absolute summation of the EMG signal throughout a window length of EMG samples is what the Integrated EMG (IEMG) value represents. The following is a description of the mathematical equation:

$$\text{IEMG} = \sum_{i=1}^{N} |x_i| \tag{2}$$

The average value of the EMG signal's power is known as the EMG signal's variance, or EMG (VAR). The formula for VAR is as follows:

$$\mathrm{VAR} = \frac{1}{N-1}\sum_{i=1}^{N} x_i^2 \tag{3}$$

The average of the EMG signal's absolute value throughout a window length of N is known as the Mean Absolute Value (MAV). The formulation of the MAV is

$$\mathrm{MAV} = \frac{1}{N}\sum_{i=1}^{N} |x_i| \tag{4}$$

The EMG signal's non-linear feature is measured by the logarithm (LOG) parameter. The average logarithm of the EMG signal is used to calculate the LOG value. The following defines the LOG value:

$$\mathrm{LOG} = \exp(\frac{1}{N}\sum_{i=1}^{N} \log(|x_i|) \tag{5}$$

The signal's length between two successive samples, $xi + 1$ and xi, is measured using the Waveform Length (WL). The formula for WL is as follows:

$$\mathrm{WL} = \sum_{i=1}^{N-1} |x_{i+1} - x_i| \tag{6}$$

The average value of the waveform length within a window of length N is known as the Average Amplitude Change (AAC). AAC looks like the following:

$$\mathrm{AAC} = \frac{1}{N}\sum_{i=1}^{N-1} |x_{i+1} - x_i| \tag{7}$$

The Distinction Based on the standard deviation between $xi + 1$ and xi, the absolute standard deviation value (DASDV) is computed. Here is how DASDV is described:

$$\mathrm{DASDV} = \sqrt{\frac{1}{N-1}\sum_{i=1}^{N-1} (x_{i+1} - x_i)^2} \tag{8}$$

The number of times the signal crosses a particular threshold value is known as the Zero Crossing (ZC) value. ZC is determined as:

$$\mathrm{ZC} = \sum_{i=1}^{N-1} [f(x_i \times x_{i+1}) \cap |x_i - x_{i+1}| \geq \mathit{threshold}$$
$$f(x) = \begin{cases} 1, \mathit{if} \rightarrow x \geq \mathit{threshold} \\ 0, \mathit{otherwise} \end{cases} \tag{9}$$

The number of times the slope of the signal changes its sign inside a window of length N is known as the Sign Slope Change (SSC). The formulation is as follows:

$$\mathrm{SSC} = \sum_{i=1}^{N-1} [f[(x_i - x_{i-1}) \times (x_i - x_{i+1})]]$$
$$f(x) = \begin{cases} 1, \mathit{if} \rightarrow x \geq \mathit{threshold} \\ 0, \mathit{otherwise} \end{cases} \tag{10}$$

The Wilson Amplitude (WAMP) measures how frequently a threshold value is exceeded by the absolute value of the difference between two successive samples ($xi + 1$ and xi). This is how it is explained:

$$\mathrm{WAMP} = \sum_{i=1}^{N-1} [f(|x_i - x_{i+1}|)]$$
$$f(x) = \begin{cases} 1, \mathit{if} \rightarrow x \geq \mathit{threshold} \\ 0, \mathit{otherwise} \end{cases} \tag{11}$$

The average of the number of times the EMG signal exceeds a predetermined threshold is known as the MyoPulse Percentage (MYOP) Rate. MYOP is characterized by:

$$\mathrm{MYOP} = \frac{1}{N} \sum_{i=1}^{N} [f(x_i)]$$
$$f(x) = \begin{cases} 1, \mathit{if} \rightarrow x \geq \mathit{threshold} \\ 0, \mathit{otherwise} \end{cases} \tag{12}$$

In addition to using time domain feature extraction, several developers of prosthetic hands based on EMG pattern recognition also use frequency domain features. This frequency domain includes mean frequency (MNF), median frequency (MDF), and mean power (MP) which can be calculated using the following equation.

MNF, or mean frequency, is determined by multiplying the EMG power spectrum by the frequency and then dividing the result by the total sum of the spectrum intensity.

It can be computed as:

$$\text{MNF} = \sum_{j=1}^{M} f_j P_j / \sum_{j=1}^{M} P_j \tag{13}$$

MDF, or half of the TTP (Total Power) feature, is a frequency at which the spectrum is split into two sections of equal amplitude. It can be said to be:

$$\text{MDF} = \sum_{j=1}^{MDF} P_j = \sum_{j=\text{MDF}}^{M} P_j = \frac{1}{2}\sum_{j=1}^{M} P_j \tag{14}$$

MNP is the EMG power spectrum's average power. The formula for the computation is

$$\text{MNP} = \sum_{j=1}^{M} P_i / M \tag{15}$$

where f indicates the frequency, P shows the EMG power, and M is the length of frequency.

In the development of prosthetic hands with the application of EMG pattern recognition, several conventional supervised machine learning methods have been successfully applied to the classification of basic movements. The supervised machine learning methods include artificial neural network (ANN), linear discriminant analysis (LDA), Simple logistic regression (SLR), decision tree (DT), logistic model tree (LMT), Support vector machine (SVM), k-nearest neighbor (k-NN), Naive Bayes (NB), and support vector machine (SVM) [13, 23, 29–31]. In addition, several researchers have developed EMG pattern recognition by applying modern machine learning, including deep learning based on convolution neural network (CNN), and deep learning based on transfer learning [32]. At this stage, the conventional classifier is still often used as EMG pattern recognition because it has low computational complexity. However, proper feature extraction exploration is needed to obtain maximum performance, and it will affect the increasing of the time computation. Deep learning using a convolution neural network (CNN) basis is a solution for implementing EMG pattern recognition for prosthetic hand control. The CNN process is the implementation of feature engineering on the CNN deep learning architecture. Therefore, researchers do not require external feature extraction. However, the convolution process requires sufficient time so that it requires layers that are not too many but are effective in classifying gestures.

Several studies related to EMG pattern recognition for prosthetic hands apply feature extraction and classifier algorithms on micro-controller platforms, Raspberry Pi, and computer systems [31]. On the microcontroller platform, the author uses the Tensorflow lite library for machine learning implementation. The development of

Table 1 The keywords of prosthetic hand-based EMG pattern recognition. The keywords are clustered into five areas

Cluster	Keywords
1	Artificial intelligence, deep learning, electromyography, machine learning, myo-control, myoelectric prosthesis, prosthesis control, prosthetic control, prosthetic, rehabilitation robotics, semg
2	Classification, myoelectric control, pattern recognition, support vector machine, surface electromyography,
3	Emg, gesture recognition, neural network, prosthetic hand, surface electromyography
4	Electromyogram, feature extraction, real-time extraction, signal processing
5	Eeg, prosthetic, rehabilitation

a Raspberry Pi-based prosthetic hand applies Python programming by utilizing the ScikitLearn and Keras libraries for machine learning implementation. The limited memory space and clock speed of the processor are weaknesses in the implementation of machine learning on the microcontroller and Raspberry Pi platforms, especially during the training process. Therefore, some researchers who are still in the machine learning evaluation stage are still using the computer platform. The development of prosthetic hands with the implementation of machine learning on the microcontroller, FPGA, Raspberry Pi and computer devices is shown in Table 1.

Several researchers of prosthetic hands based on EMG pattern recognition have developed various methods to produce high accuracy [39, 43]. Several conventional machine learning has been applied to the development of prosthetic hands, including decision tree (DT), k-nearest neighbor (KNN), support vector machine (SVM), random forest, linear discriminant analysis (LDA), artificial neural network (ANN). and Gaussian. In addition, modern machine learning is also widely applied in the development of prosthetic hands, including using deep learning, both convolution neural network models. Accuracy generated by machine learning, apart from being determined by the choice of the right classifier and feature extraction, is also determined by the type of electrode used. Some researchers use only one type of EMG sensor electrode, voice sensor, or a combination of both [44]. As shown in Table 2.

Regarding the analog hardware section, both EMG amplifiers and prosthetic hand actuators, several authors have developed prosthetic hands using DC motors, servo motors and linear actuators. The use of a DC motor as a finger motion controller in a prosthetic hand device has easier power and speed settings compared to a linear actuator. However, the use of a DC motor requires an additional circuit as a motor power control unit, as described in Table 3. On the other hand, some researchers emphasize the recognition of hand gestures to be applied to machine learning. Some researchers are pursuing in terms of movement accuracy so that the prosthetic hand design only recognizes two hand gestures, namely open and close hand movements [13, 55–61]. Furthermore, several other researchers have developed prosthetic hands that can recognize up to 8 gestures [62–65].

Table 2 Machine learning and hardware platform for prosthetic hand development

Author	Feature extraction	Type of machine learning	Platform
Akhtar [29]	Root mean square	Linear Discriminant Analysis (LDA)	Teensy 3.1 microcontroller (PJRC, Sherwood, OR)
Wilson [23]	Feature: MAV, WL, ZC, SSC	Artificial neural network (ANN) classifier [6]	16-bit PIC microcontroller from Microchip Technology Inc. the
Geethanjali [13]	Time domain (TD), frequency-domain (FD), and time–frequency domain (TFD) features TD features: mean absolute value (MAV), number of zero crossings (ZC), number of slope sign changes (SSC), waveform length (WL), and fourth- order ARcoefficient	Simple logistic regression (SLR), decision tree (DT), logistic model tree (LMT)	TMS320F28335 microcontroller
Fajardo [30]	Variance, WL, IEMG, ZC, SSC, and WAMP	Multilayer Feedforward Neural Network	TI TM4C12x microcontrollers
Qin [32]	Without feature extraction	CNN 1D and CNN 2D	Arduino nano 33 BLE sense microcontroller
Cabegin [31]	ZC, VAR, MAD, and WAMP	Support vector machine (SVM) and principal component analysis (PCA)	Raspberry Pi 3 model B+
Lonsdale [21]	Without feature extraction	Deep learning model, Inception-v3, with transfer learning to	Raspberry Pi 3 model B+
Souza [33]	ZC, VAR, MAD, and WAMP	Multi layer perceptron	Raspberry Pi 3 model B+
Akmal [34]	ZC, VAR, MAD, and WAMP	Support vector machine (SVM)	Raspberry Pi 3 model B+
Triwiyanto [35]	RMS, VAR, MAV, and SSI features	k-nearest neighbor (k-NN), Naive Bayes (NB), decision tree (DT), and support vector machine (SVM)	Raspberry Pi 3B+
Gautam [4]	Without feature extraction	Deep learning CNN	Virtex-7 Xilinx field-programmable gate array (FPGA)

(continued)

Table 2 (continued)

Author	Feature extraction	Type of machine learning	Platform
Chrapka [36]	IAV, ZC, VAR, WAMP, v-order detector, LOG, AR model, histogram	SVM	FPGA Altera DE2-70
Roy [37]	Cross-Wavelet transform (XWT)	Deep learning CNN	Computer
Raurale [38]	D-MAV, MAV, VAR, ZC, SSC, and WL	Linear Discriminant Analysis (LDA)	Computer
Young [39]	RMS, VAR, IAV, SSI, WL, MAV, MAV1, MAV2, TM3, TM4, TM5, AAC, SSC, ZC, DASDV, WAMP and MYOP	DT, k-NN, Random Forest, AdaBoost, Gradient Boosting, LDA, QDA, SVM, Gaussian (Naïve Bayes and Process) and NN	Computer, Core™ i7-8550U CPU
Parque [40]	Without feature extraction	Deep learning, GoogLeNet-based	Intel i7, Ubuntu 14.04, and GPU GeForce GTX TITAN
Nahid [41]	Continuous Wavelet Transform (Scalogram)	Transfer learning, AlexNet, and ResNet-18	Computer system
Jafarzadeh [42]	Without feature extraction	Deep convolution neural network (CNN)	Embedded GPGPU developer kit (NVIDIA Jetson TX2)

4 Discussion

A prosthetic device based on real-time EMG pattern recognition and classification is very dependent on the platform system used. Several platforms such as microcontrollers, Raspberry Pi, FPGAs and computer systems have been proposed to run feature extraction, machine learning and prosthetic hand control. Akhtar et. al has developed a prosthetic arm using the Teensy 3.1 microcontroller as the main brain which integrates the process of data acquisition, feature extraction and machine learning on the platform. Linear discriminant analysis (LDA) was used to recognize hand gestures. Furthermore, servo motor movement speed control is carried out proportionally based on the amplitude of the mean absolute value (MAV) of the EMG signal. Research conducted by Akthar is equipped with MPL115A2 barometric pressure sensors to prevent slippage when the prosthetic hand holds the object. However, from the aspect of accuracy, this research has not explored much so that this is still an opportunity for readers to develop a microcontroller-based EMG pattern recognition model. The design of a prosthetic hand with a minimal design will be an advantage because in the design of a prosthetic hand for the transradial amputee, there is not much space available in the socket. Wilson et al. proposes a prosthetic hand design with the development of electrode integration, EMG signal processing, feature

Table 3 State of the art method for prosthetic hand development

Author	Electrode	Method	Accuracy
Sam [39]	Myo EMG sensor	DT, kNN, Random Forest, AdaBoost, Gradient Boosting, LDA, (QDA), SVM, Gaussian (Naïve Bayes and Process) and NN; features RMS, VAR, IAV, SSI, WL dan MAV	94.8%
Julio [43]	Voice and EMG signal	Artificial neural network (ANN)	98.89%
Rasouli [45]	Tactile sensor array from piezo resistive	Extreme Learning Machine (ELM)	98.75
Cabegin [31]	2 EMG electrodes	Support Vector Machine (SVM)	99.72%
Nazmun [41]	2 channel EMG electrodes	Continuous Wavelet Transform (CWT), CNN dan LSTM	99.72%
Valentina [46]	12 EMG electrodes	Least-Squares Support Vector Machine (LS-SVM)	70%
Mohsen [47]	4 EMG electrodes	CNN 2D	91.26%
Arvind [4]	EMG electrodes	CNN	91.1%
Mehrshad [48]	EMG electrodes and Camera	RMS, MAV dan Variable EMG (VAR), R-CNN	95.3%
Jing-Yi [49]	Ultrasound sensor and electrogoniometer	SVM, BP ANN dan FBP ANN	RMSE: 13%
Yu Wu [50]	Electrode array wristband, bioimpedance	SVM, KNN	98.5%
R. Meattini [51]	EMG electrodes	SVM	96.3%
Morten [52]	16 EMG electrodes active (Otto Bock)	Inter-class Distance Nearest Neighbour (IDNNtotal), Inter-class Distance All Neighbours (IDAN)	Error: 7,613
Jingdong [53]	2 EMG active electrodes	Neural network berbasis Levenberg–Marquardt (LM), Autoregressive (AR)	980.46%
Manfredo [54]	22 sensor glove, inclinometer, linear force sensor, EMG electrodes	CNN	660.59 ± 60.40%

extraction and LDA classifier using a 16-bit PIC micro-controller. This research puts forward a portable model and low resource requirements. Furthermore, by using CAN-bus technology, the data communication system can be integrated with other devices.

The integration model of data acquisition, feature extraction and classifier were also developed in [13]. Geethanjali [13] applied the proposed model to the TMS320F28335 DSP controller using C++ programming. At the initial stage, feature extraction and classifier were evaluated using MATLAB application to get the best performance model. Feature extraction that is evaluated are time, frequency and time-domain feature extraction. The time domain features used in this study are the mean absolute value (MAV), zero crossings (ZC), number of slope sign changes (SSC), waveform length (WL), and fourth-order AR coefficients. Furthermore, the classifiers evaluated in this study were simple logistic regression (SLR), J48 algorithm for decision tree (DT), and logistic model tree (LMT). Machine learning that is applied to the microcontroller or processor platform is an added value in the development of prosthetic hands based on EMG pattern recognition. Therefore, in order for the prosthetic hand system to be effective, several researchers have developed an online training and testing process on the microcontroller platform. Fajardo developed a prosthetic arm based on EMG pattern recognition by applying machine learning to the IT platform TM4C12x microcontrollers [30]. The back-propagation-based artificial neural network is implemented into the ARM Cortex-M microcontroller system with training mode carried out offline using the MATLAB application. The online-classification machine learning mode on the prosthetic hand is carried out on the microcontroller system after updating the ANN weights resulting from the training generated in the MATLAB application. The development of prosthetic hands based on EMG pattern recognition where the training and testing process is carried out online will produce an effective system. Therefore, several researchers have developed prosthetic hands based on EMG pattern recognition using the Raspberry Pi platform with the Raspbian operating system. The process of training and testing machine learning can be done online on the Raspberry Pi platform. Cabegin mengembangkan prosthetic hand dengan mengimplementasikan machine learning ke platform Raspberry Pi tipe B + 3 [31]. Sinyal EMG diekstraksi dengan menggunakan feature zero crossing (ZC), variance (VAR), mean absolute deviation (MAD), and Wilson amplitude (WAMP). Proses klasifikasi gesture dilakukan dengan menggunakan support vector machine (SVM) yang diimplementasikan ke platform Raspberry Pi.

The test results show that the accuracy of the prosthetic hand varies for testing intervals at different times. The development of a prosthetic hand with EMG pattern recognition based on the Raspberry Pi platform with the Raspbian operating system was also proposed by Akmal [34]. In this system, the researcher applies a feature extraction process and machine learning using Python programming which is implemented on the Raspberry Pi machine. In this study, Akmal applied a classifier support vector machine (SVM) to classify hand gestures to move the prosthetic hand. By utilizing an operating system-based platform, the system can conduct online training and testing processes. From the evaluation results, the SVM machine classifier is able to distinguish movements with an accuracy of 78%. In addition to applying machine learning to the microcontroller, FPGA, and Raspberry Pi platforms, several other researchers have implemented the system (feature extraction and classifier) into computer systems.

According to the result reported in previous studies, embedded machine learning is still a challenge for previous research to be developed. A prosthetic hand based on EMG pattern recognition with a compact and portable engine is still the main focus of this research. Furthermore, an embedded machine learning into hardware-based platforms such as microcontrollers, Raspberries and FPGAs is expected to be able to implement online training and testing processes so that there is no need to run the system on two different platforms. On the other hand, the implementation of prosthetic hands should be not only applied in a laboratory environment but has been applied in the actual environment, namely using amputee subjects. Some other challenges that need to be done are the implementation of machine learning into embedded hardware systems that can run fully online both during training and testing. The implementation of the deep learning convolution neural network (CNN) model will be an added value if it can be fully implemented because CNN-based deep learning does not require a feature extraction stage.

5 Conclusion

The purpose of this study is to review papers related to the EMG pattern recognition, analog part, feature extraction and classifier methods to get the best prosthetic hand design recommendations. Based on review results, a prosthetic hand based on pattern recognition which embedded in the microcontroller devices and Raspberry Pi system are recommended. Furthermore, the conventional time domain feature and classifier is still used a lot in the development because the computation time is fast enough to process the EMG gesture. Additionally, in the actuator part, mostly several studies used a DC motor to drive the fingers in the prosthetic hand and some others used a servo motor. This review paper has given a guidance to develop an effective prosthetic hand. In the future, online training and testing embedded machine learning for prosthetic hands should be studied in order to make a smart prosthetic hand which able to adapt to any kind of user.

References

1. Triwiyanto T, Rahmawati T, Pawana IPA, Lamidi L (2021) State-of-the-art method in prosthetic hand design : a review. J Biomim Biomater Biomed Eng 50:15–24. https://doi.org/10.4028/www.scientific.net/JBBBE.50.15
2. Lenzi T, Lipsey J, Sensinger JW (2016) The RIC arm—a small anthropomorphic transhumeral prosthesis. el 21:2660–2671. https://doi.org/10.1109/TMECH.2016.2596104
3. Toledo C, Simon A, Muñoz R, Vera A, Leija L, Hargrove L (2012) A comparison of direct and pattern recognition control for a two degree-of-freedom above elbow virtual prosthesis. In:

Proceedings annual international conference of the IEEE engineering in medicine and biology society. EMBS. 60611, pp 4332–4335. https://doi.org/10.1109/EMBC.2012.6346925
4. Gautam A, Panwar M, Wankhede A, Arjunan SP, Naik GR, Acharyya A, Kumar DK (2020) LoCoMo-Net: a low-complex deep learning framework for sEMG based hand movement recognition for prosthetic control. IEEE J Transl Eng Heal Med 1–12 (2020). https://doi.org/10.1109/JTEHM.2020.3023898
5. Van Der Niet O, van der Sluis CK (2013) Functionality of i-LIMB and i-LIMB pulse hands: case report. J Rehabil Res Dev 50:1123
6. Alazrai R, Abuhijleh M, Alwanni H, Daoud MI (2019) A deep learning framework for decoding motor imagery tasks of the same hand using EEG signals. IEEE Access 7:109612–109627. https://doi.org/10.1109/ACCESS.2019.2934018
7. Oppus CM, Prado JRR, Marinas AG, Reyes RSJ (2016) Brain-computer interface and voice-controlled 3D printed prosthetic hand. In: 2016 IEEE region 10 conference (TENCON), pp 2689–2693
8. Pratomo MR, Irianto BG, Triwiyanto T, Utomo B, Setioningsih ED, Titisari D (2020) Prosthetic hand with 2-dimensional motion based EOG signal control. IOP Conf Ser Mater Sci Eng 850
9. Triwiyanto T, Yulianto E, Wisana IDGH, Mak'ruf MR, Guruh Irianto B, Setioningsih ED, Herdinanta DS (2021) Electromyography feature analysis to recognize the hand motion in a prosthetic hand design. J Biomimetics Biomater Biomed Eng 50:25–37. https://doi.org/10.4028/www.scientific.net/JBBBE.50.25
10. Phinyomark A, Phukpattaranont P, Limsakul C (2012) Feature reduction and selection for EMG signal classification. Expert Syst Appl 39:7420–7431. https://doi.org/10.1016/j.eswa.2012.01.102
11. Bigliassi M, Scalassara PR, Kanthack TFD, Abrão T, Moraes ACD, Altimari LR (2014) Fourier and wavelet spectral analysis of EMG signals in 1 km cycling time-trial. Appl Math 05:1878–1886. https://doi.org/10.4236/am.2014.513181
12. Kaplanis PA, Pattichis CS, Roberts CV (2002) Influence of isometric voluntary contraction on time and frequency domain parameters of surface EMG. Annu Int Conf IEEE Eng Med Biol Proc 3:2408–2409
13. Geethanjali P, Ray KK (2015) A low-cost real-time research platform for EMG pattern recognition-based prosthetic hand. IEEE/ASME Trans Mechatron 20:1948–1955. https://doi.org/10.1109/TMECH.2014.2360119
14. Shi WT, Lyu ZJ, Tang ST, Chia TL, Yang CY (2018) A bionic hand controlled by hand gesture recognition based on surface EMG signals: a preliminary study. Biocybern Biomed Eng 38:126–135. https://doi.org/10.1016/j.bbe.2017.11.001
15. Triwiyanto T, Rahmawati T, Pawana IPA (2019) Feature and muscle selection for an effective hand motion classifier based on electromyography. Indones J Electr Eng Inform 7:303–313. https://doi.org/10.11591/ijeei.v7i2.867
16. Eisenberg DG, Fyvie K, Abdul-khaaliq G (2017) Real-time segmentation and feature extraction of electromyography: towards real-time segmentation and feature extraction of electromyography : towards real-time segmentation and feature of electromyography: towards control prosthetic hand control of a P. In: IFAC-papers on line. Elsevier B.V., pp 151–156. https://doi.org/10.1016/j.ifacol.2017.12.028
17. Gini G, Arvetti M, Somlai I, Folgheraiter M (2012) Acquisition and analysis of EMG signals to recognize multiple hand movements for prosthetic applications. Appl Bionics Biomech 9:145–155. https://doi.org/10.3233/ABB-2011-0024
18. Pamungkas D, Ward K (2015) Electro-tactile feedback system for a prosthetic hand. In: 22nd annual international conference on mechatronics and machine vision in practice M2VIP, pp 27–38
19. Arozi M, Caesarendra W, Ariyanto M, Munadi M, Setiawan JD, Glowacz A (2020) Pattern recognition of single-channel sEMG signal using PCA and ANN method to classify nine hand movements. Symmetry (Basel). 12:1–18
20. Warden P, Situnayake D (2019) TinyML: machine learning with TensorFlow Lite on Arduino and ultra-low-power microcontrollers

21. Lonsdale D, Zhang L, Jiang R (2020) 3D printed brain-controlled robot-arm prosthetic via embedded deep learning from sEMG sensors. In: 2020 international conference on machine learning and cybernetics (ICMLC), pp 247–253. https://doi.org/10.1109/ICMLC51923.2020.9469532
22. Triwiyanto T, Caesarendra W, Purnomo MH, Sułowicz M, Wisana IDGH, Titisari D, Lamidi L, Rismayani R (2022) Embedded machine learning using a multi-thread algorithm on a Raspberry Pi platform to improve prosthetic hand performance. Micromachines 13. https://doi.org/10.3390/mi13020191
23. Wilson AW, Losier YG, Parker PA, Lovely DF (2011) A bus-based smart myoelectric electrode/amplifier—system requirements. IEEE Trans Instrum Meas 1–10. https://doi.org/10.1109/MEMEA.2010.5480204
24. Li H, Xu S, Yang P, Chen L (2010) A research and design on surface EMG amplifier. In: 2010 international conference on measuring technology mechatronics automation, ICMTMA 1:306–309. https://doi.org/10.1109/ICMTMA.2010.256
25. Li Y, Zhang W, Zhang Q, Zheng N (2021) Transfer learning-based muscle activity decoding scheme by low-frequency sEMG for wearable low-cost application. IEEE Access 9:22804–22815. https://doi.org/10.1109/ACCESS.2021.3056412
26. Triwiyanto T, Wahyunggoro O, Nugroho HA, Herianto H (2017) Evaluating the performance of Kalman filter on elbow joint angle prediction based on electromyography. Int J Precis Eng Manuf 18:1739–1748. https://doi.org/10.1007/s12541-017-0202-5
27. Triwiyanto T, Wahyunggoro O, Nugroho HA, Herianto H (2017) Quantitative relationship between feature extraction of sEMG and upper limb elbow joint angle. In: Proceedings—2016 international seminar on application of technology for information and communication, ISEMANTIC 2016. https://doi.org/10.1109/ISEMANTIC.2016.7873808
28. Triwiyanto T, Oyas W, Hanung AN, Herianto H (2018) Adaptive threshold to compensate the effect of muscle fatigue on elbow-joint angle estimation based on electromyography. J Mech Eng Sci 12:3786–3796
29. Akhtar A, Choi KY, Fatina M, Cornman J, Wu E, Sombeck J, Yim C, Slade P, Lee J, Moore J, Gonzales D, Wu A, Anderson G, Rotter D, Shin C, Bretl T (2016) A low-cost, open-source, compliant hand for enabling sensorimotor control for people with transradial amputations. In: IEEE 2016 38th annual international conference of the IEEE engineering in medicine and biology society (EMBC). IEEE, Orlando, pp 4642–4645. https://doi.org/10.1109/EMBC.2016.7591762
30. Fajardo J, Lemus A, Rohmer E (2015) Galileo bionic hand: sEMG activated approaches for a multifunction upper-limb prosthetic. In: 2015 IEEE thirty fifth central American and panama convention (CONCAPAN XXXV). IEEE, pp 1–6. https://doi.org/10.1109/CONCAPAN.2015.7428468
31. Cabegin KRL, Fernan MAVML, Tia DMR, Santos RGG, Magwili GV (2019) Electromyography-based Control of Prosthetic Arm for Transradial Amputees using Principal Component Analysis and Support Vector Machine Algorithms. In: 2019 IEEE 11th international conference on humanoid, nanotechnology, information technology, communication and control, environment, and management (HNICEM), pp 1–6. IEEE. https://doi.org/10.1109/HNICEM48295.2019.9073353
32. Qin S, Zhang J, Shen H, Wang Y (2021) Arm movements recognition by implementing CNN on microcontrollers. In: 2021 9th international conference on control, mechatronics and automation (ICCMA), pp 171–176. https://doi.org/10.1109/ICCMA54375.2021.9646200
33. de Souza JODO, Bloedow MD, Rubo FC, de Figueiredo RM, Pessin G, Rigo SJ (2021) Investigation of different approaches to real-time control of prosthetic hands with electromyography signals. IEEE Sens J 21:20674–20684. https://doi.org/10.1109/JSEN.2021.3099744
34. Akmal M, Qureshi MF, Amin F, Rehman MZU, Niazi IK (2021) SVM-based real-time classification of prosthetic fingers using Myo armband-acquired electromyography data. In: 2021 IEEE 21st international conference on bioinformatics and bioengineering (BIBE), pp 1–5. https://doi.org/10.1109/BIBE52308.2021.9635461

35. Triwiyanto T, Caesarendra W, Purnomo MH, Sułowicz M (2022) Embedded machine learning using a multi-thread algorithm on a Raspberry Pi platform to improve prosthetic hand performance
36. Chrapka P (2010) EMG controlled hand prosthesis : EMG classification system EMG controlled hand prosthesis : EMG classification system by
37. Roy SS, Samanta K, Chatterjee S, Dey S, Nandi A, Bhowmik R, Mondal S (2020) Hand movement recognition using cross spectrum image analysis of EMG signals—a deep learning approach. In: 2020 national conference on emerging trends on sustainable technology and engineering applications NCETSTEA 2020, pp 1–5 https://doi.org/10.1109/NCETSTEA48365.2020.9119911
38. Raurale SA (2014) Acquisition and processing real-time EMG signals for prosthesis active hand movements. In: 2014 international conference on green computing communication and electrical engineering (ICGCCEE). IEEE, pp 1–6. https://doi.org/10.1109/ICGCCEE.2014.6922225
39. Young S, Stephens-Fripp B, Gillett A, Zhou H, Alici G (2019) Pattern recognition for prosthetic hand user's intentions using EMG data and machine learning techniques. In: IEEE/ASME international conference on advanced intelligent mechatronics (AIM), pp 544–550. https://doi.org/10.1109/AIM.2019.8868766
40. Parque V, Miyashita T (2020) Estimation of grasp states in prosthetic hands using deep learning. In: Proceedings of 2020 IEEE 44th annual computers software and application conference (COMPSAC), pp 1285–1289. https://doi.org/10.1109/COMPSAC48688.2020.00-79
41. Nahid N, Rahman A, Ahad MAR (2020) Deep learning based surface EMG hand gesture classification for low-cost myoelectric prosthetic hand. In: 2020 joint 9th international conference informatics, electronics and vision; 2020 4th international conference on imaging, vision pattern recognition, ICIEV (icIVPR). https://doi.org/10.1109/ICIEVicIVPR48672.2020.9306613
42. Jafarzadeh M, Hussey DC, Tadesse Y (2019) Deep learning approach to control of prosthetic hands with electromyography signals. In: 2019 22nd IEEE international symposium on measurement and control in robotics (ISMCR). Benefit Humanit ISMCR A1-4-1–A1-4-11. https://doi.org/10.1109/ISMCR47492.2019.8955725
43. Fajardo J, Lemus A, Rohmer E (2015) Galileo bionic hand: sEMG activated approaches for a multifunction upper-limb prosthetic. In: 2015 IEEE thirty fifth central American and panama convention (CONCAPAN XXXV), pp 1–6. IEEE
44. Asyali MH, Yilmaz M, Tokmakçi M, Sedef K, Aksebzeci BH, Mittal R (2011) Design and implementation of a voice-controlled prosthetic hand. Turkish J Electr Eng Comput Sci 19:33–46. https://doi.org/10.3906/elk-0912-315
45. Rasouli M, Ghosh R, Lee WW, Thakor NV, Kukreja S (2015) Stable force-myographic control of a prosthetic hand using incremental learning. Proc Annu Int Conf IEEE Eng Med Biol Soc EMBS 4828–4831. https://doi.org/10.1109/EMBC.2015.7319474
46. Gregori V, Gijsberts A, Caputo B (2017) Adaptive learning to speed-up control of prosthetic hands: a few things everybody should know. In: IEEE international conference on rehabilitation robotics, pp 1130–1135 (2017). https://doi.org/10.1109/ICORR.2017.8009401
47. Zhu Z, Gao X, Cao L, Pan D, Cai Y, Zhu Y (2018) Analysis on the adaptive filter based on LMS algorithm Optik Analysis on the adaptive filter based on LMS algorithm. Opt Int J Light Electron Opt 127:4698–4704. https://doi.org/10.1016/j.ijleo.2016.02.005
48. Zandigohar M, Han M, Sharif M, Ya S, Furmanek MP, Yarossi M, Bonato P, Onal C, Schirner G (2022) Multimodal fusion of EMG and vision for human grasp intent inference in prosthetic hand control, vol XX, pp 1–10
49. Guo J, Zheng Y, Xie H, Koo TK (2012). Towards the application of one-dimensional sonomyography for powered upper-limb prosthetic control using machine learning models. https://doi.org/10.1177/0309364612446652
50. Wu Y, Jiang D, Liu X, Bayford R, Demosthenous A (2018) A human-machine interface using electrical impedance tomography for hand prosthesis control. IEEE Trans Biomed Circuits Syst 12:1322–1333. https://doi.org/10.1109/TBCAS.2018.2878395

51. Meattini R, Benatti S, Scarcia U, De Gregorio D, Benini L, Melchiorri C (2018) An sEMG-based human-robot interface for robotic hands using machine learning and synergies. IEEE Trans Compon Packag Manuf Technol 8:1149–1158. https://doi.org/10.1109/TCPMT.2018.2799987.
52. Kristoffersen MB, Franzke AW, Van Der Sluis CK, Bongers RM, Murgia A (2020) Should hands be restricted when measuring able-bodied participants to evaluate machine learning controlled prosthetic hands? IEEE Trans Neural Syst Rehabil Eng 28:1977–1983. https://doi.org/10.1109/TNSRE.2020.3007803
53. Zhao J, Xie Z, Jiang L, Cai H (2005) Levenberg-marquardt based neural network control for a five-fingered prosthetic hand *. In: 2005 IEEE international conference on robotics automation. Spain, pp 4482–4487. https://doi.org/10.1109/ROBOT.2005.1570810
54. Atzori M, Cognolato M, Müller H (2016) Deep learning with convolutional neural networks applied to electromyography data: a resource for the classification of movements for prosthetic hands. Front Neurorobot 10:1–10. https://doi.org/10.3389/fnbot.2016.00009
55. Engeberg ED (2013) Biomedical signal processing and control a physiological basis for control of a prosthetic hand. Biomed Signal Process Control 8:6–15. https://doi.org/10.1016/j.bspc.2012.06.003
56. Polisiero M, Bifulco P, Liccardo A, Cesarelli M, Romano M, Gargiulo GD, McEwan AL, D'Apuzzo M (2013) Design and assessment of a low-cost, electromyographically controlled, prosthetic hand. Med Dev Evid Res 6:97–104. https://doi.org/10.2147/MDER.S39604
57. Borisov II, Borisova OV, Krivosheev SV, Oleynik RV, Reznikov SS (2017) Prototyping of EMG-controlled prosthetic hand with sensory system. IFAC-Papers OnLine 50. https://doi.org/10.1016/j.ifacol.2017.08.1915
58. Belov AA (2021) Science direct prosthetic hand signals ∗ hand controlled by by by by. IFAC Pap. 54:299–304. https://doi.org/10.1016/j.ifacol.2021.10.463
59. Prakash A, Sharma S, Sharma N (2019) A compact-sized surface EMG sensor for myoelectric hand prosthesis. Biomed Eng Lett 9:467–479. https://doi.org/10.1007/s13534-019-00130-y
60. Yang D, Jiang L, Huang Q, Liu R, Liu H (2014) Experimental study of an EMG-controlled 5-DOF anthropomorphic prosthetic hand for motion restoration. J Intell Robot Syst Theory Appl 76:427–441. https://doi.org/10.1007/s10846-014-0037-6
61. Abdhul AA, Subramani D, Ganesan J, Subramaniam S, Dharani KG (2020) Design and development of EMG based prosthetic arm. In: 2020 6th international conference advanced computing and communication systems ICACCS 2020, pp 502–504. https://doi.org/10.1109/ICACCS48705.2020.9074206
62. Tavakoli M, Benussi C, Lourenco JL (2017) PT US CR Expert Syst Appl. https://doi.org/10.1016/j.eswa.2017.03.012
63. Pasquina PF, Evangelista M, Carvalho AJ, Lockhart J, Griffin S, Nanos G, Mckay P, Hansen M, Ipsen D, Vandersea J, Butkus J, Miller M, Murphy I, Hankin D (2014) First-in-man demonstration of a fully implanted myoelectric sensors system to control an advanced electromechanical prosthetic hand. J Neurosci Methods 1–9. https://doi.org/10.1016/j.jneumeth.2014.07.016.
64. Wang N, Lao K, Zhang X (2017) Design and myoelectric control of an anthropomorphic prosthetic hand. J Bionic Eng 14:47–59. https://doi.org/10.1016/S1672-6529(16)60377-3
65. Abdul-khaaliq G, Abdul-khaaliq G (2017) Real-Time segmentation and feature extraction of electromyography: towards real-time segmentation and feature extraction of electromyography: towards real-time segmentation and feature of electromyography: towards control prosthetic hand control of a P. IFAC-PapersOnLine. 50:151–156. https://doi.org/10.1016/j.ifacol.2017.12.028

Recognizing Face Using the Combination of Singular Value Decomposition and Hidden Markov Model Algorithms

Henry Candra and Susan Sulaiman

Abstract Face recognition as a biometric system is a development of an authentication system based on the face's natural characteristics. Face recognition needs to be further researched because it has been applied to various fields. After all, this system does not require direct physical contact between humans and computer input sensors. However, problems in face recognition systems are pretty dynamic and complex. This study proposed a face recognition system using Singular Value Decomposition (SVD) for feature extraction and Hidden Markov Model (HMM) for classification. It is expected that this research may contribute to developing the method of face recognition. The recognition process is based on a frontal face image which is divided into seven areas, and each area is assigned to a state in a one-dimensional HMM. 100 images are used for database creation. Image acquisition is made 10 times for each of 10 different people with different expressions. Half of the images are used for training and the rest for the testing process. In this study, the moving probability from one state to the state itself and the next state is not the same. Still, it depends on the average value of the height of the area covered by a particular state, and the result shows that it can increase the recognition rate from 94 to 96%.

Keywords Face recognition · Feature extraction · Singular value decomposition · Classifier · Hidden Markov model

1 Introduction

Humans can recognize other people's faces even though they have not seen each other for a long time, and there have been changes in the face, such as the use of glasses, hairstyle, or aging. This human visual ability is attempted to be imitated by using a machine (computer) and various algorithms [1, 2]. The face is the most essential part of the human body that is needed in the detection process for multiple

H. Candra · S. Sulaiman (✉)
Faculty of Industrial Technology, Electrical Engineering Department, Trisakti University, Jalan Kyai Tapa No 1, Grogol, Jakarta 11440, Indonesia
e-mail: susan@trisakti.ac.id

T. Triwiyanto et al. (eds.), *Proceeding of the 3rd International Conference on Electronics, Biomedical Engineering, and Health Informatics*, Lecture Notes in Electrical Engineering 1008, https://doi.org/10.1007/978-981-99-0248-4_38

applications. Face recognition is one of the biometric technology identifications using an individual's face as the main parameter. It has an advantage over some other biometric techniques, especially in this pandemic situation, because it does not require particular physical contact such as placing the hand on the fingerprint recognition process or the geometric location of the hand [3–5]. A human face is unique and complete. Its features are changing over time, therefore it is very important to have a robust face recognition system that could able to operate under a variety of conditions.

Much research on face recognition has been done, yet some problems are still unresolved [6]. Several factors may degrade the face recognition accuracy; those are intrinsic factors that are related to a human's physical condition such as facial aging and expression, and extrinsic factors which can change the face appearance such as low resolution and illumination [7, 8]. Another researcher has tried to combine different biometrics such as face and speech to improve the accuracy, however, the result comes with another drawback of larger dimensionality [9].

Face recognition has rapid progression in the last few decades due to the interests in computer vision, smart environments, and even as a means of payment. Although face recognition systems have very rapidly improved, basically the approach methods for human face recognition can be grouped into three categories, namely holistic matching methods, feature-based (structural) methods, and hybrid methods [10].

In the holistic approach, all parts or global facial features are used as data for face recognition, one of which is the Eigenface method. This method was pioneered by Turk and Pentland by using Principal Component Analysis (PCA) which is a linear technique used to project high-dimensional data into lower-dimensional subspaces. The Eigenface algorithm gives the characteristic value of a face in the form of eigen-vector values. At the identification stage, the eigenvector values in the training data are compared with the eigen vector values from the test data and the smallest distance for similarity is determined by the Euclidean distance method. R. Kosasih used the PCA method for face recognition on the Olivetti Research Laboratory (ORL) database and achieved a 96.6% recognition rate [11]. Speech, Vision, and Robotics Group of the Cambridge University, Department of Engineering has supported this ORL database for implementation in a face recognition project [12]. The Romi Mulyadi Yusni developed the PCA method to recognize the faces of smokers using 8 faces of smokers each with 5 different poses tested with 40 test images resulting in a recognition rate of 92.5% [13].

In the feature-based method, faces are divided based on local facial features such as nose, mouth, eyes, and others that are used as input data, including that used in this method known as the Hidden Markov Model (HMM). The number of states depends on the system's requirements. The face recognition performance has been enhanced by using 7-State HMM [14]. Nur Widya Pratiwi and colleagues in Face detection using Matlab-based HMM can detect facial images with 95.9% success [15]. Other research using SVD and 7 states HMM resulted in a recognition rate of 96.6% for the ORL database and 82.7% for the YALE database [16]. A study of SVD and five states of HMM were applied to process employee data consisting of 400 images and achieved a recognition rate of 99% [17]. SVD and 5 states of HMM were also applied in further research using 160 training images and 120 test images which consist of 80 still object images and 40 moving object images and gave an overall recognition rate of 80.83% [18].

Methods based on the hybrid approach use both the entire face and the local facial features as input data, some examples using this method are the modular eigenface and the hybrid local feature. H. Cho and colleagues in An Efficient Hybrid Face Recognition Algorithm using PCA and Gabor Wavelets were inspired by facial recognition methods used by humans, namely both holistic and local features. This method employs a holistic and local feature-based recognition algorithm in two stages, PCA is used to identify the test image in the first stage and Gabor wavelets in the next stage [19]. In [20], a hybrid face recognition system method is used using SURF (Speed Up Robust Features), HOG (Histogram of Oriented Gradient), and MSER (Maximally Stable Extremal Regions) algorithms.

In this pandemic situation that reduces contact as much as possible is a requirement, and face recognition plays an important role. The purpose of this study is to build a face recognition system based on features by using the SVD method in the feature selection process, and 7 states HMM as the classifier. The database is formed from 100 images that have been taken from 10 people, half of them were used as training images and the rest as test images. In previous research, the initial value of the transition probability matrix was carried out by assuming equal probability for moving from one state to the state itself or to the next state, each of which is 0.5. To increase the recognition rate, in this study, the transition probability matrix is calculated by assuming that the moving probability depends on the average value of the height of the area covered by a particular state.

2 Research Method

In this study, SVD coefficients of each sampling window of the face image are computed and used as features [21]. The model of the system is assumed to be a discrete first-order Markov chain with hidden states, where the model parameters are adjusted to find the maximum likelihood estimate of the parameters of the HMM given the set of output sequences using the Baum-Welch algorithm. All experiments and tests are carried out by using MATLAB as the programming language because the basic calculation in the process is a matrix.

2.1 Singular Value Decomposition

The main purpose of performing feature extraction is to have the characteristics or important features of an object or an image. The most reputable algorithm for its ability to extract face features is SVD which is usually combined with other algorithms [22, 23]. SVD can approximate the original data points using fewer dimensions, hence it can be seen as a method for data reduction [24]. A systematic way to determine a low-dimensional approximation to high-dimensional data in terms of dominant patterns is provided by SVD [25]. A process of decomposition in a matrix means factoring a matrix into more than one matrix. SVD is one of the decomposition techniques related to the singular value which is one of the characteristics of a matrix.

SVD is based on the theory of linear algebra, that an $m \times n$ rectangular matrix can be factored into the multiplication of 3 matrices, namely orthogonal matrix U, diagonal matrix Σ, and the transpose of orthogonal matrix V as follows:

$$A_{mn} = U_{mm} \sum_{mn} V_{nn}^{T} \tag{1}$$

where $U^T U = \mathrm{I}$ and $V^T V = \mathrm{I}$.

The column of U is an orthonormal eigenvector of AAT and the column of V is an orthonormal eigenvector of ATA. Σ is a diagonal matrix whose elements are singular or square root values of the U or V eigenvalues and arranged in descending order.

For a square matrix A_{mn}, there is a nonzero vector x and a scalar λ, such that $Ax = \lambda x$, $x \neq 0$, or it is equivalent to

$$(A - \lambda I)x = 0 \tag{2}$$

λ is the eigenvalue or the characteristic roots of A and x is the eigenvector corresponding to λ.

U_{mm} matrix can be found by calculating the eigenvalues and the corresponding eigenvectors of AA^T as follows

$$\det\left|\lambda I - AA^T\right| = 0 \tag{3}$$

$$AA^T x = \lambda x \tag{4}$$

Finally, the orthonormalization process of Gram Schmidt is used to convert it into an orthonormal matrix

$$\overline{u}_1 = \frac{u_1}{|u_1|} \tag{5}$$

where the column of U is the orthonormal eigenvector of AA^T.

The same method is applied to the $A^T A$ matrix to obtain the V matrix. The Σ diagonal matrix is formed from the singular value or the square roots of the non-zero eigenvalues of the U or V matrix (Nonzeros eigenvalues of U and V are always the same) with $\sigma_{ij} = 0$, $i \neq j$, and $\sigma_{ii} > 0$. The largest singular value is placed on Σ_{11}, the second largest on Σ_{22}, and so on.

SVD has become an important tool because SVD can be used to express image data in several singular values. Smaller storage in the memory is used because the data will be reduced by only taking some of the largest singular values which are the most important features of the image [26]. The small singular values and part of the image that corresponds to these singular values will not significantly contribute to building the original image. By ignoring these values along with the columns in the U and V matrices that have been factored by these singular values, the original image will be reconstructed or reduced quite precisely by a data set that is much smaller than the original image matrix.

2.2 Hidden Markov Model

Processes in the real world generally produce an output that can be observed as a signal and the most important thing is how to observe the signal as a signal model because the signal model can solve many things in practice such as prediction systems, recognition systems, and identification system in a very efficient way [27]. The signal model consists of deterministic models, which can be assumed to be characterized as a parameter of a random process, for example, the Markov and Hidden Markov processes [28]. HMM has been used in many types of research in various fields [29], especially in biomedical engineering, such as breast cancer recurrence prediction based on sequential patterns through gene expression profiles using HMM [30], Gray matter segmentation of brain MRI using modified K means, expected maximization and Hidden Markov random field was done to provide better spatial correlation that overcomes in-homogeneity, noise and low contrast [31].

Consider $\{q_t, t = 0, 1, 2, 3, \ldots\}$ is a discrete parameter (time) stochastic process with state space $\{S_1, S_2, S_3, \ldots S_N\}$.

$$\begin{aligned} If\ P\left(q_{t+1} = S_j \mid q_t = S_i, q_{t-1} = S_k, \ldots q_0 = S_1\right) \\ = P\left(q_{t+1} = S_j | q_t = S_i\right) = a_{ij} \end{aligned} \tag{6}$$

then the process is called a discrete-time Markov chain. The A matrix whose elements are a_{ij} is called the transition probability matrix from state S_i to S_j.

The elements of HMM are as follows.

1. N is the number of states, $S = \{S1, S2 \ldots\ldots S_N\}\ qt \in S$
2. M is the number of observation symbols for each state, with an observation space $V = \{v_1, v_2, \ldots v_M\}$.
3. $A = [a_{ij}]$ is the state transition probability matrix

$$\begin{aligned} a_{ij} = P[q_{t+1} = S_j q_t = S_i] \\ \text{The} \sum_{j=1}^{N} a_{ij} = 1, 1 \le i \le N \end{aligned} \tag{7}$$

4. $B = [b_j(k)]$ is the observation symbol probability distribution in state j

$$b_j(k) = P\left[o_t = v_k | q_t = S_j\right],\ 1 \le j \le N,\ 1 \le k \le M \quad (8)$$

5. $\pi = \{\pi_1, \pi_2, ..., \pi_N\}$ is the initial state distribution

$$\pi = P[q_1 = S_i], 1 \le i \le N \quad (9)$$

6. HMM can be written using

$$\lambda = (A, B, \pi) \quad (10)$$

HMM can be used as a generator to give an observation sequence $O = O_1, O_2, ..., O_t$ by determining the values of N, M, A, B, and π.

2.3 Data Set

There are 100 images from 10 different people with different expressions, image acquisition was done 10 times for each of them. Each picture of size 112 × 92 pixels contains only a face image of 1 person with a camera-to-face distance between 48 and 61 cm and white wall background.

2.4 Experimental Procedure

In this study, there are two main parts to the face recognition system, the training process, and the testing process. The overall system block diagram can be seen in Fig. 1 which illustrates a series of stages of the system. Some stages in both the training process and the testing process are the same, namely image acquisition, transformation, image quality improvement, and feature extraction. For the testing process, there is a phase called the recognition process which matches the test images with the training images that have been stored in the database. The result is the recognition rate or faces recognition level.

2.5 Data Processing

The training phase used five images from each person, while the remaining images went to the testing phase. To facilitate and accelerate the recognition process, the image is transformed into a grayscale one, resized to 56 × 46 pixels, and stored in the pgm format. The image quality improvement process consists of two stages,

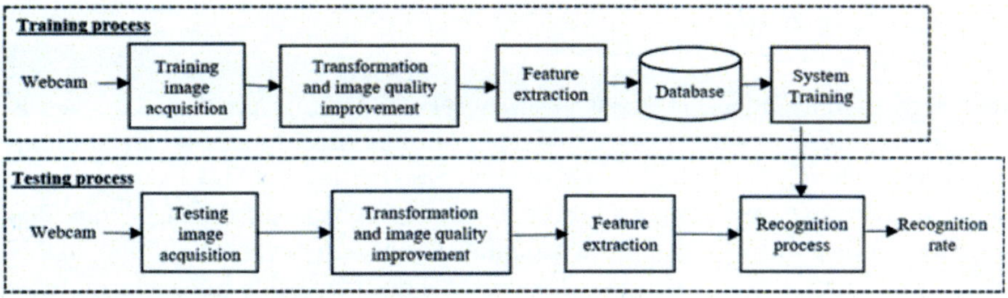

Fig. 1 Block diagram of the face recognition system

namely histogram equalization and filtering using a two-dimensional minimum order statistics filter which aims to find the darkest points in the image and reduce the effect of salt noise or white spots on the image.

Feature extraction's purpose is to select only the important features of an image. This study consists of block extraction, feature selection, and quantization. The block extraction process transforms the two-dimensional into a one-dimensional image to create the one-dimensional HMM observation sequence. At this stage, each image of width W and height H is divided into overlapping blocks of height L and the same width shifted from top to bottom. P is the overlapping size and T is the number of blocks as a result of extraction from each image which can be calculated by (11) [32].

$$T = \frac{H - L}{L - P} + 1 \tag{11}$$

In this study, $W = 46$, $H = 56$, $L = 5$, $P = 4$ and the number of blocks is 52. This means that each image produced a series of sequential blocks consisting of 52 elements, where each block has 5×46 pixels, thus each block will have $5 \times 46 = 230$ Gy level values, obtaining 52×230 Gy level values for an image. The next step is feature selection, which selects a set of features so that a subset with a smaller size is obtained which will result in minimal misclassification and the smallest computational costs. In this study, the feature selection process was carried out using the SVD method. The three features taken are the first coefficient from the U matrix and the first two coefficients from the Σ matrix (U_{11}, $\Sigma_{11,}$ and Σ_{22}) of each block while the other coefficients are ignored because these three coefficients give the best facial recognition level results. Thus, the 230 Gy level values from each block will only be represented by three values, meaning that the data is significantly reduced and at the same time simplifies the complexity of the calculation. The next stage is the quantization process which aims to change the value of the SVD coefficient which was originally continuous into discrete. This is done because for the next stage, namely the training and introduction stage, modeling is carried out with discrete HMM. If U11 is quantized in a level, Σ_{11} in b level, and Σ_{22} in c level, then we get a b c of different combinations for each block.

2.6 Training Process

After each training image is stated in the observation sequence, the next stage is the system training process using the Hidden Markov Model method. The training process consists of several stages, namely modeling with the HMM method, determining initial values, and parameter estimation using the Baumwelch algorithm. The modeling process with HMM aims to formulate HMM into facial recognition. In this study, facial images are divided into 7 states or areas, consisting of hair/head, forehead, eyebrows, eyes, nose, mouth, and chin. If the blocks formed in block extraction are shifted every time one pixel from top to bottom, then the block will always be in one of the 7 states. Based on these assumptions, a one-dimensional HMM can be formed for left–right facial recognition with 7 states.

$$\begin{aligned} N &= \text{number of states} = 7 \\ M &= a\,b\,c \end{aligned} \tag{12}$$

M is the number of observation symbols from each state or the number of combinations obtained from the quantization results, and a, b, and c are the quantization coefficients of the matrix U_{11}, $\Sigma_{11,}$ and Σ_{22}.

Determining the initial value is one of the most important stages in modeling with HMM. The initial state is always "hair or head" which probability is equal to one and the final state is always "chin". The blocks are shifted sequentially from top to bottom.

a. Same moving probability from one state to the state itself and to the next state except for the last state, the transition probability matrix can be formed as follows

$$A_1 = \begin{bmatrix} 0.5 & 0.5 & 0 & 0 & 0 & 0 & 0 \\ 0 & 0.5 & 0.5 & 0 & 0 & 0 & 0 \\ 0 & 0 & 0.5 & 0.5 & 0 & 0 & 0 \\ 0 & 0 & 0 & 0.5 & 0.5 & 0 & 0 \\ 0 & 0 & 0 & 0 & 0.5 & 0.5 & 0 \\ 0 & 0 & 0 & 0 & 0 & 0.5 & 0.5 \\ 0 & 0 & 0 & 0 & 0 & 0 & 1 \end{bmatrix} \tag{13}$$

b. The moving probability depends on the average value of the height of the area covered by a particular state. The average (mean) height of each state is calculated for the 7 states from all people in the database. One state is taken as a reference, in this case, the eye state whose height is the smallest is taken as a basis. The height of the other six states is compared to the height of the eye state. The moving probability from the eye state to the state itself and to the next state is considered equal to 0.5, while the moving probability for other states than the eye is calculated based on the ratio of the average height of the state to the eye state. The result is the A_1 transition probability matrix as seen in (14)

$$A_1 = \begin{bmatrix} 0.6 & 0.4 & 0 & 0 & 0 & 0 & 0 \\ 0 & 0.8 & 0.2 & 0 & 0 & 0 & 0 \\ 0 & 0 & 0.5 & 0.5 & 0 & 0 & 0 \\ 0 & 0 & 0 & 0.5 & 0.5 & 0 & 0 \\ 0 & 0 & 0 & 0 & 0.8 & 0.2 & 0 \\ 0 & 0 & 0 & 0 & 0 & 0.6 & 0.4 \\ 0 & 0 & 0 & 0 & 0 & 0 & 1 \end{bmatrix} \tag{14}$$

$$B = \frac{1}{abc} \begin{matrix} 1 \\ 2 \\ 3 \\ 4 \\ 5 \\ 6 \\ 7 \end{matrix} \begin{bmatrix} 1\,1 \ldots 1 \\ 1\,1 \ldots 1 \\ 1\,1 \ldots 1 \\ 1\,1 \ldots 1 \\ 1\,1 \ldots 1 \\ 1\,1 \ldots 1 \\ 1\,1 \ldots 1 \end{bmatrix} \tag{15}$$

$$\pi = \begin{bmatrix} 1\,0\,0\,0\,0\,0\,0 \end{bmatrix} \tag{16}$$

A_1 the state transition probability matrix.
B the observation symbol probability distribution.
π the initial state distribution.

The next stage is the training process or parameter estimation with the Baumwelch algorithms. Each training image is represented by its observation vector and the initialization has to be done as in (14), (15), and (16) for the first image. The iteration process is carried out so that the probability of the series of observations obtained is maximized. The reiteration process is executed for all images and the estimated value of the last image of each person becomes the final value of the HMM as seen in (17).

$$\lambda^* = \max_{\lambda} P(O|\lambda) \tag{17}$$

Each face is associated with an HMM. There were 10 people in this study and 10 HMM models were obtained.

2.7 *Testing and Recognition Process*

Each testing image, like training image, experiences the feature extraction process and is represented by its observation vector. Then, the probability of the observation vector for every incoming face image is calculated for each HMM. A face image m is recognized as face d if it meets the condition in (18).

$$P\left(O^{(m)}|\lambda_d\right) = \max_n P\left(O^{(m)}|\lambda_n\right) \tag{18}$$

The recognition rate is obtained based on the number of misclassified images as seen in (19).

$$\text{Recognition rate} = \frac{\text{number of correctly recognized images}}{\text{number of testing images}} \times 100\%. \tag{19}$$

3 Results

Image acquisition was done with different levels of variations of facial expression, orientation, and rotation as well as the distance of the camera from the face. The purpose is to see the effect of the degree of variation on the system's ability to recognize faces.

3.1 Preprocessing Process

All images in the database will go through the preprocessing process whose result is shown in Table 1. The original image is resized to 56 × 46 pixels, then the quality is improved by the histogram equalization and filtered by a minimum order statistical filter.

Table 1 shows that the image quality has enhanced its contrast after the histogram equalization. By the purpose of the minimum order statistical filter to find the darkest points in the image and reduce the effect of salt noise or white spots on the image, it can be seen from the filtering process that the slightly shiny parts of the face, especially the eyes, become shadier.

Table 1 Preprocessing steps

Original image in pgm (112 × 92)	Resized (56 × 46)	After histogram equalization	After filtering
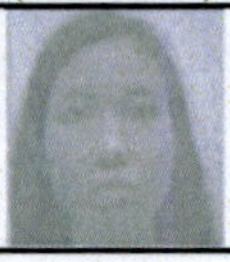	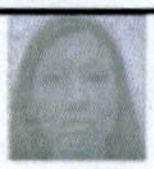	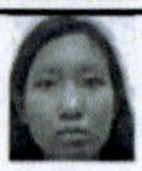	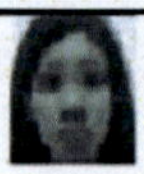

3.2 Results of the Recognition Process

The input of the feature extraction process is in the form of the image while the output is in matrix form. Each image consists of 52 blocks and each block is represented by 3 SVD features namely U_{11}, $\Sigma_{11,}$ and Σ_{22}. They are then quantized in 18, 10, and 7 levels, leaving 1260 possible distinct vectors for each block. Labeling is given to any combination of quantized U_{11}, $\Sigma_{11,}$ and Σ_{22} values, and the sequence of those numbers obtained from each image is considered as observation vectors that can be used by HMM for classification. System training is carried out using the Baumwelch algorithm with a maximum of 10 iterations or 0.01 tolerance. The output of the training process is the HMM or the model for every person in the database. The estimation results are applied to each test image which will be recognized as one of the people in the database using (18).

3.3 Results Using the a Transition Probability Matrix

Using A transition probability matrix as shown in (13), 47 from 50 face images were correctly recognized, so the face recognition rate was 94%. Here are some examples of training images, test images, and the results of the recognition process of 5 people included in the database as shown in Tables 2a, b, c, d, and e.

This face recognition system has performed very well which an achievement is 94% of recognition rate. Errors occurred in the recognition of the second test image on behalf of SH (Table 2a) and the third test image on behalf of SS (Table 2b) due to the extreme changes in orientation and rotation and on the fourth test image on behalf of N (Table 2c) due to the change of distance from the camera to the face.

3.4 Results Using the A_1 Transition Probability Matrix

Changes in the initial value of the transition probability matrix adjusted to the average value of the height of the area covered by a certain state as shown in (14) have improved the system performance because it was able to increase the face recognition rate from 94 to 96%. Compared with the results obtained using the value of A in (13), there is an improvement in image recognition, namely the fourth test image on behalf of N can be recognized correctly while the same error occurs in the other two images. The average time needed to run each stage in the entire face recognition process can be seen in Table 3.

Table 2 Training images, testing images, and recognition results

(a) Images on behalf of SH

Training images				
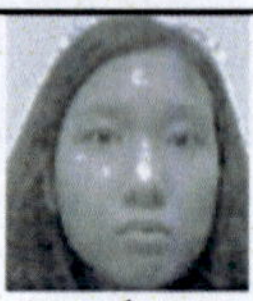	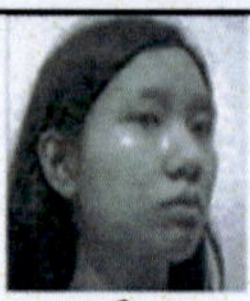	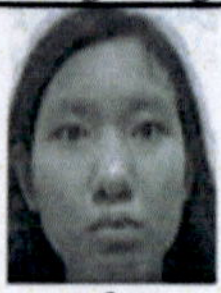	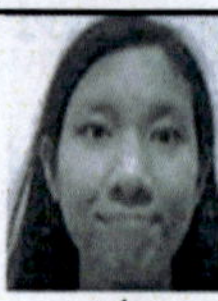	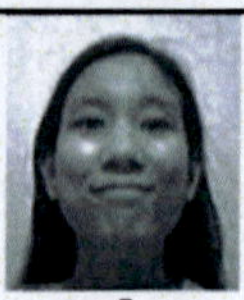
1	2	3	4	5
Testing images and Recognition results				
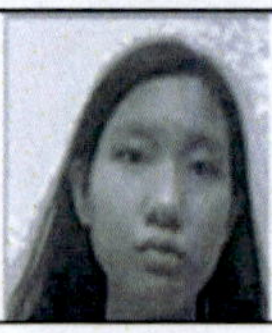	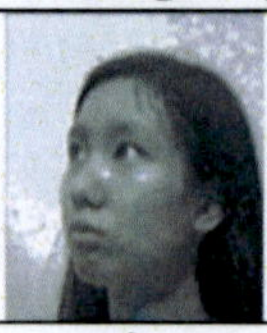	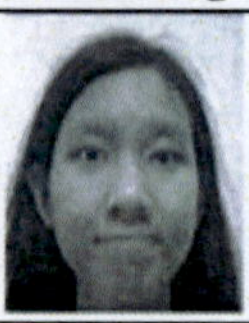	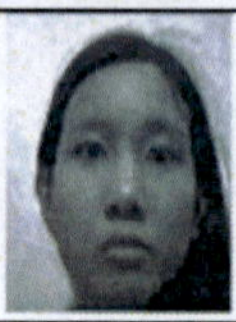	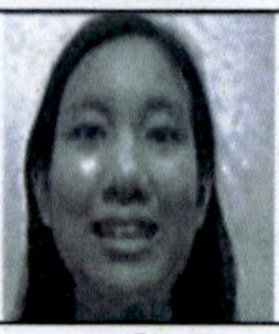
1	2	3	4	5
True	False	True	True	True

(b) Images on behalf of SS

Training images				
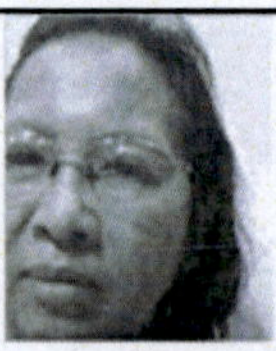	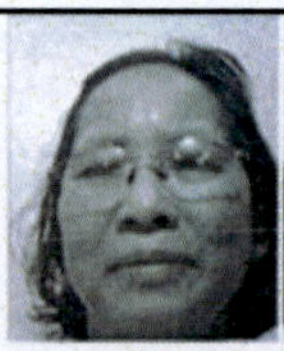	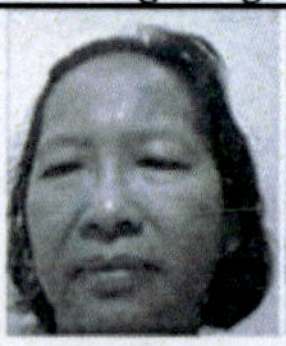	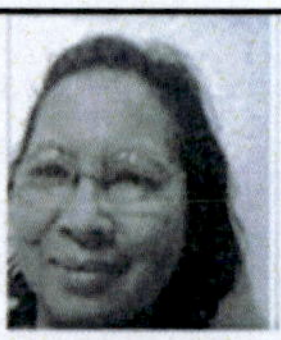	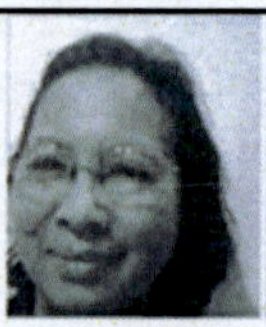
1	2	3	4	5
Testing images and Recognition results				
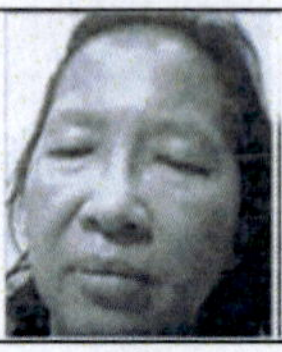	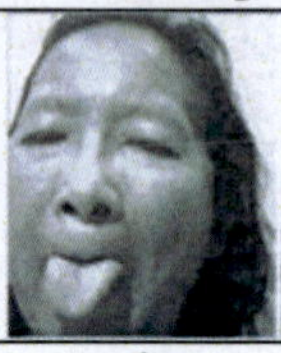	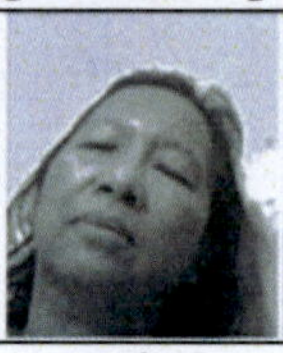	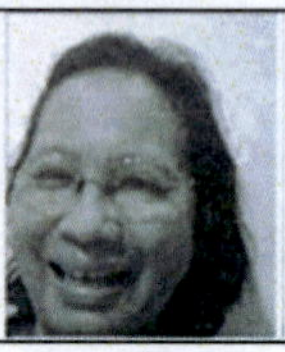	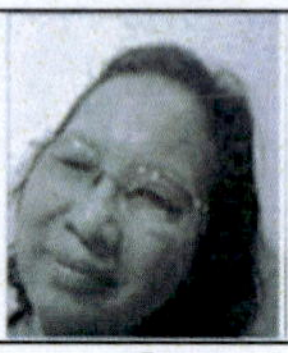
1	2	3	4	5
True	True	False	True	True

(c) Images on behalf of N

Training images				
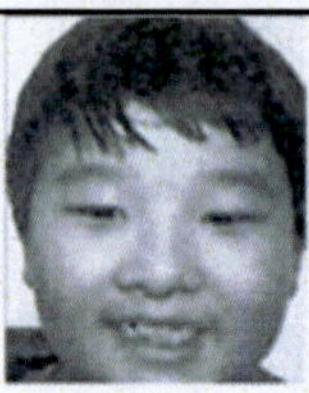	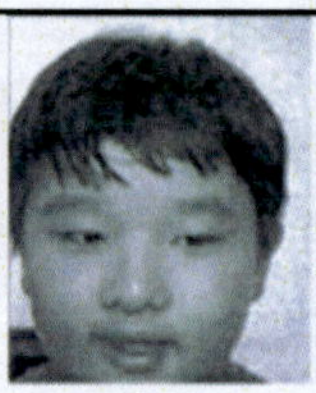	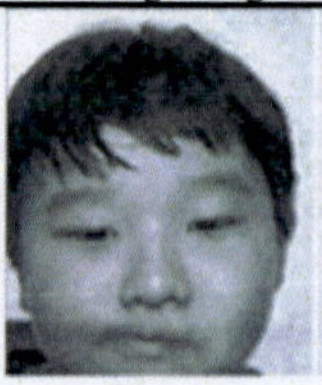	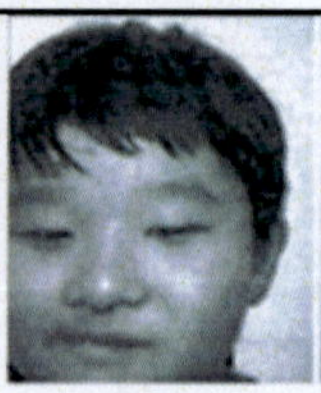	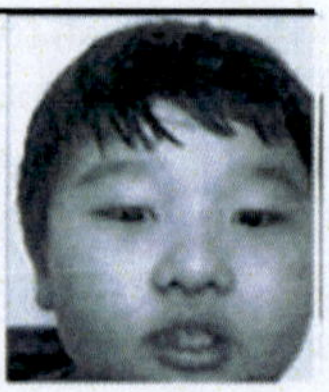
1	2	3	4	5

(continued)

Table 2 (continued)

Testing images and Recognition results				
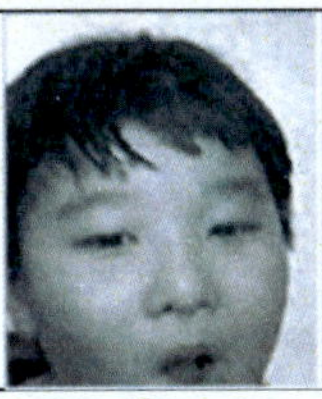	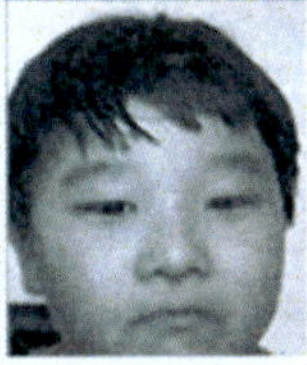	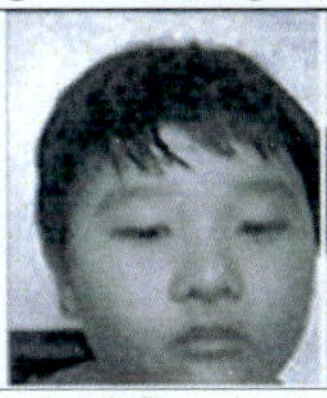	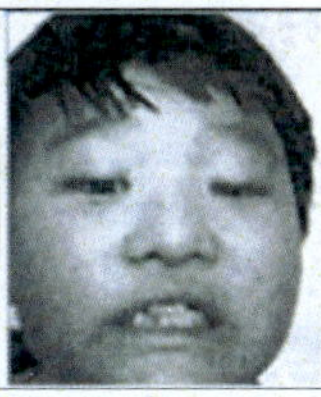	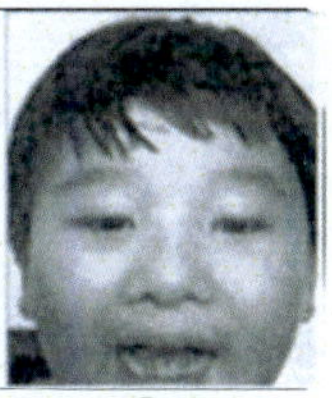
1	2	3	4	5
True	True	True	False	True

(d) Images on behalf of V

Training images				
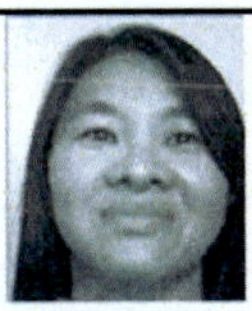	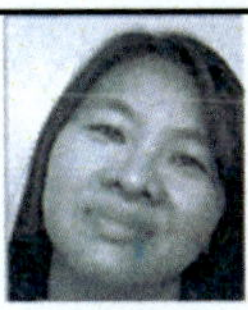	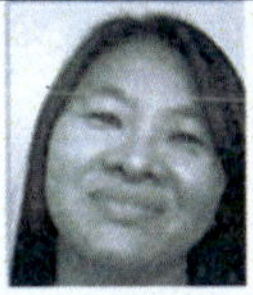	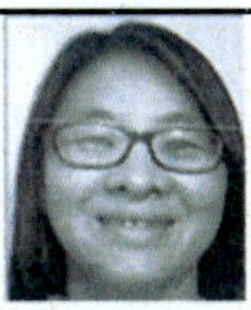	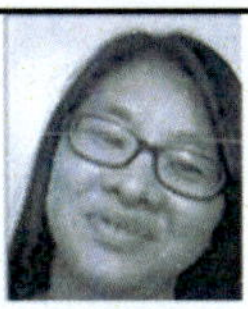
1	2	3	4	5
Testing images and Recognition results				
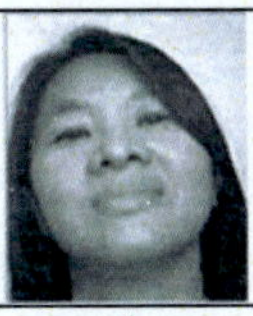	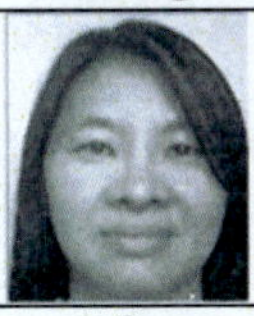	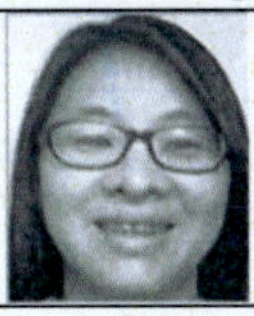	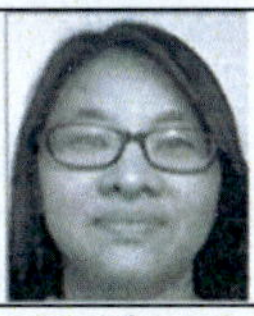	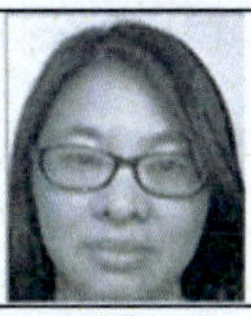
1	2	3	4	5
True	True	True	True	True

(e) Images on behalf of O

Training images				
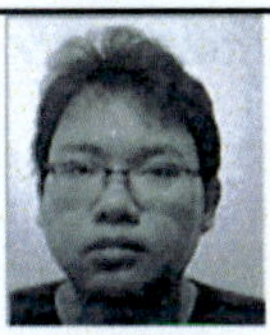	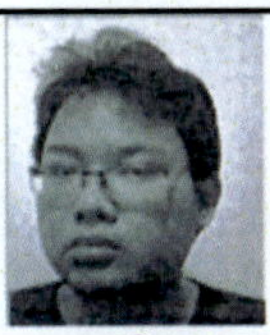	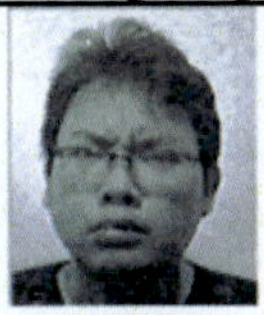	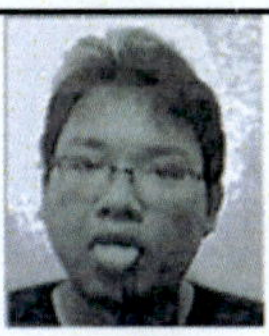	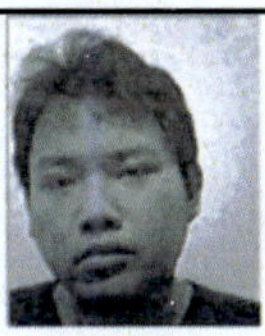
1	2	3	4	5
Testing images and Recognition results				
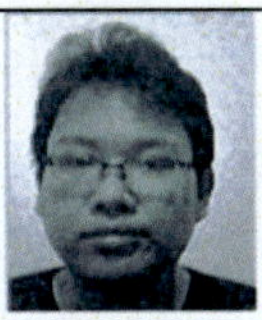	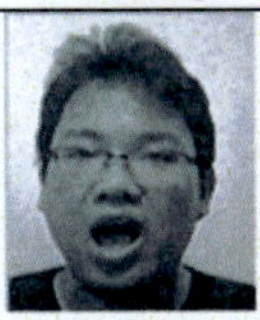	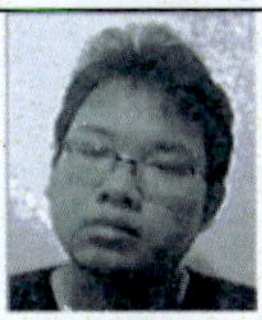	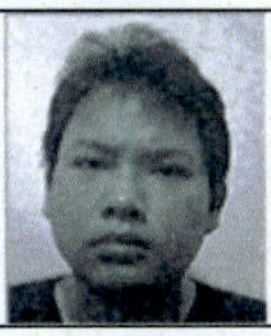	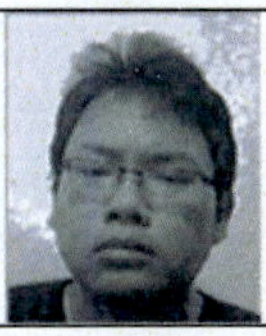
1	2	3	4	5
True	True	True	True	True

Table 3 Average time to run the process

Process	Average time (s)
Creating database	1.96
Loading	0.75
Training system	22.39
Recognition and counting recognition rate	8.74

Table 4 Influence of changing SVD coefficients on the recognition rate

1st SVD coefficient	2nd SVD coefficient	3rd SVD coefficient	Recognition rate (%)
U_{11}	$\sum_{11}$	$\sum_{22}$	96
$\sum_{11}$	$\sum_{22}$	$\sum_{33}$	10
V_{11}	$\sum_{11}$	$\sum_{22}$	22
U_{11}	$\sum_{11}$	V_{11}	14
U_{22}	$\sum_{11}$	$\sum_{22}$	34
U_{11}	$\sum_{11}$	U_{22}	20

3.5 *Influence of Changing the SVD Coefficients*

Table 4 shows the effect of changing the SVD coefficient features by taking several different SVD coefficient values while the other parameters remain the same.

It can be concluded that U_{11}, Σ_{11}, and Σ_{22} provide much better results than the other SVD coefficients combination. This is because Σ_{11} and Σ_{22} derived from each block are the largest singular values associated with the largest eigenvalues that form the principal components of each block in the image and U_{11} is the first element of u_1, corresponding to the largest singular value Σ_{11}, where U is the matrix, whose columns are left singular vectors to the corresponding eigenvalues.

3.6 *Influence of Changing the Quantization Level*

Table 5 shows the effect of changing the value of the quantization level on the recognition rate.

The results show that the values 18, 10, and 7 corresponding to a, b, c or U_{11}, Σ_{11}, and Σ_{22} quantization coefficient have given the best recognition rate. The addition of the quantization level will increase the number of combinations or the value of M, which means increasing the number of columns in the emission matrix, thus slowing down the process of making the database and training process.

Table 5 Influence of changing the quantization level on the recognition rate

a	b	c	M	R (%)	Creating a database (s)	Training system (s)
18	10	7	1260	96	1.96	22.39
10	10	10	1000	92	1.91	16.19
6	6	6	216	86	1.76	6.12
20	20	20	8000	78	2.32	134.25
15	10	10	1500	92	2.02	26.16
25	20	15	7500	84	2.16	128.21

a = U_{11} qc, b = Σ_{11} qc, c = Σ_{22} qc, q c = quantization coefficient, M = number of combinations
R = recognition rate

4 Discussion

This proposed face recognition system has shown good performance. All testing images with low and moderate levels of variation can be recognized correctly. The system can also recognize properly even though the testing images show different expressions on their faces.

Compared to the previous studies, changes in the initial value of the transition probability matrix adjusted to the average value of the height of the area covered by a certain state turned out to be successful in improving the system performance because it was able to increase the face recognition rate from 94 to 96%. Errors occurred only in the recognition of the test image with a high level of variation, namely an extreme change in the orientation and rotation of the face.

The weakness of the system is in choosing the right SVD coefficient and quantization level, however, it can be well handled when the right values are chosen. The selection of SVD coefficient is very significant, and the coefficient corresponding to the largest eigenvalue plays an important role because it has a great contribution to the formation of an image. A combination of the quantization level must also be considered. The greater the number of combinations of the quantization level, the longer the time taken in the process, and the system becomes too sensitive which decreases the facial recognition rate. Conversely, if the combination numbers are too small, the time required for processing becomes shorter but the system becomes less sensitive so that the facial recognition rate also decreases. This system is expected to have very good implications in the society, especially in this pandemic situation, where minimal contact becomes a requirement, face recognition is very useful to be applied in various fields.

5 Conclusion

The proposed system succeeded in recognizing a recognition rate of 94% when the transition probability matrix was based on equal opportunities to move from one state to the state itself and to the next state. Meanwhile, it provides a better recognition rate of 96% when the transition probability matrix was based on the moving probability that depends on the average value of the height of the area covered by a particular state. The time required for the recognition process to calculate the face recognition rate is 8.74 s on average. The numbers in the face recognition level are not absolute, because the level of accuracy is strongly influenced by existing data related to variations in poses, orientations, and rotations as well as facial expressions. The greater the variation, the level of face recognition will tend to decrease. For further development, it is recommended to use a two-dimensional HMM to improve the system performance.

References

1. Li J, Chen HF, Wang LJ, Zhang CY (2013) Face recognition method based on multi-level histogram sequence of Gabor fused features. In: Advanced materials research. Trans Tech Publications Ltd., pp 2348–2352. https://doi.org/10.4028/www.scientific.net/AMR.718-720.2348
2. Ding BY, Tang YY, Zhang ZC, Wang XW, Fang C (2013) Sparse representation frontal facial recognition algorithm based on eigenface. In: Instruments, measurement, electronics and information engineering. Trans Tech Publications Ltd., pp 3629–3633. https://doi.org/10.4028/www.scientific.net/AMM.347-350.3629
3. Mou D (2010) Fundamentals and advances in biometrics and face recognition. In: Machine-based intelligent face recognition. Springer Berlin Heidelberg, Berlin, Heidelberg, pp 13–70. https://doi.org/10.1007/978-3-642-00751-4_2
4. Nídlová V, Hart J (2015) Reliability of identification based on fingerprints in dual biometric identification systems. In: Applied mechanics and materials. Trans Tech Publications Ltd., pp 1040–1044. https://doi.org/10.4028/www.scientific.net/amm.752-753.1040
5. Zhang MH, Zhang YY (2013) The application of biometric identification technology in ATM system. In: Instruments, measurement, electronics and information engineering. Trans Tech Publications Ltd., pp 3419–3421. https://doi.org/10.4028/www.scientific.net/AMM.347-350.3419
6. Erwin E, Azriansyah M, Hartuti N, Fachrurrozi M, Tama B (2019) A study about principle component analysis and eigenface for facial extraction. J Phys Conf Ser 1196:12010. https://doi.org/10.1088/1742-6596/1196/1/012010
7. Anwarul S, Dahiya S (2020) A comprehensive review on face recognition methods and factors affecting facial recognition accuracy. In: Lecture notes in electrical engineering, vol 597, pp 495–514. https://doi.org/10.1007/978-3-030-29407-6_36
8. Gross R, Baker S, Matthews I, Kanade T (2011) Face recognition across pose and illumination. In: Li SZ, Jain AK (eds) Handbook of face recognition. Springer London, London, pp 197–221. https://doi.org/10.1007/978-0-85729-932-1_8
9. Kala R, Vazirani H, Shukla A, Tiwari R (2010) Fusion of speech and face by enhanced modular neural network. In: Prasad SK, Vin HM, Sahni S, Jaiswal MP, Thipakorn B (eds) Information systems, technology and management. Springer, Berlin, Heidelberg, pp 363–372

10. Parmar DN, Mehta BB (2014) Face recognition methods & applications. Int J Comput Technol Appl 4:84–86
11. Kosasih R (2021) Pengenalan Wajah Menggunakan PCA dengan Memperhatikan Jumlah Data Latih dan Vektor Eigen. J Inform Univ Pamulang 6:1. https://doi.org/10.32493/informatika.v6i1.7261
12. Lal M, Kumar K, Arain RH, Maitlo A, Ruk SA, Shaikh H (2018) Study of face recognition techniques: a survey. Int J Adv Comput Sci Appl 9:42–49. https://doi.org/10.14569/IJACSA.2018.090606
13. Yusni, Mulyadi R, Zaini (2020) Identifikasi Pengenalan Wajah Perokok Menggunakan Metode principal component analysis. J. RESTI (Rekayasa Sist dan Teknol Informasi) 4:892–898. https://doi.org/10.29207/resti.v4i5.2272
14. Sharif M, Naz F, Yasmin M, Shahid MA, Rehman A (2017) Face recognition: a survey. J Eng 10:166–177
15. Pratiwi NW, Fauziah F, Andryana S, Gunaryati A (2018) Deteksi Wajah Menggunakan Hidden Markov model (HMM) Berbasis Matlab. STRING (Satuan Tulisan Ris dan Inov Teknol) 3:44. https://doi.org/10.30998/string.v3i1.2538
16. Dinkova P, Georgieva P, Milanova M (2014) Face recognition using singular value decomposition and Hidden Markov models. In: 16th international conference on mathematical methods, computational techniques and intelligent systems (MAMECTIS). World Scientific and Engineering Academy and Society, pp 144–149
17. Rana N, Pancholi B (2018) HMM-based face recognition system with SVD parameter. Int J Trend Sci Res Dev 2:369–373. https://doi.org/10.31142/ijtsrd12938
18. Tjahyanto A, Hidayat N, Shahab ML, Adzkiya D, Nisa AK (2018) Individual recognition system through face identification using Hidden Markov model. In: The 2018 international conference on information technology. Engineering, science, and its applications (ITES 2018), Yogyakarta, pp 21–27
19. Cho H, Roberts R, Jung B, Choi O, Moon S (2014) An efficient hybrid face recognition algorithm using PCA and GABOR wavelets. Int J Adv Robot Syst 11:1–8. https://doi.org/10.5772/58473
20. Shoba VBT, Sam IS (2020) A hybrid features extraction on face for efficient face recognition. In: Multimedia tools and applications, vol 79, pp 22595–22616. https://doi.org/10.1007/s11042-020-08997-1
21. Liu TT, Yang C (2012) Review on singular-value-decomposition-based digital watermarking algorithm in combination with image features. In: Advanced research on engineering materials, energy, management and control. Trans Tech Publications Ltd., pp 452–463. https://doi.org/10.4028/www.scientific.net/AMR.424-425.452
22. Fronckova K, Prazak P, Slaby A (2019) Singular value decomposition and principal component analysis in face images recognition and FSVDR of faces. In: Świ\katek J, Borzemski L, Wilimowska Z (eds) Information systems architecture and technology: proceedings of 39th international conference on information systems architecture and technology—ISAT 2018. Springer International Publishing, Cham, pp 105–114
23. Wang J-W, Chen T-H (2017) Face recognition based on adaptive singular value decomposition in the wavelet domain. In: Stephanidis C (ed) HCI international 2017—posters' extended abstracts. Springer International Publishing, Cham, pp 413–418
24. Zhang Y, Xu G (2016) Singular value decomposition. In: Encyclopedia of database systems, pp 1–3. https://doi.org/10.1007/978-1-4899-7993-3_538-2
25. Brunton SL, Kutz JN (2019) Data-driven science and engineering. Cambridge University Press. https://doi.org/10.1017/9781108380690
26. Sulaiman S, Agoes S (2017) Analisis Reduksi Data Citra Menggunakan Metode Dekomposisi Nilai Singular. In: Citee. In: The 9th national conference on information technology and electrical engineering, Yogyakarta, pp 21–25
27. Shi FF, Cheng XY, Chen X (2013) The summarize of improved HMM model. In: Information technology applications in industry, computer engineering and materials science. Trans Tech Publications Ltd., pp 3384–3388. https://doi.org/10.4028/www.scientific.net/AMR.756-759.3384

28. Rabiner LR (1989) A tutorial on Hidden Markov models and selected applications in speech recognition. Proc IEEE 77:257–286. https://doi.org/10.1109/5.18626
29. Ali S, Bouguila N (2022) A roadmap to Hidden Markov models and a review of its application in occupancy estimation. In: Bouguila N, Fan W, Amayri M (eds) Hidden Markov models and applications. Springer International Publishing, Cham, pp 1–31. https://doi.org/10.1007/978-3-030-99142-5_1
30. Momenzadeh M, Sehhati M, Rabbani H (2020) Using Hidden Markov model to predict recurrence of breast cancer based on sequential patterns in gene expression profiles. J Biomed Inform 111. https://doi.org/10.1016/j.jbi.2020.103570
31. Basheera S, Sai Ram MS (2020) Gray matter segmentation of brain MRI using hybrid enhanced independent component analysis in noisy and noise free environment. J Biomimetics Biomater Biomed Eng 47:75–103. https://doi.org/10.4028/www.scientific.net/JBBBE.47.75
32. Miar-Naimi H, Davari P (2008) A new fast and efficient HMM-based face recognition system using a 7-state HMM along with SVD coefficients. Iran J Electr Electron Eng 4

Analysis of Receive Signal Strength Indicator (RSSI) on Pulse Oximetry Data Delivery via Bluetooth Low Energy (BLE)

Pandu Arsy Filonanda, I. Dewa Gede Hari Wisana, Priyambada Cahya Nugraha, Farid Amrinsani, Triwiyanto, Lusiana, and Faheem Ahmad Reegu

Abstract The concept of using short range radio technology is to connect small devices to the internet or other functions that play a very important role in the development of IoT (Internet of Things). One of the new short range radio technologies at this time is Bluetooth Low Energy (BLE). This technology has considerable potential because of its low cost, very low energy consumption, and long range. This study aimed to analyze the RSSI value of the speed of data transmission on SPO2 and BPM via Bluetooth Low Energy by using several parameters, such as distance and baud rate, to see whether there is any lost data on receiving SPO2 and BPM data that have been sent by a pulse oximetry using several parameters measured. This study was conducted using the MAX30100 sensor as BPM and SPO2 data, and the ESP32TTGO T-Display microcontroller as a Bluetooth Low Energy module. In this study, the output of the MAX30100 sensor will be processed on the ESP32TTGO T-Display microcontroller, which will then be sent to Android using Bluetooth Low Energy. Then the data will be displayed on Android and on the OLED ESP32TTGO T-Display. The data collection process was carried out at a distance of 0 to 1.5 m for 10 repetitions for each distance with a time of 1 trial for 60 s. The highest lost data was obtained at a distance of 1.5 m with a value of 8.0%. The highest time delay value was obtained at a distance of 1.5 m with a value of 2.3%, while the lowest time delay value was obtained at a distance of 0 cm with a value of 0%. At a measurement distance of 2 m, the Android application captures the RSSI value of −76 dBm, with a constant A value of −69 dBm and a constant n value of 2. The distance results obtained from the RSSI calculation are 2.24 m away. From this study, it can be concluded that the pulse oximetry module can be used using an android application that uses Bluetooth low energy communication equipped with the RSSI value, and the database of BPM and SPO2 measurement results on the android application. The

P. A. Filonanda · I. D. G. H. Wisana (✉) · P. C. Nugraha · F. Amrinsani · Triwiyanto · Lusiana
Department of Medical Electronics Technology, Poltekkes Kemenkes Surabaya, Surabaya, Indonesia
e-mail: dewa@poltekkesdepkes-sby.ac.id

F. A. Reegu
College of Computer Science and Information Technology, Jazan Unversity, Jizan, Saudi Arabia

T. Triwiyanto et al. (eds.), *Proceeding of the 3rd International Conference on Electronics, Biomedical Engineering, and Health Informatics*, Lecture Notes in Electrical Engineering 1008, https://doi.org/10.1007/978-981-99-0248-4_39

findings of this study are expected to be used as a tool for monitoring the health of patients in hospitals, without worrying about the data network to monitor the results.

Keywords RSSI · Lost data · Delay data · Pulse oximetry MAX30100 · Bluetooth low energy

1 Introduction

The concept of using short range radio technology is to connect small devices to the internet or other functions that play a very important role in the development of IoT (Internet of Things). One of the new short range radio technologies at this time is Bluetooth Low Energy (BLE) [1–4]. Bluetooth Low Energy (BLE) is one of the most widely used wireless communication technologies. BLE has been extensively used in most contemporary electronic devices, such as personal computers and smartphones, like Raspberry Pi, smart watches, fitness trackers, and many others. One example of an instrument in the medical field that can be developed using Bluetooth Low Energy technology is a pulse oximetry. Pulse oximetry is a test used to monitor (measure) the heart rate and oxygen saturation of the blood (arterial), to assist the patient's physical assessment, without having to go through blood test analysis. One of the parameters of organ health that is of serious concern is the heart. The simplest representation of heart health can be depicted through oxygen saturation (SpO2) and heart rate. SpO2 measurement is used for early detection of hypoxemia [5]. SpO2 and heart rate are used as standards of healthy heart performance and as measurement of abnormal condition (hypoxemia) in the intensive care unit to guide the administration of oxygen therapy, especially in critically ill patients. Continuous monitoring of SpO2 is also required for physiologic trauma management [5]. Monitoring the pulse oximetry is crucial if there are symptoms of a disease that must be treated quickly so that the patient's condition does not worsen [6]. This is because the lack or excess of oxygen in the blood will cause diseases or disorders of the body, and at a certain level, it can cause the risk of death. Therefore, it is crucial to monitor the pulse oximetry.

BLE is used in pulse oximetry because it begins with the detection of indoor proximity and close distance [7, 8], thus BLE technology has become popular for use in medical instrumentation. Also, BLE technology has high data transmission speed, low power consumption, strong signal strength, mini size, and low cost [4, 8–12], making it is very suitable for use in pulse oximetry that transmits small data.

Although BLE technology has been well studied and there have been previous studies on BLE, in reality BLE used for reliable and secure data transmission still faces challenges, especially in overcoming lost data. Lost data in wearable health services is complicated by various factors, including. first, larger package sizes are preferred in the medical field [3, 13]. Second, the chipset used in BLE and the operating system used, in reality, is very diverse. Finally, third, the connection between the chipset and BLE driver that is not suitable can also cause lost data. Besides, environmental differences can also cause the risk of lost data. The effect of lost data on BLE delivery can also be caused by the RSSI values on the BLE network. RSSI is a technology used to measure the signal strength indicator received by a wireless device [14]. Usually, the user never checks the RSSI values; when the device is connected to the Bluetooth the user immediately sends data without seeing the RSSI value received, and the small RSSI value received by the device causes the delivery to be unstable. This is what causes lost data on sending using BLE. The closer RSSI is to 0, the higher the signal strength received by the system. To get a good performance from a wireless sensor network, it is necessary to measure network parameters. RSSI (Received Signal Strength Indicator) [15, 16] is one of the network parameters that states the signal strength received by a radio device on the communication module.

In 2014, a study has been carried out by Yanchen Dai from the University of Electronic Science and Technology of China, on pulse oximetry using an analog circuit with Bluetooth 4.0 delivery [5]. In the study, Dai analyzed the effectiveness of the pulse oximetry designed using analog circuits such as LED and Infrared, AD623 amplifier, as well as Bluetooth communication with the CC2540 module. As a result, Dai obtained accurate and stable values on the pulse oximetry, reliable data transmission using smartphones, reduced power consumption, and simplified hardware circuits. The disadvantage is that this study does not provide the results of the pulse oximetry after delivery using BLE and does not export more deeply on the use of BLE. Then, in 2018, another study has also been carried out by RR Adiputra, S. Hadiyoso, and Y. Sun Hariyani from Telkom University, on a low-cost pulse oximetry using IOT communication, namely MySQL [17]. The study analyzed the manufacture of a low-cost pulse oximetry using BPM and SPO2 sensors and nodeMCU as the microcontroller. The results obtained show that the data sent to the Internet cloud can be accessed online and in real time through the website for further analysis. The disadvantage is that the error value is still quite high, namely the BPM measurement is ± 2.8 BPM and the (SpO2) measurement is $\pm 1.5\%$. Also, the delay between the device and IOT is 3 s. Furthermore, the shape of the designed device still consists of 2 devices, namely as BPM and SPO2 sensors and connected to other devices as a display. Also, because the device uses the internet, it is clearly constrained by the internet network in the area. Next, in 2013, a study has been conducted by Jeremy Christoputra from Universita Brawijaya on the effect of RSSI value on distance on BPM and SPO2 monitoring devices in the elderly using LoRa communication. As a result, Christoputra et al. were able to make a monitoring module using LoRa communication and connected it to IoT using SQL [18]. The designed device is equipped with a measurement of the RSSI value of the measured distance. The disadvantage is that the shape of the module (device) is large and tends to take up a lot of space. Also, LoRa communication is only used as a notification for the patient's condition, and it is not used to send data continuously to see the effectiveness of LoRa as a communication. And there is still a 3-s delay for sending from the device to the IoT [19, 20].

Based on these previous studies, the researchers were interested to conduct a study in the health sector entitled, "Analysis of Receive Signal Strength Indicator (RSSI) on Pulse Oximetry Data Delivery via Bluetooth Low Energy (BLE)" which is a subsequent development of studies that have been conducted previously. The development of the device that was used by the researchers was to analyze the RSSI value in sending pulse oximetry data by using several parameters, such as varying distance and baud rate to see the amount of lost data in sending and receiving SPO2 and BPM data that have been sent by the pulse oximetry. BLE was used as a communication because there are network constraints when using the internet.

2 Materials and Methods

This study was conducted at the Department of Medical Electronics Technology, Poltekkes, Kemenkes, Surabaya. The research design used in making the module (device) was Pre-experimental with the After Only Design type. In this design the researchers only used one group of subjects and only saw the results without measuring and knowing the initial conditions, but there was already a comparison group.

The independent variable in this study was the effect of distance and baud rate which varied on the RSSI value on data transmission. However, the dependent variable was the result of the RSSI value on sending pulse oximetry data on Bluetooth low energy. And, the controlled variable was the microcontroller board used, namely ESP32TTGO.

2.1 Theoretical Background

RSSI (Received Signal Strength Indicator)

The received signal strength value is often referred to as the Received Signal Strength Indicator (RSSI). RSSI [21, 22] is a measure of signal strength when it reaches a receiving device whose value depends on the distance and strength of the beacon. RSSI is a relative indicator whose value fluctuates/is not fixed, but if the RSSI value is greater, it can be said that the received signal is stronger [8]. But on the other hand, the received signal strength is very vulnerable to noise, multi-path fading, and other disturbances [9]. The farther the device is from the beacon, the more unstable the RSSI value will be. The RSSI value can be converted to estimate the distance between the connected devices using the measured power value and the formula defined by the BLE Serial and iBeacon [14, 22, 23] standards.

$$d = \frac{10\hat{}(A - (RSSI))}{(10 * n)} \quad (1)$$

where, A is the measured power 1 m RSSI with a constant value of −69dBm. n is a constant value that occurs when the data/signal passes through the air medium from the antenna to the receiver within a certain distance. d is the Distance which is the path length between the coordinating node and the end device node. From Eq. (1), it is assumed that A is the received signal strength within 1 m with units of dBm and n is the signal propagation constant or exponent (path loss exponent). BLE uses Rated Power which is also known as RSSI 1 m. So, the value of Rated Power of −69 needs to be paid attention to.

Packet Delay (Data Delay)

From Eq. (2), Packet delay is the difference between the time of sending data packets and the time of receiving data packets. This test is carried out by sending the number of data packets with a fixed data packet size, which is 84 Bytes using XCTU software. The value of the difference in the delivery of the resulting data packets is then recorded for each experiment carried out [22].

$$delay = \frac{\sum \text{delivery time data}}{\sum \text{time to receive data}} \tag{2}$$

where, delay is the difference between the time of sending data and the time of receiving data. Data delivery time is the length of time it takes to send a large amount of data. Time to receive data is the length of time it takes to receive data that have been sent.

Packet Loss (Lost Data)

From Eq. (3), Packet Loss is the amount of lost data during the data packet transmission process. This test is carried out by sending the number of data packets with different sizes, which are taken from the BPM and SPO2 data on the pulse oximetry. The value of the difference in the delivery of the resulting data packets is then recorded for each experiment carried out [4].

$$Packet\ loss = \frac{data\ send - data\ received}{data\ send} \times 100\% \tag{3}$$

where, data send is data sent by the ESP32 TTGO microcontroller, data received is data received by Android from sending the microcontroller, packet loss is the amount of lost data in a data transmission.

The researchers modeled a conditional packet loss probability p of any station i in an arbitrary network. Conditional packet loss probability is the most critical and complicated variable to be computed for predicting per-flow throughout in multihop WMN [24]. Previous literature ignored comprehensive behavior of the CSMA-based MAC protocol and geometric location of the interfering links, and these cause stations to have large values of packet loss probability p. Conditional packet loss probability depends on geometric configuration of flows in the immediate neighborhood. When all the stations are within the transmission range of each other, then DCF is able to coordinate among stations and transmission attempts are within well-defined time durations. From Eq. (4), Conditional packet loss probability of such scenario is given by $1 - (1 - \tau)n - 1$, here n is the number of stations in the network. But there is inherent problem in DCF when employed in a multi-hop network scenario, where DCF is unable to synchronize all stations in the network. With an objective to clearly differentiate between interference from transmission and carrier sense range, the researchers identified and modeled four possible types of packet losses that can occur due to CSMA-based MAC behavior in multi-hop wireless network, including losses because of (i) sender sensing with probability pss; (ii) asymmetric incomplete state with probability pais; (iii) symmetric incomplete state with probability psis; and (iv) destination connected with probability pdc. In the following subsections, the researchers analyzed each type and describe the exact geometric configuration. The probability of each identified type is calculated independently and then combined to compute the total packet loss probability. Transmissions which do not suffer from any of these losses are successful, as shown in the following Eq. (4).

$$p(i) = 1 - \frac{[1 - Pss(i, i')][1 - Pais(i, i')]}{[1 - Psis(i, i')][1 - Pdc(i, i')]} \tag{4}$$

where, Pss is lost data because the sender sensing with probability, Pais is lost data because the incomplete state is asymmetrical with probability, Psis is lost data because the incomplete state is symmetrical with probability, and Pdc is lost data because the destination is connected with probability. The value of i is the transmitter and receiver of a data with a receiver of a link, and i' is the transmitter and receiver of a data with a receiver of another link. Figure 1 describes modelling topology in which there are two contending flows l and l', where i and j are the transmitter and receiver of link l, and i' and j' are transmitter and receiver of link l'. Each flow transmitter and receiver are within the transmission range of each other to comprise a flow, and how packet loss probability models link l' interfering the transmission of link l in different geometrical configurations.

2.2 Experimental Procedure

The MAX30100 sensor is an integration of pulse oximetry, monitoring heart rate signals and blood oxygen levels. This sensor consists of 2 LEDs and a photodetector with parallel positions. The oximetry uses the property of hemoglobin to absorb light and the natural pulse of blood flow in the arteries to measure oxygen levels in the body. A device called a probe has a light source, a light detector, and a microprocessor that can compare and calculate the difference between oxygen-rich and oxygen-deficient hemoglobin.

As shown in Fig. 2, it is explained that the input of the BPM and SPO2 parameters is from the MAX30100 sensor. If the MAX30100 sensor takes BPM and SPO2 data then the data will be processed on the ESP32TTGO. On the ESP32TTGO microcontroller, the BPM and SPO2 data will be processed and will be sent using

Fig. 1 Two-flow topology

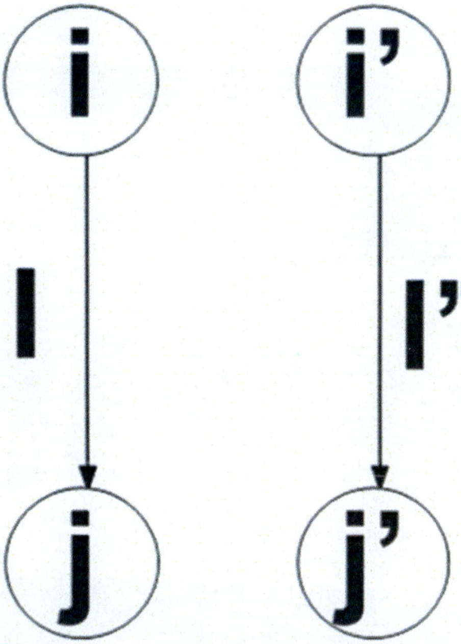

BLE (Bluetooth low energy), before the ESP32TTGO microcontroller sends BPM and SPO2 data, Android will first ask for BPM and SPO2 data to the microcontroller, after getting approval from the microcontroller, then the microcontroller will send BPM and SPO2 data to Android. After the data is sent by the microcontroller, then Android will receive the data first, before displaying it. In addition to displaying it on Android, the BPM and SPO2 values will also be displayed via the OLED in the ESP32TTGO.

2.3 Data Processing

Figure 3 is the microcontroller program flowchart explaining that when the device is turned on in the initial conditions, the initialization process occurs. After the initialization process is carried out, the MAX30100 sensor will read the SPO2 and BPM values and will display them on the ESP32TTGO OLED screen. Then Android will search for BLE (Bluetooth low energy) devices in the vicinity, and after there is a suitable BLE device, Android will connect the Bluetooth low energy device. After Bluetooth low energy has been connected to Android, Android will first ask for data requests on the microcontroller, then Bluetooth low energy will send the SPO2 and BPM data to the BLE server, and then the data will be processed on the Android device. Next the SPO2 and BPM data that have been processed on the Android device will be displayed on the Android device.

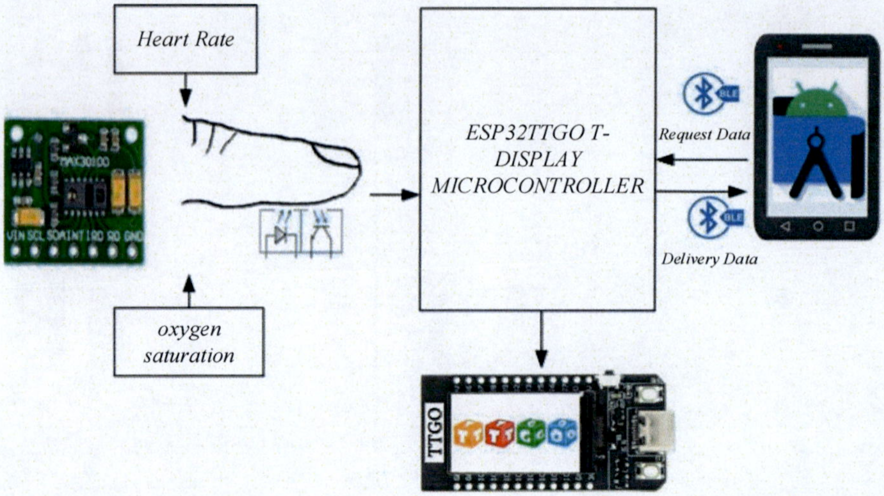

Fig. 2 System block diagram

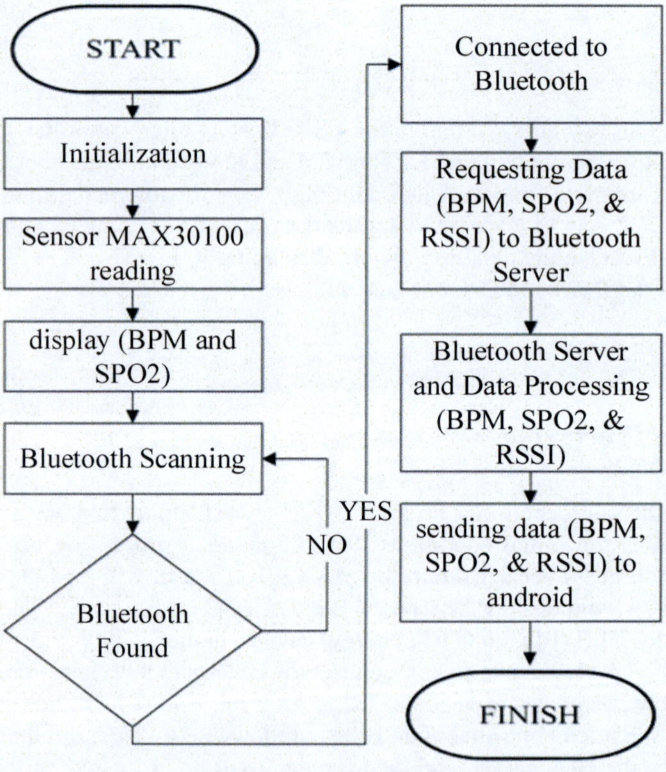

Fig. 3 Microcontroller system flowchart

Android Studio is an Integrated Development Environment (IDE) for the Android operating system, which is used to create Android applications using the Java and Kotlin programming languages. Android studio was first announced at the Google I/O conference.

Figure 4 is the Android program flowchart, explaining that when the device is turned on in the initial conditions, an initialization process occurs. After the initialization process is carried out, Android will look for BLE (Bluetooth low energy) devices in the vicinity, and once there is a suitable BLE device, Android will connect the Bluetooth low energy device. After Bluetooth low energy has been connected to Android, the latter will first request a data request on the microcontroller. Bluetooth low energy will send SPO2 and BPM data to the BLE server, and then the data will be processed on the Android device. Then Android will receive data from Bluetooth low energy and the data will be displayed on the Android device. For the BPM and SPO2 sensors, the MAX30100 sensor module has analog data output. And the microcontroller uses ESP32TTGO which is also a BLE module and an OLED display on the oximetry module. Data that have been obtained can be sent via the WhatsApp application. Then, the application will send 3 types of files, namely heart rate data, SPO2, and RSSI value in CSV form. Then, there is a screenshot of the Android application, and the location of Google maps where the tool is used.

2.4 Data Analysis

The data collection process was carried out at a distance of 0 to 1.5 m for 10 repetitions for each distance with a time of 1 trial for 60 s. The average value of the measurement is obtained by using the mean or the average by applying the following Eq. (5).

$$\overline{X} = \frac{x1 + x2... + xn}{n} \tag{5}$$

where, $\overline{x}$ is the average (mean) for the n-measurements, ×1 is the first measurement, ×2 is the second measurement, and xn is the nth measurements. Standard deviation is a value indicating the degree of variation in a data set or a measure of the standard deviation of the mean. The formula for standard deviation (SD) is as shown in the following Eq. (6):

$$SD = \sqrt{\frac{\sum (xi - \overline{X})^2}{(n - 1)}} \tag{6}$$

where, xi is the number of desired values, x is the mean (average) of the measurement results, n is the number of measurement data. Uncertainty (UA) is a doubt that appears in each measurement result. The formula for uncertainty is as shown in the following Eq. (7):

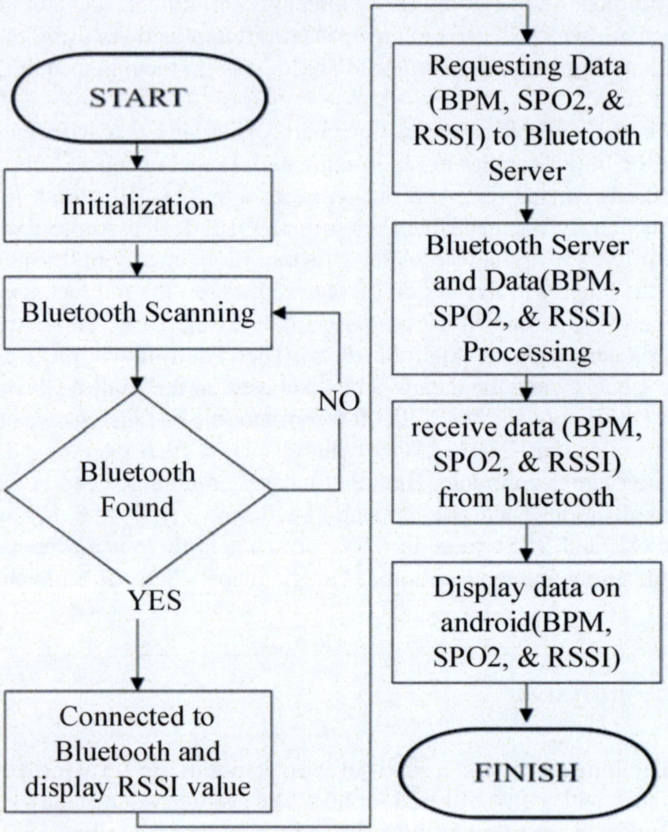

Fig. 4 Android flowchart

$$UA = \frac{SD}{\sqrt{n}} \tag{7}$$

where, UA is the uncertainty value of the total measurement, SD is the resulting standard deviation, and n is the number of measurement data. Percentage (%) of error indicates a system error. The lower Error value is the average difference of each data. Errors indicates deviations between the standard and the design or model. The % error formula is as shown in the following Eq. (8).

$$Error = \frac{(xn - x)}{xn} \times 100\% \tag{8}$$

where, xn is the measured value of the machine calibrator. X is the measured value of the design.

3 Results

3.1 SpO2 and BPM Measurement

In this study, the designed device (module) has been tested using a comparison tool, namely a pulse oximetry. The data collection process was carried out at a distance of 0 to 1.5 m for 10 repetitions for each distance with 1 trial time for 60 s. The design is shown in Figs. 5, 6. The digital part consists of an ESP32TTGO microcontroller, which is the main board of the device as well as delivery communication using BLE (Bluetooth low energy) and an OLED display that is integrated with the microcontroller. The MAX30100 sensor is an integration of pulse oximetry with heart rate and temperature parameters, monitoring heart rate signals and blood oxygen levels. This sensor consists of 2 LEDs and a photodetector with parallel positions. Figure 7 is the display on the android application. The application shows various names of devices that use Bluetooth as communication. Next to the device name, there is also the RSSI value which is the value of the strength and weakness of the Bluetooth signal of a device. The smaller the RSSI value, the farther the device is from the Android application, and vice versa. Also, the farther the distance and the smaller the RSSI value, the longer and weaker the delivery and communication between the Android application and the device will be.

Fig. 5 Results of device

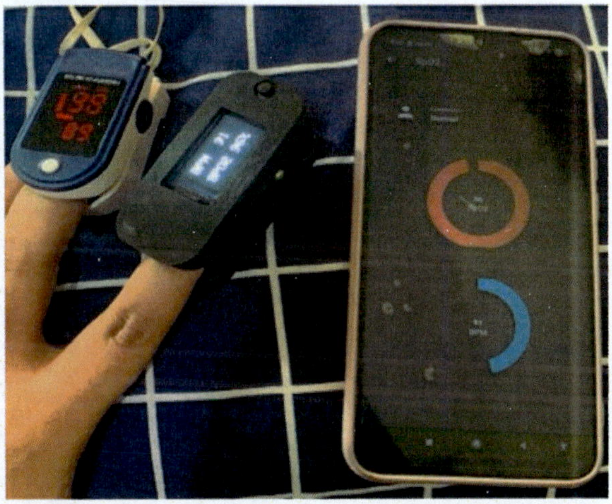

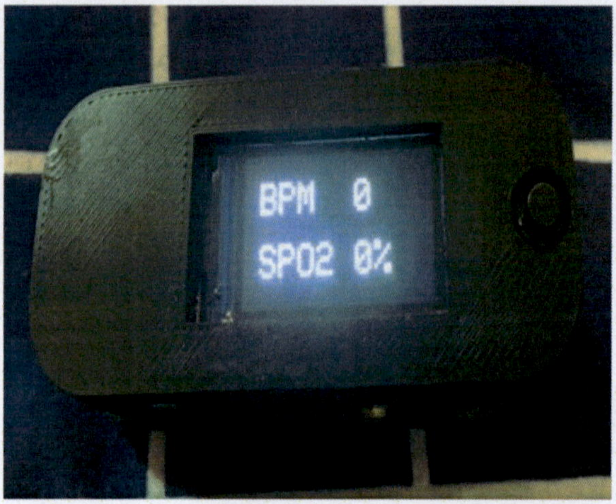

Fig. 6 Design of BPM sensor and temperature

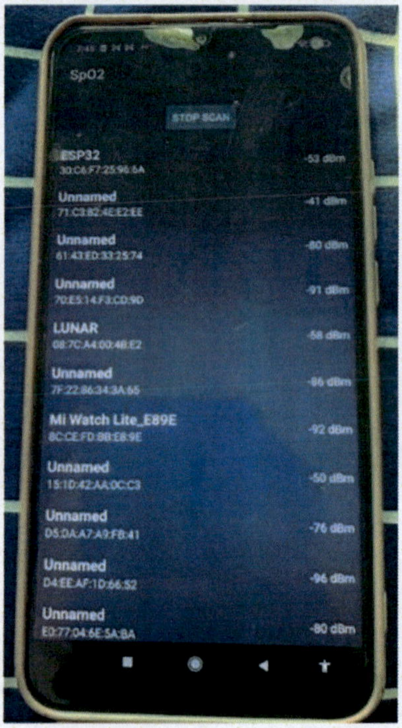

Fig. 7 Display of RSSI and device name on the android application

3.2 Results of RSSI Data Measurement on the Android Application

Figure 8 is the data collection process to determine the effect of distance on the RSSI value carried out at a distance of 0 to 1.5 m for 10 repetitions for each distance with a time of 1 trial for 60 s using BLE (Bluetooth low energy) communication on the ESP32TTGO microcontroller with the Android application comparison device that already has the RSSI value. It can be seen in Fig. 8 that the table and graph are data obtained from the results of RSSI measurements using the Android application.

RSSI is a relative indicator whose value fluctuates/is not fixed, but if the RSSI value is greater, it can be said that the received signal is stronger [5]. The closer the value to 0, the better the quality of the RSSI.

An example of distance measurement is obtained from the RSSI value at a distance of 2 m. BLE uses Rated Power which is also known as RSSI 1 m. So, the value of Rated Power of −69 needs to be paid attention to. The following is the approximate distance calculation on the obtained RSSI value, d = 2.24 m. The calculation in Eq. 6 is an example of a calculation to find the approximate distance with the obtained RSSI value, where the value of A is a constant RSSI signal strength at a distance of 1 m with a value of −69. The value of n is the constant for the missing path—the exponential value for the data collection environment conditions with the constant value for the free space environment is 2. The RSSI value of −76 is the approximate RSSI value that has been obtained through data retrieval on the Android application. Here, the calculation is done by trying at a distance of 2 m. In a measurement made at a distance of 2 m, the RSSI value is −76, but in the calculations that have been carried out, it turns out that the RSSI value of −76 is obtained at a distance of 2.24 m.

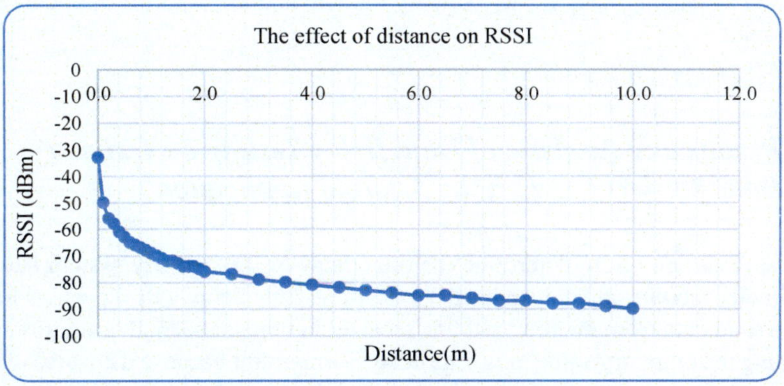

Fig. 8 Graph of RSSI data measurement results on the android application

3.3 Results and Analysis of Lost Data Testing on Oximetry Data Retrieval and on the Android Application

Packet Loss (lost data) is the amount of lost data during the data packet transmission process. This test is carried out by sending the number of data packets with different sizes, which are taken from the BPM and SPO2 data on the pulse oximetry. The value of the difference in the delivery of the resulting data packet is then recorded for each experiment carried out. This test aims to determine the lost data from the delivery system between the oximetry module and the Android application. Lost data is how much data is lost during the data transmission process. This lost data indicates a failure in data packet transmission that can be caused by many factors, such as noise on the network, errors in physical media, failure on the receiving side, and so on. The following are the standard categories for lost data:

The data collection process was carried out at a distance of 0 to 1.5 m for 10 repetitions for each distance with a time of 1 trial for 60 s using the Android application.

In this oximetry module data, lost data is considered important because it will affect the value that will be displayed on the Android application and the value that will be stored in the Android application database. The greater the value of lost data, the greater the lost data. This causes the value of the data received and the data sent to experience a significant difference.

It can be seen in Fig. 9 that new lost data occurs when the distance between the oximetry module and the Android application is 1 m. The farther the distance between the oximetry module and the Android application, the greater the lost data that will occur in the measurement. The highest lost data was obtained at a distance of 1.5 m with a value of 8.0%. Thus, it can be said that the delivery system on the module is very good at sending data, if the oximetry module and the Android application are not far apart.

3.4 Results and Analysis of Data Delay Testing on Oximetry Data Retrieval and on the Android Application

This test is carried out to determine the time delay of the delivery system between the oximetry module and the Android application. Time delay will show how long it takes to send data from the sender to the receiver in units of second or microsecond. In sending the oximetry value, this time delay is important because it ensures that the system can monitor the signal in real-time. The data collection process was carried out at a distance of 0 to 1.5 m for 10 repetitions for each distance with a time of 1 trial for 60 s using the Android application.

It can be seen in Fig. 10, the highest time delay value was obtained in data collection at a distance of 1.5 m with a value of 2.3 s, while the lowest time delay value was obtained at a distance of 0 cm with a value of 0 s. This happens because

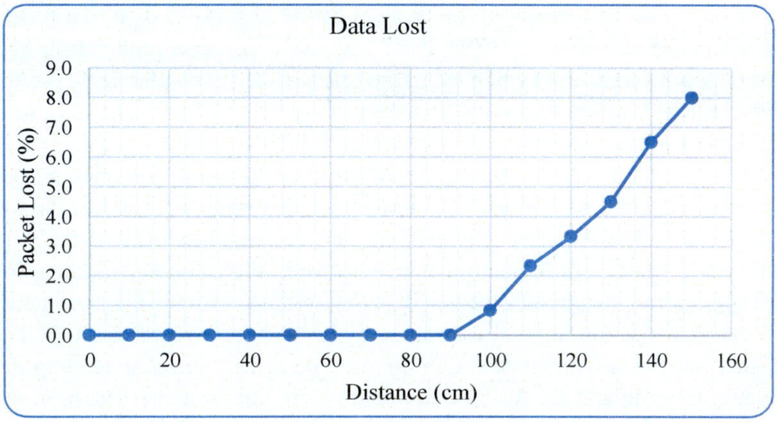

Fig. 9 Results of data lost testing on oximetry data retrieval and on the android application

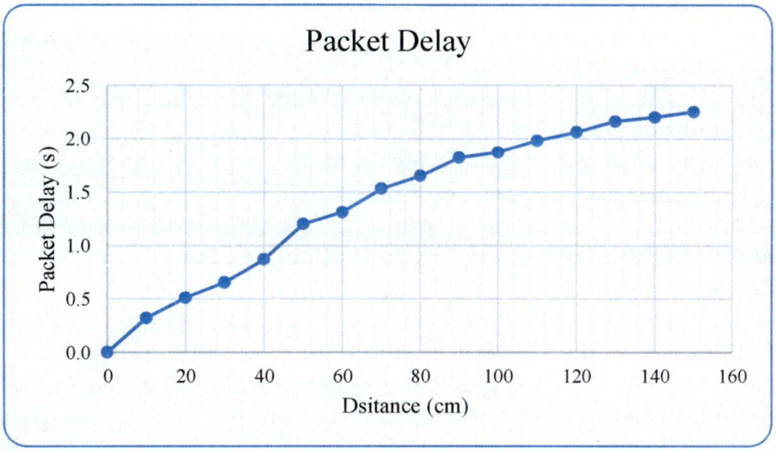

Fig. 10 Results of data delay testing on oximetry data retrieval and on the android application

the distance and the RSSI value greatly affect the sending and receiving of data by Bluetooth low energy. The farther the distance, the smaller the RSSI value, causing the ability to send and receive data to slow down and resulting in a large time delay.

4 Discussion

After taking data and measuring the oximetry module, data collection and analysis were carried out to analyze the RSSI value in sending pulse oximetry data by using several parameters, such as varying distance [2, 25, 26]and baud rate to see the amount of lost data in sending and receiving SPO2 and BPM data that have been sent by the pulse oximetry [27–29]. BLE was used as a communication because there are network constraints when using the internet. After conducting experiments to obtain the RSSI value, lost data, and data delay [30, 31] with the data retrieval process carried out at a distance of 0 to 1.5 m for 10 repetitions for each distance with a time of 1 trial for 60 s using the Android application, the results obtained on the oximetry module are as follows: In the measurements of new lost data value, lost data occurs when the distance between the oximetry module and the Android application is 1 m. The farther the distance between the oximetry module and the Android application, the greater the lost data that will occur in the measurement. The highest lost data was obtained at a distance of 1.5 m with a value of 8.0%. Thus, it can be said that the delivery system on the module is very good at sending data, if the oximetry module and the Android application are not far apart. The highest time delay value was obtained in data collection at a distance of 1.5 m with a value of 2.3 s, while the lowest time delay value was obtained at a distance of 0 cm with a value of 0 s. This happens because the distance and the RSSI value greatly affect the sending and receiving of data by Bluetooth low energy. The farther the distance, the smaller the RSSI value, causing the ability to send and receive data to slow down resulting in a large time delay.

For the calculation of the distance obtained from the calculation of the RSSI formula, the results are not far from the distance at the time of measurement. At a measurement distance of 2 m, the Android application captures the RSSI value of −76 dBm, with a constant A value of −69 dBm and a constant n value of 2. The distance results obtained from the RSSI calculation are 2.24 m away. It can be concluded that the distance measurement obtained from the RSSI formula has a small error with the actual distance.

Then, the experiment with different types of baud rate obtained results which show no difference in the RSSI value, as well as the BPM and Spo2 data values from the oximetry module. This is because the Arduino program has added a smoothing program, so the data from BPM and Spo2 on the oximetry module have good and stable values. Also, the Android application as monitoring and database storage, can only store 1 data/second, indicating no matter how much the sample rate is at the baud rate, the oximetry will perform smoothing and will display the BPM and SPO2 values with a stable value.

The implication of this study is to analyze the RSSI value in sending pulse oximetry data by using several parameters, such as varying distance and baud rate to see the amount of lost data in sending and receiving SPO2 and BPM data that have been sent by the pulse oximetry.

Due to various factors, the designed module by the researchers is still far from perfect, both in terms of planning, manufacturing, and how the module works. So, there are several limitations that have been analyzed from the designed device by the researchers, including the capacity of the battery used that is still small, leading to a short usage time. BPM and SPO2 sensors are used for further research in order to use BPM and SPO2 sensors with medical grade standards. Also, the shape of the

Table 1 Standard category on lost data

Lost data category	Target (%)
Very good	0–2
Good	3–14
Medium	15–24
Bad	>25

oximetry module can still be made as small as possible to make it more comfortable to use for patients.

5 Conclusion

This research was conducted to analyze the RSSI value in sending pulse oximetry data by using several parameters, such as varying distance and baud rate to see the amount of lost data in sending and receiving SPO2 and BPM data that have been sent by the pulse oximetry. The data collection process was carried out at a distance of 0 to 1.5 m for 10 repetitions for each distance with a time of 1 trial for 60 s. From the results and discussion of this study, the following conclusions can be drawn, namely, first, a pulse oximetry module can be made using the MAX30100 module with BPM and SPO2 parameters. Second, communication can be made using Bluetooth low energy using the ESP32TTGO microcontroller. Third, the pulse oximetry module can be used using the Android application that uses Bluetooth low energy communication equipped with RSSI values, and a database of BPM and SPO2 measurement results on the Android application. Fourth, the experiment with different types of baud rate obtained results which show no difference in the RSSI value, as well as the BPM and Spo2 data values from the oximetry module. This is because the data obtained from the sensor will be smoothed on the microcontroller, so the result on the BPM and SPO2 values will come out 1 data per second. Finally, the ESP32TTGO microcontroller module can be used as a data processor, and produce the output generated by the MAX30100 sensor to be used as BPM and SPO2 values, and send data to the Android application, which will then be displayed on the ESP32TTGO OLED screen in the form of BPM and SPO2 values.

References

1. Chen Q, Tang L (2020) A wearable blood oxygen saturation monitoring system based on bluetooth low energy technology. Comput Commun 160:101–110. https://doi.org/10.1016/j.comcom.2020.05.041
2. Putra RD, Putri RE (2021) Prototype physical distancing distance detector bracelet man to man. Chipset 2:15–22. https://doi.org/10.25077/chipset.2.02.15-22.2021

3. Bulić P, Kojek G, Biasizzo A (2019) Data transmission efficiency in bluetooth low energy versions. Sensors (Switzerland) 19. https://doi.org/10.3390/s19173746
4. Wu T, Wu F, Qiu C, Redoute JM, Yuce MR (2020) A rigid-flex wearable health monitoring sensor patch for IoT-connected healthcare applications. IEEE Internet Things J 7:6932–6945. https://doi.org/10.1109/JIOT.2020.2977164
5. Dai Y, Luo J (2015) Design of noninvasive pulse oximeter based on bluetooth 4.0 BLE. Proc 2014 7th Int Symp Comput Intell Des Isc 1:100–103. https://doi.org/10.1109/ISCID.2014.45
6. Prayogo I, Alfita R, Wibisono KA (2017) Monitoring system for heart rate and body temperature as an IOT (Internet of Thing)-based patient health level indicator using the fuzzy logic method using android. J Electr Comput Eng TRIAC 4. https://doi.org/10.21107/triac.v4i2.3257
7. Kalbandhe AA, Patil SC (2017) Indoor positioning system using bluetooth low energy. Int Conf Comput Anal Secur Trends CAST 2016 451–455. https://doi.org/10.1109/CAST.2016.7915011
8. Tipparaju VV, Mallires KR, Wang D, Tsow F, Xian X (2021) Mitigation of data packet loss in bluetooth low energy-based wearable healthcare ecosystem. Biosensors 11. https://doi.org/10.3390/bios11100350
9. Tosi J, Taffoni F, Santacatterina M, Sannino R, Formica D (2017) Performance evaluation of bluetooth low energy: a systematic review. Sensors (Switzerland) 17:1–34. https://doi.org/10.3390/s17122898
10. Williamson J, Liu Q, Lu F, Mohrman W, Li K, Dick R, Shang L (2015) Data sensing and analysis: challenges for wearables. In: 20th Asia and South pacific design automation conference ASP-DAC 2015, pp 136–141. https://doi.org/10.1109/ASPDAC.2015.7058994
11. Jiang H, Chen X, Zhang S, Zhang X, Kong W, Zhang T (2015) Software for wearable devices: challenges and opportunities. In: IEEE computer society's international computer software and applications conference, vol 3, pp 592–597. https://doi.org/10.1109/COMPSAC.2015.269
12. Zhang T, Lu J, Hu F, Hao Q (2014) Bluetooth low energy for wearable sensor-based healthcare systems. In: 2014 IEEE healthcare innovation conference HIC 2014, pp 251–254. https://doi.org/10.1109/HIC.2014.7038922
13. Giovanelli D, Milosevic B, Farella E (2015) Bluetooth low energy for data streaming: application-level analysis and recommendation. In: Proceedings of the 2015 6th IEEE international workshop on advances in sensors and interfaces, IWASI 2015, pp 216–221. https://doi.org/10.1109/IWASI.2015.7184945
14. Sahu PK, Wu EHK, Sahoo J (2013) DuRT: dual RSSI trend based localization for wireless sensor networks. IEEE Sens J 13:3115–3123. https://doi.org/10.1109/JSEN.2013.2257731
15. Rssi P, Wifi K, Strength S, Ap D, Edimax AP, Rmad AP, Kualitas H, Zte AP, Zte AP, Wifi A, Pada A, Analyzer W, Analyzer W (2014) Radio (received) signal strength indicator. Helsinki Metrop Univ Appl Sci 1–4
16. Dharmawan WW, Kurnianto A, Ar-Rasyiid A (2016) Improvement of Rssi distance estimation accuracy with normal log model using Kalman filter method on bluetooth low energy. Pros Semnastek 1–5
17. Adiputra RR, Hadiyoso S, Sun Hariyani Y (2018) Internet of things: low cost and wearable SpO2 device for health monitoring. Int J Electr Comput Eng 8:939–945. https://doi.org/10.11591/ijece.v8i2.pp939-945
18. Christoputra J (2021) Design of a data receiver module on a health monitoring system for the elderly who live alone at home
19. Rani S (2021) Modern health monitoring and analysis using Iot technology Turkish online. J Qual Inq 12:4961–4972
20. Krishnan DSR, Gupta SC, Choudhury T (2018) An IoT based patient health monitoring system. In: Proceedings 2018 international conference on advanced electronic materials, computers and materials engineering ICACCE 2018, vol 1, pp 1–7. https://doi.org/10.1109/ICACCE.2018.8441708
21. Botta M, Simek M (2013) Adaptive distance estimation based on RSSI in 802.15.4 network. Radioengineering 22:1162–1168

22. Iswara IBI, Wibisono W (2013) Selection of reliable neighbor node by taking signal strength and link quality into account in zone routing protocol in MANET environment. J Comput Sci 6:35–48
23. Shofi AYA (2017) Analysis of RSS and discovery time values on distance and number of beacons in bluetooth low energy-based smart key systems
24. Zeeshan M, Ali A, Naveed A, Liu AX, Wang A, Qureshi HK (2016) Modeling packet loss probability and busy time in multi-hop wireless networks. Eurasip J Wirel Commun Netw 2016. https://doi.org/10.1186/s13638-016-0664-7
25. Hammam RKN, Isnianto HN, Lestari S, Setiyono YW (2021) Bluetooth performance analysis on abandoned item reminder alarm system with android smartphone. J Rekayasa Elektr 17. https://doi.org/10.17529/jre.v17i3.20648
26. Firmansyah RA, Bambang GI, Sumber (2019) Monitoring heart rate and temperature based on internet of things. J Electron Electromed Eng Med Inf 1:1–7. https://doi.org/10.35882/jeeemi.v1i2.1
27. Mohan PM, Nagarajan V, Nisha AA (2018) A frame work to estimate heart rate and arterial oxygen saturation (Spo2). In: Proceedings of the 2017 international conference on communication and signal processing ICCSP 2017. 2018–Janua, pp 1645–1648. https://doi.org/10.1109/ICCSP.2017.8286669
28. Puspitasari AJ, Famella D, Sulthonur Ridwan M, Khoiri M (2020) Design of low-flow oxygen monitor and control system for respiration and SpO2 rates optimization. J Phys Conf Ser 1436. https://doi.org/10.1088/1742-6596/1436/1/012042
29. Canu A, Canu M, Marinkovic S, Faul S, Popovici E (2011) Respiration rate calculation using low power DSP processor and SpO 2 sensor. In: MeMeA 2011—Proceedings 2011 IEEE international symposium on medical measurements and applications, pp 517–520. https://doi.org/10.1109/MeMeA.2011.5966757
30. Pratama RC, Pramukantoro ES, Basuki A (2018) Development of bluetooth low energy (BLE) interface on IoT middleware to support network interoperability. J Inf Technol Comput Sci Dev Univ Brawijaya 2:4020–4026
31. Nahar L, Zafar SS, Rafiq FB (2020) IOT based ICU patient health monitoring system. In: 11th IEEE annual information technology, electronics and mobile communication conference IEMCON 2020, pp 407–413. https://doi.org/10.1109/IEMCON51383.2020.9284900

Web-Based Incubator Analyzer Effectiveness and Efficiency Analysis Using ISO:IEC 25022

Friza Servile, Andjar Pudji, Muhammad Ridha Mak'ruf, Triwiyanto, Syaifuddin, Tribowo Indrato, and Phuoc-Hai Huynh

Abstract In calibrating a baby incubator, it is necessary to calibrate the values of temperature, humidity, airflow, and noise level. However, in the conventional calibration process, it has several disadvantages such as data loss, unreadable writing, and longer time to write and copy data until the certificate is issued. Therefore, the researchers were interested to develop a web-based incubator analyzer device to support the tele-calibration feature, where the sensor reading results, besides being displayed on the TFT screen, will also be sent directly to a web application, so it can be monitored remotely and accessed by several devices at once. The data will be stored in a MySQL database and measurement reports can be printed via the web application. The designed device was compared with the standard measuring instrument using the Fluke brand incu tester II and the largest errors were obtained, namely at T1 of 0.22%, T2 of 0.38%, T3 of 1.2%, T4 of 1.68%, T5 of 0.33%, mattress temperature of 0.37%, humidity of 3.24%, and noise level of 2.09%. At the airflow velocity, the researchers treated the sensor using a mini fan with three-speed levels as high as the sensor at a distance of 30 cm and obtained the largest error of 3.26% at the low-level fan speed. Based on the evaluation results, this device can be used to verify the environmental conditions in the baby incubator compartment, and the measurement results can be monitored remotely by several devices to support tele-calibration procedures. It is hoped that this study can facilitate and accelerate the calibration process and be used to support industry 4.0 in the field of health technology.

Keywords Incubator analyzer · Temperature · Noise level · Airflow · Web

F. Servile · A. Pudji (✉) · M. R. Mak'ruf · Triwiyanto · Syaifuddin · T. Indrato
Department of Medical Electronics Technology, Poltekkes Kemenkes Surabaya, Surabaya, Indonesia
e-mail: andjar@poltekkesdepkes-sby.ac.id

P.-H. Huynh
Faculty of Information Technology, An Giang University, Long Xuyen, Vietnam

Vietnam National University, Ho Chi Minh, Vietnam

T. Triwiyanto et al. (eds.), *Proceeding of the 3rd International Conference on Electronics, Biomedical Engineering, and Health Informatics*, Lecture Notes in Electrical Engineering 1008, https://doi.org/10.1007/978-981-99-0248-4_40

1 Introduction

Premature babies require extra attention and health care in the intensive care unit. Congenital anomalies and the inability of newborn babies to regulate their body temperature are the main causes of premature infant mortality [1]. A baby incubator is needed to maintain the warmth and humidity of the baby's body [2]. Since the introduction of a baby incubator and advances in technology, the survival rate of premature and newborn babies has increased significantly [3]. However, in some cases, it was found that babies died due to excess heat in the baby incubator [4]. For this reason, it is important to verify the correctness of sensor readings on each parameter of the environmental conditions of the baby incubator. The incubator nalyser is a portable device used to verify the operation and environmental conditions of baby incubators, transport incubators, and baby warmers. The incubator nalyser verifies several important parameters for baby care such as temperature, airflow, sound/noise, and humidity [5]. The conventional calibration process has several disadvantages, including data collection of measurement recordings that is still done by manually recording the sensor reading values on the worksheet. Then, analysis and observations are carried out using Microsoft Excel, after which a measurement certificate is issued. This, of course, takes time and costs quite a lot of money [6]. Several testing and calibration bodies have tried to digitize calibration certificates by scanning worksheets into PDF format. However, instead of speeding up the process, they are actually slowing the data presentation. In the study conducted, Digitalising the calibration certificate (DCC), can be applied if the device supports sending metadata for computerized processing [7, 8].

Wang Zhihu pointed out that the conventional calibration process has a complicated operation. It requires personnel who have sufficient skills and expertise. And on a large calibration project, the calibration service unit will have difficulty in data management. Wang Zhihu designed an internet-based calibration system using the Visual Studio 2008 software platform. The system implements the automation of the calibration process instrument, and to store recorded data, a database is used so that it can be reprocessed. Through the internet, calibration data can be monitored remotely. This is very good for saving time and increasing efficiency significantly [9]. Irfan Asfy Fakhry Anto stated that there are several problems in the conventional calibration process. For example, data collection from measurements is still recorded using manual paper, then analysis and observations are carried out using Microsoft Office, after which a new calibration certificate is issued. This causes low data integrity because it can be changed (data-tampering) unilaterally. Irfan Asfy Fakhry Anto applied blockchain technology to a digital multimeter calibration system. The calibration data of each device cannot be controlled or changed unilaterally because it uses blockchain technology which applies a distribution system to every node in the network. Thus, it can increase the credibility and security of data consistently [10]. This is in line with Mohammed S. Gadelrab and Reham A. Abouhogail that in the calibration certificate system, the problem is not only the use of paper but also the data management system. A conventional management system is very slow and difficult to manage and process. In the conventional system, verifying traceability is very difficult and time-consuming [8]. For this reason, it is very important to develop an incubator nalyser that can transmit measurement data, as well as a management software that can process measurement data into digital data. The use of a web system may be considered in a measurement data processing system.

The researchers have conducted research on several previous studies regarding incubator analyzers that can transmit measurement data. The incubator nalyser with measurement data transmission was developed by Hidayah Nur Annisa Samputri and Vina Nadhirotul Azkiyak in 2019. The incubator nalyser measurement results can be displayed on Android, and then stored in the internal memory on Android, so the technician can review the measurement data that has been carried out. However, the disadvantage of this device is that measurement data is only for 1 android device so it cannot be seen by the baby incubator owner or the baby incubator operator in the hospital, and the data displayed is only the sensor reading numbers [11, 12]. In the same year, Agistya Ananda Charisa developed a portable Incubator Analyzer based on virtual-programming with SD card storage. Sensor reading data is displayed on a computer via Bluetooth using a Delphi-based application. The advantage of this device compared to the one in the previous study is that, sensor data is repeated 5 times for each parameter, and can be stored in the SD card memory. Meanwhile, the disadvantage of this device is in terms of portability and multi-access because it uses a local computer, and there is no measurement report [13]. Jaroonrut Prinyakupt and Kittipan Roongprasert in 2019 also developed a temperature and humidity verification device in a baby incubator that can transmit sensor reading to the Thingspeak platform. The disadvantage of this device is the use of the Thingspeak platform, where the platform cannot be further developed as needed [14]. In 2020, Syarifattul Ainiyah and Laily Nurrohmah developed an incubator nalyser using a computer which is equipped with a measurement certificate. The measurement data are displayed on the computer via Bluetooth and the Delphi platform. Measurements are repeated 6 times and a T1-T5 temperature graphs are also displayed. The advantage of this device is that, it can store measurement data as a measurement certificate in Microsoft Excel format, so it can be processed further. Whereas, the disadvantage of this device is the use of computer equipment, which has less portability and accessibility, also the measurement certificate that does not contain administrative data [15, 16].

Based on several problems in the incubator analyzers that have been developed in the previous study, including portability and low accessibility, this study aimed to design a portable incubator nalyser that can send measurement data to the web, and process measurement data into a digital calibration certificate. The researchers also nalyse the effectiveness and efficiency of the system and software according to the ISO:25022 standard. With the designed incubator nalyser, it is hoped that it can speed up the recording process of the baby incubator, and speed up the calibration unit in presenting digital calibration certificates without complicated procedures, and wasting a lot of time and resources.

2 General Information

2.1 Data Transfer Method

Data transfer requires a data processing unit. This unit must be programmable by considering several criteria, such as portability, effectiveness, and compatibility [17]. Internet of things (IoT) includes autonomous devices that are proficient in censorship and data processing [18]. The use of IoT continues to increase, and Gartner estimates that IoT will reach 26 billion units by 2020 [19]. In this study, the researchers used ESP32 as a microcontroller, which can also be connected to the internet network via a Wi-Fi router. The data transfer model is presented in the following Fig. 1 [20].

In general, the data transmission design is divided into 2 parts; A module as the transmitter containing a circuit that processes sensor readings and sends it to the receiver and a web service as the receiver functioning as a receiver and data processor to be displayed to users or stored in a database [21]. The environmental conditions of the baby incubator can be measured using several sensors according

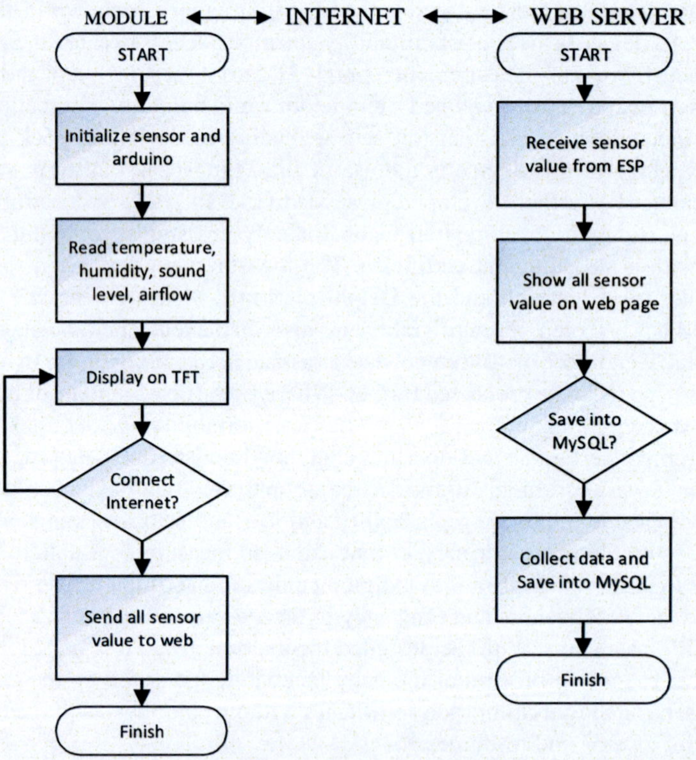

Fig. 1 Flowchart of the entire system of measuring parameters (air temperature, mattress temperature, humidity, noise, and airflow) and sending sensor readings to web pages via the internet

to measurement parameters carried out. Then the readings of each sensor will be processed by a module containing a microcontroller to be converted into numbers or raw data. These raw data are then given an appropriate delivery protocol to be displayed on other devices that support it via an internet connection. Various kinds of delivery protocols have been used in the previous incubator analyzer designs, including serial interface, Bluetooth to PC, Bluetooth to Android, IoT, and Hypertext Transfer Protocol (HTTP) using the internet as a communication medium. HTTP was introduced by Tim Berners-Lee in 1994, which is used as a navigator in web browsers. The Internet has become a revolutionary invention in the world of communication that promises speed and flexibility in data access [22]. IoT can be used to monitor data in real-time, where measurement parameters can be monitored via the website, or Android by accessing the browser [23].

The most popular language used by developers nowadays is Hypertext Preprocessor (PHP). PHP can be used for both client and server and can relate very well to cross-platform such as Apache, MySQL, and XAMPP [24]. One of the important rules in software development is to separate the user interface from application coding and other important algorithms. Currently, web-based programming has also used a lot of a Model View Controller (MVC) design to support writing programs that are systematic, and can be used repeatedly without having to rewrite them [25]. In the MVC model, the system is divided into 3 parts, each of which is independent of each other. Application data is managed by the model responsible for data storage and retrieval. The view's job is to visually present the model to the user and get a response. The controller is the core part that acts between the model and the view [26]. The data transfer interface model using the MVC design is presented in the Fig. 2.

First, the user accesses the web page through a browser and is redirected to the index. On the index page, the user needs to instruct the controller to select the

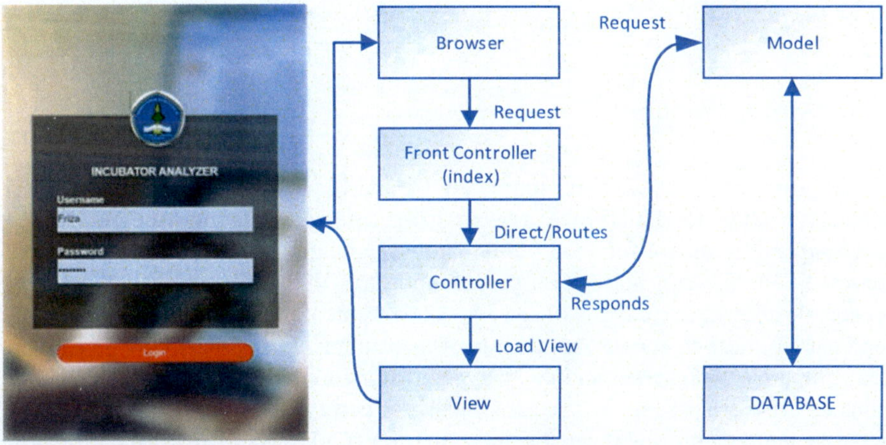

Fig. 2 User interface web application

appropriate model they want, including sending a request to the model for data access. Then, the model sends a response to the controller. Finally, the controller sends the result to the interface via the browser view. The *view* contains HTML, CSS, and JavaScript for user interface purposes [27]. The advantages of using the MVC design include [28]:

1. MVC component is modulated, which facilitates reuse of business logic.
2. A web designer or user interface (UI) developer can work on designing web pages or UIs without worrying about the business model or logic. Also, data operator can work on the model without worrying about the UI.
3. Tasks mentioned above can be performed concurrently, resulting in lower interdependence and good time utilization.

In this study, visual studio code was used to develop a web-based application that supports the built incu analyzer. Visual studio code supports several programming languages such as HTML, PHP, CSS, JavaScript and others. And in this study, the MVC (Model-View-Controller) design, which is popular because it makes web development better and more structured, was used. Besides, the use of the MVC design also has an impact on increasing development productivity because there is no need to write from scratch for commonly used tasks [24].

3 Material and Methods

This study was conducted as an experimental research. The researchers designed a web-based incu analyzer to measure the conditions of the baby incubator, consisting of several parameters including air temperature T1-T5, mattress temperature, humidity, noise, and airflow velocity. The materials and methods are explained in the following sections.

3.1 Data Collection

In this study, the researchers compared the designed device (web-based Incu analyzer) and the standard (Fluke) as a comparison device. This study used DS18B20 as a temperature sensor for T1-T5 and mattress temperature, DHT22 as a humidity sensor, SEN0232 as a noise level sensor, and D6F-V03A1 as an airflow velocity sensor. Besides, this study also used ESP32 as a microcontroller and (a device) to send data to the web server. At the time of measurement, the incu analyzer (Fluke) as a comparison is inserted into the baby incubator and the position of the sensors is adjusted according to Fig. 3. The baby incubator is set at a set temperature of 32°C. After the temperature stabilized, the incu analyzer (Fluke) is turned on and measurements are carried out for 30 min. After that, the incu analyzer (Fluke) is removed and the incu analyzer (design) is inserted. When the temperature stabilized at 32°C,

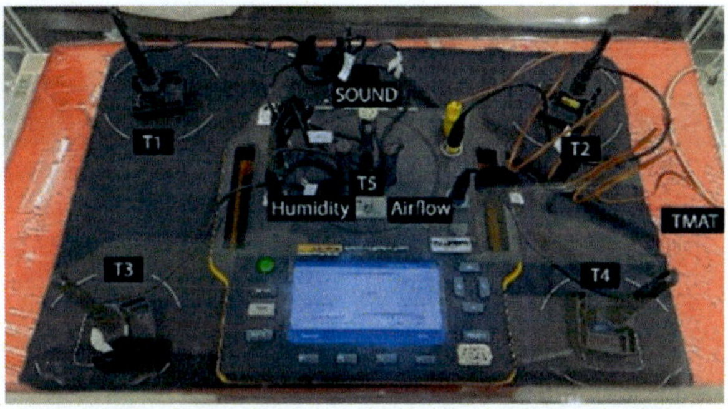

Fig. 3 Measurement points T1, T2, T3, T4, T5, and TM

the incu analyzer (design) is turned on and enters the Web mode. The measurement value will be sent to the web server and can be monitored via mobile or laptop. Measurements are also varied out for 30 min and the measurement data will be saved to the MySQL database. The second measurement is carried out in the same way but at a set temperature of 36°C.

Figure 4 shows a block diagram (flowchart) of the incu analyzer design used to measure temperatures T1, T2, T3, T4, T5, TM, noise level, and airflow velocity in a baby incubator. The sensor reading results are displayed on a TFT screen and sent to a web page. Measurement data can be stored in MySQL database in web mode or on SD card in device mode. Figure 3 shows two flow charts. The flow chart on the left shows the design of the microcontroller software and the flow chart on the right shows the design of the web application software. After the Arduino initializes, the program will read the sensor readings and display them on the TFT screen. If there is an internet connection, the program will send sensor reading data to the web server. On the web server side, the data sent by ESP32 will be saved to a MySQL database and displayed on a web page. If the operator presses the add data button, the data will be saved to the measurement table according to the incubator temperature setting (32°C or 36°C). The operator must repeat 3 times at each set point. If the operator presses the finish button, the web program will save the measurement data to MySQL.

3.2 *Data Analysis*

Based on the description of the ISO:25010 standard, compliance with a standard or regulation, which is a sub-characteristic in ISO/IEC 9126–1, is now outside the scope of the quality model as it can be identified as part of the requirements for a system. Compliance with a standard is still carried out by comparing the designed incu analyzer device with the standard measuring instruments (Incu Fluke II Tester). Measurement of each parameter (temperature, humidity, and noise) was repeated 50 times every 30 s at each setting of 32°C and 36°C incubator temperature. And in the measurement of airflow velocity, a fan with three-speed levels was used, data

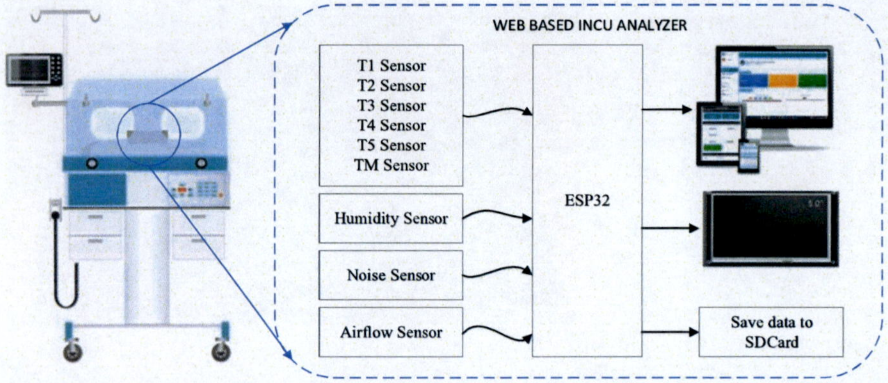

Fig. 4 The designed incu analyzer block diagram

collection was carried out to obtain as much as 500 data. The mean value is determined by the following Eq. 1:

$$\frac{\overline{x} = x1 + x2 \ldots + xn}{n} \tag{1}$$

where, x is the mean for n measurements, × 1 is the value of the first measurement, × 2 is the value of the second measurement, and xn is the value of the nth measurement. Standard deviation is a value indicating the degree of variation in a data set or a measure of the standard deviation of the mean. The formula for standard deviation (SD) is as shown in the following Eq. 2:

$$\text{SD} = \sqrt{\frac{\sum_{i=1}^{n} (Xi - \overline{x})^2}{(n-1)}} \tag{2}$$

where, xi is the number of desired values, x is the mean (average) of the measurement results, n is the number of measurement data. Percentage (%) of error is a value indicating a device error compared to the standard device. The % error formula is as shown in the following Eq. 3:

$$\%\text{Error} = \frac{x_{std} - x_{uut}}{x_{std}} \text{x } 100\% \tag{3}$$

where, x_{std} is the standard tool (Fluke) reading value and x_{uut} is the design reading value.

After the device was compared with a standard instrument, the incu analyzer was used to measure the baby incubator. Then, the device was measured for quality in its use according to the ISO:25022 standard which consists of Task completion, Task effectiveness, Error Frequency, and Time efficiency [29, 29].

Task completion is the percentage of tasks completed correctly. Each completed measurement will be calculated with a score of 1. The task completion formula is as shown in the following Eq. 4 [30]:

$$X = \frac{A}{B} \tag{4}$$

where, X is the value of task completion, A is the number of tasks that can be completed, and B is the total number of assigned tasks.

Task effectiveness means that a goal can be achieved correctly. Each potential missing or incomplete component is given a weight. The task effectiveness formula is as shown in the following Eq. 5 [30]:

$$\mathrm{X} = 1 - \Sigma Ai \tag{5}$$

where, X_i is the proportional value of each missing or incomplete component in the task output.

Error frequency shows the number of times an error or mistake occurs during the operation of the device. The error frequency formula is as shown in the following Eq. 6 [30]:

$$X = \frac{A}{B} \tag{6}$$

where, X is the value of error frequency, A is the number of errors that occurs when the device is operated, and B is the total number of assigned tasks. Time efficiency is calculated by comparing the time required to complete a task with the target time of 150 min. The time efficiency formula is as shown in the following Eq. 7 [30]:

$$\mathrm{X} = (\mathrm{Tt} - \mathrm{Ta}) / \mathrm{Tt} \tag{7}$$

where, X is the value of time efficiency, Tt is the target time, and Ta is the actual time required to complete the task. Based on the calibration work method, the standard time required to calibrate the baby incubator is 150 min.

4 Result

4.1 The Web-Based Incu Analyzer

In this study, the design of a web-based incu analyzer was used to verify the conditions of the baby incubator, which consisted of several measurement parameters such as air temperature T1 to T5, mattress temperature, humidity, noise, and airflow velocity. The design consisted of DS18B20 as a temperature sensor for T1–T5 and mattress

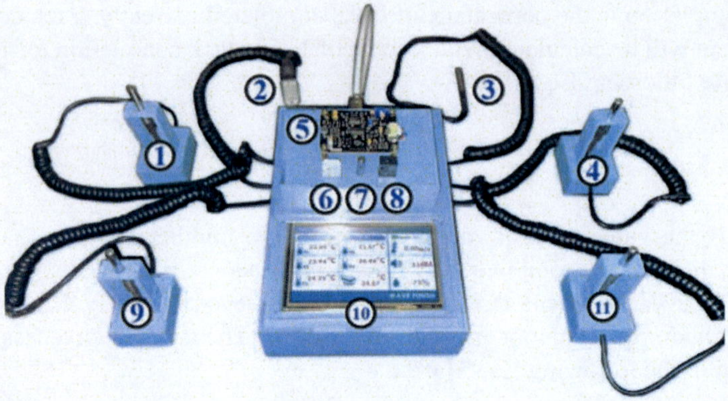

Fig. 5 The designed web-based INCU Analyzer design

temperature, DHT22 as a humidity sensor, SEN-0232 as a noise sensor, and D6F-V03A1 as an airflow velocity sensor. More details regarding the designed device are shown in the following Fig. 5.

Figure 5 shows the designed incubator analyzer device, which consists of:

1. T1 temperature sensor
2. External humidity sensor
3. Mattress temperature sensor
4. T2 temperature sensor
5. Noise sensor
6. Internal humidity sensor,
7. T5 temperature sensor
8. Airflow velocity sensor
9. T3 temperature sensor
10. TFT display
11. T4 temperature sensor

In this study, a web application was made to receive measurement data from ESP32 to be then displayed to a web page. Verification of the environmental conditions in the baby incubator can be done by operating the incubator analyzer as usual. First, the operator places the incubator analyzer in the baby incubator compartment, then the operator can view a graph of the sensor readings via a web page. After the temperature is stable, the operator can record the measurement results via the web and the system will automatically save the measurement results to the database. After the measurement result data are saved, the operator can print the report result or download the report result into a PDF file. The display of the web application is as shown in the Fig. 6.

Section (a) displays a page for adding sensor readings to the measurement worksheet. The page displays the measurement values, which consists of air temperature

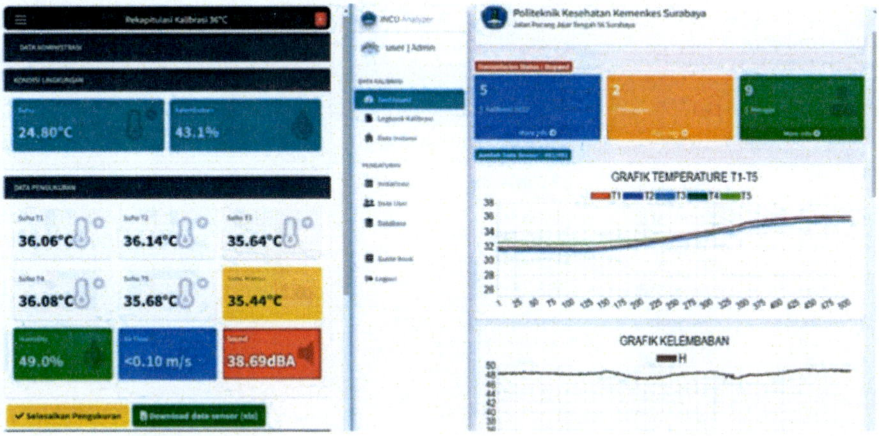

(a) (b)

Fig. 6 The display of web application

T1-T5, mattress temperature, humidity, noise, and airflow velocity. There is a button to add measurement results to the database table.

Section (b) displays a graph of the temperature sensor readings T1–T5 and humidity in real-time. This page is also equipped with an indicator when the web page receives data from ESP32. The indicator will be green if data are received and red if transmission is not in progress.

4.2 Compliance with Standards

In measuring air temperature, mattress temperature, humidity, and noise, the Fluke INCU II Tester was used as a comparison device. And in measuring airflow velocity, a DC fan with three-speed levels was used, which was focused at a distance of 30 cm to the sensor as an air flow generator, and an anemometer was used as a comparison device. Table 1 and Fig. 4 show the mean (average) of the measurement results of the design and the standard incu analyzer. The largest errors were obtained, namely at T1 of 0.22%, T2 of 0.38%, T3 of 1.2%, T4 of 1.68%, T5 of 0.33%, TM of 0.37%, humidity of 3.24%, and noise level of 2.09%. Meanwhile, at airflow velocity parameter, the largest error of 3.26% was obtained at level I (low) fan speed. The percentage of error obtained is still less than 5%. Complete data related to module compliance with the standard are presented in the Table 1.

Figure 7 shows the average temperature sensor measurement values T1 to T7 and the mattress temperature of the module and standard at 32°C and 36°C temperature settings. The highest difference value is T4 at 32°C temperature setting, which is

Table 1 Comparison of measurements of T1, T2, T3, T4, T5, T mattress, humidity, and noise between the design and the standard incu analyzer at two incubator temperature settings (32 °C and 36 °C)

Parameter		Set point of 32 °C		Set point of 36 °C	
		Mean	Error(%)	Mean	Error(%)
T1	Design	32.40	−0.22	35.53	0.11
	Standard	32.33		35.57	
T2	Design	31.77	−0.02	34.87	0.38
	Standard	31.76		35.01	
T3	Design	31.54	0,37	34.53	1.20
	Standard	31.66		34.95	
T4	Design	31.70	1,68	35.13	−0.58
	Standard	32.24		34.93	
T5	Design	32.38	−0.33	34.76	−0.17
	Standard	32.27		34.70	
TM	Design	32.42	−0.25	35.39	0.37
	Standard	32.34		35.53	
Humidity	Design	32.40	3.24	35.53	0.51
	Standard	32.33		35.57	
Noise	Design	31.77	0.77	34.87	2.09
	Standard	31.76		35.01	

0.54°C or 1.68% of the standard value. the error value is less than 5%. So it can be concluded that the sensor module accuracy value is good.

Figure 8 shows the average humidity measurement values of the module and standard at 32°C and 36°C temperature settings. The highest difference value is at the temperature setting of 32°C which is 1.42%RH or 3.24% of the standard value. However, the error value is less than 5%. So it can be concluded that the sensor module accuracy value is good.

Figure 9 shows the average noise measurement values of the module and standard at 32°C and 36 temperature settings. The highest difference value is at the 36°C temperature setting, which is 0.92dBA or 2.09% of the standard value. However, the error value is less than 5%. So it can be concluded that the accuracy of the noise sensor module is good.

In testing the air flow velocity, a DC fan with 3 speed levels is used. The mModule reading value is compared to an anemometer. The largest error was obtained at 3.26% in the level 1 fan speed setting. The complete data is shown in Table 2.

Figure 10 shows the average value of the airflow velocity measurement of the module and the standard fan speed settings for level 1 (low), 2 (medium) and 3 (high). The highest value difference is the fan speed setting level 1, which is 0.05 m/s or 3.26% of the standard value. However, the error value is less than 5%. So it can be concluded that the accuracy of the airflow velocity sensor module is good.

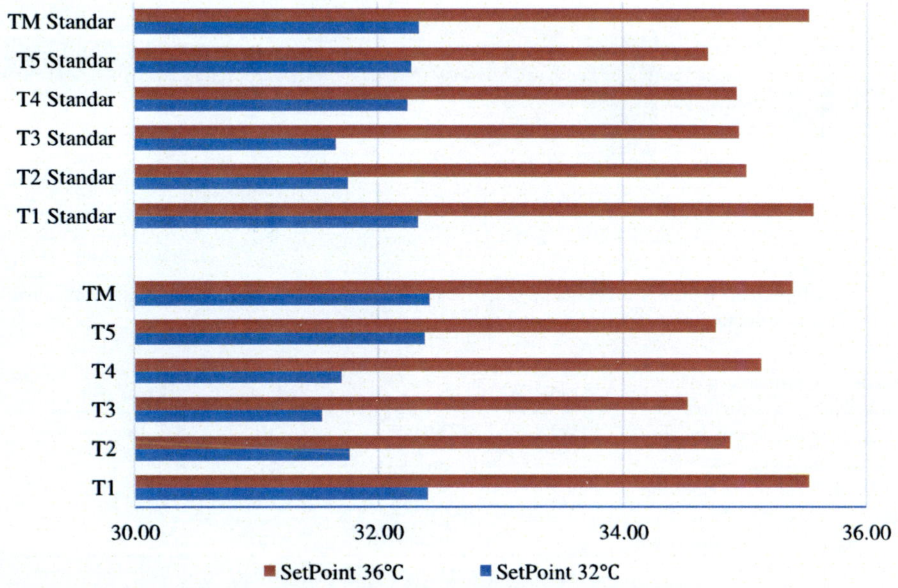

Fig. 7 Comparison of measurements of T1, T2, T3, T4, T5 and T mattress between the design and the standard incu analyzer at two incubator temperature settings (32 °C and 36 °C)

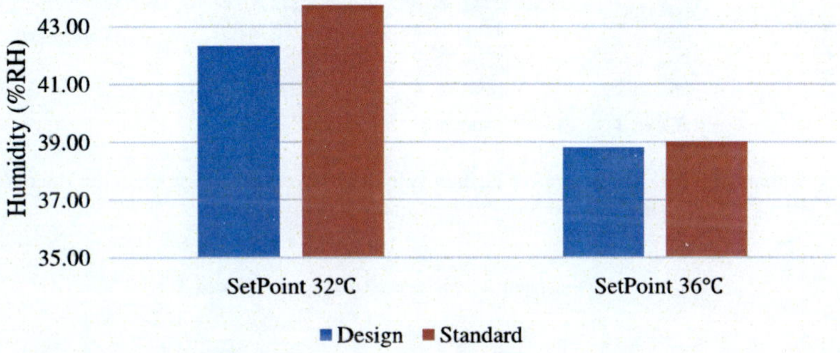

Fig. 8 Comparison of measurements of humidity between the design and the standard incu analyzer at two incubator temperature settings (32°C and 36°C)

The results of the readings of the incu analyzer module on the airflow velocity parameter are shown in Fig. 11. It can be seen that the sensor reading values are unstable, where the reading values fluctuate significantly.

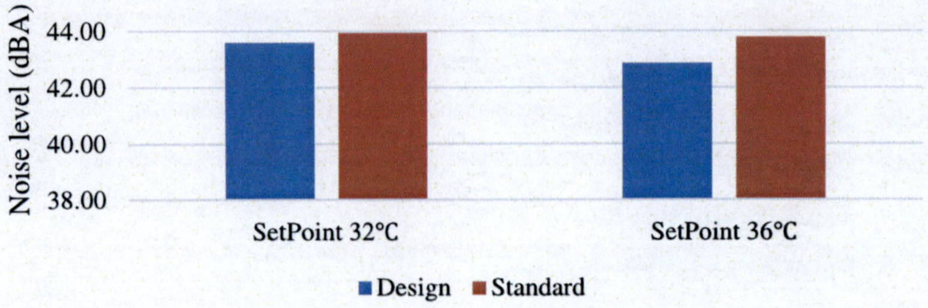

Fig. 9 Comparison of measurements of noise level between the design and the standard incu analyzer at two incubator temperature settings (32°C and 36°C)

Table 2 Comparison of measurements of airflow velocity between the design and the standard incu analyzer using a DC fan with three-speed levels. Note: In this study, the calibrator used was an anemometer

Parameter		Mean	Error (%)
Level 1	Design	1.36	3.26
	Standard	1.41	
Level 2	Design	1.758	−0.11
	Standard	1.756	
Level 3	Design	1.97	1.37
	Standard	2.00	

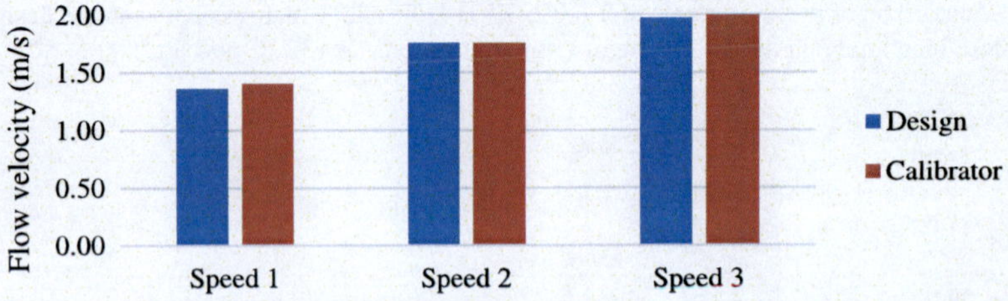

Fig. 10 Comparison of measurements of airflow velocity between the design and the standard incu analyzer (anemometer) using a DC fan with three-speed levels

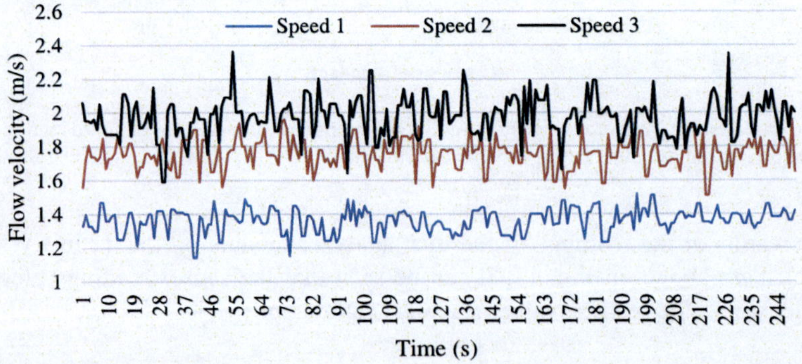

Fig. 11 The results of measurements of airflow velocity value using the INCU Analyzer module at three fan speed levels

Table 3 percentage interpretation criteria

Percentage (%)	Category
<40	Low
40–70	Medium
>70	High

Table 4 Results of measurements of quality in use

Indicator	Percentage (%)	Category
Task completion	100	High
Task effectiveness	95	High
Error frequency	1,54	Low
Time efficiency	77,13	High

4.3 *Effectiveness and Efficiency*

After obtaining the results of the compliance measurements, the researchers asked 10 people to be the participants in the module test. Participants were asked to measure the baby's incubator using the designed incu analyzer module. From the measurement results of each participant, an analysis of effectiveness and efficiency was carried out using the ISO:25022 standard with quality measurement indicators including Task completion, Task Effectiveness, Error Frequency, and Time Efficiency. After the analysis, the percentage of each quality measurement indicator was obtained. Based on the percentage obtained, the results are interpreted into 3 categories (low, medium and high) according to the ISO:25022 standard with 3 ordinal scales (1–3: Low, 4–6: Medium, 7–9: High) [30]. So, the interpretation of the percentage of effectiveness and efficiency of the test results can be made as shown in the Table 3.

After the analysis of the experimental results by 10 participants for testing the baby incubator using the designed module (device), the results of measurements of quality in use are as shown in the Table 4.

All tasks assigned to 10 participants were completed. So, the percentage obtained was 100%. Based on the classification table, task completion is included in the high category.

Based on the experimental results by 10 participants, there were writing errors or typos, so each point was deducted by 5% and from the whole task, the percentage of task effectiveness was 95%. Based on the classification table, task effectiveness is included in the high category.

In measuring error frequency, out of 130 assigned tasks, only 2 errors occurred, so the % error frequency was 1.54%. Based on the classification table, error frequency is included as the low category.

Time efficiency relates the level of effectiveness achieved with the quantity of resources expended. Efficiency is generally assessed by comparing the average time required to complete a task with a target time of 150 min. So, based on the time efficiency calculation, the percentage obtained was 77.13%. Based on the classification table, time efficiency is included in the high category.

5 Discussion

The results showed that the designed module (device) can be used to measure the parameters of the baby incubator. This module used DS18B20 to measure air and mattress temperatures, DHT22 to measure humidity, SEN0232 to measure noise level, and D6F-V03A1 to measure airflow velocity. All parameters are displayed on a 5 inch TFT screen and measurement data is sent to a web server using an internet connection so it can be monitored by several devices directly. The measurement results are displayed on a web page in the form of real-time graphs. Furthermore, the user can record the condition of the baby incubator by adding measurement data to the calibration menu as shown in Fig. 10. The results of the recording will be displayed in the form of a measurement report, as shown in Fig. 11.

The designed device was then compared with the Fluke INCU II Tester unit calibrator to validate measurements of air temperature, mattress temperature, humidity, and noise. The smallest error in measurements of air temperature is -0.02% at parameter T2 with a temperature setting of 32°C and the largest error is 1.68% at parameter T4 with a temperature setting of 32°C. Whereas, the smallest error in measurement of mattress temperature is -0.08% at a temperature setting of 32°C and the largest error is 0.37% at a temperature setting of 36°C. In the measurement of humidity, the smallest error is 0.51% at a temperature setting of 36°C and the largest error is 3.24% at a temperature setting of 32°C. Meanwhile, in the measurement of noise level, the smallest error is 0.34% at a temperature setting of 32°C and the largest error is 2.09% at a temperature setting of 36°C. Finally, in measurement of airflow velocity, the designed device was compared with an anemometer to measure three-speed levels of the DC fan and obtained the smallest error of -0.11% at medium speed levels and the largest error of 3.26% at low-speed levels. From measurement of compliance with the standard, the error value obtained is not more than 5%, so it can be stated that the designed incu analyzer device has met the standard requirements.

The ISO:25022 standard was used to measure the quality of the web-based incu analyzer system. The test was conducted by 10 participants who were asked to complete measurements of the baby incubator. There are several indicators to measure effectiveness and efficiency according to the ISO:25022 standard. First, Task Completion, which is the percentage of tasks completed correctly. Of the 10 tasks given, participants could complete all of them. So, measurement of task completion obtained a value of 100%. Second, Task Effectiveness, which is a measurement of the level of success and correctness of an assignment goal. The measurements of the designed incu analyzer aimed to record the conditions of the baby incubator into a measurement report form. Each parameter was verified to see whether any data is missing, misplaced, or mistyped (typo). If there is a missing, the value is reduced by

50%, if there is a misplacement, the value is reduced by 20%, and if there is only a typo or writing error, the value is reduced by 5%. From 10 measurements, there was a writing error in the noise parameter where the decimal value was written as 2 digits where it should only be 1 digit. For this reason, measurement of task effectiveness obtained a value of 95%. Third, Error Frequency, which is calculated based on errors that occur during the operation of the device. From a total of 130 program steps, only 2 errors occurred. So, measurement of error frequency only obtained a value of 1.54%. Finally, Time Efficiency, where the time from each task completion is measured and averaged. The time is then compared with the target time of 150 min. From 10 trials, the average task completion time of 34.3 min was obtained. From the calculation exemplified by the ISO:25022 standard, measurement of time efficiency obtained a value of 77.13%. From the results of quality testing, the designed incu analyzer has met the quality test requirements for effectiveness and efficiency.

The limitation of this study is that the results of measurement of airflow velocity are still unstable, where the reading values fluctuate significantly. Also, sending sensor readings to a web server requires an internet connection, so if the internet connection is lost, the sensor readings cannot be sent. Then, the system can only be used for 1 incu analyzer device. Moreover, the incu analyzer device is also not equipped with a real-time clock.

The web-based incu analyzer design can be applied to verify the conditions of the baby incubator both during calibration and routine inspections. The implementation of web can speed up the process of recording the conditions of the baby incubator. The calibration unit can present digital calibration certificates more quickly without complicated operations compared to the conventional calibration system.

6 Conclusion

In this study, a web-based incu analyzer was designed to verify the conditions of the baby incubator. This study aimed to measure the effectiveness and efficiency of the web system applied to the incubator analyzer when compared to the conventional calibration system. To achieve this objective, a hardware design was developed using an ESP32 microcontroller so that the device can send measurement data to the web. The use of a web system helps speed up the recording process of the baby incubator. Measurement of effectiveness and efficiency carried out also yielded good values. For further development, other procedures can be added according to the working method of the baby incubator, such as reviewing the physical condition and electrical safety [31], so the system can be applied to the baby incubator calibration process. The web system must also be developed further, so it can be used in more than 1 incu analyzers simultaneously. The addition of a real-time clock will be very useful for displaying real-time on the TFT screen and entering time data on each data sent to the web-server.

References

1. Niversity IU (2016) Science and engineering M . Sc . Thesis
2. Akhir ST (2014) Incubator temperature and body temperature monitoring. 1–10
3. Oyebola B (2017) Development of a microcontroller based temperature and humidity controller for infant incubator. J Ind Technol 2:78–89
4. Koli M, Ladge P, Prasad B, Boria R, Balur NJ (2018). Intell Baby Incubator. https://doi.org/10.1109/ICECA.2018.8474763
5. fluke Coporation (2015) Incu II incubator analyzer. 15
6. Brown C, Elo T, Hovhannisyan K, Hutzschenreuter D, Kuosmanen P, Maennel O, Mustapaa T, Nikander P, Wiedenhoefer T (2020) Infrastructure for digital calibration certificates. In: 2020 IEEE International Workshop on Metrology for Industry 4.0 and IoT, MetroInd 4.0 and IoT 2020—Proceedings. 485–489. https://doi.org/10.1109/MetroInd4.0IoT48571.2020.9138220
7. Nummiluikki J, Mustapaa T, Hietala K, Viitala R (2021) Benefits of network effects and interoperability for the digital calibration certificate management. In: 2021 IEEE International Workshop on Metrology for Industry 4.0 & IoT (MetroInd4.0&IoT). IEEE. pp 352–357. https://doi.org/10.1109/MetroInd4.0IoT51437.2021.9488562.
8. Gadelrab MS, Abouhogail RA (2021) Towards a new generation of digital calibration certificate: Analysis and survey. Meas: J Int Meas Confed. 181, 109611. https://doi.org/10.1016/j.measurement.2021.109611
9. Wang Zhihu (2012) Design of an internet-based calibration system. In: IET International Conference on Information Science and Control Engineering 2012 (ICISCE 2012). Institution of Engineering and Technology. pp 1.65–1.65. https://doi.org/10.1049/cp.2012.2322
10. Fakhry IA, Bagus Baskara Nugraha IG (2018) Blockchain-Based for calibration of digital multimeter system design. In: Proceeding—2018 International Conference on ICT for Smart Society: Innovation Toward Smart Society and Society 5.0, ICISS 2018. 1–6. https://doi.org/10.1109/ICTSS.2018.8549924
11. Samputri HNA, Syaifudin S, Titisari D (2019) Incubator analyzer using android app. Jurnal Teknokes. 12, 14–20. https://doi.org/10.35882/teknokes.v12i1.3
12. Azkiyak VN, Syaifudin S, Titisari D (2020) Incubator analyzer using bluetooth android display (Humidity & Air Flow). Indones J Electron, Electromed Eng, Med Inform. 1, 71–77. https://doi.org/10.35882/ijeeemi.v1i2.5
13. Charisa AA, Utomo B, Syaifudin S (2019) Visual programming based portable analyzer incubator equipped with storage to Sd Card. J Teknokes. 12, 29–35. https://doi.org/10.35882/teknokes.v12i2.5.
14. Prinyakupt J, Roongprasert K (2019). Verification device for temperature and relative humidity inside the infant incubator via IoT. https://doi.org/10.1109/BMEiCON47515.2019.8990351
15. Laily Nurrohmah, Dwi Herry Andayani, Andjar Pudji (2020) Development of incubator analyzer using personal computer equiped with measurement certificate. J Electron, Electromed Eng, Med Inform. 2, 74–79. https://doi.org/10.35882/jeeemi.v2i2.6
16. Syarifatul Ainiyah, Andayani DH, Pundji A, Shaib M (2020) Development of incubator analyzer based on computer with temperature and humidity parameters. J Electron, Electromed Eng, Med Inform. 2, 48–57. https://doi.org/10.35882/jeeemi.v2i2.3
17. Tukade TM, Banakar RM (2018) Data Transfer Protocols in IoT-An Overview. Int J Pure Appl Math. 118:121–138
18. Venusamy K, Musannah AS (2021) Renewable energy with IoT and biomedical applications
19. Lee I, Lee K (2015) The internet of things (IoT): Applications, investments, and challenges for enterprises. Bus Horiz 58:431–440. https://doi.org/10.1016/j.bushor.2015.03.008
20. Shin DI, Huh SJ, Lee TS, Kim IY (2003) Web-based remote monitoring of infant incubators in the ICU. Int J Med Informatics 71:151–156. https://doi.org/10.1016/S1386-5056(03)00095-9
21. Ding L, Wang X (2011) Design of a web-based temperature and humidity monitoring system. In: 2011 2nd International Conference on Artificial Intelligence, Management Science and Electronic Commerce, AIMSEC 2011—Proceedings. 2028–2030. https://doi.org/10.1109/AIMSEC.2011.6010968

22. Nimodiya AR, Ajankar SS (2022) A Review on Internet of Things. Int J Adv Res Sci, Commun Technol. 113, 135–144. https://doi.org/10.48175/ijarsct-2251
23. Firmansyah R, Widodo A, Romadhon AD, Hudha MS, Saputra PPS, Lestari NA (2019) The prototype of infant incubator monitoring system based on the internet of things using NodeMCU ESP8266. In: Journal of Physics: Conference Series. 1171. https://doi.org/10.1088/1742-6596/1171/1/012015
24. Adam Stenly, Andolo S (2019) In: 1st International Conference on Cybernetics and Intelligent System (ICORIS) : Institut Teknologi dan Bisnis (ITB) STIKOM Bali, Indonesia, 22nd-23rd August 2019. 2019 1st International Conference on Cybernetics and Intelligent System (ICORIS). 1, 18–22
25. Sa'Adah U, Akhmad J, Hisyam M (2016) Implementing singleton method in design of MVC-based PHP framework. In: Proceedings—2015 International Electronics Symposium: Emerging Technology in Electronic and Information, IES 2015. 212–217. https://doi.org/10.1109/ELECSYM.2015.7380843
26. Zhao H, Zhang H, Chen Q (2014) The research of dynamic statistics chart based on MVC design pattern. In: Conference Proceedings—2014 International Conference on System Science and Engineering, ICSSE 2014. 56–59. https://doi.org/10.1109/ICSSE.2014.6887904
27. Tongbai J, Nuratch S (2020) Temperature-Controlled enclosures using networked measurement and Real-time. In: 2020 the 5th International Conference on Control and Robotics Engineering Design. 95–98.
28. Singh A, Chawla P, Singh K, Singh AK (2018) Formulating an MVC framework for web development in java. In: Proceedings of the 2nd International Conference on Trends in Electronics and Informatics, ICOEI 2018. 926–929. https://doi.org/10.1109/ICOEI.2018.8553746
29. Standard N (2011) CAN / CSA-ISO/IEC 25010 : 12 National standard of Canada. 12
30. Jtc, I.E.C. (2012) Systems and software engineering—systems and software quality requirements and evaluation (SQuaRE)—measurement of quality in use

Effectiveness Analysis of Infinite Impulse Response Digital Filter on Electrocardiogram Signal to Extract Respiration Rate Signal

Halida Hasrifah, Muhammad Ridha Mak'ruf, Andjar Pudji, Levana Forra Wakidi, Bambang Guruh Irianto, Triwiyanto, and Anilkumar Suthar

Abstract Respiration Rate (RR) is the number of respirations or movements that determine inspiration and expiration calculated in breaths per minute (BrPM). The Respiration Rate Signal can be extracted from an electrocardiogram signal (ECG-Derived Respiration). There have been many studies to extract the respiration rate signal from the ECG signal but there has been no study on the effectiveness of extracting the respiration rate signal with a digital filter, therefore, this study aimed to determine the effectiveness of the Infinite Impulse Response (IIR) digital filter in the design of the Butterworth Filter and the Chebyshev I filter based on the selection of different orders, namely orders 4, 6, and 8 to extract the Lead II Electrocardiogram signal-based Respiration Rate signal. This study used the AD8232 ECG module, Arduino Nano, Ms. Excel, and MATLAB. The method used to analyze the signal was the Fast Fourier Transform (FFT) method. The tricks were to determine the components of the mean frequency, the mean power frequency, and the mean power frequency respiration rate obtained from the use of the IIR digital filter on respondents which would be compared with the gold standard in the form of phantom. The results were analyzed using a correlation analysis where in the Butterworth filter, the highest correlation value is 0.996 in order 6 while in the Chebyshev I filter, the highest correlation value is 0.999 in order 8. It can be concluded that the Chebyshev I digital filter of order 8 has the best effectiveness value.

Keywords Electrocardiogram · Infinite impulse response · AD8232 · Respiration rate

H. Hasrifah · M. R. Mak'ruf (✉) · A. Pudji · L. F. Wakidi · B. G. Irianto · Triwiyanto
Department of Medical Electronics Technology, Poltekkes Kemenkes Surabaya, Surabaya, Indonesia
e-mail: ridha@poltekkesdepkes-sby.ac.id

A. Suthar
New LJ Institute of Engineering and Technology, Gujarat Technological University, S.G. Highway, Ahmedabad, Gujarat, India

T. Triwiyanto et al. (eds.), *Proceeding of the 3rd International Conference on Electronics, Biomedical Engineering, and Health Informatics*, Lecture Notes in Electrical Engineering 1008, https://doi.org/10.1007/978-981-99-0248-4_41

1 Introduction

Carbon dioxide and oxygen are exchanged in the body during respiration, a crucial physiological activity [1, 2]. Respiration Rate (RR) is the number of respirations or movements that determine inspiration and expiration calculated in breaths per minute (BrPM) [3, 4]. Normal breathing for adults is in the range of 12–20 times per minute [5], if there is a condition of RR > 27 then it indicates abnormalities in the heart system [6, 7]. Chronic obstructive pulmonary disease (COPD), congestive heart failure (CHF), and abnormal respiratory waveforms are a few disorders that can be detected early using respiration rate [6, 8–10].

The respiration rate signal can be obtained from the extraction of ECG or PPG signal [4, 11–15]. Signal extraction from ECG is called the ECG-derived respiration (EDR) technique. This EDR technique utilizes from single lead (Lead II) ECG signal leads by using gel electrodes when mounting on subjects [6, 10, 16, 17]. In this study, the focus was on extracting the respiration rate signal from the ECG signal (EDR) by utilizing the filter process. The filter functions to pass the cool signal frequencies and withstand unwanted signal frequencies. In the process of extracting, the filter signal used can be analog filters or digital filters. In analog filters, there is a disadvantage, namely, there is still much noise during the filtering process of the respiration rate signal from the ECG signal. Whereas, in digital filters, the noise produced is not as much as in analog filters [18, 19]. Digital filters are better in the use of the process of decreasing the signal respiration rate of the ECG, and in terms of the level of accuracy and precision, digital filters are more accurate and precise.

Heman Sharma, et al., in 2015, conducted a study on respiration rate signal subduction from a single lead ECG using homomorphic filtering methods (discrete Fourier transform (DFT) and discrete cosine transform (DCT)) with a frequency from 0.2 to 0.8 Hz. The results obtained based on the Kaiser window on the extraction of respiration rate signal showed that the use of the Butterworth filter was better than those of the Chebyshev I and FIR filters. This study still needs to be continued to carry out further analysis regarding the selection of filters and orders in the extraction of respiration rate signal [20].

Next, Preeti Jagadev, et al., in 2019 [21], conducted a study by using thermal cameras to monitor respiration rate with the algorithm method of Ensemble of regression trees, which is a method of comparing the performance of several IIR digital filters and an FIR filter. The results obtained showed that the extraction of respiration rate using the Butterworth filter was better, and the filter performance is good every time there is an increase in the filter order. A study by Christna Orphannidou in 2016, used the algorithm method of EEMD in IMF2 and IMF3 to retrieve EDR/PDR signal. An FIR filter was set on a band pass filter with a frequency from 0.1 to 0.6 Hz. The results obtained showed that the performance of the ECG was better than the PPG, although there was no significant difference. Respiration rate showed a mean absolute error of 1.8 bpm and a mean average error of 10% [4]. A study by Subhadeep Basu, et al., in 2020, compared the Butterworth digital filter with the Chebyshev I filter to see the effect of orders and cut off frequency on the ECG signal [18]. However, these filters have not been applied to analyze the respiration rate signal.

Based on the previous studies, the researchers of this study were interested in conducting a study on ECG-free respiration rate signal extraction using the Infinite Impulse Response (IIR) digital filter in the design of the Butterworth filter and the Chebyshev I filter in orders 4, 6, and 8 with the Baseline Wander method using a Band Pass Filter with a Cut Off frequency from 0.1 to 0.5 Hz, based on the frequency of respiration rate signal [22]. The data would be processed on a personal computer using MATLAB software and analyzed using frequency-based features such as mean frequency and mean power, and median frequency of the signal. This study aimed to investigate the IIR filter performance to extract the EDR signal.

2 Material and Methods

2.1 Theoretical Background

ECG-derived respiration. ECG-derived respiration (EDR) is an ECG-based respiration rate signal extraction technique and is a non-invasive method for monitoring respiratory activity when the respiration rate signal is not recorded [16, 20]. In the clinical world, this method provides convenience because it allows for simultaneous monitoring of cardiac and respiratory signals from the ECG signal that has been recorded. The EDR technique has a category of methods, namely the multiple lead method based on the Angle of Mean Electrical Axis variation, the single lead method based on the R-wave amplitude (AM) frequency modulation (FM), and the baseline wander (BW), in addition to the heart rate-based method, discrete wavelet transform method, and band pass filter method [9, 22–25].

Of the several categories of methods used by the EDR technique above, the researchers applied the single lead method based on the baseline wander (BW) [2, 11, 12]. This baseline wander method uses a band pass filter with a cut off frequency from 0.1 to 0.5 Hz [10, 22, 23]. The following Fig. 1 shows the ECG-Derived Respiration (EDR).

Figure 1 shows the Approach to the Baseline Wander method as a way to obtain a respiration rate signal from an ECG (EDR) signal. Baseline wander is when expansion and contraction of the chest cavity occur in the breathing process, resulting in the

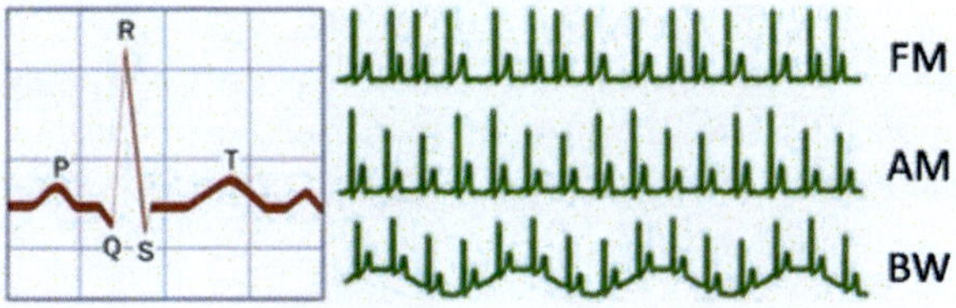

Fig. 1 ECG-derived respiration (EDR)

movement of the electrodes relative to the heart that will cause baseline wander on the ECG signal [15, 26, 27].

Electrocardiogram Leads. Leads using 3 electrodes are commonly used for simple monitoring, while leads using 2 electrodes are for active monitoring. The Lead II configuration can be obtained by placing the electrodes using the Einthoven triangle system, namely, the electrodes are placed at the torso, namely the Right arm (RA), Right Leg (RL), and Left Leg (LL) [26, 28, 29].

Filter Infinite Impulse Response. Digital filters of a certain type, such as the infinite impulse response (IIR) filter, are employed in DSP applications. The benefit of using IIR filters is that they demand less efficiency for steep frequency response, which cuts down on the amount of processing time [30]. Therefore, a digital filter is needed to extract the respiration rate signal based on the ECG signal from the IIR filter design type, namely the Butterworth filter (BF) and the Chebyshev type I filter (CT1F). The following Eqs. 1 and 2 show the formula for BF and CT1F [21]:

$$\begin{aligned} y(n) = {} & b_0 x(n) + b_1 x(n-1) + \cdots \\ & + b_M x(n-M) - a_1 y(n-1) - \cdots - a_N y(n-N) \end{aligned} \quad (1)$$

And, the IIR filter transfer function given is

$$H(z) = \frac{Y(z)}{X(z)} = \frac{b_0 + b_1 z^{-1} + \cdots + b_M z^{-M}}{1 + a_1 z^{-1} + \cdots + a_N z^{-N}} \quad (2)$$

where the M numerator and N denominator coefficients, respectively, are b_i and a_i. The *z*-transform functions of the filter input $x(n)$ and filter output $y(n)$ are $Y(z)$ and $X(z)$, respectively.

$$|H_n(j\omega)| = \frac{1}{\sqrt{1 + E^2\left(\frac{\omega}{\omega_c}\right)^{2n}}} \quad (3)$$

where, n is the filter order, ω is the angular frequency, ω_c is the cut off angular frequency, and E is the maximum band pass gain. The CT1F filter transfer function given is

$$|H_n(j\omega)| = \frac{1}{\sqrt{1 + R_f^2 T_n^2\left(\frac{\omega}{\omega_c}\right)}} \quad (4)$$

where, R_f is the ripple factor, and T_n is the Chebyshev polynomial of order n.

Fast Fourier Transform. In the sectors of education, business, and the military, the Fast Fourier Transform (FFT) is a crucial method for solving all sorts of issues.

This technique was first introduced by Gauss in 1805. However, FFT received attention during a seminar by Cooley and Tukey in 1965, where they found the main disciplines of digital signal processing [31]. The Fast Fourier Transform (FFT) transforms an analog time-domain signal into various frequencies using a complex exponential function [27]. Fast Fourier Transform can be defined by the following Eq. 5.

$$S(f) = \int_{-\infty}^{\infty} s(t)e^{-j2\pi ft}dt$$
$$S(f) = \int_{-\infty}^{\infty} s(t)\cos(2\pi ft)dt - j\int_{-\infty}^{\infty} s(t)\sin(2\pi ft)dt \quad (5)$$

where, $S(f)$ is a signal in the frequency domain, $s(t)$ is a signal in the time domain, and $s(t)e^{-j2\pi ft}dt$ is the signal value constant.

Fast Fourier Transform has an effective algorithm for computing Discrete Fourier Transform (DFT). The time it takes to evaluate the DFT on a computer mainly depends on the number of multiplications involved. DFT requires $N2$ multiplication. FFT only takes $N\log2$ (N). This algorithm's fundamental idea is the understanding that a discrete Fourier transform of a series of N points can be represented in two discrete Fourier transforms of length $N/2$. So, if N is a power of two, it is possible to apply this decomposition recursively until a Discrete Fourier Transform of single point is obtained.

In digital signal processing (DSP) software, there are three classes of FFT commonly used, namely Decimation in Time (DIT), Decimation in Frequency (DIF) and Split Radix. Another type of FFT that has been used is parallel FFT uses parallel computing to sequence data so that the transformation process will be faster. FFT has a resolution of f_s/N where f_s is the value of the sampling rate and N is the number of sampled data. With computer limitations, the above equation, especially for the real part, can be approximated by the following Eq. 6.

$$\int_{-\infty}^{\infty} s(t)\cos(2\pi ft)dt \rightarrow \sum_n x(n\Delta t)\cos(2\pi fn\Delta t)\Delta t$$
$$= \sum_n x(n\Delta t)\cos(2\pi nm\Delta t\Delta f)\Delta t$$
$$= \sum_n x(n\Delta t)\cos(2\pi \frac{nm}{N})\Delta t \quad (6)$$

where, m and n are integers, in the time domain, the signal is defined as $T = N\Delta t$, while in the frequency domain, $\Delta f = \frac{f_s}{N}$ where Δf is the value of interval between frequency and $f_s = \frac{1}{\Delta t} = N\Delta f$. Thus, the equation $\Delta t\Delta f = \frac{1}{N}$ is the link between the time domain and the frequency domain. If the number of data N is smaller than the sampling frequency, the resulting frequency will not be precise. The sampling frequency value must be greater than or equal to 2 times the maximum frequency value to avoid frequency aliasing [31].

Power Spectrum Density (PSD). The power present in a signal as a function of frequency is described by its power spectral density (PSD). When the signal is described just in voltage and there is no specific power connected with the amplitude, a PSD is typically stated in watts per Hertz (W/Hz). In this case, "power" is only considered in terms of the square of the signal, as its value will always be proportional to the actual power delivered by that signal within a given impedance. So, one can use the units $V^2\ Hz^{-1}$ for PSD and $V^2s\ Hz^{-1}$ for ESD (Energy Spectrum Density) even though no power or energy is defined. Signal power intensity in the frequency domain is measured by a power spectral density, or PSD. The FFT spectrum of a signal is used to calculate a PSD. The amplitude and frequency content of a random signal can be characterized using information from a PSD [32]. A PSD can be defined using the following Eq. 7.

$$S_{xx}(\omega) = \lim_{\tau \to \infty} E \frac{\left[|\widehat{x_T}(\omega)|^2\right]}{\tau} \tag{7}$$

where, $S_{xx}(\omega)$ is the result of a power spectral density, $\widehat{x_T}(\omega)$ is the fast fourier transform of the Respiration Rate signal.

Frequency Domain Feature. Power Spectral Density is commonly used to extract the frequency domain information (PSD). Welch is employed in this study to calculate the power spectral density. The frequency domain features employed are represented by the mathematical Eqs. (8), (9), and (10).

Mean Frequency. The mean frequency is the average (mean) frequency calculated as the sum of the power spectrum products of the Respiration Rate signal and the frequency divided by the total number of spectrum intensities. The mean frequency defined using the following Eq. 8.

$$\mathrm{MNF} = \sum_{j=1}^{M} f_j P_j / \sum_{j=1}^{M} P_j \tag{8}$$

where, f_j is the spectrum frequency, P_j is the power of the Respiration Rate signal, and M is the length of the signal frequency.

Median Frequency. The median frequency is the frequency at which the spectrum is divided into two regions of equal amplitude. The median frequency can be defined using the following Eq. 9.

$$\sum_{j=1}^{\mathrm{MDF}} P_j = \sum_{j=\mathrm{MDF}}^{M} P_j = \frac{1}{2} \sum_{j=1}^{M} P_j \tag{9}$$

where, MDF is the median frequency value, P_j is the power of the Respiration Rate signal, and M is the length of the Respiration Rate signal.

Mean Power. The Mean Power (MNP) is the average (mean) value of the power spectrum of the Respiration Rate signal, defined by the following Eq. 10.

$$\mathrm{MNP} = \sum_{j=1}^{M} P_j / M \tag{10}$$

where, MNP is the mean power value, P_j is the power of the Respiration Rate signal, and M is the length of the Respiration Rate signal.

2.2 Data Set

This study was carried out by taking data on the phantom as a gold standard signal, data retrieval on the phantom was carried out with settings of 15, 20, and 30 brpm and heart settings of 80, 90, and 100 bpm, in each respiration rate setting with 10 recordings of each setting. The amount of data obtained from the recording of phantom signal was 90 data, the time required was approximately 2 h. Then, data on 10 respondents with an age range of 20–30 years for 10 times per respondent was taken. Respondents were positioned to sleep on their backs with a relaxed state without speaking, gel electrodes were placed in the Lead II ECG position on the chest, namely RA, RL, and LL [6, 26, 28, 29]. Figure 2 shows how data were taken on the phantom and respondents.

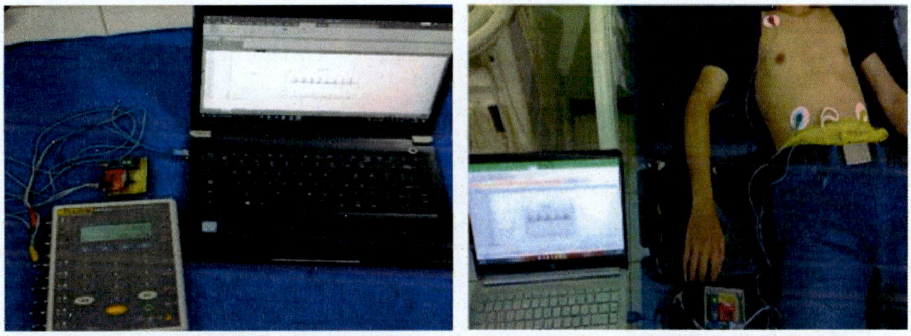

(a) (b)

Fig. 2 Data collection **a** phantom **b** respondent

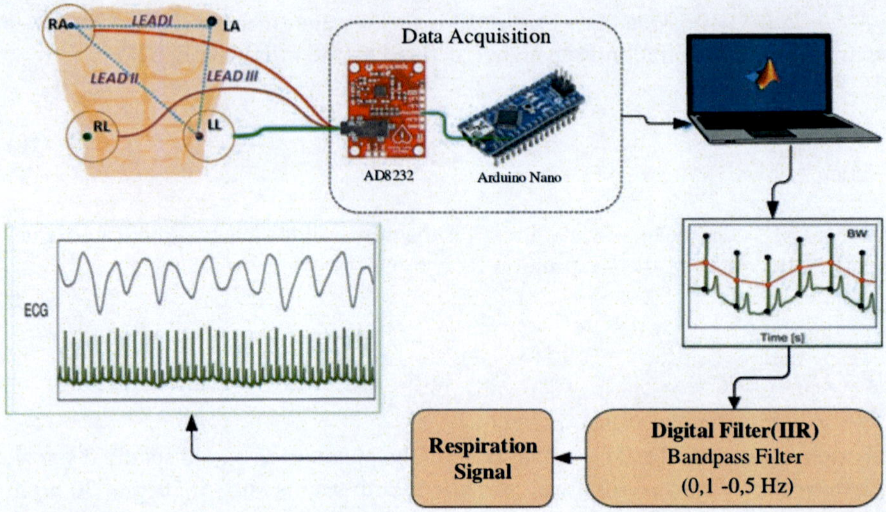

Fig. 3 Flowchart of experimental procedure

2.3 Experimental Procedure

This study used the AD8232 ECG Module to generate an ECG signal, Arduino Nano to be used as a microcontroller, MS. Excel to be used for signal recording, and MATLAB to be used for signal data processing [27, 33].

Figure 3 shows the research flowchart, where the output of the signal recorder by the AD8232 ECG Module is in the form of an ECG signal in the form of analog data that were processed on the Arduino. Arduino was used in this study as a microcontroller to forward the ANALOG ECG signal to a computer or PC to be displayed, recorded, and stored on MS. Excel. The stored analog signal was then be processed using MATLAB to extract the respiration rate signal based on the ECG signal using the Infinite Impulse Response (IIR) digital filter in the design of the Butterworth filter and the Chebyshev I filter in orders 4, 6 and 8.

2.4 Data Processing

Figure 4 shows the research framework, where the AD8232 ECG module output generates a lead II ECG signal. The ECG signal was recorded on MS. Excel with a sampling frequency of 100 Hz. Furthermore, the ECG signal was then processed in MATLAB software to go through the extraction process of the respiration rate signal.

The extraction process of the respiration rate of the ECG signal used the FFT method. This method will look at the frequency component of the ECG signal. After

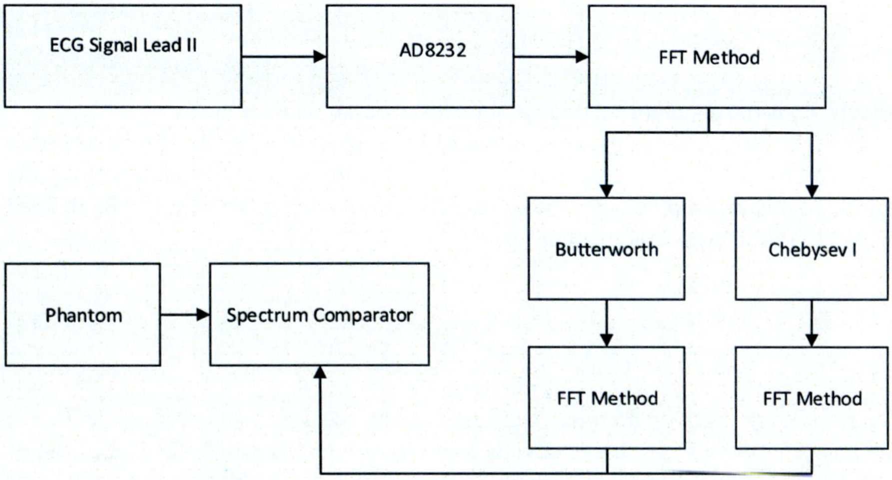

Fig. 4 Research framework

extracting the respiration rate, the signal was filtered using the IIR digital filter in the design of the Butterworth filter in orders 4, 6, 8 and the Chebyshev I filter in orders 4, 6 and 8. The signal that has been processed using the filters was then be reanalyzed by the frequency component using the FFT method. Furthermore, the results from the FFT analysis were processed using a spectrum comparator to see the effectiveness of the filters in extracting the respiration rate signal from the ECG. The effectiveness analysis process was carried out by comparing the shape and components of the respiration rate signal from the Butterworth filter and the Chebyshev I filter with the reference respiration rate signal derived from the phantom using a spectrum comparator.

2.5 *Data Analysis*

Mean. The calculation of the mean value is carried out to determine the trend of the heart rate measurement value and the respiration rate on the drowsiness level. The following Eq. 10 shows the mean value formula to be used in the data analysis process. In this equation, $\overline{x}$ is the mean data, $\sum x_n$ is the data value, and n is the total data.

$$\text{mean}(\overline{x}) = \sum \frac{x_n}{n} \tag{11}$$

Relative Error. The relative error is used to determine the level of accuracy of the sensor reading to the actual value. The formula for the percent error or relative can be defined in the following Eq. 11.

$$\varepsilon_e = \frac{x_n - \overline{x}}{x_n} \times 100\% \tag{12}$$

where, X_n is the standard mean and $\overline{X}$ is the research module mean.

Correlation. A correlation is intended to explore the degree of relationship between two variables. A correlation coefficient is the measure for determining the degree of relationship between variables. The correlation coefficient can be defined using the following mathematical Eq. 13.

$$R = \frac{n(\sum XY) - (\sum x).(\sum y)}{\sqrt{n\sum x^2 - (\sum x)^2 . n(\sum y^2) - (\sum y^2)}} \tag{13}$$

where, n is the sum of the observations, x is the measurement of variable 1, y is the measurement of variable 2, Σxy is the sum of both variables, Σx is the sum of variable 1, Σy is the sum of variable 2, Σx^2 is the sum of the squared values of variable 1, and Σy^2 is the sum of the squared values of variable 2.

3 Results

3.1 Module Test Result

The results of the tool making are presented in Fig. 5, namely the front of the tool and the inside of the tool consisting of the AD8232 ECG Module and Arduino Nano. The ECG module used in this study is the type of "Fully integrated single-lead ECG front end" AD8232. The circuit of the AD8232 module has 3 inputs that can later be utilized for input from the electrodes. The 3-electrode configuration used is designed to monitor ECG waveform which operates at a voltage of 2.0–3.5 V. The Arduino Nano is a small, complete, and breadboard-friendly board based on the ATmega328 (Arduino Nano 3.x). It lacks only a DC power jack and works with a Mini-B USB cable instead of a standard one. An ADC (Analog to Digital Converter) is a type of analog-to-digital converter that converts a continuous analog waveform into a digital representation. The ADC pins on the Arduino Nano are 8 pins used in the study, namely the analog pin A4, the input voltage used is between 7 and 12 V, and the maximum current is 40 mA [33].

Figure 6 shows the sensor output in the form of an ECG signal displayed on the Digital Oscilloscope with a Time/DIV setting of 500 ms and Volt/DIV of 100 mv, so a sensor output amplitude of 120 mV is obtained. Figure 7 shows the testing of sampling frequency to determine the size of the Arduino sampling frequency. Testing is important, considering that the data from this testing are needed in the filter design process that will be used on the tool. To find out the sampling frequency, the researchers used the ADC reading program using analog pins and DigitalWrite

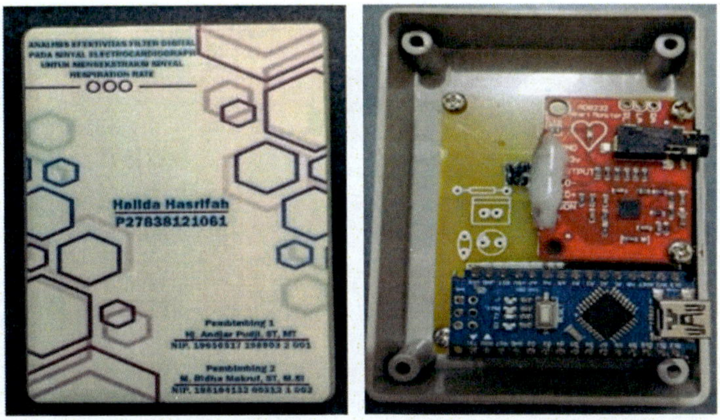

(a) (b)

Fig. 5 **a** Module **b** inside of module

on the digital pin as output which will be measured by a digital oscilloscope with a Time/DIV setting of 5 ms and Volt/DIV of 2 V, so an Arduino sampling frequency of 100.148 Hz is obtained.

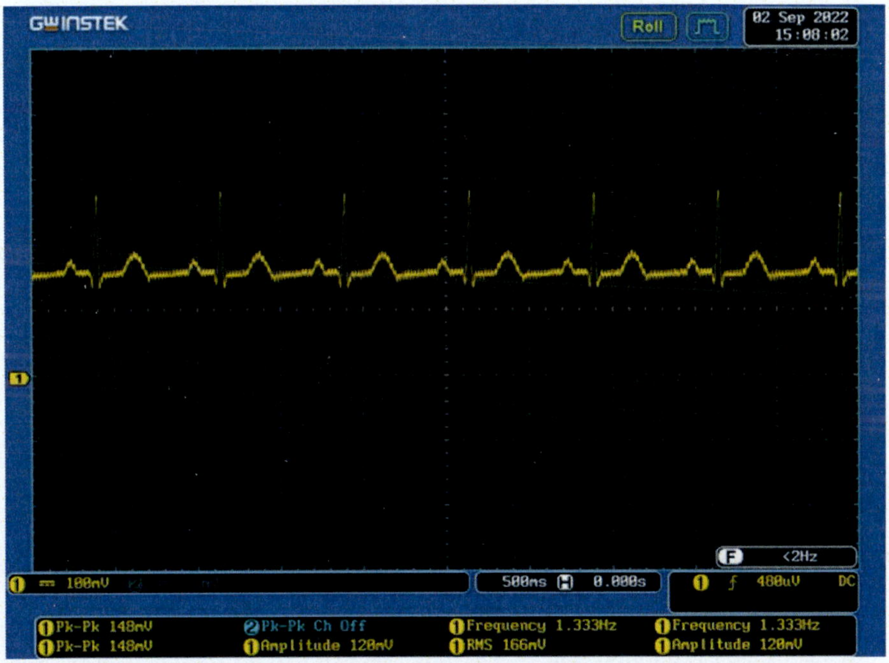

Fig. 6 Output of AD8232 ECG module on the oscilloscope

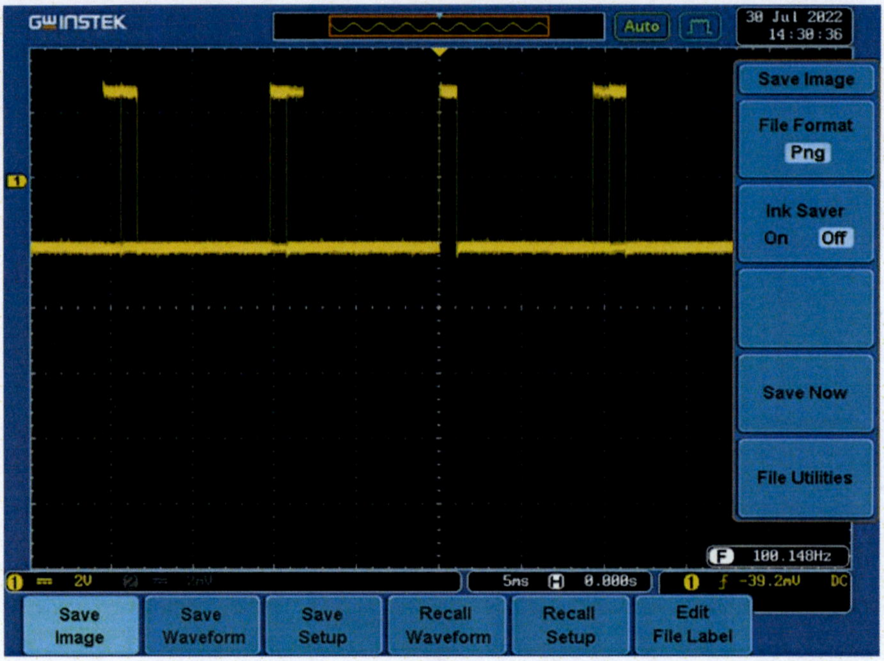

Fig. 7 Testing of sampling frequency on the oscilloscope digital

3.2 Research Results

Results of the Butterworth filter on the phantom

Figure 8 shows a graph of the mean dominant frequency yielded from the analysis using the FFT method on the phantom data with respiration rate settings of 15, 20, and 30 Brpm of the Butterworth filter in orders 4, 6, and 8.

Results of the Chebyshev I filter on the phantom

Figure 9 shows a graph of the mean dominant frequency yielded from the analysis using the FFT method on the phantom data with respiration rate settings of 15, 20, and 30 Brpm of the Chebyshev I filters in orders 4, 6, and 8.

The shape of Respiration Rate signal on the phantom

Figure 10a shows the shape of the ECG signal before filtering and Fig. 10b shows the shape of the Respiration Rate signal based on the extraction from the lead II ECG signal using the Butterworth filter in orders 4, 6, and 8.

Figure 11a shows the shape of the ECG signal before filtering and Fig. 11b shows the shape of the Respiration Rate signal based on extraction from the lead II ECG signal using the Chebyshev I filter in orders 4, 6, and 8.

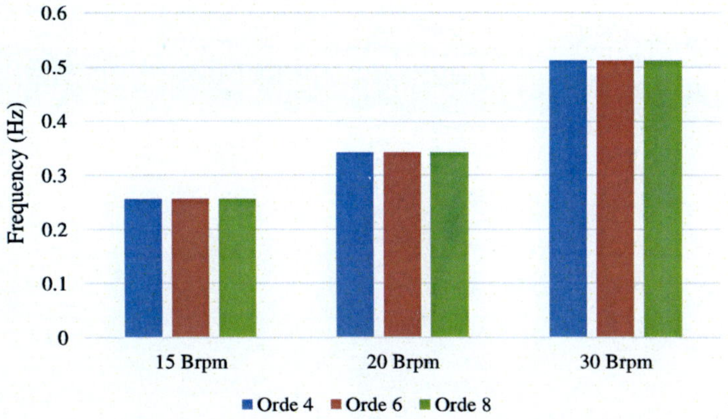

Fig. 8 Mean frequency FFT of the Butterworth filter on the phantom

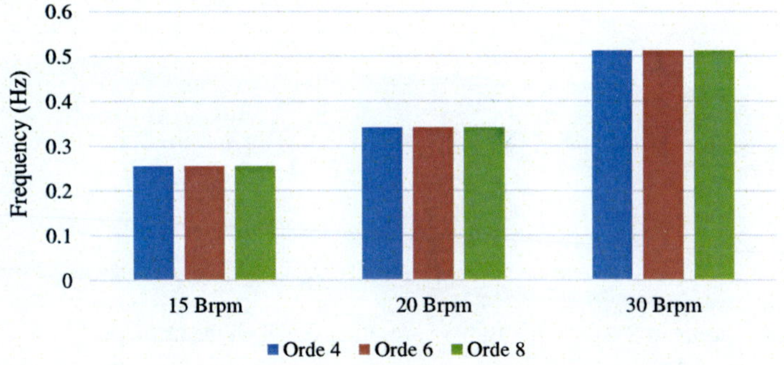

Fig. 9 Mean frequency FFT of the Chebyshev I filter on the phantom

Table 1 shows the results of the number of Respiration Rate signal, error values, standard deviations, and type values of the Butterworth and Chebyshev I filters in Order 4. Then, Table 2 shows the results of the number of Respiration Rate signal, error values, standard deviations, and type values of the Butterworth and Chebyshev I filters in Order 6. Finally, Table 3 shows the results of the number of Respiration Rate signal, error values, standard deviations, and type values of the Butterworth and Chebyshev I filters in Order 8.

Results of the Butterworth filter on respondents

Figure 12 shows a graph of the mean dominant frequency yielded from the analysis using the FFT method on Respondent data using the Butterworth filter in orders 4, 6, and 8.

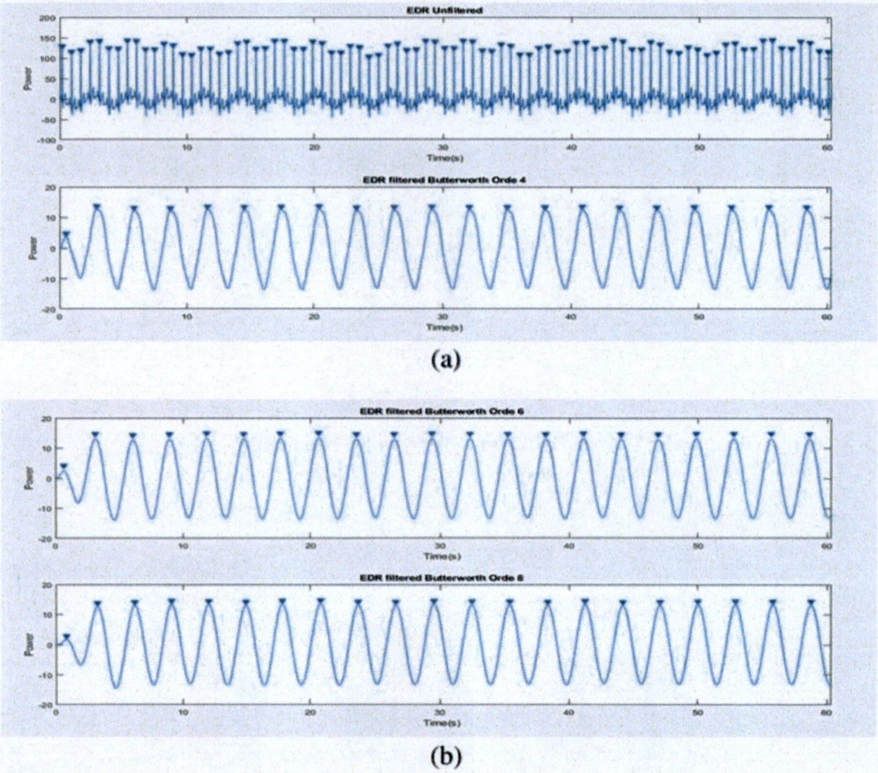

Fig. 10 **a** ECG signal. **b** Shape of the Butterworth filter signal on the phantom

Results of the Chebyshev I filter on respondents

Figure 13 shows a graph of the mean dominant frequency yielded from the analysis using the FFT method on Respondent data using the Chebyshev I filter in orders 4, 6, and 8.

The shape of Respiration Rate signal on respondents

Figure 14a shows the shape of the ECG signal before filtering on Respondents and the filter result of order 4. Figure 11b shows the shape of Respiration Rate signal based on the extraction from the lead II ECG signal using the Butterworth filter in orders 4, 6, and 8.

Figure 15a shows the shape of the ECG signal before filtering on respondents and the filter result of order 4. Figure 15b shows the shape of Respiration Rate signal based on the extraction from the lead II ECG signal using the Chebyshev I filter in orders 6 and 8 (Fig. 15).

Table 4 shows the results of the number of Respiration Rate signal and error values of the Butterworth and Chebyshev I filter in each order. The data were obtained from the calculation of the peak count signal EDR. From the data, information was

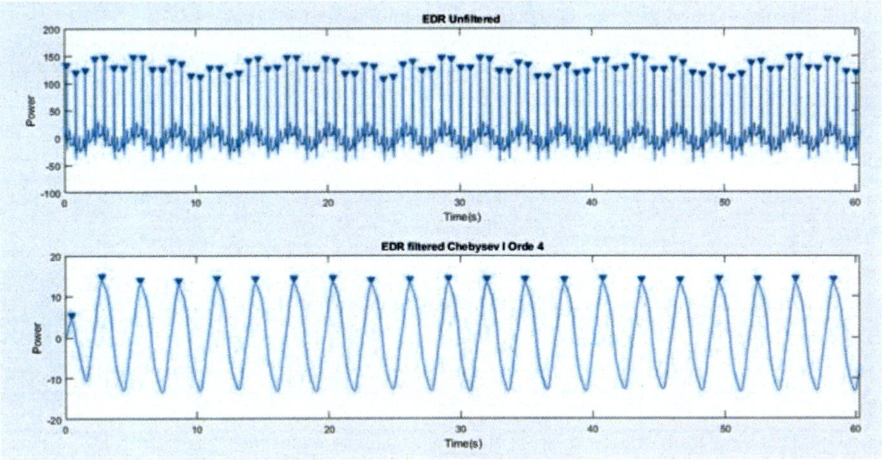

(a)

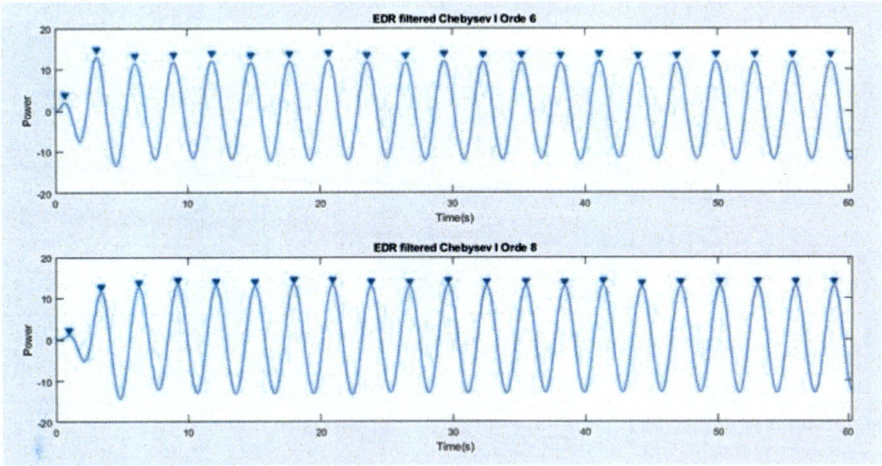

(b)

Fig. 11 Shape of the Chebyshev I filter signal on the phantom

Table 1 Results of the respiration rate on the phantom in order 4

Phantom (BPM)	Order 4		Error	
	BF	CT1F	BF (%)	CT1F (%)
15	27.17	29.97	81.1	99.8
20	20.97	24.17	4.8	20.8
30	30.27	30.60	0.9	2.0
Mean	26.13	28.24	28.9	40.9

Table 2 Results of the respiration rate on the phantom in order 6

Phantom (BRPM)	Order 6		Error	
	BF	CT1F	BF (%)	CT1F (%)
15	15.73	15.63	4.89	4.22
20	20.57	20.33	2.83	1.67
30	30.33	30.23	1.11	0.78
Mean	22.21	22.07	2.94	2.22

Table 3 Results of the respiration rate on the phantom in order 8

Phantom (BRPM)	Order 8		Error	
	BF	CT1F	BF (%)	CT1F (%)
15	15.57	15.53	3.78	3.56
20	20.47	20.23	2.33	1.17
30	30.17	30.13	0.56	0.44
Mean	22.07	21.97	2.22	1.72

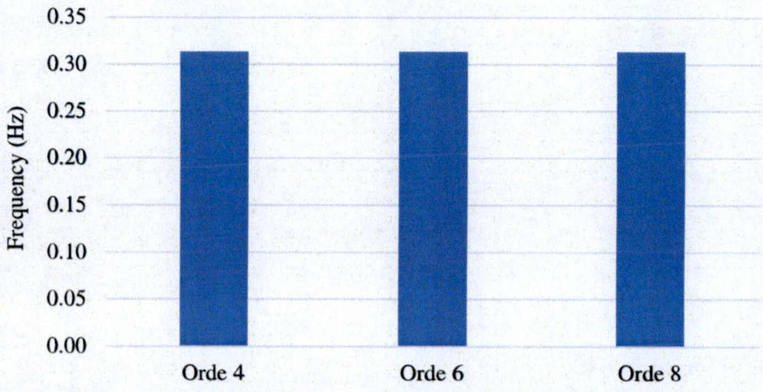

Fig. 12 Mean frequency FFT of the Butterworth filter on respondents

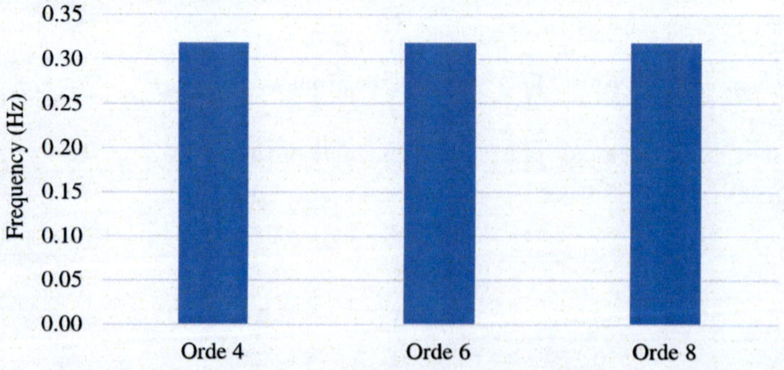

Fig. 13 Mean frequency FFT of the Chebyshev I filter on respondents

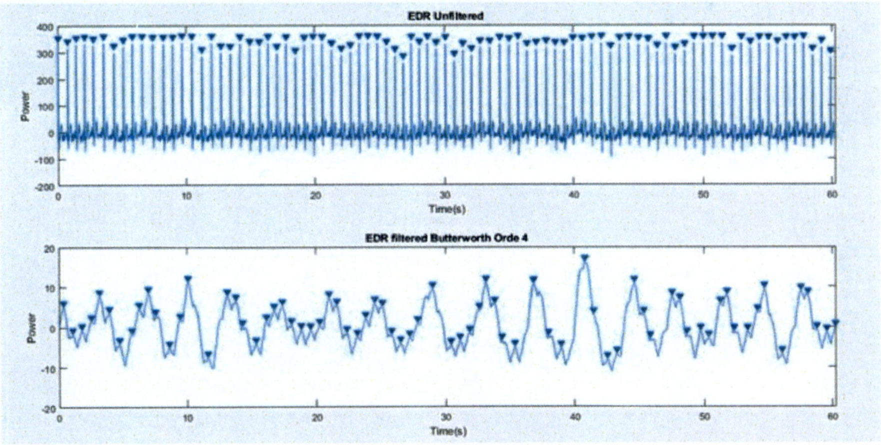

(a)

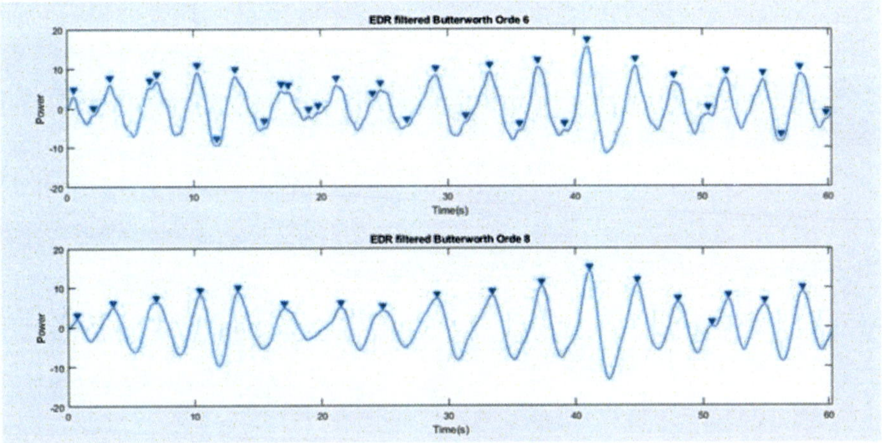

(b)

Fig. 14 **a, b** The shape of Butterworth filter signal on respondents

obtained that the smallest error value of the Chebyshev I filter in order 8 was 4%, and the largest error value was obtained in order 4. This is because in order 4, the resulting signal has a lot of noise so that the peak count has a large error value. This proves that the higher the order of the signal, the better the results, so the error of measuring the respiration rate using the peak count is smaller. Figure 16 shows the graph (boxplot) of the value of the respiration rate signal in respondents, and it can be seen from the graph that order 8 data distribution is more centralized from both the Butterworth and the Chebyshev I filter.

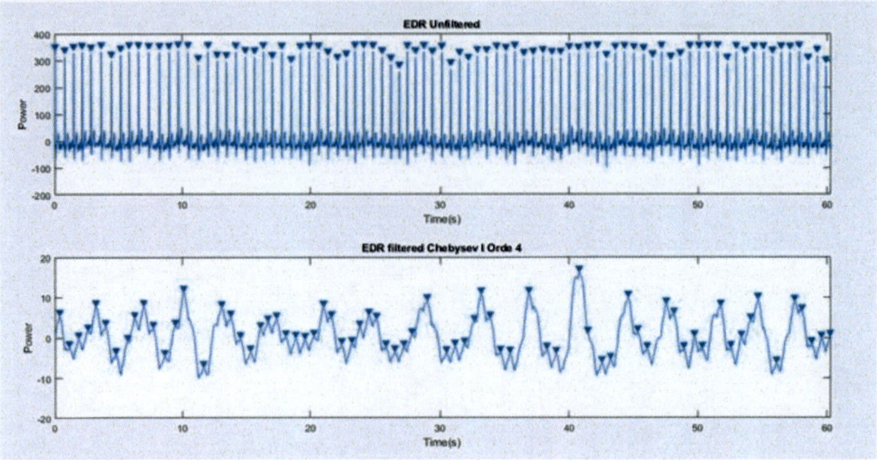

(a)

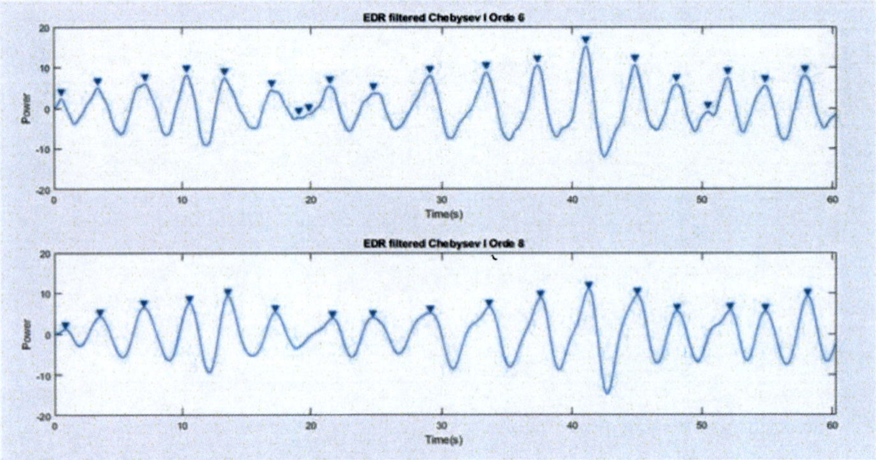

(b)

Fig. 15 **a**, **b** The shape of Chebyshev I filter signal on respondents

Table 4 Respiration rate error value on respondents

Order	Setting (BRPM)	Filter type		Error %	
		BF	CT1F	BF (%)	CT1F (%)
4	21.1	71.4	70.1	238.4	232.2
6		36.3	27.3	72.0	29.4
8		23	21.9	9.0	3.8

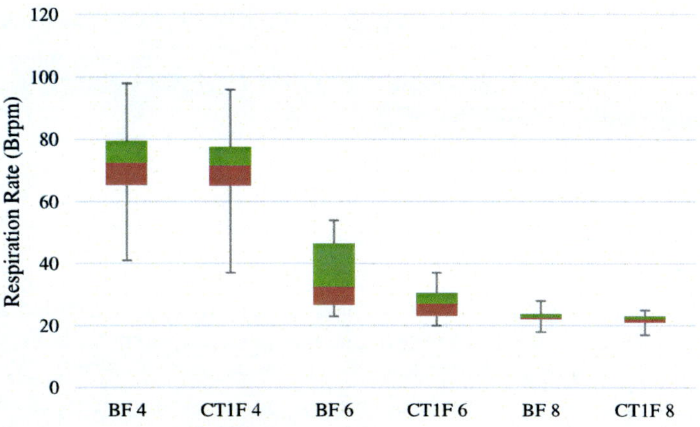

Fig. 16 Respiration rate error value on respondents

3.3 *Correlation Analysis*

The correlation value (r) ranges from 1 to -1; the value closer to 1 or -1 means that the relationship between the two variables is getting stronger, on the contrary the value closer to 0 means that the relationship between the two variables is getting weaker. A positive value indicates a unidirectional relationship (X goes up then Y goes up) and a negative value indicates an inverse relationship (X goes up then Y goes down). According to Sugiyono [34], the guidelines for providing interpretation of the correlation coefficient are 0.00–0.199 for very low, 0.20–0.399 for low, 0.40–0.599 for medium, 0.60–0.799 for strong and 0.80–1.000 for very strong.

Butterworth filter. The PSD components were yielded from the phantom and respondents signals using the Butterworth filter with different orders, namely orders 4, 6, and 8 with Respiration Rate settings of 15, 20, and 30 brpm and heart rate settings of 80, 90, and 100 bpm. Furthermore, the component values taken include Mean F, which is a table of mean frequency value, Mean P, which is a mean power value, and Median F, which is a middle value of frequencies. Then, the data were analyzed using a correlation analysis between the phantom values and respondent values. Table 7 shows the results of correlation between the phantom and respondents in orders 4, 6, and 8. Based on the results of the correlation analysis values for the phantom and respondents using the Butterworth filter, the highest (strongest) correlation value is 0.996982309 in order 6.

Chebyshev, I filter. The PSD components were yielded from the phantom and respondent signals using the Chebyshev I filter with different orders, namely orders 4, 6, and 8 with Respiration Rate settings of 15, 20, and 30 brpm and heart rate settings of 80, 90, and 100 bpm in Orders 4, 6 and 8. Furthermore, the component values taken include Mean F, which is a table of mean frequency values, Mean P, which is a mean power value, and Median F, which is a middle value of frequencies. Then, the data were analyzed using a correlation analysis between the phantom values and respondent values. Table 8 shows the results of correlation between the phantom and respondents in orders 4, 6, and 8. Based on the results of the correlation analysis values for the phantom and respondents using the Chebyshev I filter, the highest (strongest) correlation is 0.999669555 in order 8.

4 Discussion

Figures 8 and 9 show graphs of the mean dominant frequency yielded from the FFT method after using the Butterworth and Chebyshev I filters with a respiration rate of 15 Brpm on the phantom, showing the same result of 0.2563 Hz in each order. Furthermore, a respiration rate of 20 Brpm on the phantom showed a result of 0.3418 Hz in each order. Then, a respiration rate of 30 Brpm on the phantom also showed the same result of 0.5127 Hz in each order. Figure 12 shows a graph of the mean dominant frequency of the respiration rate signal yielded from the FFT method after using the Butterworth filter on respondents, showing the same result of 0.31 Hz and Fig. 13 shows a graph of the mean dominant frequency of the respiration rate signal yielded from the FFT method after using the Chebyshev I filter on respondents, showing the same result of 0.32 Hz in each order. In the Butterworth and Chebyshev, which I filter in each order, both from the phantom and respondents' data, it is shown the frequency value of the respiration rate signal that had been extracted from the ECG signal, namely the frequency range of 0.1–0.5 Hz.

Tables 1, 2, and 3 show the results on MATLAB processing based on the phantom data in the form of a Respiration Rate signal extracted from an ECG signal, showing the smallest error value in the Chebyshev I (CT1F) filter in order 8 of 1.72%. Then Tables 4, 5, and 6 show the results on MATLAB processing based on respondents' data in the form of a Respiration Rate signal extracted from the ECG signal, showing the smallest error value in the Chebyshev I (CT1F) filter in order 8 of 3.8%. It can be concluded that the extraction results of the Respiration Rate signal based on the ECG signal with the Butterworth and Chebyshev I filter in orders 4, 6, and 8, the best result was found in the Chebyshev I (CT1F) filter in order 8 from both the phantom and respondents' data.

The correlation between the phantom and respondents with Mean *F*, Mean *P*, and Median *F* components in the Butterworth filter, namely in Table 7, showed the highest (strongest) correlation result, namely in order 6 of 0.996982309. Meanwhile,

Table 5 Correlation coefficient in the Butterworth filter

Correlation between the phantom and respondents	Correlation coefficient	Correlation category
Order 4	0.568053032	Medium
Order 6	0.996982309	Very strong
Order 8	0.415058226	Medium

Table 6 Correlation coefficient in the Chebyshev I filter

Correlation phantom and respondents	Correlation coefficient	Correlation category
Order 4	0.95936178	Very strong
Order 6	0.99858902	Very strong
Order 8	0.999669555	Very strong

the correlation between the phantom and respondents with Mean *F*, Mean *P*, and Median *F* components in the Chebyshev I filter, namely in Table 8, showed the highest (strongest) correlation result, namely in in order 8 of 0.999669555. This suggests that the Chebyshev I filter of order 8 is better than the Butterworth filter because the correlation value obtained reaches 0.999.

The results of this correlation are positive results (positive correlations), which means the correlation between the two variables, in this case are the phantom and respondents, is in the same direction. That is, if variable *X* increases then variable *Y* also increases or vice versa. It can be concluded that the correlation value is very strong. It can prove the effectiveness in extracting the Respiration Rate signal based on the ECG signal, namely the Chebyshev I filter in order 8.

When compared to the previous studies [20, 21], this study has succeeded in comparing the effectiveness of the use of IIR digital filters with an increase in orders where the most effective filter to extract respiration rate signal from ECG signal was obtained, namely the Chebyshev I filter of order 8. This is shown from the results of the error value of the respiration signal from a gold standard and respondents which are smaller than the previous studies [4].

5 Conclusion

This study was conducted to determine the effectiveness of the use of the Infinite Impulse Response (IIR) digital filter in the design of the Butterworth Filter and the Chebyshev I filter with an increase in orders 4, 6, and 8 in extracting the respiration rate signal based on the ECG signal. The results of this study showed that the Chebyshev I filter of order 8 was better than the Butterworth filter based on the analysis of the highest (strongest) correlation from the phantom to respondents, and based on the smallest error values of both the phantom and respondents' respiration rate signals.

The disadvantage of the research that has been carried out is that, it has not been able to calculate the Respiration Rate in real time and there is no display in the form of a signal processing software on MATLAB. It is hoped that this study can add insight and knowledge about the Respiration Rate Signal extraction Method, especially using the digital filters on MATLAB, and can be used as a reference for subsequent studies.

References

1. Jagadev P, Giri LI (2020) Non-contact monitoring of human respiration using infrared thermography and machine learning. Infrared Phys Technol 104:103117. https://doi.org/10.1016/j.infrared.2019.103117
2. Charlton PH, Bonnici T, Tarassenko L, Clifton DA, Beale R, Watkinson PJ (2016) An assessment of algorithms to estimate respiratory rate from the electrocardiogram and photoplethysmogram. Physiol Meas 37:610–626. https://doi.org/10.1088/0967-3334/37/4/610
3. Miyagi SA, Mak'ruf MR, Setioningsih ED, Das T (2020) Design of respiration rate meter using flexible sensor. J Electron Electromed Eng Med Inform 2:13–18. https://doi.org/10.35882/jeeemi.v2i1.3
4. Orphanidou C (2017) Derivation of respiration rate from ambulatory ECG and PPG using ensemble empirical mode decomposition: comparison and fusion. Comput Biol Med 81:45–54. https://doi.org/10.1016/j.compbiomed.2016.12.005
5. Sarotama A (2019) Melyana: Implementasi Peringatan Abnormalitas Tanda-Tanda Vital pada Telemedicine Workstation. J Nas Sains dan Teknol 21:1–9
6. Bao X, Howard M, Niazi IK, Nlandu Kamavuako E (2020) Comparison between embroidered and gel electrodes on ECG-derived respiration rate. In: Proceedings of the annual international conference of the IEEE engineering in medicine and biology society EMBS, 2020 July, pp 2622–2625. https://doi.org/10.1109/EMBC44109.2020.9176485
7. Maghfiroh AM, Arifin A, Sardjono TA (2019) Wavelet-based respiratory rate estimation using electrocardiogram. In: Proceedings of the 2019 international seminar on intelligent technology and its applications ISITIA 2019, pp 354–359. https://doi.org/10.1109/ISITIA.2019.8937201
8. Lázaro J, Reljin N, Bailón R, Gil E, Noh Y, Laguna P, Chon KH, Member S (2020) Electrocardiogram derived respiratory rate using a wearable armband. IEEE Trans Biomed Eng 9294. https://doi.org/10.1109/TBME.2020.3004730
9. Sarkar S, Bhattacherjee S, Pal S (2015) Extraction of respiration signal from ECG for respiratory rate estimation. IET Conf Publ 2015:336–340. https://doi.org/10.1049/cp.2015.1654
10. Varon C, Morales J, Lázaro J, Orini M, Deviaene M, Kontaxis S, Testelmans D, Buyse B, Borzée P, Sörnmo L, Laguna P, Gil E, Bailón R (2020) A comparative study of ECG-derived respiration in ambulatory monitoring using the single-lead ECG. Sci Rep 10:1–14. https://doi.org/10.1038/s41598-020-62624-5
11. Pimentel MAF, Charlton PH, Clifton DA (2015) Probabilistic estimation of respiratory rate from wearable sensors. Smart Sensors Meas Instrum 15:241–262. https://doi.org/10.1007/978-3-319-18191-2_10
12. Otrokov MM, Klimovskikh II, Calleja F, Vilkov O, Rybkin AG, Estyunin D, Mu S, Vázquez de Parga AL, Miranda R, Guinea F, Cerdá JI, Chulkov EV (2018) Extraction of respiratory signals from the electrocardiogram and photoplethysmogram: technical and physiological determinants. 0–13
13. Raquel G, Laguna P (2013) Deriving respiration from photoplethysmographic pulse width. 233–242. https://doi.org/10.1007/s11517-012-0954-0
14. Charlton PH, Villarroel M, Salguiero F (2016) Waveform analysis to estimate respiratory rate. Second Anal Electron Heal Rec 377–390. https://doi.org/10.1007/978-3-319-43742-2
15. Jan HY, Chen MF, Fu TC, Lin WC, Tsai CL, Lin KP (2019) Evaluation of coherence between ECG and PPG derived parameters on heart rate variability and respiration in healthy volunteers with/without controlled breathing. J Med Biol Eng 39:783–795. https://doi.org/10.1007/s40846-019-00468-9
16. Sarkar S, Bhattacherjee S, Pal S (2015) Extraction of respiration signal from. Michael Faraday IET Int Summit 336–340
17. Sharma H, Sharma KK, Bhagat OL (2015) Respiratory rate extraction from single-lead ECG using homomorphic filtering. Comput Biol Med 59:80–86. https://doi.org/10.1016/j.compbiomed.2015.01.024
18. Basu S (2020) Comparative study on the effect of order and cut off frequency of Butterworth low pass filter for removal of noise in ECG signal. IEEE Int Conf Converg Eng 156–160

19. Leonard C, Sabrina NH, Bayuntara PGA, Ariel Y (2020) Analisis Keefektifan Penggunaan Filter FIR dan IIR pada Sinyal Pernapasan EMGdi dengan Simulasi MATLAB. Ultim Comput XII
20. Sharma H, Sharma KK, Bhagat OL (2015) Respiratory rate extraction from single-lead ECG using homomorphic filtering. Comput Biol Med (Elsevier) 59:80–86. https://doi.org/10.1016/j.compbiomed.2015.01.024
21. Jagadev P, Giri LI (2020) Non-contact monitoring of human respiration using infrared thermography and machine learning. Infrared Phys Technol (Elsevier) 104:103117. https://doi.org/10.1016/j.infrared.2019.103117
22. Zhuang S, Li F, Zhuang Z, Rao W, Joseph Raj AN, Rajangam V (2021) Improved ECG-derived respiration using empirical wavelet transform and Kernel principal component analysis. Comput Intell Neurosci. https://doi.org/10.1155/2021/1360414
23. Sohrt-petersen L (2014) Evaluation of algorithms for ECG derived respiration in the context of heart rate variability studies. 1–77
24. Rahman AM (2018) A comparison of three ECG-derived respiration methods for sleep apnoea detection. Biomed Phys Eng Express 0–68
25. Lenis G, Conz F, Dössel O (2015) Combining different ECG derived respiration tracking methods to create an optimal reconstruction of the breathing pattern. Curr Dir Biomed Eng 1:54–57. https://doi.org/10.1515/cdbme-2015-0014
26. Gargiulo GD, Bifulco P, Cesarelli M, McEwan AL, Moeinzadeh H, O'loughlin A, Shugman IM, Tapson JC, Thiagalingam A (2018) On the einthoven triangle: a critical analysis of the single rotating dipole hypothesis. Sensors (Switzerland) 18. https://doi.org/10.3390/s18072353
27. Kusuma DT (2020) Fast Fourier Transform (FFT) Dalam Transformasi Sinyal Frekuensi Suara Sebagai Upaya Perolehan Average Energy (AE) Musik. Petir 14:28–35. https://doi.org/10.33322/petir.v14i1.1022
28. Francis J (2016) ECG monitoring leads and special leads. Indian Pacing Electrophysiol J 16:92–95. https://doi.org/10.1016/j.ipej.2016.07.003
29. Drew BJ, Califf RM, Funk M, Kaufman ES, Krucoff MW, Laks MM, Macfarlane PW, Sommargren C, Swiryn S, Van Hare GF (2004) Practice standards for electrocardiographic monitoring in hospital settings: an American Heart Association scientific statement from the councils on cardiovascular nursing, clinical cardiology, and cardiovascular disease in the young. Circulation 110:2721–2746. https://doi.org/10.1161/01.CIR.0000145144.56673.59
30. Lidyawati L, Darlis AR, Tamba AF (2016) Implementasi Filter Infinite Impulse Response (Iir) Dengan Respon Butterworth Dan Chebyshev Menggunakan Dsk Tms320C6713. J Elektro dan Telekomun Terap 2:95–103. https://doi.org/10.25124/jett.v2i1.97
31. Sidney Burrus C, Frigo M, Johnson SG, Markus Pueschel IS (2012) Fast Fourier transforms. Texas
32. Lubis MZ, Batam PN, Manik H (2016) Signal processing for power spectral density. https://doi.org/10.13140/RG.2.1.2106.2006
33. CCA. Analog to digital converter module of ATmega328P
34. Sugiyono (2014) Metode Penelitian kuantitatif, kualitatif dan R & D. Alfabeta, Bandung

Analysis of Finite Impulse Response (FIR) Filter to Reduce Motion Artifacts of Heart Rate Signal Based on Photoplethysmography

Novita Kusherdianti, Her Gumiwang Ariswati, I. Dewa Gede Hari Wisana, Bambang Guruh Irianto, Triwiyanto, Endang Dian Setioningsih, Triana Rahmawati, and Awotunde Joseph Bamidele

Abstract Currently, heart rate monitoring method using photoplethysmography has attracted a lot of attention because of its advantages. However, the results of photoplethysmography (PPG) recordings are susceptible to interference with motion artifacts (MA) that can reduce the accuracy of their readings. This study aimed to determine the performance of the Finite Impulse Response (FIR) filter by analyzing the filter type and order in reducing the motion artifacts of the photoplethysmography heart rate signal. This research was conducted using SKU sensors: SEN0203 to get PPG signal because it has specifications to be used for reading heart rate signal, Arduino Nano, and MATLAB to design FIR filter. Furthermore, FFT and PSD which consist of frequency-based features and use skewness value were also employed in order to know the performance of the filter. The study was conducted on 10 respondents in their relax condition and moving condition in the forms of bending finger. The results showed that mean frequency and skewness value had a strong correlation to the PPG signal. By using a filter, the mean frequency error value could be reduced from 10 to 0.23% and the error skewness value could be reduced from 74.9 to 21.69%. Based on several performances, we concluded that FIR filter least square on order 50 could reduce MA with good performance among the other filter that we have been tested. This study is useful as a framework for finding out the right features in the PPG signal classification method and selecting the appropriate type of filter for future application.

Keywords Finite impulse response · Motion artifacts · Heart rate · Photoplethysmography

N. Kusherdianti · H. G. Ariswati (✉) · I. D. G. H. Wisana · B. G. Irianto · Triwiyanto · E. D. Setioningsih · T. Rahmawati
Department of Electromedical Engineering, Poltekkes Kemenkes Surabaya, Surabaya, Indonesia
e-mail: ariswatihergumiwang@gmail.com

A. J. Bamidele
Department of Computer Science, Faculty of Information and Communication Sciences, University of Ilorin, Ilorin 240003, Nigeria

T. Triwiyanto et al. (eds.), *Proceeding of the 3rd International Conference on Electronics, Biomedical Engineering, and Health Informatics*, Lecture Notes in Electrical Engineering 1008, https://doi.org/10.1007/978-981-99-0248-4_42

1 Introduction

Monitoring vital signs of the human body is very important because changes in vital signs such as heart rate can determine health conditions and can indicate several serious diseases such as heart failure, severe pneumonia [1]. The heart rate parameter can be measured using ECG and has the advantage of high accuracy and resistance values [2]. However, measurements using ECG require the placement of several electrodes on the patient's body so that it can cause discomfort, especially when the patient moves. In addition to using ECG, heart rate signals can be obtained using Photoplethysmography techniques. Photoplethysmography (PPG) is a non-invasive technique that provides an image of the pulsed peripheral blood flow waveform using an optical sensor [3]. By using Photoplethysmography, the monitoring process does not require the placement of many electrodes [4–9].

Several research and development projects of PPG-based heart rate monitoring tools have been carried out starting from research using wireless networks such as the Internet of Things (IoT) to facilitate remote monitoring [10–15]. However, the design and implementation of the system that have been made still has shortcomings where the research has not been equipped with a detection and reduction system or elimination of motion artifacts when the patient is moving. Other studies have shown that the recorded signal is susceptible to interference with motion artifacts which results in an error value of up to 10% [13] and the estimated heart rate cannot be calculated on the workstation [12]. This proves that motion artifacts can reduce the level of accuracy and validation of data from heart rate monitoring [16, 17]. Therefore, motion artifacts on heart rate monitoring tools need to be reduced so that heart rate readings have high accuracy.

Research on the reduction and cancellation of motion artifacts has been developed by applying certain methods and algorithms to the signals resulting from monitoring. In his research, Shao Hanyu uses statistical analysis methods to reduce motion artifacts and increase the accuracy of blood oxygen saturation readings. However, this method has not been applied to heart rate monitoring device [16].

Abdul Q. Javaid et al. conducted a study using Empirical Mode Decomposition (EMD) technique to perform denoising on Seism cardiography (SCG) signals. The results showed that this method can significantly increase the SNR value of SCG during running activities. However, this method only focused on denoising SCG signals; in addition the authors themselves provided input for applying this method to PPG signal denoising [6]. Another study used a fusion method to reduce motion artifacts in PPG signals. In this study, the stopband filter was designed using an FIR filter with an order of 100 and a frequency of 0.4–6 Hz. The results showed this method could reduce the heart rate error from 2.1 heart rate to 0.8 heart rate. However, this research has not been completed with the identification of the effect of the order of the stopband filter on the level of accuracy of the PPG signal and filters have not been implemented in the heart rate monitoring device [2]. Another study was also carried out to compare the performance of FIR, IIR, and adaptive digital filters to reduce motion artifacts in ECG signals. In this study, Xiang Ann used a hamming window function with a High-Pass FIR filter. However, the use of FIR obtained a delay result at a value of 1.65 s and has not been implemented on PPG signals [17].

Another study on PPG signals was conducted by Wei et al. [18]. This study aimed to find efficient pre-processing algorithms and features for PPG signal processing. In this study, the authors applied the 21st order Hamming Window FIR filter in the pre-processing process of PPG signal extraction and to remove baseline from respiratory signals. The results showed that after preprocessing the signal, noise from breathing can already be eliminated. However, this study has not conducted an analysis of the use of other types of FIR and the effect of order on MA reduction.

Based on this, the authors intended to conduct research in the form of FIR filters application to reduce motion artifacts of heart rate signals obtained, and carried out development by analyzing FIR filters performance based on certain types and orders in reducing MA on PPG signals so that monitoring results can have an accuracy above 95%. Another purpose of this study was to know a better FIR filter type to be applied on PPG Signals. The FIR filter was chosen because this type of filter has a constant level of stability and delay compared to the IIR filter [17].

2 Material and Methods

2.1 *Theoretical Background*

Photoplethysmography Signal. Photoplethysmography (PPG) is a photoelectric method for measuring tissue blood volume based on changes in blood volume. PPG is a unique non-invasive technology with the advantage of ease of use compared to the existing methods. PPG is widely used to detect various basic physiological characteristics such as detection of blood oxygen level, heart rate, respiration, and blood pressure [18]. Since the PPG signal is generated from the pulsating peripheral blood flow, the heart rate (HR) can also be calculated. In addition, blood vessel flexibility and blood viscosity can also be known from the PPG signal. As a result, PPG signals can capture a lot of cardiovascular information. In this case, the PPG signal is shown in Fig. 1 below.

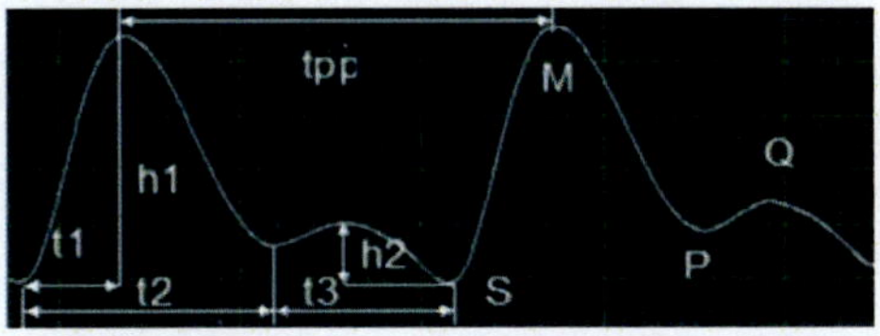

Fig. 1 Photoplethysmography signal [18]

In the PPG signal above, the part from the S to M points indicates the fast-flowing blood phase or when the heart contracts early, while the area from M to P represents the late phase. The main peak of the signal is at point M. Blood pressure (BP) is at its maximum throughout the M period. While the Q peak is a dicrotic wave that can indicate arteriolar compliance. The point P is known as the dicrotic notch. The time interval between the two main peaks (TPP) was used to calculate HR, while the time interval between M-Q was used as an indicator of arteriosclerosis. The heart rate (HR) on a clean PPG signal without motion artifacts had a dominant frequency of 0.5–3.5 Hz, while the HR on a corrupted PPG signal can have a different dominant frequency [19].

Motion Artifacts. Motion artifacts are one of the disturbances in the measurement of bio signal. This can be caused by hemodynamic effects, deformation of body tissues, and changes in sensor position [2]. In PPG signals, the most significant motion artifacts are caused by changes in skin pressure on the sensor [20]. The PPG signal contaminated by motion artifacts can be seen from the dramatic changes in the morphology of the waveform such as changes in the frequency value and wave amplitude. This can jeopardize the quality of the signal that was used as a reference in analyzing the condition of a person's body so that a signal processing algorithm system that is resistant to these motion artifacts is needed [21]. Figure 2 shows a PPG signal with motion artifacts interference and a PPG signal free from motion artifacts interference in the time domain.

In the PPG signal recorded at rest, random movements originating from the hand cause the MA value to be aperiodic [23]. Therefore, motion artifacts have various frequencies from 0.1 Hz to higher frequencies than PPG signals [16]. Meanwhile, the bending finger movement resulted in a dominant frequency in the range of 12 Hz [24].

Filter FIR. Finite impulse response (FIR) filter is a type of digital filter that has a linear phase, high stability, and steep cut-off value compared to IIR filters. FIR filters are widely applied in digital signal processing, biomedical signal processing, and image processing. There is no feedback in this type of filter, so that the impulse response is "infinite". The FIR filter can be described using the following Eq. 1 [25].

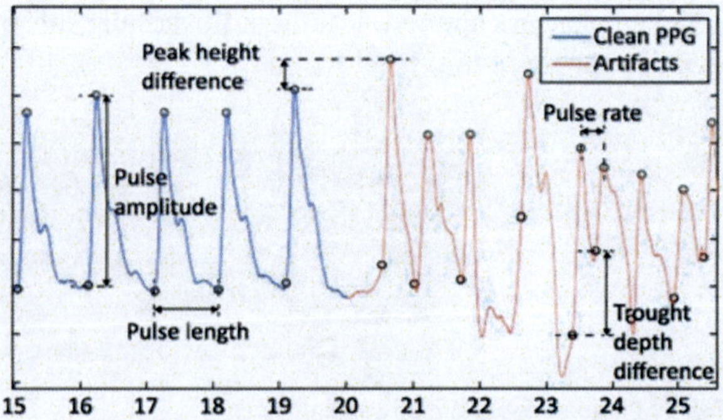

Fig. 2 PPG signal in time domain [22]

$$y(n) = \sum_{m=0}^{M-1} b_m x(n-m) \tag{1}$$

where b_m is the filter coefficient value, m—is the order value of the filter, m is the filter length, $x(n)$ is the input signal, and $y(n)$ is the filter signal.

The b_m filter coefficient can be calculated using the windowing method and the windowing selection must meet the passband and attenuation requirements, then the filter coefficient value is defined based on the relationship between the filter length and the window transition width [17]. Futhermore, by applying the Z-transform on both side of Eq. 2 leads to Eq. 2 [25].

$$y(z) = b_0 X(z) + b_1 z^{-1} X(z) + \ldots + b_k z^{-k} X(z). \tag{2}$$

where $b_0(z)$ denotes filter coefficient after Z-transform, X represents input signal, and k represents FIR filter length. By factoring out $X(z)$ on the right-hand side of Eq. 2 and then dividing $X(z)$ on both sides, we had the transfer function, which depicts the FIR filter, as Eq. 3 [25].

$$H(z) = \frac{Y(z)}{X(z)} = b_0 + b_1 z^{-1} + \ldots + b_K z^{-K} \tag{3}$$

Similarly, we can obtain FIR design equation for bandpass filter by using their ideal responses. In this case, Eq. 4 gives the formula for FIR filter coefficient calculations [25].

$$h(n) = \begin{cases} \frac{\Omega_H - \Omega_L}{\pi}, n=0 \\ \frac{\sin(\Omega_H n)}{n\pi} - \frac{\sin(\Omega_L n}{n\pi}, n \neq 0, -M \leq n \leq M \end{cases} \tag{4}$$

where $h(n)$ represents the ideal impulse response from FIR filter, Ω_H is the frequency cutoff high pass, and Ω_L denotes frequency cutoff low pass.

Fast Fourier Transform. Fast Fourier Transform (FFT) is a fundamental technique used to solve various kinds of problems in the fields of education, industry, and military. This technique was first introduced by Gauss in 1805. However, FFT just received attention during a seminar conducted by Cooley and Tukey in 1965 where the main disciplines of digital signal processing were found in this seminar paper [26]. Fast Fourier Transform (FFT) divides a time domain analog signal into different frequencies in a complex exponential function. Fourier Transform can be defined by the following Eq. 5 [27].

$$\begin{aligned} S(f) &= \int_{-\infty}^{\infty} s(t) e^{-j2\pi ft} dt \\ S(f) &= \int_{-\infty}^{\infty} s(t)\cos(2\pi ft) dt - j\int_{-\infty}^{\infty} s(t)\sin(2\pi ft) dt \end{aligned} \tag{5}$$

where $S(f)$ is a signal in the frequency domain, $s(t)$ is a signal in the time domain, and $s(t)e^{-j2\pi ft}dt$ is the signal value constant.

Fast Fourier transform has an effective algorithm for computing discrete Fourier transform (DFT). The time it takes to evaluate the DFT on a computer mainly depends on the number of multiplications involved. DFT requires $N2$ multiplication. FFT only takes *N*log2(*N*). The main insight leading to this algorithm is the realization that a discrete Fourier transform of a sequence of N points can be written in two discrete Fourier transforms of length *N*/2. So, if *N* is a power of two, it is possible to apply this decomposition recursively until we get a discrete Fourier transform of single points.

In digital signal processing (DSP) software, there are three classes of FFT commonly used, namely Decimation in Time (DIT), Decimation in Frequency (DIF) and Split Radix. Another type of FFT that has been used is parallel FFT which uses parallel computing to sequence data so that the transformation process will be faster. FFT has a resolution of *fs*/*N* where *fs* is the value of the sampling rate and *N* is the number of sampled data. With computer limitations, the above equation, especially for the real part, can be estimated using the following Eq. 6 [27].

$$\begin{aligned} \int_{-\infty}^{\infty} s(t)\cos(2\pi ft)dt &\rightarrow \sum_n x(n\Delta t)\cos(2\pi fn\Delta t)\Delta t \\ &= \sum_n x(n\Delta t)\cos(2\pi nm\Delta t\Delta f)\Delta t \\ &= \sum_n x(n\Delta t)\cos(2\pi \frac{nm}{N})\Delta t \end{aligned} \tag{6}$$

where *m* and *n* are integers, in the time domain the signal is defined as $T = N\,\Delta t$, while in the frequency domain $\Delta f = \frac{f_s}{N}$ where Δf is the value of interval between frequency and $f_s = \frac{1}{\Delta t} = N\Delta f$. Thus, the equation $\Delta t\Delta f = \frac{1}{N}$ is the link between the time domain and the frequency domain. If the number of data *N* is smaller than the sampling frequency, the resulting frequency will not be precise. The sampling frequency value must be greater than or equal to 2 times the maximum frequency value to avoid frequency aliasing [26].

Power Spectrum Density (PSD). The Power Spectrum Density (PSD) of a signal describes the power presents in the signal as a function of frequency. PSD is usually expressed in watts per hertz (W/Hz). In this case, the signal is defined only in voltage and there is no unique power associated with the amplitude. The term "power" is only considered in terms of the square of the signal, as its value will always be proportional to the actual power delivered by that signal within a given impedance. So, one can use the units V2 Hz − 1 for PSD and V2s Hz − 1 for ESD (Energy Spectrum Density) even though no "power" or "energy" is defined.

Power Spectral Density (PSD) is a measure of signal power intensity in the frequency domain. PSD is calculated from the FFT spectrum of a signal. PSD provides useful information for characterizing the amplitude and frequency content of random signals and can be defined as the following Eq. 7 [28].

$$S_{xx}(\omega) = \lim_{\tau \to \infty} E \frac{\left[|\widehat{x_T}(\omega)|^2\right]}{\tau} \tag{7}$$

where $S_{xx}(\omega)$ is the result of the power spectrum density, $\widehat{x_T}(\omega)$ represents the fourier transform of PPG signal.

Frequency Domain Feature. The frequency domain features were extracted extensively using Power Spectral Density (PSD). In this work, Welch was used to estimate Power Spectral Density. The following is a mathematical equation of the frequency domain features used.

Mean Frequency

The average frequency is the average frequency calculated as the sum of the power spectrum products of the PPG signal and the frequency divided by the total number of spectrum intensities. The mean frequency is defined in the following Eq. 8 [29].

$$MNF = \sum_{j=1}^{M} f_j P_j \Big/ \sum_{j=1}^{M} P_j \tag{8}$$

where, f_j is the frequency spectrum, P_j is the power of the PPG signal and M is the length of the signal frequency.

Median Frequency

The median frequency is the frequency at which the spectrum is divided into two regions of equal amplitude. It is defined in Eq. 9 below [30].

$$\sum_{j=1}^{MDF} P_j = \sum_{j=MDF}^{M} P_j = \frac{1}{2} \sum_{j=1}^{M} P_j \tag{9}$$

where MDF is representing the value of median frequency, P_j is the power of the PPG signal, and M is the length of the signal PPG.

Mean Power

Mean Power (MNP) is the average value of the power spectrum of the PPG signal, defined by Eq. 10 below [29].

$$MNP = \sum_{j=1}^{M} P_j \Big/ M \tag{10}$$

where MNP is the value of mean power, P_j is the power of the PPG signal, and M is the length of the signal PPG.

Time Domain Feature. The time domain feature is extracted from the clean PPG signal and comes with the MA, making it easy to implement. The time domain feature perceives the data as a stationary signal. The time domain features are calculated from the signal amplitude values; the following are the widely used time domain features.

Skewness

Skewness measures signal asymmetry or a cumulative measure of a signal, and is defined as Eq. 12 [30].

$$skew = \frac{\frac{1}{n}\sum_{i=1}^{n}(x_i - \overline{x})^3}{std^3} \tag{11}$$

where *skew* mean skewness value, *n* represents PPG signal length, *std* means standard deviation, $\overline{x}$ represents mean of signal PPG, and x_i denotes PPG signal in a segment *i*.

2.2 Dataset

The research was conducted on the data sampled collected from 10 people 10 times per data type, namely the data type for clean PPG and motion PPG. In order to get the appropriate value, the respondents were positioned to sit relaxed, and the sensor was attached to the index finger. Furthermore, the data collection was carried out for 10 min, then the respondent will be conditioned to move the index finger vertically for 10 min. This data collection took about 30 min per respondent.

2.3 Experimental Procedure

The research used the PPG SKU sensor: SEN0203 as a heart rate value reader sensor, OLED TFT to display the readable heart rate value, Arduino Nano as a microcontroller, and MATLAB for signal data processing. Figure 3 below shows a block diagram for the experimental procedure where the bio signal was obtained from the results of the respondent's finger leads.

The output of recording the bio signal by the SKU: SEN0203 sensor in the form of a PPG signal in the form of analog data was further processed on the Arduino. In this case, Arduino functions as a controller that forwarded PPG analog signals to a personal computer or PC to be displayed, recorded, and stored. The stored analog signal was then processed using MATLAB to determine the best FIR filter design to use. After the author obtained the appropriate filter, the filter was applied to the Arduino nano and the signal after the filter will be converted to a digital form to be displayed on the OLED display in the form of heart rate values.

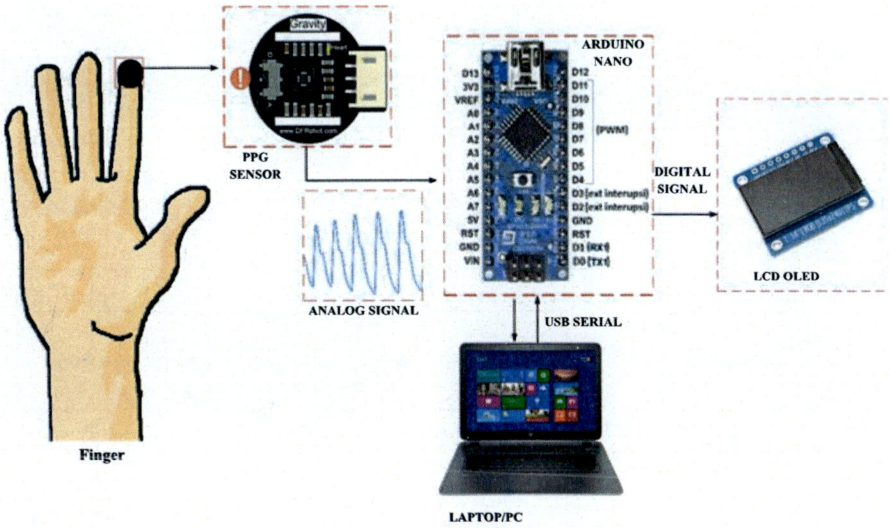

Fig. 3 Block diagram of experimental procedure

2.4 Data Processing

Figure 4 shows the research framework for data processing where the output of the SKU: SEN0203 sensor in the form of an analog PPG signal will be processed in the pre-processing signal block. At this stage, the signal was adjusted to the value of the sampling frequency by 100 Hz according to Nyquist frequency [25].

Furthermore, the signal was processed in the MATLAB application; the signal was then divided into signals without motion artifacts and signals with motion artifacts. Each signal was processed using FFT to determine the heart rate and MA frequencies contained in the signal. Signals with motion artifacts were processed using an FIR bandpass filter cut off 0.7 Hz according to the frequency of Motion signal from previous research [18] and 4 Hz according to the frequency of pulsatile component in the PPG signal [16]. Furthermore, in order to analyze the result of the research, the authors calculated the frequency-based features from the FFT method clean PPG signal as a control and from PPG signal before and after the filter. However, the signals before the FFT method were also processed by calculating the time domain-based features.

2.5 Data Analysis

Data analysis was carried out to find out the results of the data that had been obtained and ensured that these results could answer the objectives of this study. Stages of analysis were carried out from Frequency features domain using the PSD method

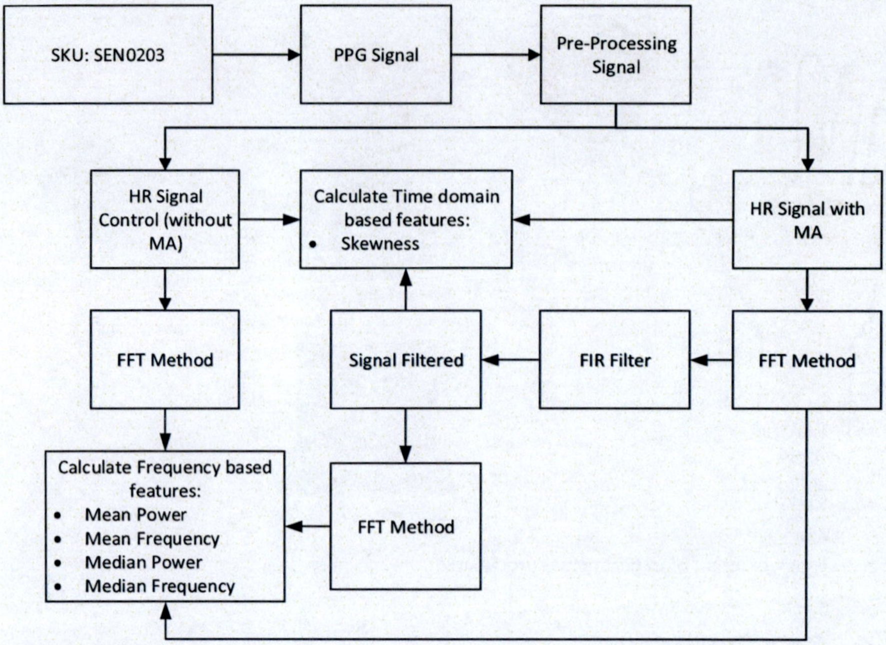

Fig. 4 Framework data processing

and time domain feature using the skewness value. The data were then processed using the equation of the relative error value and the average value per feature before and after the filter process both in a relaxed and gesticulate state. Stages of analysis were carried out using the following method.

Mean. The calculation of the mean value was carried out to determine the trend of feature measurement values in the clean PPG signal and PPG accompanied by Motion by the tool module obtained by the author. Equation 13 shows the average formula that will be used in the data analysis process.

$$mean(\overline{x}) = \sum \frac{x_n}{n} \tag{12}$$

where $\overline{x}$ represents mean data, $\sum x_n$ is the value of data, and n is the amount of data.

Relative error. The relative error was used to determine the level of accuracy of the sensor reading to the actual value. The formula for the percent error or relative error is given in Eq. 14.

$$\varepsilon_e = \frac{x_n - \overline{x}}{x_n} \times 100\% \tag{13}$$

where x_n is the mean of clean PPG and $\overline{x}$ is the mean of PPG with MA.

Correlation. Correlation was intended to explore the degree of relationship between the variables. The Correlation Coefficient is a measure for measuring the degree of relationship between the variables. The correlation coefficient can be written in mathematical equations 14.

$$R = \frac{n(\sum XY) - (\sum x).(\sum y)}{\sqrt{n\sum x^2 - (\sum x)^2 \cdot n(\sum y^2) - (\sum y^2)}} \tag{14}$$

where n is the sum of the observations, x is the measurement of variable 1, y is the measurement of variable 2, Σxy is the sum of both variables Σx is the sum of variable 1, $\Sigma y =$ sum of variable 2, Σx^2 is the sum of the squared values of variable 1 and Σy^2 is the sum of the squared values of variable 2.

3 Results

3.1 *System Evaluation*

Figure 5 shows a tool that has been designed on the front view where the tool consists of an OLED LCD that functions to display the readable heart rate value, and a heart rate sensor. Meanwhile, Fig. 6 shows the inside of the tool which consists of Arduino nano, connectors for sensors, and connectors to OLED.

Figure 6 shows the sensor output in the form of a PPG signal displayed on an oscilloscope.

Meanwhile, in order to determine the exact value of the sampling frequency, the author also conducted a test using an oscilloscope and the mean value of the sampling frequency was ±100 Hz as shown in Fig. 7.

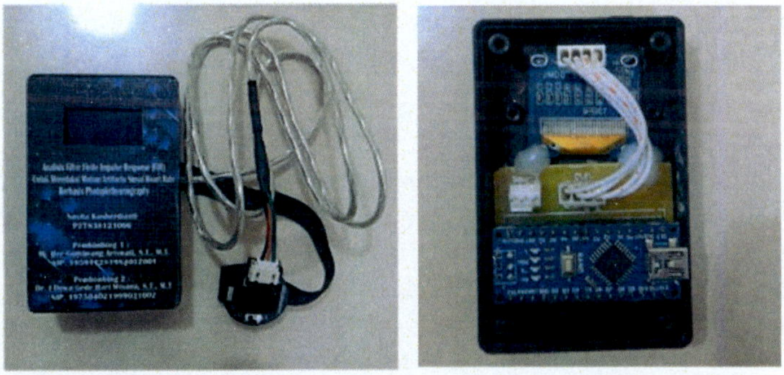

(a) (b)

Fig. 5 **a** Module of heart rate monitoring based on PPG signal. **b** Inside of module

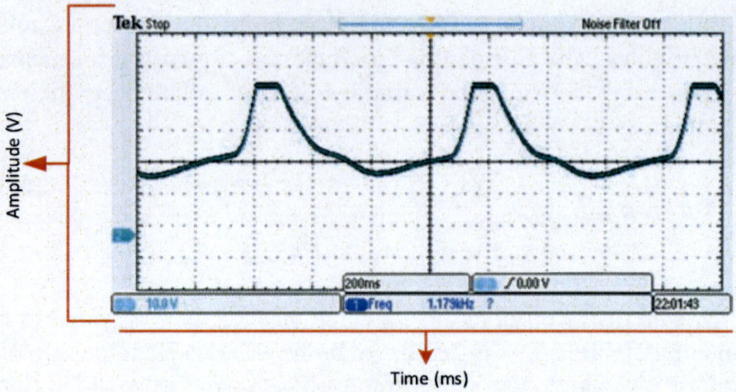

Fig. 6 Output PPG sensor on oscilloscope

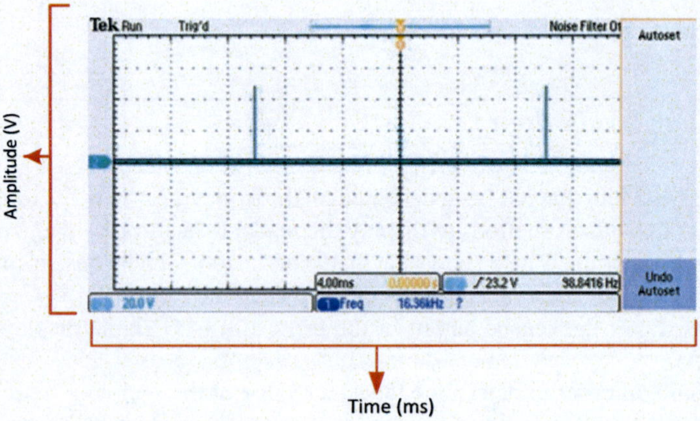

Fig. 7 Frequency sampling test result

3.2 *Motion Artifact Test Results*

The results of the study were obtained from the respondent's PPG recording signal processing. The results obtained from the value of the frequency domain feature (FFT) of the signal included the mean frequency, mean power, median frequency, median power, standard deviation [31], and skewness or signal tendency[32]. Based on the results obtained, the mean frequency and median frequency components had quiet strong correlation value to signal classification and the skewness value had a strong correlation value to the determination of signal classification with a correlation value of 0.58 [33]. The correlation value is shown in Table 1.

Meanwhile, in order to find out the value of motion caused by movement, a test was carried out using PSD and the obtained results as shown in the following Fig. 8. Based on Fig. 8, the MA obtained from the vertical movement of the fingers was at a

Table 1 Correlation between features and classification signal

	Mean F	Mean P	Median F	Median P	Skewness	Class
Mean F	1.000					
Mean P	0.204	1.000				
Median F	0.760	0.324	1.000			
Median P	0.333	0.393	0.256	1.000		
Skewness	−0.270	−0.294	−0.397	−0.186	1.000	
Class	0.338	0.007	0.216	0.116	−0.580	1.000

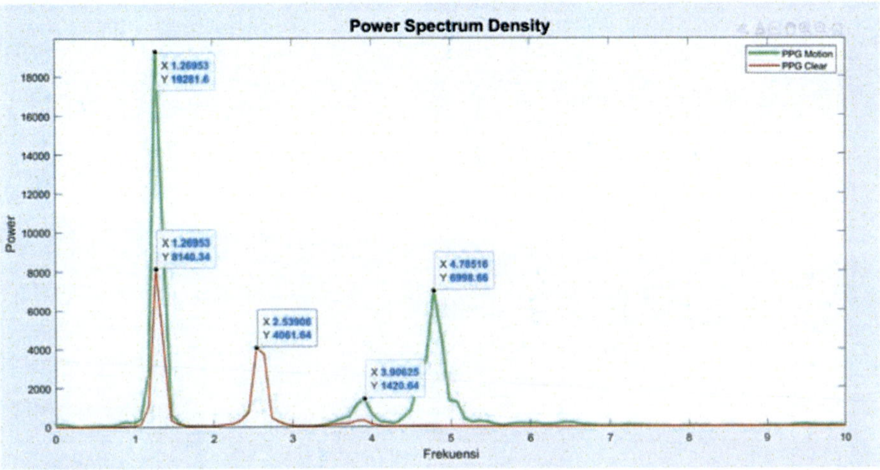

Fig. 8 PSD of MA on PPG signal

frequency of more than 4 Hz. Furthermore, based on all data, the average MA value is 4,524 Hz.

Figure 9 shows images of FFT motion, clear, and filtered signal. The Fig. 9 indicates that the implementation of the filter can reduce the range of MA frequency, so that the FFT filtered approaches the Clean FFT.

Furthermore, Fig. 10 shows the images of PPG signals without motion and with motion artifacts. From Fig. 10 we can see that MA intervenes and changes the morphology of the signal so that the shape of the signal becomes aperiodic [34].

Other data are shown in Table 2 which contains the average value of the clean PPG signal components, PPG signal components with motion artifacts and error value. Mean F is a table of the average frequency value, Mean P is the average power value, the median F is the center frequency value, and the median P is the power center value. Based on the table, the clean PPG signal has an average mean frequency of 0.128, an average mean power of 86.05, a median frequency of 0.094, a median power of 0.05, and a signal skewness of 0.95. The signal with motion artifact has a mean frequency value greater than the clean PPG signal with a value of 0.14, the

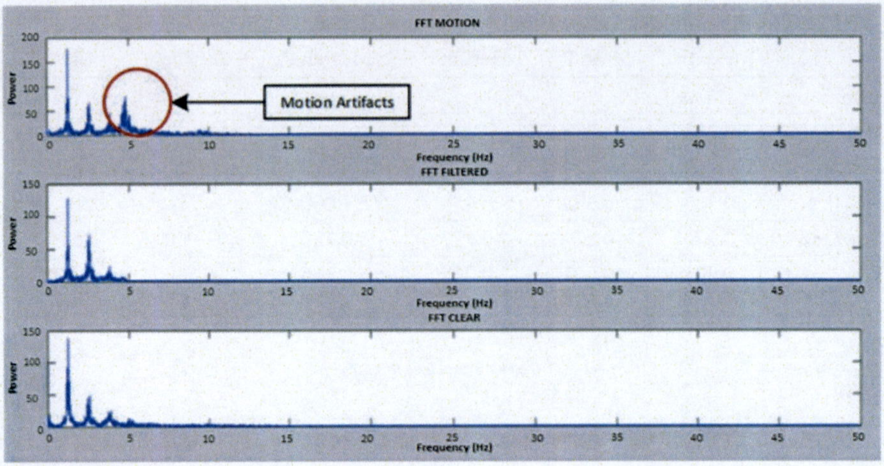

Fig. 9 FFT clear, motion and filtered PPG signal

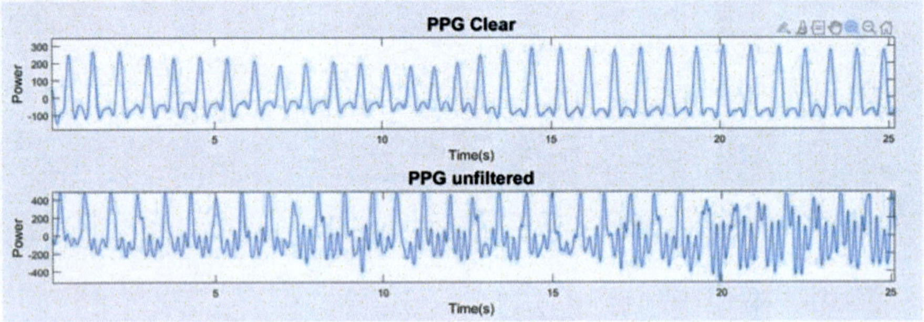

Fig. 10 Effect of motion on PPG signal

mean power 86.55, median frequency 0.1, median power 0.08, while skewness value decreased to 0.23.

If we make the mean value of the clean PPG signal as a reference value, then we can obtain the relative error value for each component of the PPG signal caused by the presence of motion artifacts. The mean power was 21.74%, the median frequency was 9.92%, the median power was 168.15%, and the skewness was 74.94%.

Table 2 Relative error value of MA signal

PPG type	Mean F	Mean P	Median F	Median P	Skewness
Clean	0.128	86.05	0.094	0.050	0.95
Motion	0.14	86.55	0.10	0.08	0.23
% Error	10.10	21.74	9.92	168.15	74.94

Table 3 Relative error value of each feature after filtered order 20

Filter	% Error				
	Mean F	Mean P	Median F	Median P	Skewness
Windowing	16	−33	0.372	96	82
Constrained least square	−0.51	98.85	−7.79	97.90	54.90
Least square	15.13	40.26	−0.37	98	79.44

3.3 Filter Test Result

Table 3 shows the value of the signal component after filter order 20. According to these data, the constrained least square filter had the lowest error value for signal skewness where the error value of 77% can be reduced to 54.9%. However, the mean power value increases from 21.74 to 98.85%. Meanwhile, in the windowing type filter, the mean frequency error value increases from 10 to 16%; in this filter the relative error value that can be reduced only on the median frequency and median power features. This situation is like the results on the least square filter of order 20 but, at least square of order 20, the skewness of the signal can still be reduced from 74.94 to 74.44%.

Table 4 shows the signal features values after filter order 50. In this order, filter windowing can reduce the relative mean frequency error to 0.23%. However, the relative error is in the mean power, median frequency is high while the skewness error value was 41%, indicating a lower value compared when using order 20.

For the constrained least square type of filter, the mean frequency value was not much different from using order 20 where the relative error value obtained was 0.37%. However, in this order the relative error of other components was lower compared to order 20. For the least square filter of order 50, the error value in the mean frequency can be reduced to -8.32%. In other components, there was also a decrease with a significant decrease in the error value in the skewness component from 74.94 to 21, 69%.

Figure 11 shows a boxplot of the mean frequency of the net PPG signal, PPG with motion and after filter. From the diagram, the PPG signal with motion had a median frequency value above the clear PPG. The application of the filter on the PPG signal with motion can affect the value of the data distribution where, in the Windowing filter, the least square of order 20 and the median value of the PPG signal can be

Table 4 Relative error value of each feature after filtered order 50

Filter	% Error				
	Mean F	Mean P	Median F	Median P	Skewness
Windowing	0.23	33	−11	98	41
Constrained least square	0.37	17.58	−10.54	62.7	42.05
Least square	−8.32	14.57	−31.34	97.22	21.69

lowered so that it is below the net PPG value. The use of the Least square filter of order 50 also makes the median of the PPG signal with downward motion but the median of the data is still above the net PPG signal. Meanwhile, the use of filter constrained least square order 20, 50 and windowing order 50 was able to reduce the median value and data from PPG with motion approaching the data on clean PPG.

Figure 12 shows a boxplot of the frequency median. In the figure, the data distribution of the median frequency of the PPG signal with motion had a data outlier value that was higher than the net PPG signal. In addition, the median value of the data was also above the net PPG signal. These obtained data show that the use of filter windowing 20 and least square 20 made the data distribution closest to the clean PPG signal but, in this filter, there were no outlier values. Meanwhile, the use of the least square 50 filter made the data distribution widen with a median value higher than the PPG motion signal.

Figure 13 shows a boxplot diagram of the signal's tendency or skewness. In the figure, the PPG signal with motion had a skewness value below the clean PPG signal.

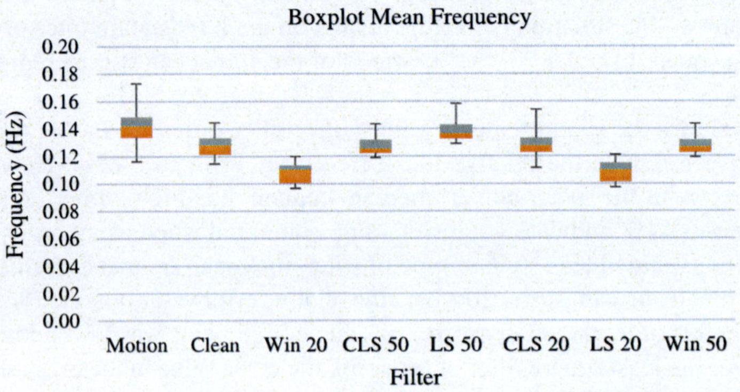

Fig. 11 Boxplot of mean frequency

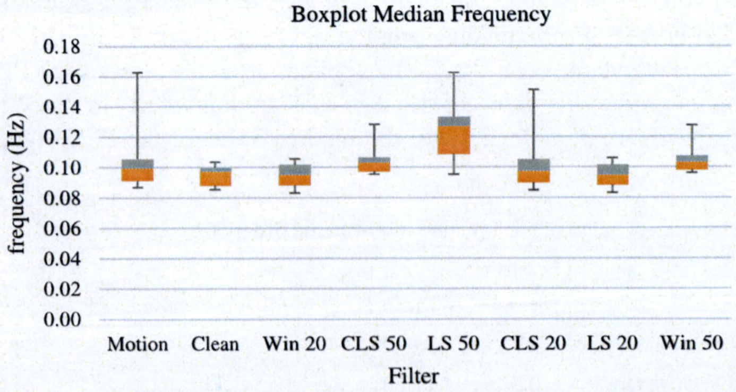

Fig. 12 Boxplot median frequency

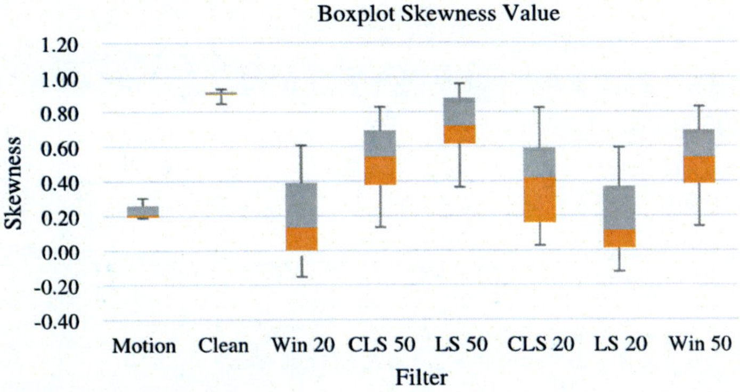

Fig. 13 Boxplot of skewness signal

The use of filters made the distribution of the data wider, and from the data it can also be seen that the use of a least square filter of order 50 made the median of the data closer to the data on a clean PPG signal compared to other filters.

Figures 14, 15, 16, 17, 18, and 19 show images of the PPG signal before and after the filter was applied. The images were taken using the same data. Based on the figure, the use of filters could reduce motion artifacts and made the PPG signal quality better. The filter could return the signal shape better at order 50 compared to order 20.

In order to find out the best filter performance, the author conducted a correlation analysis between the feature values that have been obtained from the clean PPG signal and the signal after the filter. The results are shown in Table 5 where Clean is the correlation value for clean PPG, Win is for windowing filter results, CLS is for the constrained least square filter, LS for the least square filter, and the value behind it indicates the order used.

Table 5 indicates that the highest correlation value to the clean signal was obtained by the Least square filter of order 50, constrained least square of order 50, windowing order of 50 and windowing order 20. This is also supported by the graph shown in the

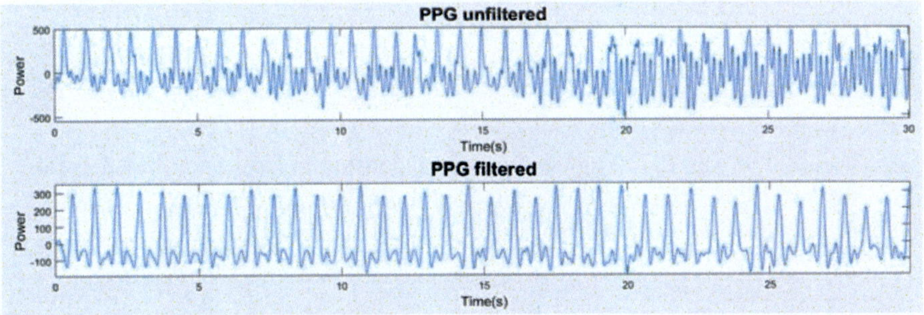

Fig. 14 PPG signal before and after windowing order 50

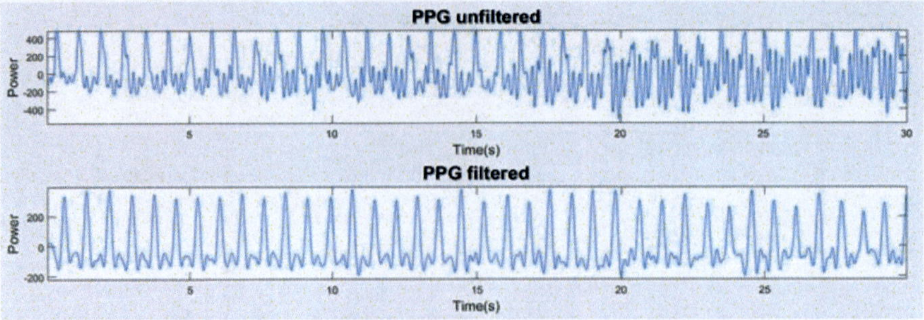

Fig. 15 PPG signal before and after filter constrained least square order 50

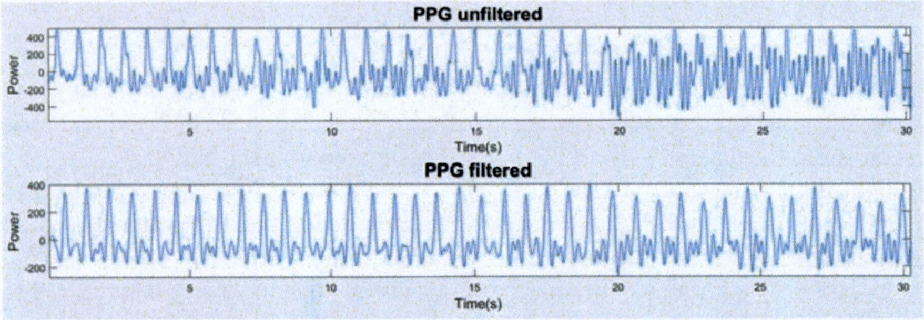

Fig. 16 PPG signal before and after filter least square order 50

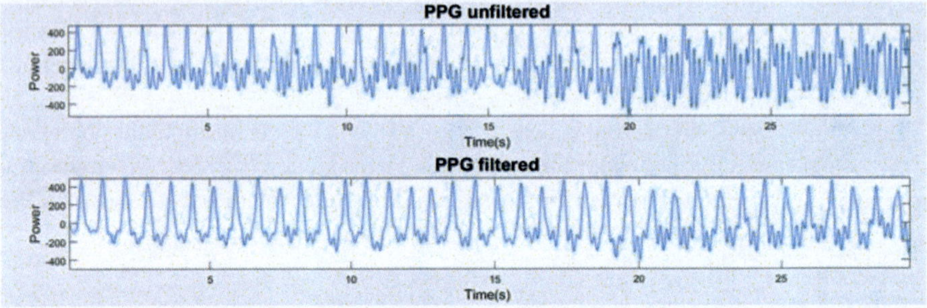

Fig. 17 PPG signal before and after filter windowing order 20

Figs. 19 and 20. While Fig. 20 gives the data according to frequency-based features domain, Fig. 21 gives the data according to the time domain feature.

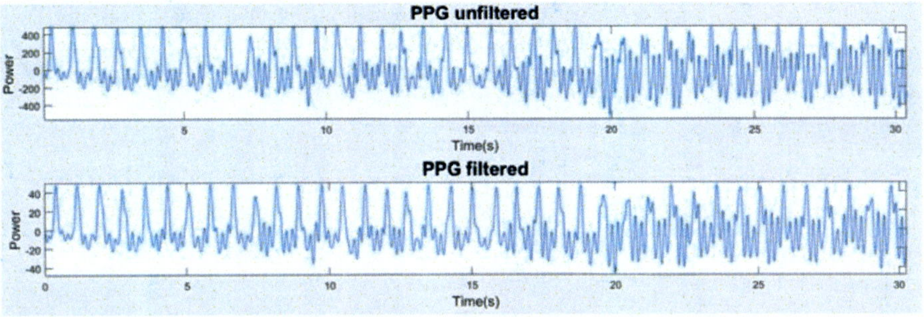

Fig. 18 PPG signal before and after filter constrained least square order 20

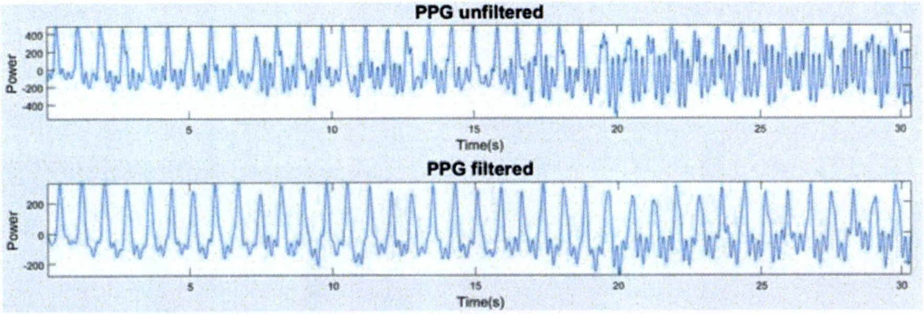

Fig. 19 PPG signal before and after filter least square order 20

Table 5 Correlation between signal after filter and PPG clean as a control signal

	CLEAN	Win 20	CLS 50	LS 50	CLS 20	LS 20	Win 50
Clean	1.000						
Win 20	0.998	1.000					
CLS 50	1.000	0.998	1.000				
LS 50	1.000	0.998	1.000	1.000			
CLS 20	0.906	0.879	0.909	0.905	1.000		
LS 20	0.997	0.991	0.998	0.997	0.936	1.000	
Win 50	0.999	0.994	0.999	0.999	0.926	1.000	1.000

4 Discussion

The data for the study were obtained from 10 respondents and each respondent was measured 20 times so that the total data obtained by the author was 200 data where respondents 1, 7, 9 and 10 were conditioned to carry out extreme movements by moving their fingers quickly. Among the 200 data recorded, the FFT results showed that the movement of the fingers had an average dominant frequency of 4,524 Hz.

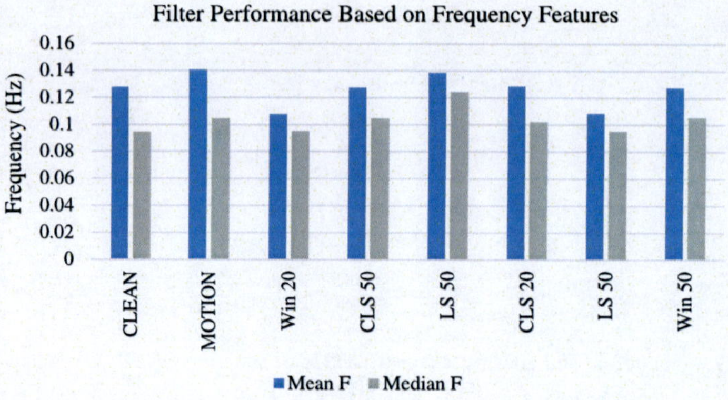

Fig. 20 Filter performance based on frequency features

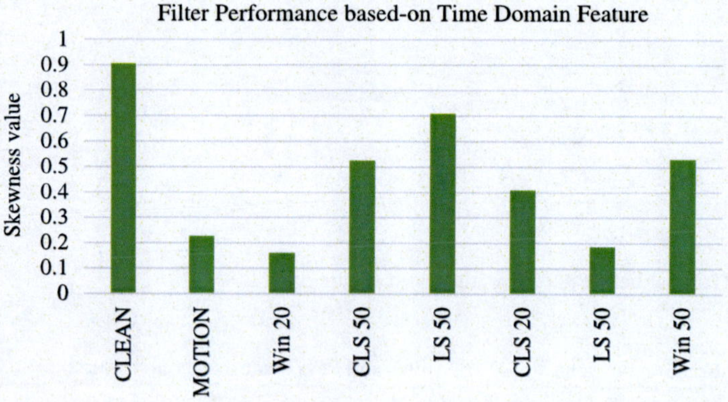

Fig. 21 Filter performance based-on time domain feature

This value was smaller than the results in the previous studies [24] where MA finger movements Up and Down or vertically have frequency in the 12 Hz range.

The results showed that by moving the hand quickly, the mean frequency and other features experienced a high increase from the rest state of 0.173–34.33 Hz in respondent 7. So, in this study, the presence of MA made an error in the relative features of the mean frequency of 10.10%, the median frequency was 21.74%, the mean power was 9.92%, and the median power was 168.15%. In addition to utilizing the features of the frequency, the authors also measured the skewness of the signal to determine the quality level of the PPG signal.

After getting the data from these features, the authors conducted a correlation test between the frequency domain features on the labeling of the PPG signal and the results obtained that the mean frequency, median frequency, and skewness values had high correlation values. This means that these three features greatly affected the PPG signal with Motion Artifacts. The skewness value had the highest correlation according to previous research which states that the skewness value is very influential with the PPG signal quality index compared to other data [30]. In the results of the study, the skewness value also had a high relative error value between the MA signal and the net PPG signal, which is 74.94%.

The results presented in "A Survey on Big Data Analytics for Load Prediction in Smart Grids" chapter also show that FIR digital filters could reduce motion artifacts in PPG signals and can reduce the relative error frequency features of the signal. The FIR constrained least square filter had the same performance to reduce the mean frequency error value both on order 20 and order 50 where, at order 20 the relative error value could be reduced to −0.51% and on order 50–0.37%. However, the results of Fig. 17 present that at order 20, the shape of the signal did not change significantly before and after the filter and the skewness value was less than filter order 50. The windowing type filter on order 20 has not been able to reduce MA because in some features there is an increase in the error value, such as the mean frequency from 10.10 to 16%. At order 50, the filter has been able to reduce MA well, seen from the mean error frequency which has decreased to 0.23%, in other features there has also been a decrease in the error value. For the Least Square filter, the frequency feature has a high value of reduction in order of 50. However, from Fig. 20 we can see that least square order 50 has the great performance to normalize the skewness value of the signal according to another filter.

By using a filter of order 20, the time delay value was 0.63 radians/Hz and in order 50, the time delay value was 1.57 radians/Hz. This value was smaller than the previous study which reached a delay of 1.65 radians/Hz [17].

Although the filter could reduce MA, using a filter alone is not enough to remove MA noise, especially if there was an MA signal that had the same frequency value as the heart rate frequency. Therefore, a better algorithm system is needed to eliminate MA.

5 Conclusion

This study aims to determine the performance of FIR digital filters Windowing, Least Square and Constrained Least Square order 20 and order 50 in reducing Motion Artifacts on PPG Signals. We use frequency-based features such as mean frequency, median frequency, and skewness value to conclude the performance of filter.

Based on the research that has been done, FIR filters can be used to reduce MA and reduce the value of the relative error frequency feature (PSD) in the signal. FIR filter can also increase the value of the PPG signal quality index by reducing the skewness error value. The results of the MA relative error to the Clean PPG signal for the mean frequency value of 10.10%, median frequency of 9.92%, mean power of 21.74%, median power of 168.15%, and skewness value of 74.94%, respectively. Windowing filter 50 can reduce the relative error value until it reaches 0.23% at the mean frequency value, while the least square filter can reduce the error value on skewness to 21%, and the constrained least square filter works stably to reduce the relative error of the mean frequency on order 20 to −0.51% and order 50–0.37%. Referring to several data features, the author concludes that the least square filter can improve the quality of the PPG signal index better than other filters. The windowing filter has the quality to reduce the relative error of the mean frequency better than other filters on order 50 and the constrained least square filter has a stable performance where all features have decreased the relative error value well.

Research can be developed further by conducting a deeper analysis of the accuracy of the tool equipped with a digital filter, conducting a deeper analysis of machine learning to be able to detect Motion Artifacts better and adding a gyroscope, accelerometer, or piezoelectric sensor to be a reference for the MA value formed from motion.

References

1. Pan F, Ye T, Sun P, Gui S, Liang B, Li L, Zheng D, Wang J, Hesketh RL, Yang L, Zheng C (2020) Time course of lung changes at chest CT during recovery from coronavirus disease 2019 (COVID-19). Radiology 295:715–721. https://doi.org/10.1148/radiol.2020200370
2. Nabavi S, Bhadra S (2020) A robust fusion method for motion artifacts reduction in photoplethysmography signal. IEEE Trans Instrum Meas 69:9599–9608. https://doi.org/10.1109/TIM.2020.3006636
3. Alqudah AM, Qananwah Q, Dagamseh AMK, Qazan S, Albadarneh A, Alzyout A (2020) Multiple time and spectral analysis techniques for comparing the PhotoPlethysmography to PiezoelectricPlethysmography with electrocardiography. Med Hypotheses 143:109870. https://doi.org/10.1016/j.mehy.2020.109870
4. Valsalan P, Ahmed T, Baomar B, Hussain A, Baabood O (2020) IOT based health monitoring system. J Crit Rev 7:739–743. https://doi.org/10.31838/jcr.07.04.137
5. Piuzzi E, Pisa S, Pittella E, Podesta L, Sangiovanni S (2019) Low-cost and portable impedance plethysmography system for the simultaneous detection of respiratory and heart activities. IEEE Sens J 19:2735–2746. https://doi.org/10.1109/JSEN.2018.2887303
6. Javaid AQ, Ashouri H, Dorier A, Etemadi M, Heller JA, Roy S, Inan OT (2017) Quantifying and reducing motion artifacts in wearable seismocardiogram measurements during walking to assess left ventricular health. IEEE Trans Biomed Eng 64:1277–1286. https://doi.org/10.1109/TBME.2016.2600945
7. Kumar G, Shilpa Maurya K, Goyal G, Professor A (2017) Design and development of heart rate and temperature measuring device using MATLAB. In: International conference on computer and communication engineering, pp 11–13. https://doi.org/10.1109/ICCCE.2010.5556841
8. Biswas D, SimoesCapela N, Van Hoof C, Van Helleputte N (2019) Heart rate estimation from wrist-worn photoplethysmography: a review. IEEE Sens J 19:6560–6570. https://doi.org/10.1109/JSEN.2019.2914166
9. Tamura T (2019) Current progress of photoplethysmography and SPO2 for health monitoring. Biomed Eng Lett 9:21–36. https://doi.org/10.1007/s13534-019-00097-w
10. Chooruang K, Mangkalakeeree P (2016) Wireless heart rate monitoring system using MQTT. Procedia Comput Sci 86:160–163. https://doi.org/10.1016/j.procs.2016.05.045
11. Bathilde JB, Then YL, Chameera R, Tay FS, Zaidel DNA (2018) Continuous heart rate monitoring system as an IoT edge device. In: 2018 IEEE sensors applications symposium (SAS). IEEE, pp 1–6. https://doi.org/10.1109/SAS.2018.8336777
12. Xiao N, Yu W, Han X (2020) Wearable heart rate monitoring intelligent sports bracelet based on Internet of things. Meas J Int Meas Confed 164:108102. https://doi.org/10.1016/j.measurement.2020.108102

13. Zhou D (2020) Design and implementation of heart-rate monitoring circuit. J Phys Conf Ser 1654. https://doi.org/10.1088/1742-6596/1654/1/012002
14. Hamidi EAZ, Effendi MR, Ramdani F (2019) Heart rate monitoring system based on website. J Phys Conf Ser 1402. https://doi.org/10.1088/1742-6596/1402/4/044003
15. Gregoski M, Vertegel A, Treiber F (2011) Photoplethysmograph (PPG) derived heart rate (HR) acquisition using an Android smart phone. In: Proceedings—wireless health 2011, WH'11, pp 5–6. https://doi.org/10.1145/2077546.2077572
16. Hanyu S, Xiaohui C (2017) Motion artifact detection and reduction in PPG signals based on statistics analysis. In: 2017 29th Chinese control and decision conference (CCDC). IEEE, pp 3114–3119. https://doi.org/10.1109/CCDC.2017.7979043
17. An X, Stylios GK (2020) Comparison of motion artefact reduction methods and the implementation of adaptive motion artefact reduction in wearable electrocardiogram monitoring. Sensors (Switzerland)
18. Wei C, Sheng L, Lihua G, Yuquan C, Min P (2011) Study on conditioning and feature extraction algorithm of photoplethysmography signal for physiological parameters detection. In: Proceedings—4th international congress on image and signal processing, CISP 2011, vol 4, pp 2194–2197. https://doi.org/10.1109/CISP.2011.6100581
19. Bashar SK, Han D, Soni A, McManus DD, Chon KH (2018) Developing a novel noise artifact detection algorithm for smartphone PPG signals: preliminary results. In: 2018 IEEE EMBS international conference on biomedical & health informatics (BHI). IEEE, pp 79–82. https://doi.org/10.1109/BHI.2018.8333374.
20. Dubey H, Kumaresan R, Mankodiya K (2018) Harmonic sum-based method for heart rate estimation using PPG signals affected with motion artifacts. J Ambient Intell Humaniz Comput 9:137–150. https://doi.org/10.1007/s12652-016-0422-z
21. Couceiro R, Carvalho P, Paiva RP, Henriques J, Muehlsteff J (2012) Detection of motion artifacts in photoplethysmographic signals based on time and period domain analysis. In: 2012 annual international conference of the IEEE engineering in medicine and biology society. IEEE, pp. 2603–2606. https://doi.org/10.1109/EMBC.2012.6346497
22. Couceiro R, Carvalho P, Paiva RP, Henriques J, Muehlsteff J (2014) Detection of motion artifact patterns in photoplethysmographic signals based on time and period domain analysis. Physiol Meas 35:2369–2388. https://doi.org/10.1088/0967-3334/35/12/2369
23. Khan E, Al Hossain F, Uddin SZ, Alam SK, Hasan MK (2016) A robust heart rate monitoring scheme using photoplethysmographic signals corrupted by intense motion artifacts. IEEE Trans Biomed Eng 63:550–562. https://doi.org/10.1109/TBME.2015.2466075
24. Sumber Nasution A (2015) Quantifying the influence of moving artifact on the determination of pulse rate variability (PRV) from the pulse oximetry (SpO_2) signal measurements. Appl Mech Mater 771:204–208. https://doi.org/10.4028/www.scientific.net/amm.771.204
25. Tan L (2008) Digital signal processing fundamentals and applications. Elsevier, USA
26. Sidney Burrus C, Frigo M, Johnson SG, Markus Pueschel IS (2012) Fast Fourier transforms. Texas
27. Kusuma DT (2020) Fast Fourier transform (FFT) Dalam Transformasi Sinyal Frekuensi Suara Sebagai Upaya Perolehan Average Energy (AE) Musik. Petir 14:28–35. https://doi.org/10.33322/petir.v14i1.1022
28. Lubis MZ, Batam PN, Manik H (2016) Signal processing for power spectral density. https://doi.org/10.13140/RG.2.1.2106.2006
29. Phinyomark A, Phukpattaranont P, Limsakul C (2012) Feature reduction and selection for EMG signal classification. Expert Syst Appl 39:7420–7431. https://doi.org/10.1016/j.eswa.2012.01.102
30. Altın C (2016) Comparison of different time and frequency domain feature extraction methods on elbow gesture's EMG. 4138:35–44
31. Phinyomark A, Thongpanja S, Hu H (2012) The usefulness of mean and median frequencies in electromyography analysis. In: Computational intelligence in electromyography analysis—a perspective on current applications and future challenges, pp 195–220. https://doi.org/10.5772/50639

32. Liang Y, Elgendi M, Chen Z, Ward R (2018) Analysis: an optimal filter for short photoplethysmogram signals. Sci Data 5:1–12. https://doi.org/10.1038/sdata.2018.76
33. Senthilnathan S (2019) Usefulness of correlation Analysis. https://doi.org/10.2139/ssrn.3416918
34. Lee H, Chung H, Kim JW, Lee J (2019) Motion artifact identification and removal from wearable reflectance photoplethysmography using piezoelectric transducer. IEEE Sens J

Analysis of Electrocardiogram and Photoplethysmogram Signals to Detect Car Driver Drowsiness Using the Threshold Method

Ardi Oktariana, Endro Yulianto, Syaifudin, Triwiyanto, Her Gumiwang Ariswati, Anita Miftahul Maghfiroh, and Vishwajeet Shankhwar

Abstract Drowsiness in drivers can be detected through human physiological signals. Heart Rate and Respiration Rate are physiological parameters that can be used for detecting drowsiness. This study aimed to see the accuracy of the drowsiness detection system using the threshold method with heart rate and respiration rate parameters. The sensors used were a MAX86150 and a pulse sensor to get ECG and PPG signals as it uses dry electrodes so that there is no need to attach electrodes to the driver's body. To find out the drowsiness conditions in drivers, a subjective assessment with the Karolinska Sleepiness Scale (KSS) consisting of 9 sleepiness scales (levels) was used. The correlation value between the drowsiness condition levels and respiration rate is low, with a value of −0.26 and the correlation value between the drowsiness condition levels and heart rate is moderate, with a value of −0.49. The drowsiness detection system using the threshold method with heart rate and respiration rate parameters has a low accuracy value of 81% when drivers are in a condition between drowsy and not drowsy. Therefore, it is still difficult to apply to actual driving conditions. This study is very useful to find out the relationship between human physiological signals and drowsiness conditions when driving and to find out the most appropriate drowsiness classification method to apply to driving conditions, as seriously as possible, to help reduce the number of traffic accidents due to drowsiness.

Keywords ECG · PPG · Respiration rate · Heart rate · Karolinska sleepiness scale · Max86150 · XD-58C pulse sensor

A. Oktariana · E. Yulianto (✉) · Syaifudin · Triwiyanto · H. G. Ariswati · A. M. Maghfiroh
Department of Electromedical Engineering, Poltekkes Kemenkes Surabaya, Surabaya, Indonesia
e-mail: endro76@poltekkesdepkes-sby.ac.id

V. Shankhwar
Mohammed Bin Rashid University of Medicine and Health Sciences, Dubai 505055, UAE

T. Triwiyanto et al. (eds.), *Proceeding of the 3rd International Conference on Electronics, Biomedical Engineering, and Health Informatics*, Lecture Notes in Electrical Engineering 1008, https://doi.org/10.1007/978-981-99-0248-4_43

1 Introduction

One of the main causes of traffic accidents is the drowsiness conditions in drivers. The drowsiness conditions in drivers can be detected through several methods, namely monitoring the movement of the vehicle for example by measuring the speed, monitoring the movement of the steering wheel or the pressure on the gas pedal, recognition of facial characteristics such as blinking of the eyes, and detection of human physiological signals [1–3]. Generally, human physiological signals are only used for diagnosis purposes but currently they are also used for other purposes, such as for special control in wheelchairs for people with spinal Cord Injury (SCI) to operate independently [4, 5].

Human physiological signals will provide accurate information because they provide direct information on the physical conditions of humans when driving [2, 6]. Human physiological signals in the form of ECG and PPG signals will provide information related to changes in the heart rate and respiration rate which are physiological parameters to detect drowsiness [7–11]. The conventional drowsiness detection system with ECG and PPG signals uses electrodes that are instructive, or attached directly on the driver's body making it difficult to apply to actual driving conditions [12–15]. Therefore, an alternative drowsiness detection system uses non-instructive physiological signals so that the drowsiness detection system can be applied to actual driving conditions.

In 2018, a study has been conducted by Serajeddin Ebrahimian Hadi Kiashari et al. The study measured the respiration rate in drivers when they are sleepy and not sleepy. It was found that the respiration rate from normal to severe drowsiness conditions decreased by 3.5 breaths per minute with a standard deviation of 0.70 breaths per minute. However, the study did not explain further regarding the classification of the drowsiness condition levels of a person [12]. In 2019, a study has been conducted by Hyeonjeong Lee et al. The study designed a sleepiness detection system with ECG and PPG signals by analyzing the heart rate variability (HRV). Heart rate variability (HRV) is a variation of the R-R intervals (RRIs). The study used the convolutional neural network (CNN) analysis method for the classification of the driver's conditions, but the study still used sensors attached to the driver's body, and it also used many types of feature extraction that were not explained in detail whether those features could be used for the classification of drowsiness conditions [16]. In 2020, a study has been conducted by Yaacob et al. The study designed a drowsiness detection system with EEG and ECG signals. The study analyzed the sub-bands of Alpha and Delta on the EEG signal and analyzed the frequency domain of the heart rate variability (HRV) of the ECG signal. The study used the support vector machine and KNN classifier classification methods. The results of the study showed a classification accusation with the KNN classifier method of 97.2% and the SVM method of 95.85% but in this study the electrodes of both EEG and ECG were attached to the driver's body, so they caused a lot of noise. Also, the study did not show differences in the results of the EEG and ECG features and only analyzed the type of classification used [17]. In 2021, a study has been conducted by Sangho

Jo et al. The study aimed to determine the changes in the driver's heart rate when driving from not drowsy conditions to drowsy conditions. The results of the study showed a decrease in the driver's heart rate of 9.3% from not drowsy conditions to drowsy conditions [18].

Although some studies conducted have been able to detect drowsiness, these previous studies still used sensors that must be attached to the body and did not explain the advantages and disadvantages of each feature used. For this reason, the researchers were interested to conduct a study on the analysis of electrocardiogram and photoplethysmogram signals to detect car driver drowsiness using thresholding method. The sensors used were a MAX86150 sensor because it can be used to get the ECG signal with dry electrodes, and a XD-58C pulse sensor because it has a sensor output in the form of an analog signal so that the respiration signal in the PPG does not disappear [19–21].

2 Materials and Methods

2.1 Theoretical Background

Drowsiness

The drowsiness conditions in a person can be determined subjectively with the Karolinska Sleepiness Scale (KSS) method. The Karolinska Sleepiness Scale (KSS) method consists of 9 scales (levels) indicating the drowsiness conditions in a person [17, 22]. From not drowsy conditions to drowsy conditions, a person's heart rate will decrease by 9.3% and the respiration rate will decrease by 3.5 breaths/minute [18]. The Karolinska sleepness scale (KSS) is presented in the following Table 1.

Table 1 Karolinska sleepiness scale (KSS)

Description	Karolinska sleepiness scale (KSS)
Extremely alert	1
Very alert	2
Alert	3
Rather alert	4
Neither alert nor sleepy	5
Some signs of sleepiness	6
Sleepy, but no effort to keep awake	7
Sleepy, but some effort to keep awake	8
Very sleepy, great effort to keep awake, fighting sleep	9

Electrocardiogram and Photoplethysmogram

An electrocardiogram (ECG) is a simple test that can be used to check the heart's rhythm and electrical activity. ECG displays a graph of the time and voltage data that myocardium generates during one cardiac pumping cycle. From the electrical activity, it can be known that the size of the number of heartbeats per unit of time, which is called the heart rate, is usually expressed in units of beats per minute (BPM) [13, 14, 23]. A photoplethysmogram (PPG) is a photoelectric method for measuring the volumetric variations of blood circulation. PPG is a unique non-invasive technology with advantages in the form of ease of use when compared to the existing methods. PPG is widely used to detect various basic physiological characteristics, such as blood oxygen levels, heart rate, respiration rate, and blood pressure [15]. Generally, ECG and PPG signals are only used for diagnosis of heart defects or monitoring the physiological conditions of a person who has a heart defect and monitoring the physiological conditions of a person who has abnormalities in the respiration rate [24, 25].

Heart rate

Heart rate is a measure of the number of heartbeats per unit of time, usually expressed in units of beats per minute (BPM). Heart rate is an important cardiovascular parameter because it can indicate the conditions of the human body. The heart rate value is obtained from the calculation of the R-R intervals in the electrocardiogram. The hart rate value can be formulated mathematically using the following Eq. (1)

$$Heart\ Rate\ (BPM) = \frac{60}{ECG\ peak\ to\ peak\ interval} \tag{1}$$

where, 60 is seconds, and the ECG peak to peak interval is the time difference from the first R peak to the second R peak.

Respiration rate

Respiration rate is one of the important vital signs. Respiratory rate can be obtained through ECG and PPG signals [9, 10]. There are several methods for obtaining respiration signals from ECG and PPG; these methods are baseline wander, amplitude modulation, and frequency modulation. In this study, to get a respiration signal, the frequency modulation method was used. Frequency modulation is a method based on Respiratory Sinus Arrhythmia. The heart rate accelerates during inhalation and decelerates during exhalation, which will be represented as a change in the interval between the peak R in the ECG signal and a change in the peak interval to the peak of the PPG signal. The result of the interval is called heart rate variability, and from this heart rate variability, a respiration signal will be formed [26–29]. The respiration rate value is obtained from the results of the peak to peak interval of the respiration signal, which can be formulated in the following Eq. (2):

$$\text{Respiration rate(Brpm)} = \frac{60}{\text{Respiration signal peak to peak interval}} \quad (2)$$

where, 60 is seconds, and respiration signal peak to peak interval is the time difference from the first peak of respiration signal to the second peak of the respiration signal.

Digital filter (FIR)

Finite impulse response (FIR) filter is a type of digital filter that has a linear phase, high stability, and steep cut-off value compared to the IIR filter. FIR filter is widely applied in digital signal processing, biomedical signal processing, and image processing. In this type of filter, there is no feedback so that the impulse response is "infinite". The FIR filter can be described using the following Eq. (3) [30].

$$y(n) = \sum_{m=0}^{M-1} b_m x(n-m) \quad (3)$$

where, b_m is the filter coefficient value, $m - 1$ is the order value of the filter, m is the filter length, $x(n)$ is the input signal, $y(n)$ is the filter signal.

The b_m filter coefficient can be calculated using the windowing method, and the windowing selection must meet the band pass and attenuation requirements. Then the filter coefficient value is defined based on the relationship between the filter length and the window transition width [31]. Applying the Z-transform on both sides of Eq. 3 leads to the following Eq. (4) [30].

$$y(z) = b_0 X(z) + b_1 z^{-1} X(z) + \ldots + b_k z^{-k} X(z). \quad (4)$$

where, $b_0(z)$ is the filter coefficient after Z-transform, X is the input signal and k is the FIR filter length.

Factoring out $X(z)$ on the right-hand side of Eq. 4 and then dividing $X(z)$ on both sides, results in the transfer function which depicts the FIR filter, as presented in the following Eq. (5) [30].

$$H(z) = \frac{Y(z)}{X(z)} = b_0 + b_1 z^{-1} + \ldots + b_K z^{-K} \quad (5)$$

Similarly, we can obtain the FIR design equation for the band pass filter by using their ideal responses. The following Eq. (6) gives the formula for the calculation of the FIR filter coefficient [30].

$$h(n) = \begin{cases} \frac{\Omega_H - \Omega_L}{\pi}, n=0 \\ \frac{\sin(\Omega_H n)}{n\pi} - \frac{\sin(\Omega_L n}{n\pi}, n \neq 0, -M \leq n \leq M \end{cases} \quad (6)$$

where, $h(n)$ is the ideal impulse response from FIR filter, Ω_H is the cutoff frequency of high pass, Ω_L is the cutoff frequency of low pass.

Peak detection. Peak detection aims to obtain peak to peak intervals of ECG, PPG, and Respiration signals. Peak detection uses adaptive threshold where the threshold value will follow changes in the increase or decrease in the signals, where, if the signal increases by 10% from the lower limit of the signal, it will have a peak value = 1, and if the signal decreases by 10% from the upper limit of the signal, it will have a peak value = 0. The intervals from peak to peak obtained from the difference in the time of appearance of the binary = 1. The peak detection can be formulated mathematically using the following Eq. (7):

$$peak = \begin{cases} 1, if\ signal = 110\%\ of\ Upper\ Treshold \\ 0, if\ signal = 90\%\ of\ Bottom\ Treshold \end{cases} \tag{7}$$

where, the peak = 1 if the signal is above 110% of the lower threshold and the peak = 0 if the signal is below 90% of the upper threshold. The distances or intervals of peak to peak in the time domain will be calculated to obtain the peak to peak intervals, which can be formulated mathematically using the following Eq. (8).

$$\text{Interval} = T_{\text{peak}(n+1)} - T_{\text{peak}(n)} \tag{8}$$

where $T_{\text{peak}(n+1)}$ is the period time of peak (n + 1) and $T_{\text{peak(n)}}$ is the period time for peak to n.

Threshold Algorithm. Threshold Algorithm is an algorithm used to create a barrier between 2 conditions where the limiter is called the threshold value [32]. In this study, the threshold value was made based on a person's drowsiness using the heart rate and respiration rate. The result of this threshold algorithm output illustrates the conditions of drivers, whether they are drowsy or not drowsy, and which calculation is presented in the following in Eq. (9):

$$\text{Drowsiness} = \begin{cases} 1, If\ HR \le T_{HR}\ or\ RR \le T_{RR} \\ 0, If\ HR > T_{HR}\ and\ RR > T_{RR} \end{cases} \tag{9}$$

where, the system will classify into drowsy conditions if the Heart rate is below the threshold heart rate or the respiration rate is below the threshold respiration rate while if the heart rate is above the threshold heart rate and the respiration rate is above the threshold respiration rate, the system will classify into not drowsy conditions.

2.2 Dataset

This study used subjects with normal conditions as respondents. The age of these respondents ranged from 18 to 25 years old. These respondents were randomly taken from the Health Polytechnic of Surabaya. Initial testing was carried out to test the results of the prototype system with a patient monitor as a standard that has the

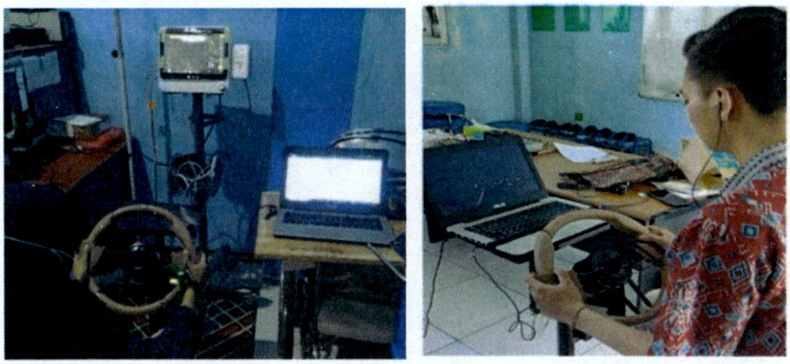

(a) (b)

Fig. 1 **a** Testing the research modul with patient monitor. **b** Testing the research modul for drowsiness detection

ability to measure the heart rate and respiration rate. Testing was performed on 15 respondents. Second testing was carried out to test the drowsiness detection system. One day before the data collection was carried out, it was confirmed that respondents have avoided factors that could affect drowsiness outside their physiological causes by conducting interviews and controlling their sleep time, which should not be less than 6 h at night so that the same sleep time was obtained for each respondent. Then, data collection was carried out in 3 different time periods, namely in the morning at 07.00, in the afternoon at 13.00, and in the evening at 22.00 in each respondent. This data collection aimed to see the correlation or relationship between the heart rate and and the respiration rate values with the KSS sleepiness scale and to determine the accuracy value of the drowsiness detection system. The data collection process is presented in the following Fig. 1.

2.3 Experimental Procedure

This study was designed to obtain data from the heart rate and respiration rate when driving in drowsy (sleepy) conditions, as well as to test the accuracy of the drowsiness detection system using the threshold method. This study used a steering wheel as a simulator of the actual driving conditions. On the steering wheel, there would be a sensor to get ECG and PPG signals. The flowchart of the module is presented in the following Fig. 2.

In this study, there were three inputs in the form of MAX86150 and XD-58C pulse sensors and the KSS scale. The MAX86150 input in the form of an ECG signal is then processed on the Arduino where the result of the sensor reading will then be given a digital filter to eliminate noise. After the digital filter, the result of the sensor reading is obtained from the R-R intervals value. The result of the R-R intervals is

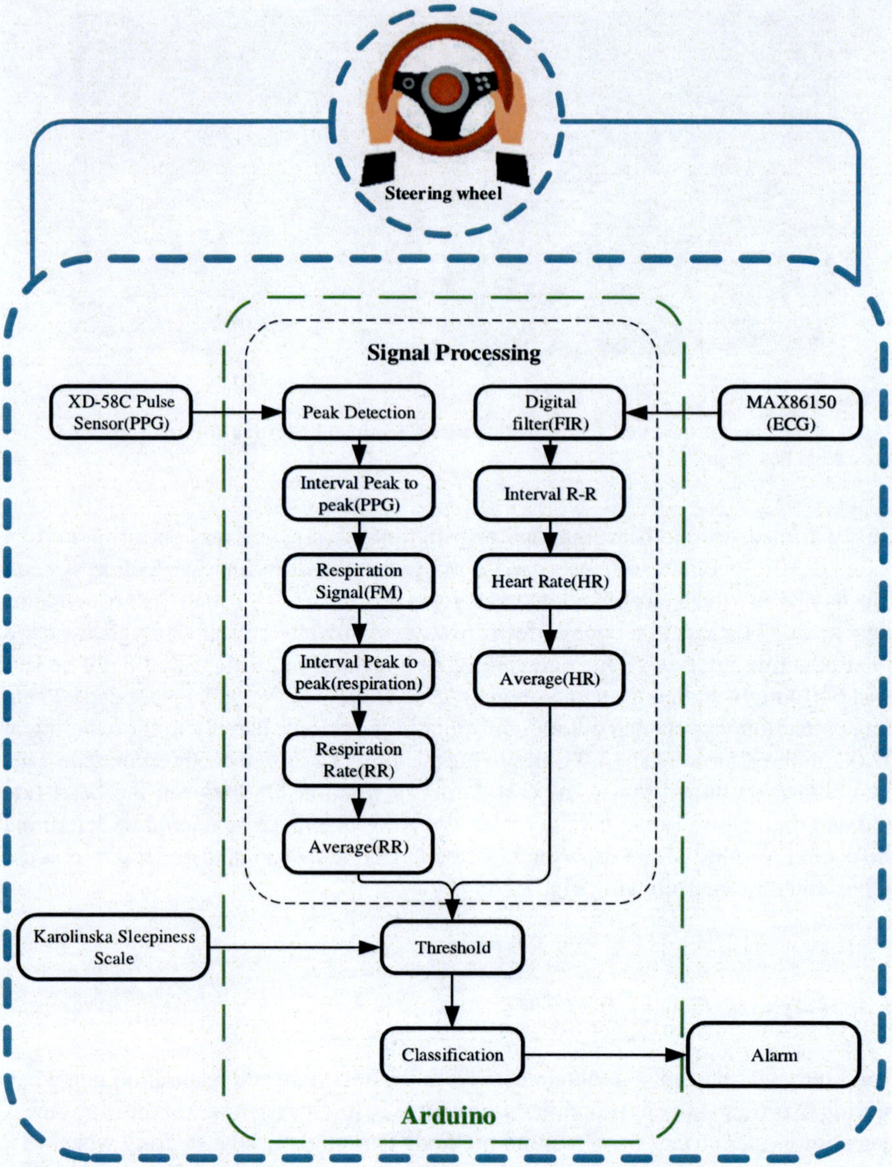

Fig. 2 Flowchart of the module

used to obtain the heart rate (HR) value so that the average (mean) heart rate value can also be obtained. The XD-58C pulse sensor input in the form of a PPG signal is then also processed on the Arduino where from the result of the sensor reading the peak to peak intervals of the PPG signal was obtained. From the peak to peak intervals there will be a modulation frequency to the heart rate due to the respiration process. From the result of the modulation frequency a respiration signal will be prepared. From the respiration signal, the peak to peak intervals of the respiration signal are obtained. The result of the peak to peak intervals of the respiration signal is used to obtain the respiration rate (RR) value so that the average respiration rate value can also be obtained. From these results, features in the form of averages of HR and RR are obtained. The features obtained, as well as the value of the KSS scale are used to determine the threshold value used for the classification of drowsiness conditions, if a person is in drowsy conditions, there will be a warning alarm as an output.

2.4 Data Processing

Figure 3 is a flowchart of Input threshold formulation. The process starts from initialization, then it is continued to entering the drowsiness level input, consisting of 1–9 sleepiness scales (levels).

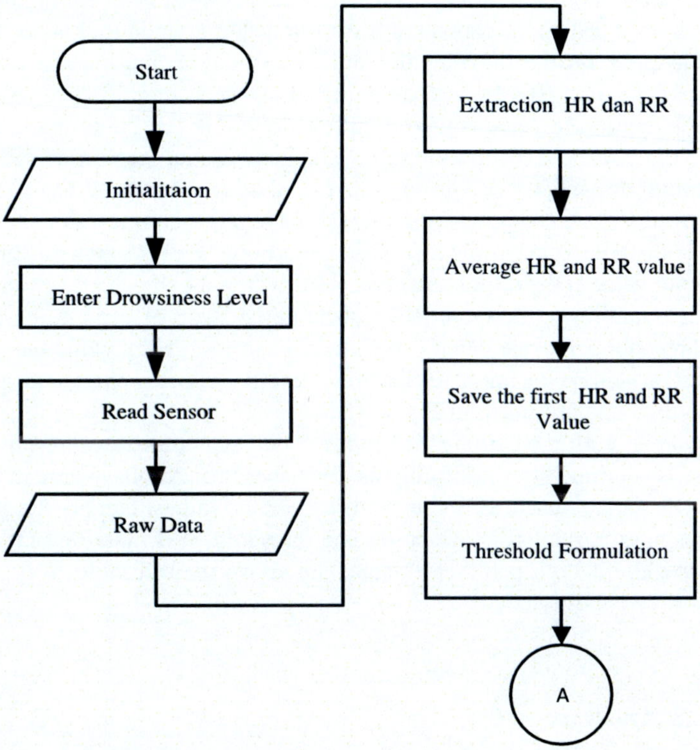

Fig. 3 Flowchart of input threshold formulation

The next process is reading the MAX86150 sensor and XD-58C sensor values and get the raw data. From the raw data, signal extraction will be carried out to obtain heart rate (HR) and respiration rate (RR) features so that the averages of heart rate (HR) and respiration rate (RR) can also be obtained. After that, the process is continued to storing the averages of heart rate and respiration rate which are used to calculate the threshold value of the drowsiness conditions. In the calculation to obtain the threshold value of the drowsiness conditions, the threshold is influenced by the initial drowsiness condition level, as well as the initial heart rate (HR) and respiration rate (RR) conditions. If the initial drowsiness condition is level 1 then the threshold heart rate value is the initial heart rate (HR)—12% the initial heart rate, while the threshold respiration rate value is the initial respiration rate (RR)—4, if the initial drowsiness condition is level 2 then the threshold heart rate value is the initial heart rate (HR) is10% the initial heart rate, while the threshold respiration rate (RR) value is the initial respiration rate (RR)—4, if the initial drowsiness condition is level 3 then the threshold heart rate value is the initial heart rate (HR)—8% the initial heart rate, while the initial threshold respiration rate value is the initial respiration rate (RR)—4, if the initial drowsiness condition is level 4 then the threshold heart rate value is the initial Heart rate (HR) is 6% of the initial heart rate, while the threshold respiration rate value is the initial respiration rate (RR)—2, if the initial drowsiness condition is level 5 then the threshold heart rate value is the initial heart rate (HR) is 4% of the initial heart rate, while the initial threshold respiration rate value is the initial respiration rate (RR)—2, if the initial drowsiness condition is level 6 then the threshold heart rate value is the initial heart rate (HR) is 2% of the initial heart rate, while the threshold respiration rate value is the initial respiration rate (RR)—2, if the initial drowsiness condition is level 7 then the threshold heart rate value is the initial heart rate (HR), while the threshold respiration rate value is the initial respiration rate (RR), if the initial drowsiness condition is level 8 then the initial heart rate threshold value is the initial heart rate (HR), while the threshold respiration rate value is the initial respiration rate (RR), if the initial sleepiness condition is level 9 then the threshold heart rate value is the initial heart rate (HR), while the threshold respiration rate value is the initial respiration rate (RR). The flowchart of the threshold value formulation is presented in Fig. 4.

Based on Fig. 5, after obtaining the heart rate and respiration rate threshold values, the process is continued to classifying the drowsiness conditions, where in this classification OR logic is used. If one or both parameter values, namely the heart rate (HR) or respiration rate (RR) are below the threshold, it is classified into drowsy conditions, while if both parameter values are above the threshold, it is classified into not drowsy conditions.

2.5 Data Analysis

Mean. The calculation of the average (mean) value was carried out to determine the trend of the measurement of the heart rate and respiration rate value on the

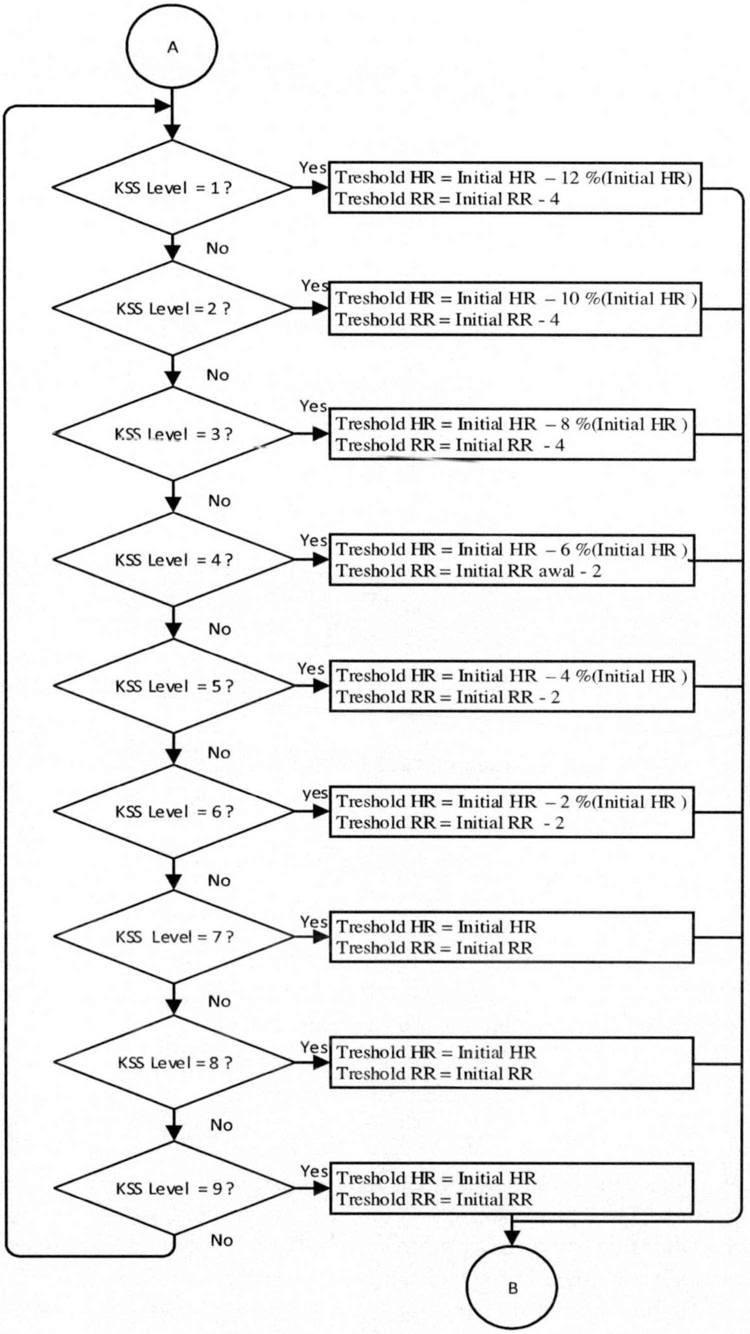

Fig. 4 Flowchart of the threshold formulation

Fig. 5 Drowsiness detection

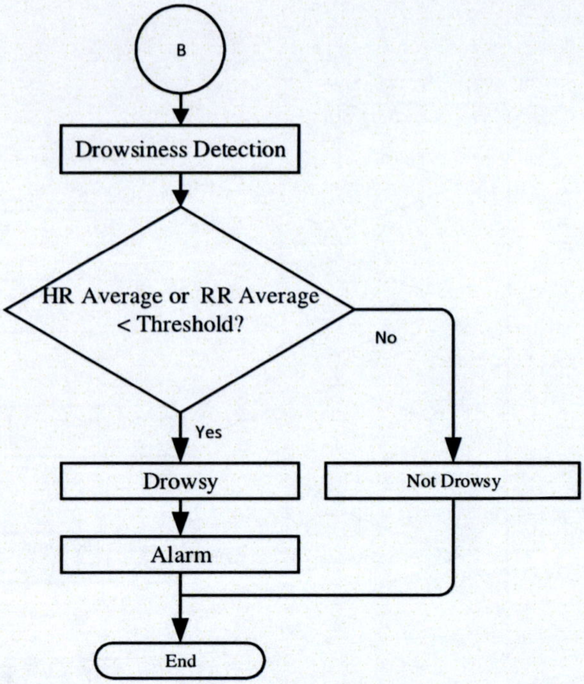

drowsiness condition level. Equation (10) shows the mean formula used in the data analysis process, where $\overline{x}$ is the data mean, $\sum x_n$ is the data value and n is the data amount.

$$mean(\overline{x}) = \sum \frac{x_n}{n} \tag{10}$$

Relative error. The calculation of relative error was carried out to determine the level of accuracy of the sensor reading to the actual value. The formula for the relative error or percent error is presented in the following Eq. (11).

$$\varepsilon_e = \frac{x_n - \overline{x}}{x_n} \times 100\% \tag{11}$$

where, X_n is the standard mean and $\overline{X}$ is the module mean.

Correlation. The calculation of correlation was carried out to determine the degree of relationship between the variables. The Correlation coefficient is a measure for determining the degree of relationship between the variables. The correlation coefficient can be formulated mathematically using the following Eq. (12):

$$R = \frac{n(\sum XY) - (\sum x) \cdot (\sum y)}{\sqrt{n\sum x^2 - (\sum x)^2 \cdot n(\sum y^2) - (\sum y^2)}} \quad (12)$$

where, *n* is the sum (total) of the observations, x is the measurement of variable 1, *y* is the measurement of variable 2, Σxy is the sum of both variables, Σx is the sum of variable 1, Σy is the sum of variable 2, Σx^2 is the sum of the squared values of variable 1 and Σy^2 is the sum of the squared values of variable 2.

Accuracy. The calculation of accuracy was carried out to determine the exact value of the drowsiness detection system classification using the threshold method. Accuracy is determined by calculating the True number of the drowsiness detection system against the entire data. The accuracy can be formulated mathematically using the following Eq. (13):

$$\text{accuracy } (\%) = \frac{\sum T}{\sum N} \cdot 100\% \quad (13)$$

where, T is the sum of True and N is the sum of the entire data

3 Results

3.1 Device Evaluation

The result of the module development consisted of two parts, namely the steering wheel of the car and the parts of the overall circuit. On the steering wheel of the car, there are 3 components, namely 1 XD-58C sensor which is a PPG sensor and 2 dry electrodes that diffuse as ECG leads on both hands of the driver. The Steering wheel of the car is presented in the following Fig. 6.

In addition to the 3 main components in the overall circuit, there are several other components, namely several buttons as inputs and battery indicators as this drowsiness detection system uses batteries, as well as an LCD display that can be seen in Fig. 7.

3.2 Results of Parameters Test

The results of the patient monitor test are presented in Table 2. The results of this test are in the form of error values of the module to the patient monitor and relative error values of the module to the patient monitor.

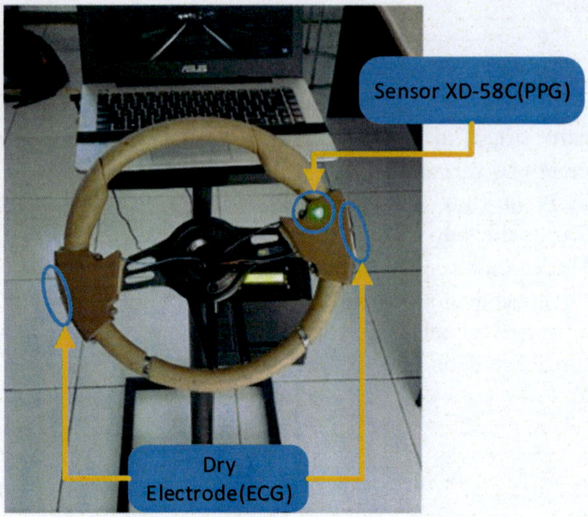

Fig. 6 Simulation of car steering wheel

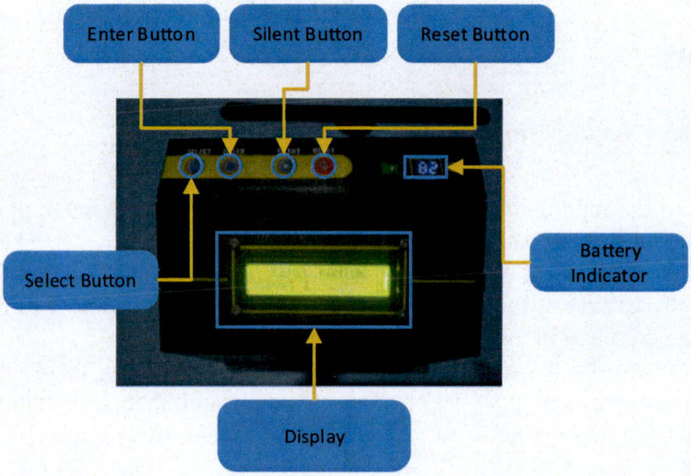

Fig. 7 Button and display

3.3 *Results of Drowsiness Test*

The results of the drowsiness detection system test were obtained from 5 respondents to get the heart rate and respiration rate values for 3 testing periods for each respondent. The results of these 5 respondent tests resulted in 1800 data on heart rate and respiration rate. The heart rate and respiration rate values obtained were seen for the value of changes and the distribution of heart rate and respiration rate data to a

Table 2 Results on the patient monitor test

No	Error values of heart rate (BPM)	Error values of respiration rate (Brpm)	Relative error values of heart rate (%)	Relative error values of respiration rate (%)
1	0.33	1.53	0.38	7.56
2	0.03	0.13	0.03	0.68
3	1.20	0.70	1.40	3.29
4	1.47	1.10	1.39	4.95
5	0.4	0.47	0.47	2.55
6	0.13	0.30	0.14	1.72
7	0.17	0.03	0.18	0.16
8	3.17	1.23	3.25	6.31
9	0.47	0.17	0.54	0.83
10	0.33	1.33	0.34	6.84
11	0.20	1.03	0.22	5.76
12	2.40	0.13	3.20	0.71
13	1.60	2.37	2.12	10.67
14	1.10	0.13	1.27	0.83
15	1.37	1.20	1.5	6.14
Mean of error values	1.002	0.927		
Relative error values (%)			1.167	4.419

person's drowsiness conditions, which is illustrated in the following box plot chart. Figure 8 shows the distribution of heart rate data.

In addition to the distribution of heart rate data in Fig. 8, there was also the distribution of respiration rate data, which is also illustrated in the form of box plot

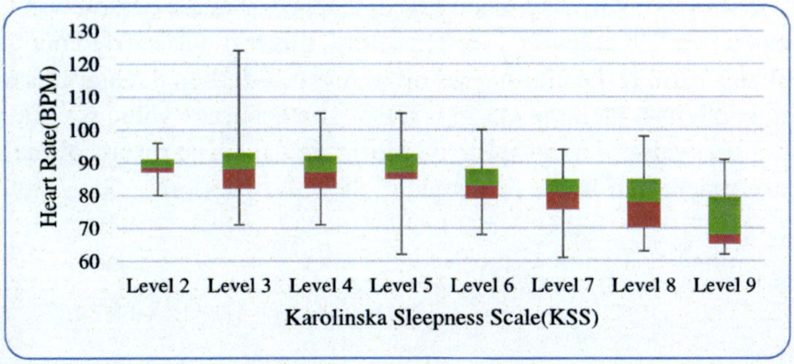

Fig. 8 Distribution of heart rate data on drowsiness condition levels

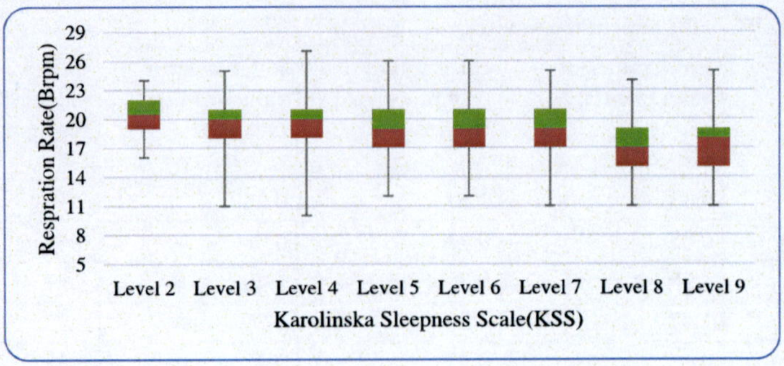

Fig. 9 Distribution of respiration rate data on drowsiness condition levels

Table 3 Correlation coefficient

Correlation relationship between-	Correlation coefficient	Correlation category
Heart rate and drowsiness condition levels	−0.49	Mid
Respiration rate and drowsiness condition levels	−0.26	Low

chart. From these box plot charts, it can see the distribution of data by looking at the maximum, minimum, lower quartile, upper quartile, and median values so that the trend line of the heart rate and respiration rate of each drowsiness condition levels can be known.

In addition to looking at the distribution of heart rate and respiration rate data, in this study, a correlation coefficient calculation was also carried out to see the degree of relationship between the heart rate and the drowsiness condition level, as well as the relationship between the respiration rate and the drowsiness condition levels (Fig. 9). The results of the calculation of the correlation coefficient are presented in the following Table 3.

Drowsiness classification testing was carried out to determine the accuracy of the drowsiness detection system, where in the test, the parameters tested were alarm sounds on the drowsiness condition levels. In this drowsiness detection system, a person will be said to be drowsy when it is at levels 7–9 and a person will be said to be not drowsy when it is at levels 1–6. Therefore, this test was carried out to find out the sound of an alarm. If the alarm goes off at levels 7–9 then the alarm is true but if it goes off at levels 1–6 then the alarm is false. The accuracy value is obtained from the number of true values on the alarm on the entire data. The results of the accuracy at each measurement period are presented in the following Fig. 10.

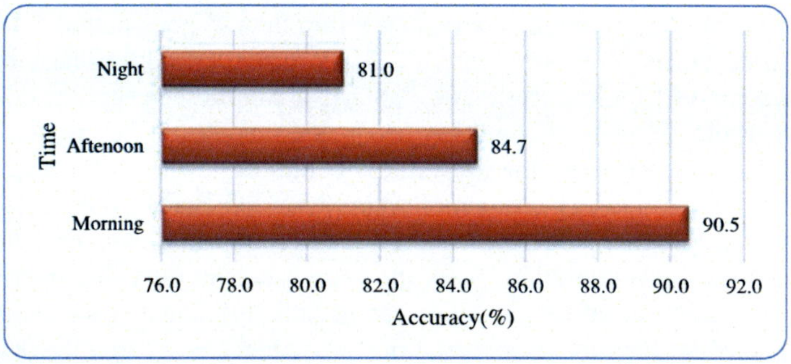

Fig. 10 Accuracy

4 Discussion

Based on the results of the patient monitor test—in which it is a standard tool where the result of the patient monitor reading is considered as the actual value—it was found that the largest absolute error value of the heart rate is 2.4 BPM and the smallest absolute error value of the heart rate is 0.03 BPM, while the average (mean) of the absolute error value is 1 BPM. Also, it was found that the largest absolute error value of the respiration rate is 2.97 Brpm and the smallest absolute error value of the respiration rate is 0.03 Brpm, while the average of the absolute error values is 0.93 Brpm. Based on these absolute error values, the relative error values were obtained where the average of the relative error value of the heart rate is 1.167% and the average of the relative error value of the respiration rate is 4.491%.

The results of the heart rate data distribution chart are presented in Fig. 6. It can be seen from the entire drowsiness condition levels, the heart rate value shows a decreasing trend line where on each drowsiness condition level the median value tends to decrease and the largest data distribution value is on the drowsiness condition level 3 because the minimum and maximum values on the KSS scale have a very long range compared to other drowsiness condition levels. Likewise with the distribution of respiration rate data chart which is presented in Fig. 4, it can be seen from the entire drowsiness condition levels, the respiration rate value shows a decreasing trend line where on each drowsiness condition level the median value tends to decrease and the largest data distribution value is on the drowsiness condition level 4 because the minimum and maximum values on the KSS scale have a very long range compared to other the drowsiness condition levels.

To determine the relationship between the drowsiness condition levels and heart rate, and the relationship between the drowsiness condition levels and respiration rate, correlation testing was carried out on these parameters. The correlation value (r) ranges from 1 to −1, the value of closer to 1 or −1 means that the relationship between the two variables is getting stronger, on the contrary, the value of closer to 0 means that the relationship between the two variables is getting weaker. A positive value indicates a unidirectional relationship (X goes up then Y goes up) and a negative value indicates an inverse relationship (X goes up then Y goes down). The results of testing the correlation of heart rate, respiration rate, and drowsiness condition levels is presented in Table 1. Based on Table 1, it can be seen that the correlation value between the drowsiness condition levels and respiration rate is −0.26 while the correlation value between the drowsiness condition levels and heart rate is of −0.49 which means that the correlation value between the drowsiness condition levels and respiration rate is in the low correlation range while the correlation value between the drowsiness condition levels and heart rate is in the medium correlation range. The two correlation relationships are negatively valued, which means that the two relationships have an inverse relationship, namely the greater the drowsiness condition levels, the smaller the respiration rate and heart rate. This results are similar to the chart of the distribution of heart rate and respiration rate data. Based on the results of correlation testing, it can be concluded that the two parameters, namely the heart rate and respiration rate, have an inverse relationship with the drowsiness condition levels even though the respiration rate correlation value is included in the low correlation range.

The next is drowsiness classification testing which was carried out to determine the accuracy of the drowsiness detection system. This test was carried out by looking at the true and false values of the output alarm in the drowsiness detection system. The results of this test are presented in Fig. 5. Based on the results of the drowsiness classification testing, it was found that the largest accuracy value was obtained at a value of 90.5% in the morning and the smallest accuracy value was obtained at a value of 81% in the evening. This was because in the morning, people are usually in a low drowsiness conditions so that the drowsiness detection system will always detect respondents as people who are not sleepy, unlike the condition found in the evening, where the drowsiness detection system will have a low level of accuracy because in the evening (at night) people usually are in a high drowsiness condition so that the drowsiness detection system often experiences misclassification when switching from a non-drowsy condition to a drowsy condition. This accuracy value is caused by the correlation values between the drowsiness condition levels and heart rate which is only moderate, and the drowsiness condition levels and respiration rate which is low.

When compared to previous studies [17], the accuracy of the drowsiness detection system with the threshold method is still much lower than with the machine learning method. But, this study has succeeded to measure the heart rate and respiration rate with sensors that are non-instructive [17, 33]. Based on these results, it can be concluded that the accuracy results of the drowsiness detection system with the threshold method have poor results if applied to their actual conditions because it still has a fairly low accuracy value.

5 Conclusion

This study was conducted to determine the accuracy of the drowsiness detection system using the threshold method with heart rate and respiration rate parameters and to create a drowsiness detection system that is not instructive in drivers. The results showed that the correlation value between the drowsiness condition levels and respiration rate is low, with a value of −0.26 and the correlation value between the drowsiness condition levels and heart rate is moderate, with a value of −0.49, but these two values show a negative correlation value which means that every increase in the drowsiness conditions will make the heart rate and respiration rate decrease. The drowsiness detection system using the threshold method with heart rate and respiration rate parameters has a low accuracy value when drivers are in a condition between drowsy and not drowsy. Therefore, it is still difficult to apply to the actual driving conditions. However, this study has succeeded to develop a non-instructive drowsiness detection system for drivers, so it is hoped that subsequent studies will use a machine learning sleepiness classification system by using non-instructive sensors so that they can improve the accuracy of the sleepiness detection system and apply it to actual driving conditions.

References

1. Siddiqui HUR, Saleem AA, Brown R, Bademci B, Lee E, Rustam F, Dudley S (2021) Non-invasive driver drowsiness detection system. Sensors 21. https://doi.org/10.3390/s21144833
2. Leng LB, Giin LB, Chung WY (2015) Based on biomedical and motion sensors. Sensors 15–18
3. Lee BG, Lee BL, Chung WY (2014) Mobile healthcare for automatic driving sleep-onset detection using wavelet-based EEG and respiration signals. Sensors (Switzerland) 14:17915–17936. https://doi.org/10.3390/s141017915
4. Yulianto E, Indrato TB, Bima TMN, Suharyati (2020) Wheelchair for quadriplegic patient with electromyography signal control wireless. Int J Online Biomed Eng 16:94–115. https://doi.org/10.3991/ijoe.vl6il2.15721
5. Yulianto E, Muzakkir HW, Triwiyanto, Nugraha PC, Moch Prastawa P, Lamidi (2022) Development of electromyography signal contraction detection using the double threshold method for controlling wheelchair. J Biomimetics Biomater Biomed Eng 55:93–106. https://doi.org/10.4028/p-04pbd2
6. Solaz J, Laparra-Hernández J, Bande D, Rodríguez N, Veleff S, Gerpe J, Medina E (2016) Drowsiness detection based on the analysis of breathing rate obtained from real-time image recognition. Transp Res Procedia 14:3867–3876. https://doi.org/10.1016/j.trpro.2016.05.472
7. Jacobé de Naurois C, Bourdin C, Stratulat A, Diaz E, Vercher JL (2019) Detection and prediction of driver drowsiness using artificial neural network models. Accid Anal Prev 126:95–104. https://doi.org/10.1016/j.aap.2017.11.038
8. Waldeck MR, Lambert MI (2003) Heart rate during sleep: implications for monitoring training status. J Sport Sci Med 2:133–138
9. Charlton PH, Bonnici T, Tarassenko L (2016) An assessment of algorithms to estimate respiratory rate from the electrocardiogram. https://doi.org/10.1088/0967-3334/37/4/610

10. Charlton PH, Bonnici T, Tarassenko L, Alastruey J, Clifton DA, Beale R, Watkinson PJ (2017) Extraction of respiratory signals from the electrocardiogram and photoplethysmogram: technical and physiological determinants. Physiol Meas 38:669–690. https://doi.org/10.1088/1361-6579/aa670e
11. Kessler V, Kächele M, Meudt S, Schwenker F, Palm G (2016) Machine learning driven heart rate detection with camera photoplethysmography in time domain. Lecture Notes in Computer Science. (including Subser. Lect. Notes Artif. Intell. Lect. Notes Bioinformatics), vol 9896 LNAI, pp 324–334. https://doi.org/10.1007/978-3-319-46182-3_27
12. Kiashari SEH, Nahvi A, Homayounfard A, Bakhoda H (2018) Monitoring the variation in driver respiration rate from wakefulness to drowsiness: a non-intrusive method for drowsiness detection using thermal imaging. J Sleep Sci 3:1–9
13. Das N, Chakraborty M (2017) Performance analysis of FIR and IIR filters for ECG signal denoising based on SNR. In: Proceedings of 2017 third international conference on research in computational intelligence and communication networks, ICRCICN 2017, pp 90–97. https://doi.org/10.1109/ICRCICN.2017.8234487
14. khandpur R (2002) Handbook of second edition biomedical instrumentation
15. Wei C, Sheng L, Lihua G, Yuquan C, Min P (2011) Study on conditioning and feature extraction algorithm of photoplethysmography signal for physiological parameters detection. In: Proceedings of 4th international congress on image and signal processing. CISP 2011, vol 4, pp 2194–2197. https://doi.org/10.1109/CISP.2011.6100581
16. Lee H, Lee J, Shin M (2019) Using wearable ECG/PPG sensors for driver drowsiness detection based on distinguishable pattern of recurrence plots. Electron 8. https://doi.org/10.3390/electronics8020192
17. Yaacob S, Izzati Affandi NA, Krishnan P, Rasyadan A, Yaakop M, Mohamed F (2020) Drowsiness detection using EEG and ECG signals. In: IEEE international conference on artificial intelligence in engineering and technology, IICAIET 2020, pp 2–6. https://doi.org/10.1109/IICAIET49801.2020.9257867
18. Jo S, Kim J, Kim DK, Jo S, Kim J (2019) Heart rate change while drowsy driving. 34:8–12
19. Maxim (2018) MAX86150 integrated photoplethysmogram and electrocardiogram bio-sensor module for mobile health. MAX86150 datasheet 49
20. Embedded Lab. Introducing easy pulse: a DIY photoplethysmographic sensor for measuring heart rate
21. Abdul H, Dalimi A, Jaafar H (2015) Detecting drowsy driver using pulse sensor. Jurnal Teknologi 3:5–8
22. Shahid A, Wilkinson K, Marcu S, Shapiro CM (2012) STOP, THAT and one hundred other sleep scales. 1–406. https://doi.org/10.1007/978-1-4419-9893-4
23. Zhang A, Liu F (2012) Drowsiness detection based on wavelet analysis of ECG and pulse signals. In: 2012 5th international conference on biomedical engineering and informatics, BMEI 2012, pp 491–495. https://doi.org/10.1109/BMEI.2012.6513058
24. Gunawan IPC, Andayani DH, Triwiyanto T, Yulianto E, Rahmawati T, Soetjiatie L, Musvika SD (2020) Design and development of telemedicine based heartbeat and body temperature monitoring tools. IOP Conf Ser Mater Sci Eng 850
25. Wardhani NV, Aulia AM, Yulianto E, Mak'Ruf MR, Indrato TB, Setioningsih ED, Sumber, Triwiyanto T (2019) A portable vital sign device with liquid crystal display TFT touchscreen. In: Proceedings of 2019 international seminar on application for technology of information and communication: industry 4.0: retrospect, prospect, and challenges, iSemantic 2019, pp 429–433. https://doi.org/10.1109/ISEMANTIC.2019.8884351
26. Varon C, Morales J, Lázaro J, Orini M, Deviaene M, Kontaxis S, Testelmans D, Buyse B, Borzée P, Sörnmo L, Laguna P, Gil E, Bailón R (2020) A comparative study of ECG-derived respiration in ambulatory monitoring using the single-lead ECG. Sci Rep 10:1–14. https://doi.org/10.1038/s41598-020-62624-5
27. Helfenbein E, Firoozabadi R, Chien S, Carlson E, Babaeizadeh S (2014) Development of three methods for extracting respiration from the surface ECG: a review. J Electrocardiol 47:819–825. https://doi.org/10.1016/j.jelectrocard.2014.07.020

28. Rahimi A, Safari A, Mohebbi M (2019) Sleep stage classification based on ECG-derived respiration and heart rate variability of single-lead ECG signal. In: 2019 26th national and 4th international Iranian conference on biomedical engineering ICBME 2019, pp 158–163. https://doi.org/10.1109/ICBME49163.2019.9030391
29. Charlton PH, Birrenkott DA, Bonnici T, Pimentel MAF, Johnson AEW, Alastruey J, Tarassenko L, Watkinson PJ, Beale R, Clifton DA (2018) Breathing rate estimation from the electrocardiogram and photoplethysmogram: a review. IEEE Rev Biomed Eng 11:2–20. https://doi.org/10.1109/RBME.2017.2763681
30. Tan L (2008) Digital signal processing fundamentals and applications. Elsevier, USA
31. An X, Stylios GK (2020) Comparison of motion artefact reduction methods and the implementation of adaptive motion artefact reduction in wearable electrocardiogram monitoring. Sensors (Switzerland)
32. Bhahri S, Rachmat (2018) Transformasi Citra Biner Menggunakan. J Sist Inf dan Teknol Inf 7:195–203
33. Sekar K, Thileeban R, Padmini TN (2022) Drowsiness and real-time road condition detection using heart rate sensor, accelerometer and gyroscope

Comparing Machine Learning and Deep Learning Approaches to Diagnose Epilepsy Disease

Shahed Salehzehi, Elyas Irankhah, and Maryam Sabet

Abstract Even though, epilepsy is recognized as a component of brain disease, and seizures in these diseases vary from person to person. This study aimed to implement some procedures based on machine learning and deep learning on EEG signal frequency, where they were compared with each other. Accordingly, to extract more accurate statistical features such as the Short-Time Fourier Transform (STFT) environment in terms of which artificial intelligent algorithms are the most effective applications for early diagnosis in epilepsy disease, is the significant point of the research. After removing the noise from the EEG signal, it entered the STFT environment, where its spectrogram was determined. In the STFT environment, the statistical features of the signal have been extracted, which are segmented at a frequency sampling rate of 173.61 Hz in the form of triangular windows. Finally, seven segmentations have been obtained, in each of which four features have been extracted, for a total of 28 statistical features. Technically, in terms of the deep learning algorithm, feature extraction is done by performing CNN models such as Xception, EfficientNetB0, ResNet50, and VGG16, which are given as inputs to a simple model with the label of being healthy or an epileptic patient, and then the classification of two classes has been applied. In addition, in the machine learning algorithm, basically, the EEG signals were transferred from the time domain to the STFT domain while they were placed next to each other, where we applied an ANOVA feature selection, and extracted 10 main features, which are given to the model as inputs. Furthermore, K-Fold Validation was performed in the dataset evaluation and division section, and eventually, the results were computed in the Support Vector Machine (SVM) model, which equaled 95%, Linear Discriminant Analysis (LDA) equaled 97.5%, and K-nearest neighbors (KNN) equaled 90%. As a conclusion, the study has been figured

S. Salehzehi (✉)
Department of Biomedical Engineering, Islamic Azad University of Mashhad, Mashhad, Iran
e-mail: Shahedsalehzehii@gmail.com

E. Irankhah
Department of Mechanical Engineering, University of Massachusetts Lowell, Lowell, MA, USA

M. Sabet
Department of Computer Engineering, Fasa University, Fasa, Iran

T. Triwiyanto et al. (eds.), *Proceeding of the 3rd International Conference on Electronics, Biomedical Engineering, and Health Informatics*, Lecture Notes in Electrical Engineering 1008, https://doi.org/10.1007/978-981-99-0248-4_44

out that the deep learning algorithm has better performance than the machine learning algorithm in order to early diagnose epilepsy disease.

Keywords Epilepsy disease · Machine learning · Deep learning · EEG signals

1 Introduction

In the human world, the impact of machine learning models is felt more than ever in human lives, which means machine learning has presented a great assistant to humans, especially in treatment environments as new sciences are being discovered [1]. Actually, by making progress in science, the deep learning model, is more complex. According to this truth, brain disorders can be different in humans, and seizures caused by epilepsy are also able to occur in several ways of spectrum. These spectra, which have been created through the electrical activities in the brain, have characteristics that can be potentially effective in either improving or diagnosing.

Nowadays, many approaches are applied to diagnose the disease, such as Machine Learning, Deep Learning, utilizing different Neural Networks, etc., although, the significant point in these procedures is how to implement them and how to extract features from them. In addition, it should be stated that, in some of the mentioned approaches, researchers are working to get the best, most optimal novel procedures. For example, Yang Li published a study that brain signals can be classified using the LPP algorithm. Of course, such a work is not able to figure out and classify epileptic seizures definitively, however, it can be increasingly effective. In addition, G. Shahraki has proposed that the mixture of EEG signals data with MRI images are practical in early diagnosis. Conversely, this study emphasized about existence of a relationship between the image and the signals, which are progressing the process of diagnosis in the disease [2–4]. One of the issues to consider in the field of artificial intelligence, which is known as deep learning, can be seen in H. Li's study that has gained the adequate results by implementing the classification of EEG signals through deep learning models [5].

Actually, how to extract the EEG signals is one of the most important points that is typically emphasized in diagnosis even in clinical works. Particularly, to obtain optimal accuracy in terms of machine learning features, some studies have focused on EEG frequency, which is the appropriate environment to extract more details [6, 7].

As regards machine learning models, it should be considered that diagnosing brain diseases require to intervene human generally, but by machine learning techniques this issue would be removed, where the machine learns how to perform with the scripts [8, 9]. Many works recently have been done by utilizing deep learning algorithms, for example, in the study of the entire part of the process implemented by Xception networks with an accuracy percentage of 98.47%, which is compared to the current study this number has reached 100% diagnosis of the epilepsy disease. These days, recent research has proven that engineers and MD doctors in the field of artificial intelligence have not yet achieved a coherent and definitive procedure in the treatment of epilepsy or its early diagnosis, and they are looking for the implementation of algorithms to achieve that as soon as possible [10, 11].

The cited studies believe that the implementation and applying of deep learning algorithm is an advantageous way to carry out diagnostic purposes in the human brain diseases. Although, this path is delighted, but benefiting from other paths such as machine learning algorithms along with deep learning have shown a proof to demonstrate the superiority of each of them.

In the continuation, it would be appeared to see how machine learning has been applied in this study by STFT, also how to take out the results by feature selection tools. Additionally, it should be noted that this issue clearly shows how, based on other studies and research, there is a relationship between the implemented methods that can improve their ideas and methods.

2 Materials and Method

2.1 Dataset

The dataset used in this work was prepared in collaboration with the University of Bonn,[1] Germany, and was analyzed in three cases. The first condition is normal people who have subtitles A and B, the second condition includes people who had epilepsy but did not have seizures, which is included in the C and D subgroups; and eventually, the third condition includes people who have epilepsy and seizures, who have been placed in the E subgroup. Technically, it has been considered only healthy people in A group with severe people in E group while we were comparing the feature extraction results with each other in these groups. Frequency sampling equaled 176.3 by a single channel in the 100 cases in each group. Figure 1 represents the EEG signal for the normal and epileptic groups in the time domain.

2.2 De-noising EEG Signal

The modification of noise removal methods has been proposed in order to reduce the distortion of the signal. Actually in these methods, the effects of frequency correction are adjusted in such a way that by leaving a certain amount of initial noise, a certain improvement in the signal-to-noise ratio is achieved, and instead, the distortion of the signal is minimized [12]. By applying a parameter, the benefits of several noise removal methods are adjusted to achieve a certain level of noise removal. In fact,

[1] https://www.ukbonn.de.

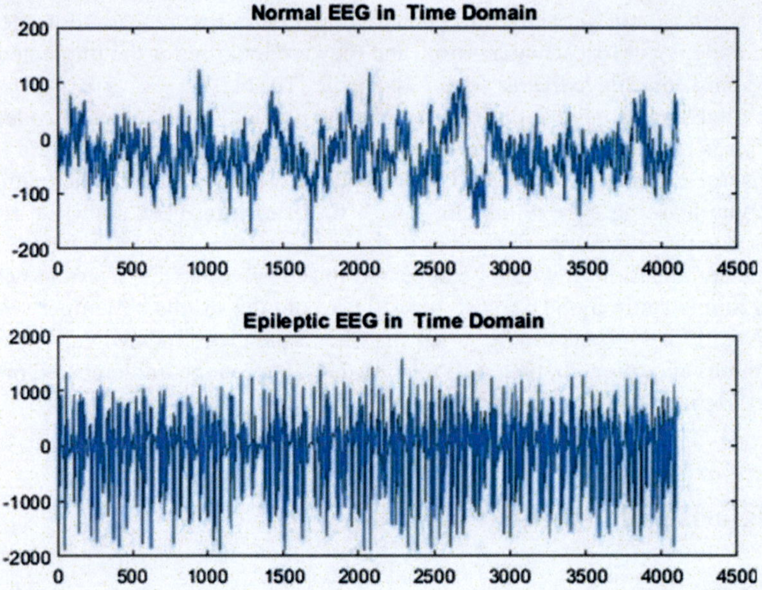

Fig. 1 Shown the frequency EEG signal in time domain (from above, respectively, normal people, epileptic people)

de-noising EEG signals by transferring them to the wavelet environment uses two filters, which are: the average filter and the detail filter [13].

2.3 Short-Time Fourier Transform (STFT)

According to the studies, one of the cons of the classical Fourier transform is that it does not reflect the local behavior of the signal. Technically, a simple way to overcome this problem is to compare the signal with basic functions localized in both time and frequency domains [14]. Actually, short-term Fourier transform, or STFT, is one of the primary methods of comparing signals with these preliminary functions, which are defined as follows (1):

$$\mathrm{STFT}(t,\omega) = \int_{-\infty}^{+\infty} s(\tau)\gamma^{*}_{t,\omega}(\tau)d\tau \tag{1}$$

where $\mathrm{STFT}(t,\omega)$ indicates the window function, $s(\tau)$ indicates the signal which is transformed. In the above expression, $\gamma(\mathrm{t})$ is a time function with limited length called the window function where the short-term Fourier transform is the windowed Fourier transform of the signal in different time intervals. This conversion is also written as follows also (2):

$$\mathrm{STFT}(t,\omega) = \int_{-\infty}^{+\infty} s(\tau)\gamma^{*}(\tau - t)e^{-j\omega\tau}d\tau = <s(t), \gamma(\tau - t)e^{j\omega\tau}>$$

$$\gamma_{t,\omega}(\tau) = \gamma(\tau - t)e^{j\omega\tau} \tag{2}$$

where the variables such as $\gamma_{t,\omega}(\tau)$ are discrete and quantized.

2.4 Spectrogram Images

Nowadays, research has shown that the power of a signal over time would be displayed at different frequencies as a waveform by a spectrograph. Thus, spectrograms are able to be displayed as two-dimensional graphs with a third variable represented by colors. Plus, the same applies to 3D graphs with a fourth color gamut. Based on the following figures, the spectrogram of normal people as well as epileptic group are plotted as shown in Figs. 2 and 3.

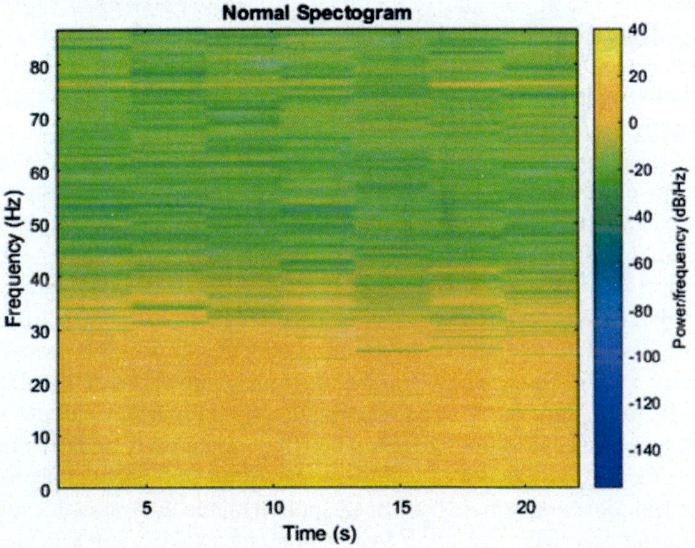

Fig. 2 Spectrogram images in normal people

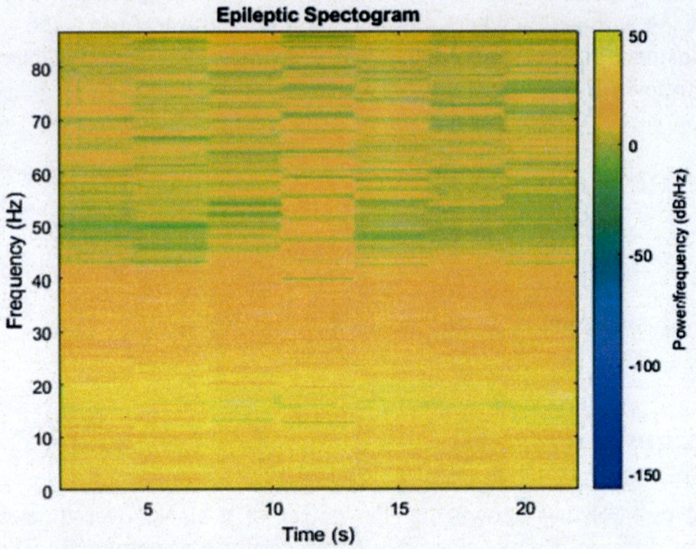

Fig. 3 Spectrogram images in epileptic patients

2.5 *Machine Learning*

Machine learning algorithms perform computational and statistical approaches to learn directly from data rather than using a predetermined equation that might operate like a model. The efficiency of machine learning algorithms improves by increasing the number of samples and data during the learning process [15–17]. For an example in this context, "deep learning" is a subset of machine learning that trains computers to imitate human characteristics. Basically, deep learning has provided better performance parameters than conventional machine learning algorithms [18, 19]. Based on the input data and issues including whether they are labeled or unlabeled, the machine learning algorithm makes an estimate of a pattern in the data. At this stage, a decision must be made regarding the type of data, the algorithm execution method, and the problem-solving approach that should be selected. In addition, if the model can correlate well with the data in the training dataset, the weights are adjusted to reduce the accuracy difference between the previously known models and the newly created model estimate [20, 21]. The machine learning algorithm iterates this optimization as well as an evaluation process where it automatically updates the weights until the desired goal is reached. Technically, based on the machine learning algorithm, three significant classifiers have been applied on the dataset which are: Linear discriminant analysis (LDA), Support Vector Machine (SVM), and k-nearest neighbors. As it mentioned clearly in the Table 1. In the result section, the highest accuracy percentage founded on dataset classification is in LDA model.

Table 1 The accuracy/sensitivity/specificity of classifiers by machine learning models

Machine learning model	Accuracy (%)	Sensitivity (%)	Specificity (%)
K-nearest neighbors algorithm (KNN)	90	85	95
Support-vector machines (SVM)	95	100	90
Linear discriminant analysis (LDA)	97.50	100	95

2.6 Deep Learning

Deep learning is a multi-layered algorithmic machine learning method inspired by the neural network of the human brain. Like the deep neural networks in our brains, deep learning architecture plays an important role in complementing the processed information in the field of artificial intelligence. Concretely, the word "deep" refers to the number of layers through which data is transformed during processes. By using deep learning, it is possible to teach machines the tasks that humans usually do [22, 23].

Since this work is applied CNN, these deep neural networks, which work specifically with things like image classification, mimic the neural network found in the brain's visual cortex. As a result, CNNs provide unique insights into the processing of specific data. CNNs are networks used when analyzing data including images, audio files, and video clips. An input and output layer as well as several hidden layers make up the structure of a CNN [24].

As mentioned before, one of the most significant deep learning models for computer vision and its applications in related fields is convolutional neural networks. Convolutional neural networks include a set of "Convolution Layers" and "Pooling Layers" that enable the deep learning model to extract relevant features (for modeling and decision-making) from "Visual Data" such as images. Due to the existence of such "multi-layer architecture" in convolutional neural networks, these networks will be able to learn powerful "hierarchical" (hierarchical) features in the image. This class of learned features is unaffected by "spatial invariant," "rotational invariant," and "translational invariant" changes; in other words, this class of methods is unaffected by these spatial factors; rotational and translational invariant [25, 26].

According to the above description, in this work, it has been attempted to perform convolutional neural network weights such as ResNet50, VGG16, EfficeintNetB0, and Xception, which are implemented so that the feature extraction process is used after the processes [27, 28]. Potentially, the input labels were imported into two classes: normal and epileptic patients, for classification into the implemented model. In Table 2, the accuracies are computed in order to compare with each other. Obviously, the highest accuracy equaled 99% for both VGG16 and EfficeintNetB0.

Table 2 The accuracy/sensitivity/specificity of classifiers by deep learning models

Pretrained network	Accuracy (%)	Sensitivity (%)	Specificity (%)
Xception	98	100	96
EfficientNetB0	99	98	98
VGG16	99	98	100
ResNet50	98	96	96

3 Results

In general, as mentioned in the previous sections, the principal goal of this study was to compare the outputs of artificial intelligence approaches, which these days are playing a significant role in the early diagnosis and treatment of brain diseases. According to the results obtained from the machine learning model, the classifiers have shown that the lowest accuracy percentage is for KNN which is equaled 90% and the highest percentage is obtained by LDA which is also equaled 97.5%.

In the deep learning model, the spectrogram photos in two classes, normal and epileptic patients, are divided into training and testing data, then using the models mentioned in Fig. 4 the weights that have already been seen on the ImageNet dataset in the form of training, features have been extracted for each image. Eventually, the features are entered with their class type as input to the two-class classification model while the training model sees, by re-calling the model for the test data, and the above evaluation results are obtained, which is the lowest percentage for Xception and ResNet50 the highest is for VGG16 as well as EfficeintNetB0. As is obvious, the performance of the deep learning algorithm has been better compared to the performance of the machine learning algorithm (Figs. 5, 6, 7, 8 and 9).

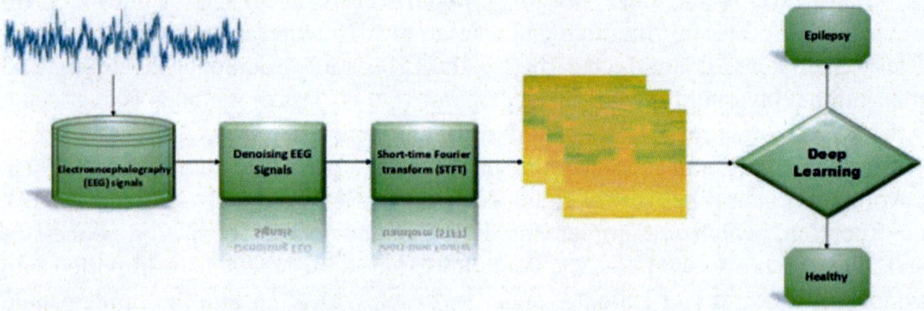

Fig. 4 Deep learning algorithm block diagram

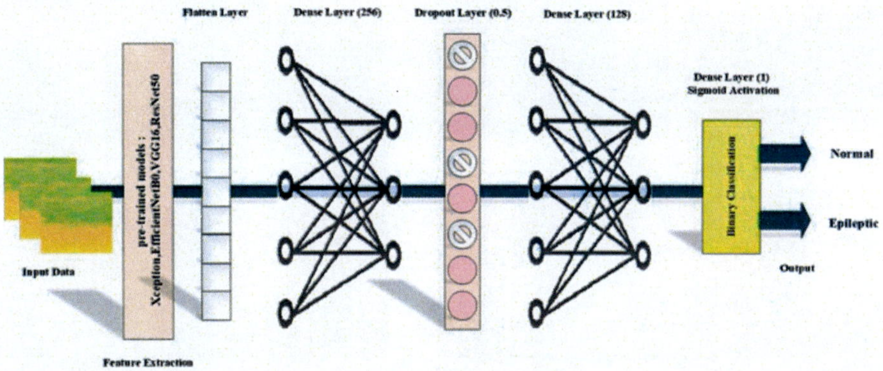

Fig. 5 Deep learning architecture

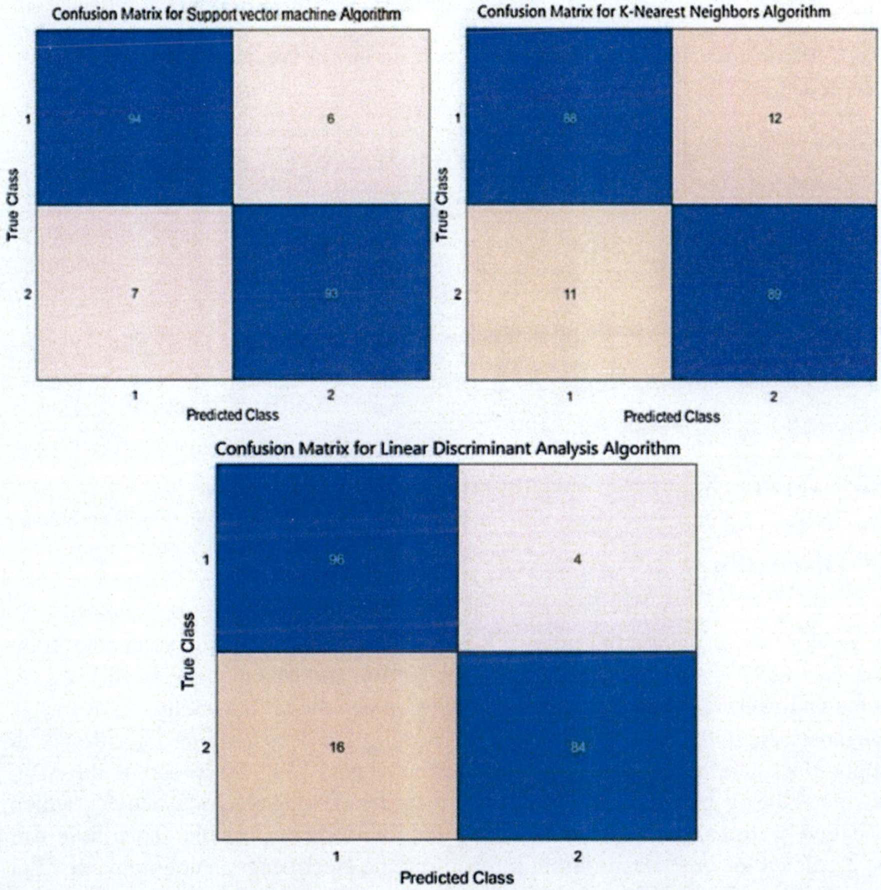

Fig. 6 Confusion matrix for machine learning models

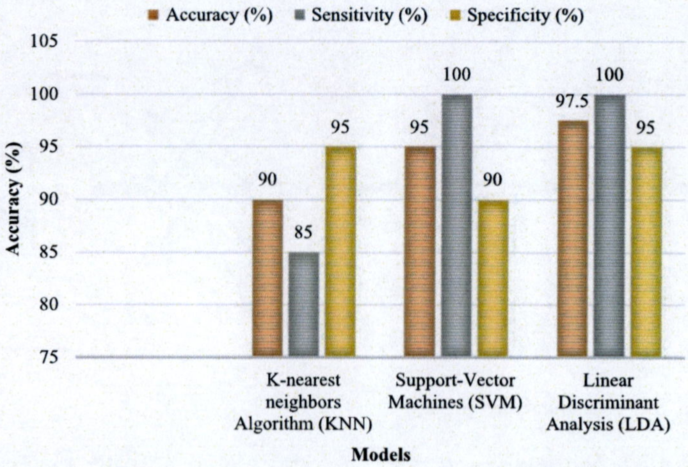

Fig. 7 The accuracy, sensitivity, specificity of classifiers by machine learning model

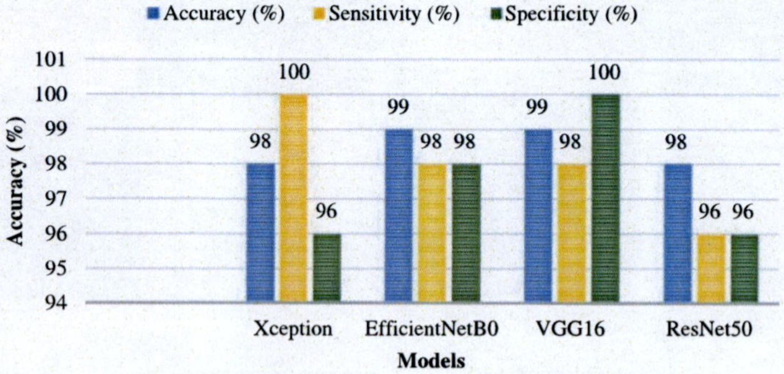

Fig. 8 The accuracy, sensitivity, specificity of classifiers by deep learning model

4 Discussion

In general, the diagnosis of epilepsy is basically one of the most challenging brain diseases and is usually discussed among scientists and MD doctors. In this regard, some engineering-science procedures would be beneficial to MD doctors for early diagnosis. As stated in the study, machine learning and deep learning algorithms that apply classifiers have shown significant effectiveness [29]. Since one of the main effects in the occurrence of epilepsy is the disorder of brain electrical activity, which is called seizures, they should be controlled as much as possible. This issue can be predicted to some extent through recording the electroencephalography, or EEG signals. Classifiers are able to be performed in line with the accuracy of data output, so that, as the study mentioned, the results have been compared with new deep learning models such as neural networks. Eventually, results were obtained for the two classes,

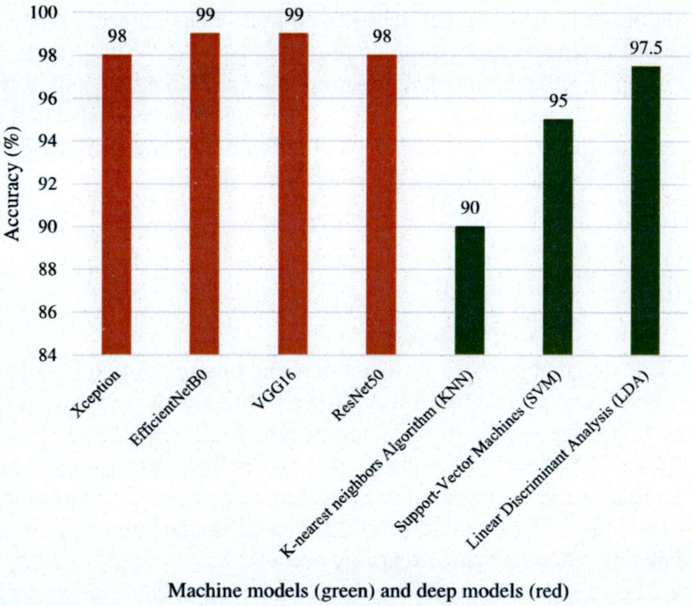

Fig. 9 Accuracy of machine learning and deep learning models

95.92, and 98.08%, respectively. In another study, applied machine learning and deep learning methods are used to diagnose psychiatric disorders including bipolar disorder by EEG signals. Overall, four models of the machine learning algorithms were implemented, which are: an extreme gradient boosting (XGB), k-nearest neighbors (KNN), decision tree (DT), Gaussian Naïve Bayes (GNB), and support vector machine (SVM), while the best percentage obtained was equal to 94% by XGB [30]. It is worth noting that based on the previous evidence and research, the studies whose accuracy percentage is above 90% have better performance in terms of processing and diagnosing the disease. On the other hand, some researchers, believe that automatic deep learning algorithms can play a significant role in clinical reports and related analyses. In this research, in addition to pointing out the important notes in this direction, the VGG-16 neural network model has been applied to validate the data for the diagnosis of epilepsy, that the output equaled 98%. It is quite clear that compared to the output of the VGG16 neural network implemented in this research, which is equal to 98.55, the performance of the trained neural network has been better. Accordingly, the study performance in comparison to the others shows the better efficiency where the authors have attempted to improve the results as well as optimize them. Finally, this issue proved that, to achieve the purpose of early diagnosis of epilepsy disease, it is necessary to develop and implement the deep learning algorithms [21]. Since the review of the implemented models in voluminous dimensions has not been done in terms of datasets, it is important to note that the diagnosis of brain diseases and disorders through artificial intelligence algorithms is highly dependent on pre-recorded clinical datasets. In fact, these algorithms are meant to facilitate the processing of high volumes of clinic data. According to the statistical community of epileptic patients, data creation is a costly method with a long duration to be able to gather the patient's clinical data in a comprehensive and complete manner. Although, today with the existence of specialized centers in these fields, this has become easier, but there are still data creation problems.

5 Conclusion

In this study, the original purpose is to compare the outputs of two substantial algorithms in artificial intelligence. As it was shown in this result comparison that in the feature extraction stage, verity of the features which are not extracted by the user, are extracted with the algorithm in which this issue shows the disadvantage of this algorithm, so that in the deep learning algorithm extraction, the feature is going to extract automatically. All these descriptions are based on the numerical results which is LDA equaled 97.5% by machine learning and 98.08% by deep learning. In future work, this will be attempted by applying algorithms such as GNN networks or graphs neural network in order to better and more accurately diagnose the disease.

References

1. Mateo-Sotos J, Torres AM, Santos JL, Quevedo O, Basar C (2022) A machine learning-based method to identify bipolar disorder patients. Circuits Syst Signal Process 41:2244–2265. https://doi.org/10.1007/s00034-021-01889-1
2. Liu Y, Jiang B, Feng J, Hu J, Zhang H (2021) Classification of EEG signals for epileptic seizures using feature dimension reduction algorithm based on LPP. Multimed Tools Appl 80:30261–30282. https://doi.org/10.1007/s11042-020-09135-7
3. Srinath R, Gayathri R (2022) Epilepsy disorder detection and diagnosis using empirical mode decomposition and deep learning architecture. Concurr Comput 34. https://doi.org/10.1002/cpe.6903
4. Li H, Wu L (2022) EEG classification of normal and alcoholic by deep learning. Brain Sci 12:778. https://doi.org/10.3390/brainsci12060778
5. Shahraki G, Irankhah E (2022) Diagnosis of epilepsy disease with MRI images analysis and EEG signal processing. https://doi.org/10.1007/978-981-19-1804-9_40
6. Gia TN, Wang Z, Westerlund T (2022) Detection of epilepsy seizures based on deep learning with attention mechanism. https://doi.org/10.1007/978-3-031-06368-8_5
7. Yin W, Li L, Wu F-X (2022) Deep learning for brain disorder diagnosis based on fMRI images. Neurocomputing 469:332–345. https://doi.org/10.1016/j.neucom.2020.05.113
8. Ibrahim FE, Emara HM, El-Shafai W, Elwekeil M, Rihan M, Eldokany IM, Taha TE, El-Fishawy AS, El-Rabaie EM, Abdellatef E, Abd El-Samie FE (2022) Deep-learning-based seizure detection and prediction from electroencephalography signals. Int J Numer Method Biomed Eng 38. https://doi.org/10.1002/cnm.3573
9. Beeraka SM, Kumar A, Sameer M, Ghosh S, Gupta B (2022) Accuracy enhancement of epileptic seizure detection: a deep learning approach with hardware realization of STFT. Circuits Syst Signal Process 41:461–484. https://doi.org/10.1007/s00034-021-01789-4

10. Sowmya N, Pradhan S, Biswal PK, Panda SK, Misra VP (2022) Epileptic seizure detection using deep learning architecture. https://doi.org/10.1007/978-981-19-2277-0_22
11. Irankhah E (2020) Evaluation of early detection methods for Alzheimer's disease. Bioprocess Eng 4:17. https://doi.org/10.11648/j.be.20200401.13
12. Qaisar SM, Hussain SF (2021) Effective epileptic seizure detection by using level-crossing EEG sampling sub-bands statistical features selection and machine learning for mobile healthcare. Comput Methods Programs Biomed 203:106034. https://doi.org/10.1016/j.cmpb.2021.106034
13. Chalaki M, Omranpour H (2022) Epileptic seizure classification using ConvLSTM deep classifier and rotation short-time Fourier transform. J Ambient Intell Humaniz Comput. https://doi.org/10.1007/s12652-022-04204-1
14. Ahmad I, Wang X, Zhu M, Wang C, Pi Y, Khan JA, Khan S, Samuel OW, Chen S, Li G (2022) EEG-based epileptic seizure detection via machine/deep learning approaches: a systematic review. Comput Intell Neurosci 2022:1–20. https://doi.org/10.1155/2022/6486570
15. Yuan J, Ran X, Liu K, Yao C, Yao Y, Wu H, Liu Q (2022) Machine learning applications on neuroimaging for diagnosis and prognosis of epilepsy: a review. J Neurosci Methods 368:109441. https://doi.org/10.1016/j.jneumeth.2021.109441
16. Ahsan MM, Luna SA, Siddique Z (2022) Machine-learning-based disease diagnosis: a comprehensive review. Healthcare 10:541. https://doi.org/10.3390/healthcare10030541
17. Brari Z, Belghith S (2021) A novel machine learning approach for epilepsy diagnosis using EEG signals based on correlation dimension. IFAC-PapersOnLine 54:7–11. https://doi.org/10.1016/j.ifacol.2021.11.018
18. Sone D, Beheshti I (2021) Clinical application of machine learning models for brain imaging in epilepsy: a review. Front Neurosci 15. https://doi.org/10.3389/fnins.2021.684825
19. Kang L, Chen J, Huang J, Zhang T, Xu J (2022) Identifying epilepsy based on machine-learning technique with diffusion kurtosis tensor. CNS Neurosci Ther 28:354–363. https://doi.org/10.1111/cns.13773
20. Asadi-Pooya AA, Kashkooli M, Asadi-Pooya A, Malekpour M, Jafari A (2022) Machine learning applications to differentiate comorbid functional seizures and epilepsy from pure functional seizures. J Psychosom Res 153:110703. https://doi.org/10.1016/j.jpsychores.2021.110703
21. Sameer M, Gupta B (2022) CNN based framework for detection of epileptic seizures. Multimed Tools Appl 81:17057–17070. https://doi.org/10.1007/s11042-022-12702-9
22. Singh K, Malhotra J (2022) Predicting epileptic seizures from EEG spectral band features using convolutional neural network. Wirel Pers Commun 125:2667–2684. https://doi.org/10.1007/s11277-022-09678-y
23. Lillo E, Mora M, Lucero B (2022) Automated diagnosis of schizophrenia using EEG microstates and deep convolutional neural network. Expert Syst Appl 209:118236. https://doi.org/10.1016/j.eswa.2022.118236
24. Rijnders B, Korkmaz EE, Yildirim F (2022) Hybrid machine learning method for a connectivity-based epilepsy diagnosis with resting-state EEG. Med Biol Eng Comput 60:1675–1689. https://doi.org/10.1007/s11517-022-02560-w
25. Sabarivani A, Ramadevi R (2022) Detection and classification of epilepsy using hybrid convolutional neural network. Concurr Eng 30:253–261. https://doi.org/10.1177/1063293X221089089
26. Dhar P, Garg VK, Rahman MA (2022) Enhanced feature extraction-based CNN approach for epileptic seizure detection from EEG signals. J Healthc Eng 2022:1–14. https://doi.org/10.1155/2022/3491828
27. Shoeibi A, Khodatars M, Ghassemi N, Jafari M, Moridian P, Alizadehsani R, Panahiazar M, Khozeimeh F, Zare A, Hosseini-Nejad H, Khosravi A, Atiya AF, Aminshahidi D, Hussain S, Rouhani M, Nahavandi S, Acharya UR (2021) Epileptic seizures detection using deep learning techniques: a review. Int J Environ Res Public Health 18:5780. https://doi.org/10.3390/ijerph18115780
28. Ouichka O, Echtioui A, Hamam H (2022) Deep learning models for predicting epileptic seizures using iEEG signals. Electronics (Basel) 11:605. https://doi.org/10.3390/electronics11040605

29. Tuncer E, Bolat ED (2022) Channel based epilepsy seizure type detection from electroencephalography (EEG) signals with machine learning techniques. Biocybern Biomed Eng 42:575–595. https://doi.org/10.1016/j.bbe.2022.04.004
30. Zhang F, Qi L, Li M, Wang B, Yang Y, Zheng G (2022) Classification of epileptic brain signals of college students based on deep learning. J Phys Conf Ser 2278:012026. https://doi.org/10.1088/1742-6596/2278/1/012026